# Orthopedics: An Evidence-Based Approach

# Orthopedics: An Evidence-Based Approach

Edited by **Newman Wagner**

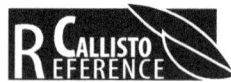

RCALLISTO REFERENCE

New York

Published by Callisto Reference,
106 Park Avenue, Suite 200,
New York, NY 10016, USA
www.callistoreference.com

**Orthopedics: An Evidence-Based Approach**
Edited by Newman Wagner

International Standard Book Number: 978-1-63239-727-0 (Hardback)

Printed in the United States of America.

# Contents

# Preface

This book has been an outcome of determined endeavour from a group of educationists in the field. The primary objective was to involve a broad spectrum of professionals from diverse cultural background involved in the field for developing new researches. The book not only targets students but also scholars pursuing higher research for further enhancement of the theoretical and practical applications of the subject.

Bones are responsible for providing a firm structure and unhindered movement to human body. Red blood cells are formed in the bone marrow and bone cells also release a hormone called osteocalcin which regulates blood sugar and fat deposition. The branch of medical science that deals with the structure, functions, diagnosis and treatment of diseases related to bones is termed as orthopedics. It unravels the recent studies in the field of orthopedics. It is a resource guide for experts as well as students. The extensive content of this book provides the readers with a thorough understanding of the subject. Modern science and technology have revolutionized the field of orthopedics. This book presents researches and studies performed by experts across the globe.

It was an honour to edit such a profound book and also a challenging task to compile and examine all the relevant data for accuracy and originality. I wish to acknowledge the efforts of the contributors for submitting such brilliant and diverse chapters in the field and for endlessly working for the completion of the book. Last, but not the least; I thank my family for being a constant source of support in all my research endeavours.

**Editor**

# Retrospective Analysis of Arthroscopic Superior Labrum Anterior to Posterior Repair: Prognostic Factors Associated with Failure

**Rachel M. Frank,**[1] **Shane J. Nho,**[1] **Kevin C. McGill,**[2] **Robert C. Grumet,**[1] **Brian J. Cole,**[1] **Nikhil N. Verma,**[1] **and Anthony A. Romeo**[1]

[1] *Division of Sports Medicine, Department of Orthopaedic Surgery, Rush University Medical Center, 1611 West Harrison Street, Suite 300, Chicago, IL 60612, USA*
[2] *Department of Diagnostic Radiology, Henry Ford Hospital, Detroit, MI, USA*

Correspondence should be addressed to Shane J. Nho; snho@hotmail.com

Academic Editor: Stephen Esses

*Background.* The purpose of this study was to report on any prognostic factors that had a significant effect on clinical outcomes following arthroscopic Type II SLAP repairs. *Methods.* Consecutive patients who underwent arthroscopic Type II SLAP repair were retrospectively identified and invited to return for follow-up examination and questionnaire. Statistical analysis was performed to determine associations between potential prognostic factors and failure of SLAP repair as defined by ASES of less than 50 and/or revision surgery. *Results.* Sixty-two patients with an average age of 36 ± 13 years met the study criteria with a mean followup of 3.3 years. There were statistically significant improvements in mean ASES score, forward elevation, and external rotation among patients. Significant associations were identified between ASES score less than 50 and age greater than 40 years; alcohol/tobacco use; coexisting diabetes; pain in the bicipital groove on examination; positive O'Brien's, Speed's, and/or Yergason's tests; and high levels of lifting required at work. There was a significant improvement in ASES at final followup. *Conclusions.* Patients younger than 20 and overhead throwers had significant associations with cases requiring revision surgery. The results from this study may be used to assist in patient selection for SLAP surgery.

## 1. Introduction

Superior labrum anterior to posterior (SLAP) lesions may occur in the athletic and working populations and represent a common source of shoulder pain in these patients. With a prevalence of approximately 6% [1, 2] in the general population and even higher in the active, military population [3], the classification, mechanisms of injury, and surgical treatment of these somewhat common injuries have been thoroughly described in the literature. The arthroscopic surgical management of SLAP tears has evolved over the years and varies depending on the type of tear, ranging from simple excision to debridement to formal repair with and without concurrent treatment to the long head of the biceps tendon (tenotomy or tenodesis).

Advancements in imaging, techniques, and instrumentation have improved our ability to perform all-arthroscopic SLAP repairs; yet significant controversy regarding diagnosis, operative indications, and treatment technique continues to exist. To further complicate the matter, substantial anatomic variation has been demonstrated in this region of the shoulder [4, 5] which may sometimes cause a nonpathologic labrum to appear injured, leading to inappropriate or even unnecessary surgery. Clinical outcomes after SLAP repair have been reported as good to excellent in 63%–100% of patients; thus, up to approximately one-third of patients are still dissatisfied after SLAP repair [6–13]. While recently some authors have analyzed the correlation between presenting symptoms and mechanism of injury [14, 15], it is unknown if there are any variables or factors that can predict the potential success or failure of SLAP repair for a given patient. The purpose of the present study was to report on potential prognostic factors that may have a significant effect on clinical outcomes following arthroscopic repair of Type II SLAP tears.

## 2. Materials and Methods

Between 2004 and 2006, all patients with a Type II SLAP lesion repair performed by senior fellowship-trained surgeons at a single institution were retrospectively identified. Inclusion criteria for participation in the study were followup greater than two years, and exclusion criteria were patients undergoing treatment for a SLAP tear other than Type II (labral fraying with detached biceps tendon anchor). Patients were not excluded for having concomitant procedures including rotator cuff repair, biceps tenodesis, subacromial decompression, or acromioplasty. Our institutional review board approved the study proposal, and informed consent was obtained for all patients prior to data collection.

Patients that met the study criteria were contacted by telephone and invited to return for followup examination and questionnaire (Table 1). At baseline and final followup, shoulder functional outcome was measured using validated, shoulder-specific outcome scores including the Simple Shoulder Test (SST), American Shoulder and Elbow Score (ASES), Single Assessment Numeric Evaluation (SANE) score, and Visual Analogue Score (VAS). Each questionnaire also contained the Short Form-12 (SF-12) health status survey (Table 1). Physical examination by a single orthopaedic research fellow was performed independent from the operating surgeon, with all components of the examination performed on both shoulders. The examination consisted of active and passive ranges of motion measured with a goniometer, including active forward elevation in the scapular plane, external rotation at the side, and internal rotation behind the back. A dynamometer (Commander Muscle, JTech Medical, Salt Lake City, UT, USA) was used to test strength in both forward elevation and external rotation at the side. In addition, several diagnostic clinical tests, including the O'Brien's [16] test, Kibler test [17], Speed's test [18], Yergason's test [19], Compression-rotation test [2], Apprehension test, and Relocation test [20], were performed.

Intraoperative information, including diagnostic information, number and type of anchors used, concomitant procedures performed at the time of surgery, labral pathology (location and size), chondral lesions (location, size, and depth), and biceps pathology (none, incomplete or complete tear) was also collected.

*2.1. Surgical Technique.* Patients in our institution undergo a combination of general anesthesia and an interscalene block for postoperative pain control. The patient is placed in either the beach chair or lateral decubitus position with shoulder suspension. The posterior portal is created 3 cm inferior and in line with the acromial angle, and a 30-degree arthroscope is introduced into the glenohumeral joint. The anterior portal is established high in the rotator interval with an outside-in technique utilizing a spinal needle. A 8.25 mm cannula is placed for instrumentation. A diagnostic arthroscopy is

TABLE 1: Prognostic factors asked on post-operative questionnaire.

| Factor | Possible Responses |
| --- | --- |
| Age | Years |
| Tobacco history | Yes or no |
| Preoperative pain | Yes or no |
| Anti-inflammatory use | Yes or no |
| Narcotic use | Yes or no |
| Extremity | Right or left |
| Dominant extremity | Yes or no |
| Trauma | Yes or no |
| Mechanism or injury | Sports, motor vehicle accident, fall, traction, insidious |
| Sport | |
| Level of sports participation | Professional, collegiate, high school, recreational, none |
| Thrower | Yes or no |
| Overhead athlete | Yes or no |
| Collision sport | Yes or no |
| Level of work | Very heavy, heavy, medium, light, sedentary |
| Worker's compensation | Yes or no |
| History of dislocation | Yes or no |
| History of subluxation | Yes or no |
| Pre-operative O'Brien's test | Positive, negative, equivocal |
| Pre-operative biceps load II test | Positive or negative |
| Pre-operative Compression-rotation | Positive or negative |
| Pre-operative Kibler test | Positive or negative |
| Pre-operative bicipital groove tenderness | Yes or no |
| Pre-operative Speed's test | Positive or negative |
| Pre-operative Yergason's test | Positive or negative |
| Pre-operative apprehension test | Positive or negative |
| Pre-operative relocation test | Positive or negative |

performed to determine the extent of the SLAP lesion as well as to assess for other concomitant pathology. Once a Type II SLAP tear is confirmed, a hooded arthroscopic burr is used to debride the superior glenoid to bleeding cancellous bone to facilitate labral healing. A spinal needle is inserted adjacent to the lateral acromial edge aiming toward the superior glenoid just below the biceps origin. A small skin incision is made, and the spear and trocar for the suture anchor are introduced into the glenohumeral joint at a 45-degree angle just medial to the glenoid articular surface. A 3.0 mm suture anchor (BioComposite SutureTak, Arthrex, Inc., Naples, FL) is positioned at 12 o'clock. Through the anterior portal, a 45 degree curved suture shuttle device (Spectrum, Linvatec, Key Largo, FL) loaded with a no. 1 PDS suture is passed posterior to the biceps tendon and underneath the labrum. The PDS suture is advanced into the joint, and the suture shuttle device is carefully withdrawn back out of the anterior cannula. Using the same cannula, a suture retriever is used to grasp both the

(a)

(b)

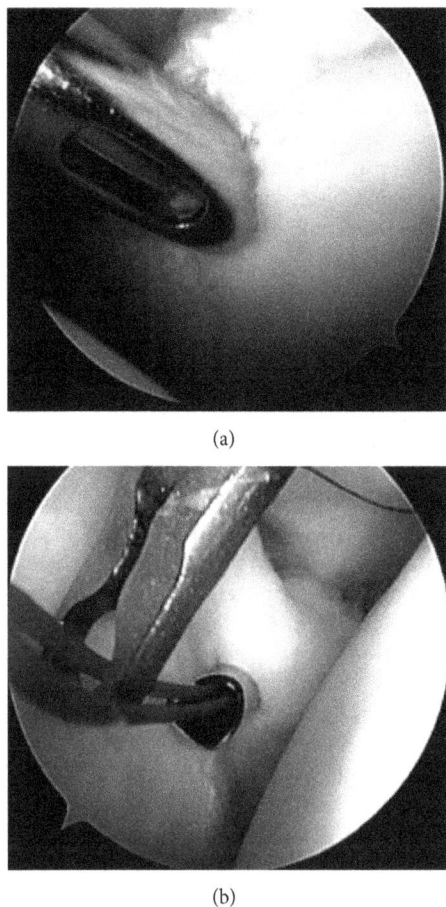

FIGURE 1: Arthroscopic figures demonstrating surgical technique of SLAP repair: (a) a hooded arthroscopic burr is used to debride the superior glenoid to bleeding cancellous bone to facilitate labral healing; (b) passage of no. 1 PDS suture posterior to the biceps tendon and underneath the labrum.

passed PDS and the FiberWire from the suture anchor and withdraws both of them to prevent suture tangling. The PDS suture is the tied to the FiberWire suture outside the joint, and the PDS limb still attached to the suture shuttle device is pulled to shuttle the FiberWire underneath the labrum and back out of the anterior cannula. The other FiberWire limb is pulled out of the anterior cannula with a crochet hook. The FiberWire suture that is passed through the labrum is the postlimb, and an arthroscopic knot using five reverse half hitches with alternating posts is tied with the knot on top of the superior labrum and away from the articular surface. Using the same steps as previously described, another suture anchor can be placed posterior to the initial anchor at 10 o'clock (right shoulder) depending on the posterior extent of the SLAP tear (Figure 1).

*2.2. Standard Postoperative Rehabilitation Protocol for All Patients.* All patients followed the same standardized rehabilitation protocol postoperatively. For the first 6 weeks, the shoulder was immobilized, with passive- and active-assisted ranges of motion permitted, including motion up to 40° of external rotation and 140° of forward flexion. From 6 to 12 weeks, the patient was advanced to active range of motion. The final 12 weeks focused on rotator cuff strengthening and conditioning. All patients were released to full activity after 6 months.

*2.3. Indicators of Surgery Failure.* Indicators of surgery failure included revision surgery on the ipsilateral shoulder related to the capsule and/or labrum, ASES less than 50, complications (stiffness, recurrent instability), and/or poor patient satisfaction.

*2.4. Statistical Analysis.* Statistical analysis was performed utilizing both parametric and nonparametric testing methods using SPSS software (SPSS, Chicago, IL, USA). Descriptive analysis consisted of frequencies and percentages for discrete data and means and standard deviations for continuous data. Paired student's $t$-test were used comparing preoperative measures with corresponding postoperative measures at final followup. Contingency table analysis using Fisher's Exact test was used for identifying correlations between potential risk factors and outcome measures. Significance was set at $P < 0.05$ for all tests.

## 3. Results

Sixty-two patients with an average age of 36 ± 13 years were available for followup from an original cohort of 100 consecutive patients (62% followup rate). The average followup duration was 3.3 years (range: 2.0 to 5.0). Forty-six patients (74%) were male, and 16 (26%) were female. Eleven patients reported either active or prior tobacco history. In addition to SLAP repair, several patients also underwent concomitant Bankart repair ($n = 9$), rotator cuff tear repair ($n = 10$), acromioplasty ($n = 8$), distal clavicle resection ($n = 2$), and biceps tenodesis ($n = 9$).

There were statistically significant improvements in the average ASES (preop: 64.8±19; postop: 83.9±18.3; $P < 0.001$), SST (preop: 8.6 ± 2.9; postop: 10.3 ± 2.3, $P = 0.004$) and VAS (preop: 3.3 ± 2.3; postop: 1.6 ± 1.9, $P < 0.001$) scores. The mean postoperative SANE score, indicating the patient's overall assessment of their shoulder function, was 86.9±16.4.

There was a statistically significant improvement in average forward flexion (preop: 156 ± 34°; postop: 172 ± 14°, $P = 0.005$) when comparing preoperative values to those postoperatively. Similarly, there were clinically relevant improvements in average, external rotation (preop: 66 ± 19°; postop: 70 ± 12°, $P > 0.05$) and abduction (preop: 155 ± 34°; postop: 169 ± 66°, $P > 0.05$); however, these results were not statistically significant.

Patients with a postoperative ASES of less than 50 and/or those who went onto revision surgery were considered failures. There were a total of 5 patients (8.1%) with a postoperative ASES less than 50. In addition, a total of 5 other patients (8.1%) went onto receive revision shoulder surgery. Thus, the overall failure rate was 16.2% for the entire cohort.

There was a significant association identified between patients with an ASES less than 50 and several factors, including age greater than 40 years ($P = 0.005$), alcohol use

($P$ = 0.033), tobacco use ($P$ = 0.002), and diabetes ($P$ < 0.001). Associations between physical examination maneuvers, including pain in the bicipital groove on examination ($P$ < 0.001), positive O'Brien's test ($P$ = 0.002), positive Speed's test ($P$ < 0.001), and positive Yergason's test ($P$ = 0.015) were also seen with ASESs less than 50. Finally, there was a significant association between ASES less than 50 and high levels of lifting required at work ($P$ = 0.004).

The 5 revision surgeries included capsular release (softball injury), 270-degree labral repair after traumatic retear of labrum (baseball injury), two revision SLAP repairs (both baseball injuries), and debridement to SLAP repair (wrestling injury). Two out of 3 patients under 20 years old were revised, as compared to 3 out of 35 patients aged 20 years and older. Four out of 10 patients who were throwers were revised, as compared to 0 out of 29 nonthrowing patients. A significant association was identified between patients requiring revision surgery and age less than 20 years ($P$ = 0.035) as well as preoperative participation in throwing activities ($P$ < 0.001). Overhead throwers were defined as patients who use their arms in an overhead position, including but not limited to baseball players (including pitchers), football players, swimmers, and tennis players.

## 4. Discussion

Although the technical aspects of arthroscopic repair of Type II SLAP tears have been well described, the clinical decision making may not be as apparent. There may be a certain subset of patients that have suboptimal clinical outcomes after surgical fixation unstable SLAP lesions. The present study suggests that arthroscopic repair of Type II SLAP tears results in a significant improvement in shoulder functional outcome and range of motion; however, there are a number of prognostic factors that may have a higher association with clinical failure. The principle findings of this study include the following: (1) when using revision surgery as an indicator of failure, the prognostic factors most associated with failure were overhead throwers and age less than 20 years, and (2) when using ASES less than 50 as an indicator of failure, the prognostic factors most associated with failure were age greater than 40 years, heavy laborers, users of tobacco and/or alcohol, diabetics, and/or patients who present with persistent anterior shoulder pain (symptoms consistent with persistent SLAP lesion or bicipital groove tenderness).

Using a poor ASES as a reflection of overall poor shoulder function, the results from the present study suggest that patients more likely to fail SLAP repair are older than 40 years old, heavy laborers, users of tobacco and/or alcohol, diabetics, and/or patients who present persistent SLAP or bicipital groove pain (tenderness over the long head of the biceps tendon, positive O'Brien's test, positive Speed's test, and/or positive Yergason's sign). These are the type of patients that one might expect to have a poor outcome due to persistent bicipital symptoms and not necessarily due to the SLAP tear or repair itself. In patients over 40 years old with a Type II SLAP lesion, the decision of whether to perform a SLAP repair, biceps tenodesis, or SLAP repair with a biceps tenodesis remains unclear as the true etiology of symptoms in this

specific patient population is extremely difficult to determine clinically. Although the cohort in the present study only evaluated patients who have had SLAP repairs, these patients may have had improved shoulder functional outcome with a biceps tenodesis with or without a SLAP repair [4, 21]. Boileau et al. [21] recently studied the clinical outcomes following arthroscopic biceps tenodesis using interference screws as an alternative to repair of isolated unstable Type II SLAP defects. The authors found that patients were subjectively more satisfied and had a significantly higher rate of return to previous level of activity in the biceps tenodesis group as compared to the SLAP repair group, including patients participating in overhead sport. Interestingly, in this study, the patients in the biceps tenodesis group were significantly older with a mean age of 52 years (range: 28–64) compared to the SLAP repair group with a mean age of 37 years (range: 19–57) ($P$ < 0.001), which clearly may be a contributing factor to the success of the biceps tenodesis procedure in this cohort.

When using revision surgery as the definition of a failed SLAP repair, age under 20 years was a significant (negative) prognostic factor. Based on these results, it is evident that greater proportions of patients under 20 years old had to be revised compared to their comparison groups (patients over 20 years old). It is possible that young patients who had SLAP repairs are less likely to tolerate these repairs, potentially due to postoperative stiffness and/or reinjury.

As proposed by Burkhart and Morgan [26] in 2001, it is possible that the mechanism of SLAP injury in overhead athletes, notable baseball pitchers, is actually related to the acceleration phase of throwing when the shoulder is in a position of extreme abduction and external rotation. Overhead athletes with high pitching/throwing volumes may develop posteroinferior shoulder stiffness, causing a deficit in internal rotation range of motion and subsequent stiffness, also known as the "dead arm syndrome" as coined by Rowe [27]. This becomes problematic when the athlete acquires a SLAP lesion, as unlike in a healthy shoulder, the patient is unable to compensate for their internal rotation deficit with a gain of external rotation. In an outcomes study of SLAP repairs comparing overhead athletes to nonoverhead athletes, Kim et al. [11] found that nonoverhead athletes had significantly better outcomes when using UCLA scores and return to preinjury level of activity as outcomes assessments. Specifically, the authors reported that only 22% of overhead athletes returned fully to their preinjury level of activity, as compared with 63% of the nonoverhead athletes. Interestingly, Pagnani et al. [28] found that 12/13 athletes (92%) were able to return to their preinjury level of overhead activity following SLAP repair. Ide et al. [25] found that 36 of 40 (90%) overhead athletes were satisfied with their SLAP repair, with 75% of the athletes returning to their preinjury level of competitiveness. Finally, Yung et al. [22] recently found that overhead athletes required a longer duration of therapy/rehabilitation in order to return to their preoperative level of activity following SLAP repair. Thus, the results represented in the literature are inconsistent, and the reason explaining why overhead athletes may be more likely to be less satisfied or take longer to return to activity after SLAP repair remains largely unknown.

TABLE 2: Outcomes and potential contributing factors following arthroscopic SLAP lesion repair.

| Authors (reference) | Number of patients | Clinical outcome measures | Outcomes | Potential factors |
|---|---|---|---|---|
| Katz et al., 2009 [14] | 40 shoulders (39 patients) | SST, patient satisfaction | 71% of those with poor outcome dissatisfied with conservative treatment | Not discussed |
| Brockmeier et al., 2009 [6] | 47 | ASES, L'Insalata | 87% good to excellent | Higher outcomes after traumatic etiology |
| Boileau et al., 2009 [21] | 10 (15 others with BT) | Constant, patient satisfaction | (i) Constant score 65 → 83 (ii) 60% dissatisfied (iii) 4 overall failures converted to BT | Not discussed |
| Yung et al., 2008 [22] | 16 | UCLA, physical exam | 31% excellent, 44% good, 25% poor | Overhead athletes required longer time to RTP |
| Park et al., 2008 [15] | 24 | UCLA, VAS | (i) UCLA: 22.7 → 29.9 (ii) VAS: 6.4 → 2.1 | Mechanism of injury did not impact outcomes |
| Oh et al., 2008 [23] | 25 (58 total in study, only 25 with isolated SLAP lesions) | VAS, ASES, UCLA, SST, constant | Significant improvements: (i) VAS pain: 1.8 (ii) ASES: 84.1 (iii) UCLA 32.6 (iv) SST: 94.7 (v) VAS: 8.9 | Not discussed |
| Voos et al., 2007 [13] | 30 (combined RCT with SLAP or Bankart) | ASES, L'Insalata | (i) 90% good to excellent (ii) 77% return to play (iii) 2 recurrent RCT | Not discussed |
| Funk and Snow, 2007 [24] | 18 | Satisfaction, time to RTP | 89% satisfaction | Isolated SLAP lesions had quickest return to play |
| Enad et al., 2007 [9] | 27 (15 with isolated tears), military population | ASES, UCLA | Excellent in 4, good in 20, fair in 3 96% return to duty | Higher outcomes scores in pts with concomitant diagnosis |
| Coleman et al., 2007 [8] | 50 (16 with concomitant acromioplasty) | ASES, L'Insalata, | (i) 65% good to excellent in SLAP only group (ii) 81% good to excellent in acromioplasty group | Not discussed |
| Cohen et al., 2006 [7] | 39 | ASES, L'Insalata, | (i) 71% satisfied (ii) 41% with continued night pain | Athletes and pts with rotator cuff piercing with worse outcomes |
| Ide et al., 2005 [25] | 40, all overhead athletes | Modified Rowe | (i) Rowe: 27.5 → 92.1 (ii) 75% return to preinjury level of activity | Traumatic etiology with better return to activity than overuse etiology |
| Kim et al., 2002 [11] | 34 | UCLA | (i) 94% satisfied (ii) 91% return to preinjury level | Overhead sports with lower ASES ($P = 0.024$) and lower return to preinjury level ($P = 0.015$) |
| O'Brien et al., 2002 [12] | 31 | ASES, L'Insalata | (i) 52% return to preinjury level (ii) L'Insalata: 87 (iii) ASES: 87.2 | Not discussed |

Abbreviations: SLAP: superior labrum anterior to posterior; BT: biceps tenodesis; ASES: American Shoulder and Elbow Society; UCLA: University of California Los Angeles; SST: Simple Shoulder Test; VAS: Visual Analog Scale; RCT: rotator cuff tear; RTP: return to play.

Recently, Katz et al. [14] performed an analysis of patients with poor outcomes following SLAP repair, with a focus on outcomes following subsequent treatment after the initial poor outcome. Overall, the authors reported that while 68% of their patient cohort was satisfied after initial SLAP failure followed by either surgical or nonoperative therapy, 32% continued to have a suboptimal response. While the authors commented on the number of patients who used tobacco (4) and had a history of diabetes (2), no statistical analysis was performed in attempt to correlate these and other similar demographic and social factors with a potential prognostic significance. In addition, there are a number of additional studies available that report on outcomes following SLAP repair, several of which report associations between poor outcomes and specific factors (Table 2 [6–9, 11–15, 21–25, 29]).

This study had several limitations, most notably its retrospective nature, lack of control group, and followup rate of 62%. Multiple attempts were made to contact all of the 100 consecutive patients in the initial cohort, and unfortunately due to missing and/or incorrect contact information, several patients were unable to be reached. Another limitation is the number of concomitant procedures performed in our patient population. One major difficulty with treating shoulders with multiple injuries is understanding which lesions are truly symptomatic and which are simply incidental. As discussed by Boileau et al. [21] and Kim et al [30], it is impossible to know if patients who had a successful outcome following, for example, both SLAP and rotator cuff repair, benefited more from one of the repairs versus the other, or if both were truly needed to produce a successful outcome. Subgroups of patients undergoing concomitant procedures could not be statistically analyzed secondary to the small number of patients undergoing these procedures as well as the overlap between patients undergoing more than one concomitant procedure. Another limitation is the lack of followup imaging, which would have provided another objective outcome as to whether or not the SLAP repairs remained intact.

This study also had several strengths. To our knowledge, this is the first study that discusses the prognostic factors affecting the clinical outcome after SLAP repair. All patients of this relatively large cohort completed questionnaires utilizing validated, shoulder-specific outcomes surveys. Additionally, all patients were examined by a single, blinded orthopaedic research fellow. There were four fellowship-trained orthopaedic surgeons, in either sports medicine or upper extremity surgery, performing all procedures at a single institution, allowing the results to be generalizable to other surgeons who focus on the shoulder. Finally, the rehabilitation protocol utilized was standardized for all patients.

## 5. Conclusion

Overall, patient selection in SLAP repairs can be difficult, and the results from this study may be used to assist with patient selection for SLAP surgery and can help predict which patients might benefit from SLAP repair and which are less likely to experience significant improvement. Further long-term studies necessary to determine the natural history of SLAP repair as well as to determine factors that may be associated with improved surgical outcomes.

## Disclosure

No sources of support in the forms of grants, equipment, or other items were received for this study. The authors report no conflict of interest.

## References

[1] F. Handelberg, S. Willems, M. Shahabpour, J. P. Huskin, and J. Kuta, "SLAP lesions: a retrospective multicenter study," *Arthroscopy*, vol. 14, no. 8, pp. 856–862, 1998.

[2] S. J. Synder, R. P. Karzel, W. Del Pizzo, R. D. Ferkel, and M. J. Friedman, "SLAP lesions of the shoulder," *Arthroscopy*, vol. 6, no. 4, pp. 274–279, 1990.

[3] R. J. Kampa and J. Clasper, "Incidence of SLAP lesions in a military population," *Journal of the Royal Army Medical Corps*, vol. 151, no. 3, pp. 171–175, 2005.

[4] F. A. Barber, L. D. Field, and R. K. Ryu, "Biceps tendon and superior labrum injuries: decision making," *Instructional Course Lectures*, vol. 57, pp. 527–538, 2008.

[5] L. D. Higgins and J. J. P. Warner, "Superior labral lesions: anatomy, pathology, and treatment," *Clinical Orthopaedics and Related Research*, no. 390, pp. 73–82, 2001.

[6] S. F. Brockmeier, J. E. Voos, R. J. Williams, D. W. Altchek, F. A. Cordasco, and A. A. Allen, "Outcomes after arthroscopic repair of type-II SLAP lesions," *Journal of Bone and Joint Surgery A*, vol. 91, no. 7, pp. 1595–1603, 2009.

[7] D. B. Cohen, S. Coleman, M. C. Drakos et al., "Outcomes of isolated type II SLAP lesions treated with arthroscopic fixation using a bioabsorbable tack," *Arthroscopy*, vol. 22, no. 2, pp. 136–142, 2006.

[8] S. H. Coleman, D. B. Cohen, M. C. Drakos et al., "Arthroscopic repair of type II superior labral anterior posterior lesions with and without acromioplasty: a clinical analysis of 50 patients," *American Journal of Sports Medicine*, vol. 35, no. 5, pp. 749–753, 2007.

[9] J. G. Enad, R. J. Gaines, S. M. White, and C. A. Kurtz, "Arthroscopic superior labrum anterior-posterior repair in military patients," *Journal of Shoulder and Elbow Surgery*, vol. 16, no. 3, pp. 300–305, 2007.

[10] L. D. Field and F. H. Savoie, "Arthroscopic suture repair of superior labral detachment lesions of the shoulder," *American Journal of Sports Medicine*, vol. 21, no. 6, pp. 783–790, 1993.

[11] S. H. Kim, K. I. Ha, and H. J. Choi, "Results of arthroscopic treatment of superior labral lesions," *Journal of Bone and Joint Surgery A*, vol. 84, no. 6, pp. 981–985, 2002.

[12] S. J. O'Brien, A. A. Allen, S. H. Coleman, and M. C. Drakos, "The trans-rotator cuff approach to SLAP lesions: technical aspects for repair and a clinical follow-up of 31 patients at a minimum of 2 years," *Arthroscopy*, vol. 18, no. 4, pp. 372–377, 2002.

[13] J. E. Voos, A. D. Pearle, C. J. Mattern, F. A. Cordasco, A. A. Allen, and R. F. Warren, "Outcomes of combined arthroscopic rotator cuff and labral repair," *American Journal of Sports Medicine*, vol. 35, no. 7, pp. 1174–1179, 2007.

[14] L. M. Katz, S. Hsu, S. L. Miller et al., "Poor outcomes after SLAP repair: descriptive analysis and prognosis," *Arthroscopy*, vol. 25, no. 8, pp. 849–855, 2009.

[15] J. H. Park, Y. S. Lee, J. H. Wang, H. K. Noh, and J. G. Kim, "Outcome of the isolated SLAP lesions and analysis of the results according to the injury mechanisms," *Knee Surgery, Sports Traumatology, Arthroscopy*, vol. 16, no. 5, pp. 511–515, 2008.

[16] S. J. O'Brien, M. J. Pagnani, S. Fealy, S. R. McGlynn, and J. B. Wilson, "The active compression test: a new and effective test for diagnosing labral tears and acromioclavicular joint abnormality," *American Journal of Sports Medicine*, vol. 26, no. 5, pp. 610–613, 1998.

[17] W. B. Kibler, "Specificity and sensitivity of the anterior slide test in throwing athletes with superior glenoid labral tears," *Arthroscopy*, vol. 11, no. 3, pp. 296–300, 1995.

[18] W. F. Bennett, "Specificity of the Speed's test: arthroscopic technique for evaluating the biceps tendon at the level of the bicipital groove," *Arthroscopy*, vol. 14, no. 8, pp. 789–796, 1998.

[19] R. Yergason, "Supination sign," *The Journal of Bone & Joint Surgery*, vol. 13, p. 160, 1931.

[20] D. L. Hamner, M. M. Pink, and F. W. Jobe, "A modification of the relocation test: arthroscopic findings associated with a positive test," *Journal of Shoulder and Elbow Surgery*, vol. 9, no. 4, pp. 263–267, 2000.

[21] P. Boileau, S. Parratte, C. Chuinard, Y. Roussanne, D. Shia, and R. Bicknell, "Arthroscopic treatment of isolated type II slap lesions: siceps tenodesis as an alternative to reinsertion," *American Journal of Sports Medicine*, vol. 37, no. 5, pp. 929–936, 2009.

[22] P. S. H. Yung, D. T. P. Fong, M. F. Kong et al., "Arthroscopic repair of isolated type II superior labrum anterior-posterior lesion," *Knee Surgery, Sports Traumatology, Arthroscopy*, vol. 16, no. 12, pp. 1151–1157, 2008.

[23] J. H. Oh, S. H. Kim, H. K. Lee, K. H. Jo, and K. J. Bae, "Trans-rotator cuff portal is safe for arthroscopic superior labral anterior and posterior lesion repair: clinical and radiological analysis of 58 SLAP lesions," *American Journal of Sports Medicine*, vol. 36, no. 10, pp. 1913–1921, 2008.

[24] L. Funk and M. Snow, "SLAP tears of the glenoid labrum in contact athletes," *Clinical Journal of Sport Medicine*, vol. 17, no. 1, pp. 1–4, 2007.

[25] J. Ide, S. Maeda, and K. Takagi, "Sports activity after arthroscopic superior labral repair using suture anchors in overhead-throwing athletes," *American Journal of Sports Medicine*, vol. 33, no. 4, pp. 507–514, 2005.

[26] S. S. Burkhart and C. Morgan, "Slap lesions in the overhead athlete," *Orthopedic Clinics of North America*, vol. 32, no. 3, pp. 431–441, 2001.

[27] C. R. Rowe, "Recurrent transient anterior subluxation of the shoulder. The "dead arm" syndrome," *Clinical Orthopaedics and Related Research*, no. 223, pp. 11–19, 1987.

[28] M. J. Pagnani, K. P. Speer, D. W. Altchek, R. F. Warren, and D. M. Dines, "Arthroscopic fixation of superior labral lesions using a biodegradable implant: a preliminary report," *Arthroscopy*, vol. 11, no. 2, pp. 194–198, 1995.

[29] J. E. Samani, S. B. Marston, and D. D. Buss, "Arthroscopic stabilization of type II SLAP lesions using an absorbable tack," *Arthroscopy*, vol. 17, no. 1, pp. 19–24, 2001.

[30] T. K. Kim, W. S. Queale, A. J. Cosgarea, and E. G. McFarland, "Clinical features of the different types of SLAP lesions: an analysis of one hundred and thirty-nine cases," *Journal of Bone and Joint Surgery A*, vol. 85, no. 1, pp. 66–71, 2003.

# Total Knee Arthroplasty Designed to Accommodate the Presence or Absence of the Posterior Cruciate Ligament

Melinda K. Harman,[1] Stephanie J. Bonin,[2] Chris J. Leslie,[3]
Scott A. Banks,[4] and W. Andrew Hodge[5]

[1] Department of Bioengineering, 301 Rhodes Engineering Research Center, Clemson University, Clemson, SC 29634-0905, USA
[2] MEA Forensic Engineers & Scientists, 23281 Vista Grande Drive, Laguna Hills, CA 92653, USA
[3] Leslie Orthopaedics & Sports Medicine, 226 East U.S. Highway 54, Camdenton, MO 65020, USA
[4] Department Mechanical & Aerospace Engineering, MAEA 318, University of Florida, P.O. Box 116250, Gainesville, FL 32611, USA
[5] Department of Orthopaedics, Eastern Maine Medical Center, 489 State Street, Bangor, ME 04401, USA

Correspondence should be addressed to Melinda K. Harman; harman2@clemson.edu

Academic Editor: Rene C. Verdonk

Evidence for selecting the same total knee arthroplasty prosthesis whether the posterior cruciate ligament (PCL) is retained or resected is rarely documented. This study reports prospective midterm clinical, radiographic, and functional outcomes of a fixed-bearing design implanted using two different surgical techniques. The PCL was completely retained in 116 knees and completely resected in 43 knees. For the entire cohort, clinical knee ($96 \pm 7$) and function ($92 \pm 13$) scores and radiographic outcomes were good to excellent for 84% of patients after 5–10 years in vivo. Range of motion averaged $124° \pm 9°$, with 126 knees exhibiting $\geq 120°$ flexion. Small differences in average knee flexion and function scores were noted, with the PCL-resected group exhibiting an average of 5° more flexion but an average function score that was 7 points lower compared to the PCL-retained group. Fluoroscopic analysis of 33 knees revealed stable tibiofemoral translations. This study demonstrates that a TKA articular design with progressive congruency in the lateral compartment can provide for femoral condyle rollback in maximal flexion activities and achieve good clinical and functional performance in patients with PCL-retained and PCL-resected TKA. This TKA design proved suitable for use with either surgical technique, providing surgeons with the choice of maintaining or sacrificing the PCL.

## 1. Introduction

Contemporary total knee arthroplasty (TKA) provides reliable pain relief and restoration of moderate function for patients suffering from severe joint degeneration. Outcomes are typically very good [1, 2], but many times patients do not regain a normal range of motion and strength. In particular, TKA designs that allow excessive anterior-posterior (AP) translation of the femur with respect to the tibia (knee instability) exhibit reduced knee flexion, diminished functional strength, and unfavorable conditions for bearing surface wear [3–13]. Excessive AP motion in well-aligned prostheses occurs with the femur sliding anterior on the tibia in flexion and posterior in extension, resulting in limited femoral

rollback and the potential of bony impingement between the femur bone and posterior rim of the tibial insert [5, 14–16]. This instability appears to result from the loss of the knee's natural intrinsic stabilizing structures after TKA, including one or both of the cruciate ligaments and the menisci [17]. Therefore, controlling AP translation of the femur, in the presence or absence of the posterior cruciate ligament (PCL), is often cited as a means for achieving optimal function in modern TKA designs [5, 16, 18–26].

Traditionally, orthopaedic surgeons have been trained to execute surgical techniques that depend on the integrity of the posterior cruciate ligament by utilizing one of two basic TKA designs, the cruciate-retaining type (CR) or the posterior-stabilized type (PS). However, joint laxity can vary

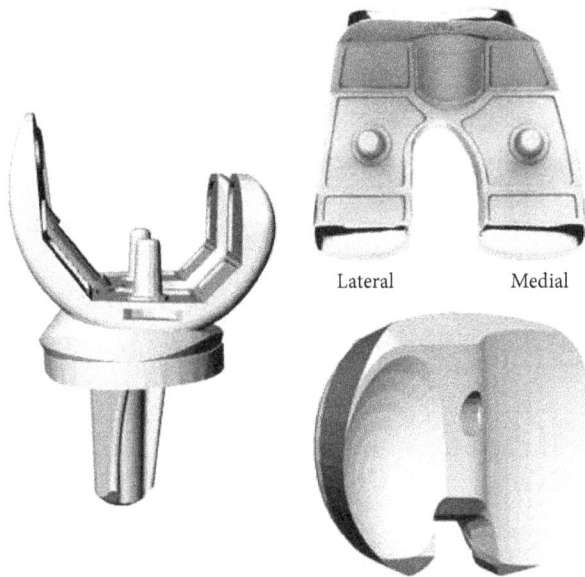

FIGURE 1: The 3D Knee is a fixed-bearing total knee prosthesis suitable for use in PCL-retained or PCL-resected TKA.

Lateral    Medial

widely after TKA due to common variations in these surgical techniques, including whether the PCL is preserved with a tibial bone block at the insertion site, recessed to the level of the tibial bone cut, or completely resected [27–29]. TKA designs incorporate different articular constraints in order to accommodate such variations [30]. While it previously has been suggested that some TKA designs are suitable for use regardless of whether the PCL is retained or resected [31], the clinical outcomes and biomechanical considerations of such designs rarely have been considered [28, 29]. Moreover, it remains unclear precisely how much conformity is required for successful TKA [30].

The current study was initiated in order to gather evidence documenting the performance of a new TKA articular design concept that incorporates progressive congruency in the lateral compartment (Figures 1 and 2). This design does not require use of a femoral cam and tibial post articulation typical of PS designs, helping to conserve femoral bone and avoiding complications associated with wear of the tibial post [32, 33]. It is implanted using a PCL-retaining surgical technique, which avoids widening of the flexion gap known to occur with PCL resection [34]. Moreover, the highly congruent lateral femoral condyle and widened medial condyle that provide for large contact areas help to optimize load distribution and lower contact stresses compared to other fixed-bearing, CR, and PS TKA designs [35]. The purpose of this study was to characterize the midterm clinical and functional outcomes of a TKA designed to improve knee function by providing more intrinsic AP stability after arthroplasty. Patient populations operated by two surgeons, one utilizing a PCL-retaining surgical technique and the other utilizing a technique with complete PCL resection, were compared.

## 2. Materials and Methods

Two clinical sites in the United States participated in this prospective IRB-approved study to record clinical results of a fixed-bearing TKA design (3D Knee, DJO Surgical, Austin, TX) implanted using two different surgical techniques; either the PCL was retained with a bone block or the PCL was completely resected. Patients with surgery dates between January, 2002 and December, 2006, were identified from TKA surgical databases provided by the two surgeons, providing for evaluation at a minimum follow-up of five years. Inclusion criteria for this study required that patients be older than 21 years, demonstrate severe arthritis with bone to bone disease in at least one knee compartment, have varus or valgus deformity not exceeding 15 degrees, not have had prior knee sepsis, and not have undergone prior knee arthoplasty for any reason. Patients were required to provide informed consent and to be willing to travel to the clinical office to undergo physical evaluation and a radiological exam. Eligible patients were contacted by telephone to schedule clinical visits and were enrolled sequentially until the enrollment target of 150 TKA was achieved.

During the four-year operative period, a total of 251 TKA were implanted by the two participating surgeons using the same implant design. A total of 134 patients (159 TKA) met the inclusion criteria and were willing to participate in the study, including 116 of 193 (60%) TKA implanted by a surgeon who preserved the PCL with a bone block and 43 of 58 (74%) TKA implanted by a surgeon who completely resected the PCL. There were 84 female patients (98 TKA) and 50 male patients (61 TKA) with an average age of 69 ± 9 (range, 33 to 89) years at the time of index TKA. Average duration of function for all TKA was 8.0 ± 1.1 (range, 5.6 to 10.3) years.

Surgical exposure for both surgeons at index TKA was a mid-vastus approach through a standard midline skin incision. Handling of the PCL followed the surgical techniques routinely used by each participating surgeon. Preservation of the PCL was accomplished with a bone block surgical technique, whereas resection of the PCL was accomplished through complete ligament removal and insertion of a Hohmann retractor for anterior tibial dislocation. All knees in both groups were implanted with the same fixed-bearing TKA design (3D Knee), including patellar resurfacing and cement fixation of all three components. All modular tibial inserts and domed patellar components were machined from compression molded polyethylene and were sterilized using gamma radiation and packaged in nitrogen gas.

Patients were followed up prospectively to record clinical and radiological outcomes. The physical evaluation included measurement of maximum knee flexion using a hand-held goniometer and assessment of clinical outcome using the Knee Society Score (KSS knee and function scores) [36]. The radiological exam included acquisition of standard-length radiographs with the patients in a standing, weight-bearing posture, which were obtained at the immediate postoperative and annual intervals. Radiolucent lines were evaluated in predefined zones about the fixation interfaces of the femoral, tibial, and patellar components [37] and graded as none,

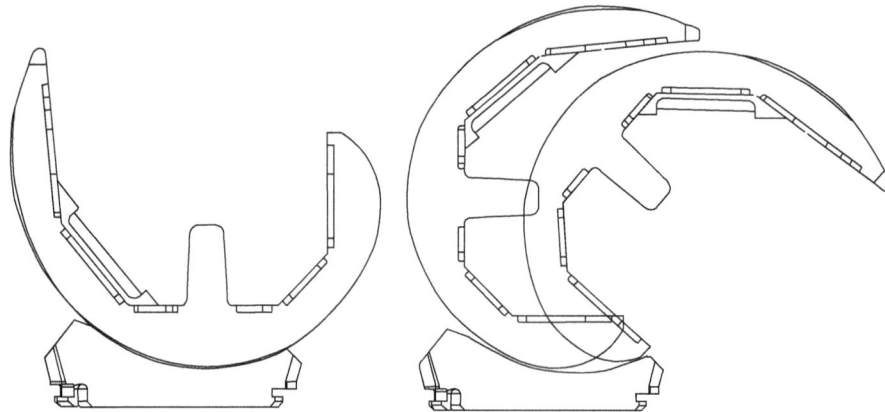

FIGURE 2: The 3D Knee fixed-bearing TKA design incorporates a hemispherical lateral condyle and tibial articulation to provide definitive AP translational control while providing for proper axial rotation. The asymmetric femoral component incorporates a constant sagittal radius from −15° to 80° while providing progressively decreasing articular constraint with higher flexion to allow femoral condyle rollback. The posterior condyles are shaped to provide maximum posterior condylar offset late in the flexion arc.

TABLE 1: Patient demographics and outcome measures for all TKA and for the PCL-retained and PCL-resected groups.

| | All TKA | PCL-retained | PCL-resected | $P^*$ |
|---|---|---|---|---|
| Patients | 159 | 116 | 43 | |
| Sex (F/M, % female) | 98/61 (62%) | 65/51 (56%) | 33/10 (77%) | |
| Age at index surgery (yrs.) | 70 ± 9 | 72 ± 7 | 64 ± 9 | <0.001 |
| Age at last follow-up (yrs.) | 76 ± 8 | 78 ± 7 | 71 ± 9 | <0.001 |
| KSS (knee) | 96 ± 7 | 96 ± 7 | 96 ± 5 | 0.76 |
| KSS (function) | 92 ± 13 | 94 ± 12 | 87 ± 14 | 0.003 |
| Maximum knee flexion (°) | 124 ± 9 | 122 ± 9 | 127 ± 9 | 0.002 |

*Significant differences between the PCL-retained and PCL-resected groups were assessed using a Student's $t$-test.

narrow (1-2 mm), and wide (>3 mm) based on the total width of any observed radiolucent line.

In addition to the clinical and radiological outcomes described above, some patients were requested to participate in a quantitative analysis of two deep flexion activities in the early follow-up period (3 to 13 months), including 20 patients from the PCL-retained group and 13 patients from the PCL-resected group. Similar to previous fluoroscopy studies [4, 5, 14–16, 38–40], included patients were recruited arbitrarily on the basis of combined KSS of >180 and willingness to provide informed consent to participate in the activities. Fluoroscopic imaging of knee kinematics was obtained during a nonweight bearing kneeling and a weight bearing lunge activities using a standardized technique that has been widely described (Figure 3) [5, 38–40]. For the kneeling activity, the patients kneeled on a padded chair with their operated knee and flexed to their maximum comfortable flexion. For the lunge activity, the subjects placed their foot upon a 30 cm riser and lunged forward with their operated knee to maximum comfortable flexion. Once the subjects had reached their maximal flexed position in each activity, one to three seconds of fluoroscopic images were digitally recorded. The subjects' postures were not constrained in any way during these activities. An investigator was always available to assist the subjects in case of misbalance by holding their hands or forearms. Using the sagittal plane images, three-dimensional knee kinematic

was analyzed using a model-image registration technique [38]. Maximum skeletal knee flexion was measured as the angle between the axes of the femoral and tibial shafts. Condylar translations were determined from the anteroposterior location of the lowest point on each femoral condyle relative to the transverse plane of the tibial baseplate, with the coordinate system defining femoral anterior translation as positive and femoral posterior translation as negative values. Standard errors for this fluoroscopic imaging process are approximately 0.5° to 1.0° for rotations and 0.5 to 1.0 mm for translations in the sagittal plane [38].

## 3. Results

Prospectively measured clinical scores and radiographic outcomes were generally good to excellent after five to ten years of in vivo function (Table 1). Among all 159 TKA, KSS knee and function scores at last follow-up averaged 96 ± 7 (range, 55 to 100) and 92 ± 13 (range, 50 to 100), respectively. Stability scores reported within the KSS knee score were perfect (25 points) for 97% and 86% of the TKA in the PCL-retained and PCL-resected groups, respectively. Passive flexion at last follow-up averaged 124° + 9° (range, 90° to 150°), with 126 TKA (79%) exhibiting 120° or more flexion. Small, but statistically significant, differences in knee flexion and function scores were also noted, with the PCL-resected group

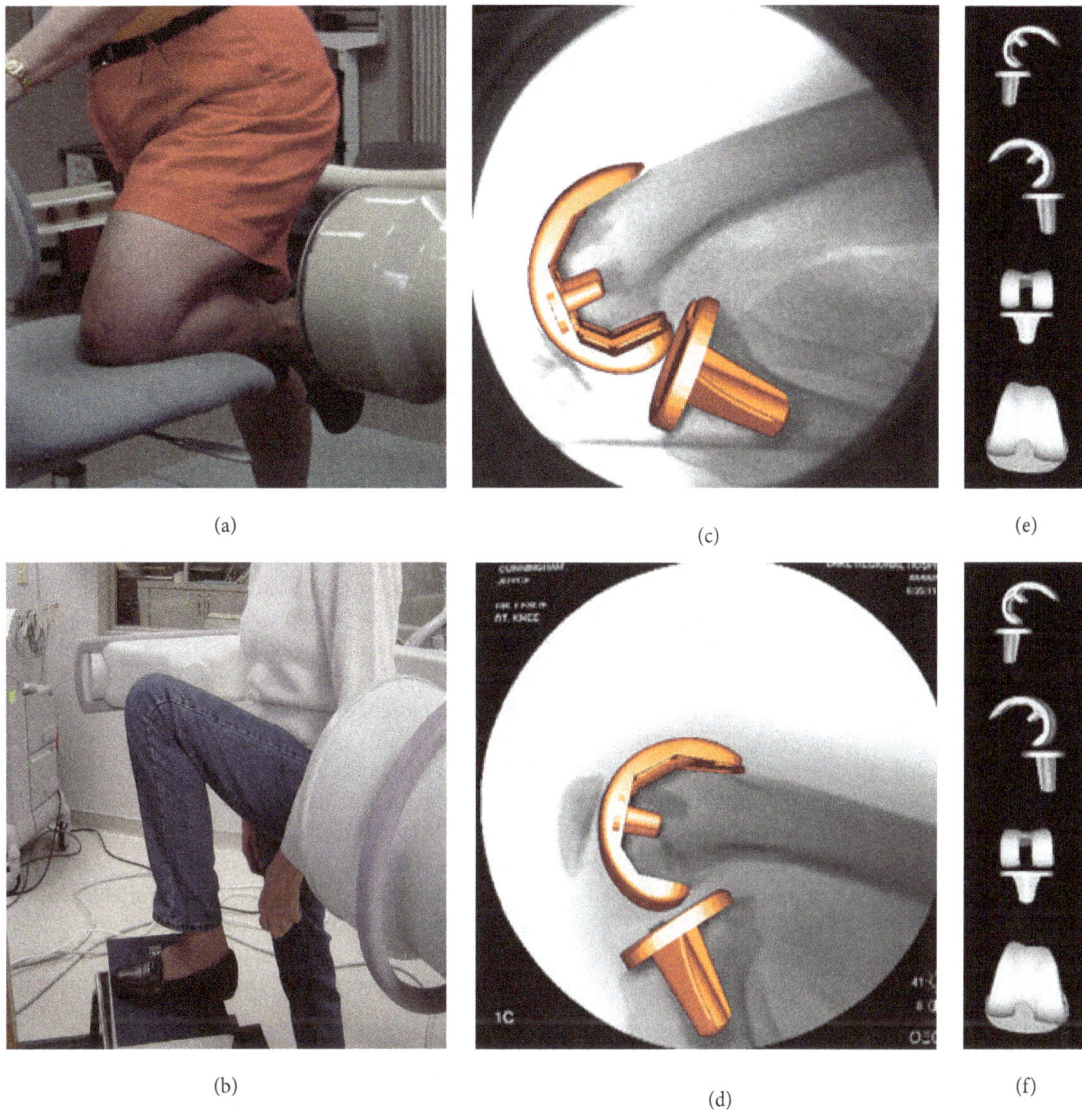

FIGURE 3: In vivo sagittal plane fluoroscopic images acquired during kneeling and lunge activities (a, b) were analyzed using a shape-matching procedure for fitting the prosthesis surface models to the image silhouettes (c, d) and calculating the position and orientation of the femoral component relative to the tibial component (e, f).

exhibiting an average of 5° more flexion ($P = 0.002$) but an average function score that was 7 points lower ($P = 0.003$) compared to the PCL-retained group (Table 1). The clinical cohort in each of the PCL-retained and PCL-resected groups had dissimilar patient ages ($P < 0.001$), which were generally representative of the diverse geographic locations of the two clinical sites.

Radiological assessments by a nonauthor third party orthopaedic surgeon were completed on 141 TKA that had sufficient follow-up films for examination. Restoration of suitable limb alignment was noted, recorded as part of the KSS knee score. Narrow (less than 2 mm), nonprogressive radiolucent lines were noted on 19% of the TKA, including 27% and 2% of the TKA in the PCL-retained and PCL-resected groups, respectively. None showed progression on the yearly radiographs. The largest proportion of radiolucent lines were noted in two femoral regions of dense cortical bone on the anterior femur (zone 1) or in sclerotic bone on the posterior femur (zone 4) and one tibial region on the medial tibial pleateau (zone 1). Three TKA in the PCL-retained group exhibited wide radiolucent lines (more than 2 mm) in one zone and were also classified as nonprogressive on serial radiographs. None of the TKA in the PCL-resected group had wide radiolucent lines.

Detailed fluoroscopic analysis revealed few significant differences between the PCL-retained and PCL-resected groups (Table 2). Maximum skeletal flexion during non-weight bearing kneeling ranged from 109° to 160°, with no statistical difference ($P = 0.15$) between the PCL-retained group measuring an average of 131°±13° and the PCL-resected group averaging 124°±11°. Tibial axial rotation averaged 10° for both groups during kneeling. Lateral femoral rollback in

TABLE 2: Kinematics during the kneeling and lunge activities for the PCL-retained and PCL-resected groups (mean ± standard deviation, range).

| | Nonweight bearing kneeling | | | Weight bearing lunge | | |
| --- | --- | --- | --- | --- | --- | --- |
| | PCL-retained | PCL-resected | $P^*$ | PCL-retained | PCL-resected | $P^*$ |
| Patients | 20 | 13 | | 20 | 10 | |
| Skeletal knee flexion (°) | 131 ± 13 (109 to 160) | 124 ± 11 (105 to 141) | 0.15 | 120 ± 11 (95 to 147) | 123 ± 17 (87 to 145) | 0.54 |
| Implant valgus (°) | −1 ± 2 (−3 to 2) | 1 ± 3 (−3 to 8) | 0.02 | −1 ± 1 (−2 to 1) | 1 ± 2 (−5 to −1) | 0.00 |
| Tibial external rotation (°) | −10 ± 4 (−18 to −3) | −10 ± 6 (−19 to −1) | 0.75 | −11 ± 4 (−16 to −3) | −9 ± 4 (−18 to −4) | 0.25 |
| Medial condyle AP (mm) | −2 ± 4 (−10 to 9) | 2 ± 4 (−3 to 9) | 0.02 | 0 ± 4 (−6 to 8) | −2 ± 4 (−9 to 3) | 0.22 |
| Lateral Condyle AP (mm) | −10 ± 4 (−20 to −1) | −5 ± 4 (−9 to 1) | 0.01 | −8 ± 4 (−15 to −1) | −9 ± 3 (−15 to −5) | 0.41 |

*Significant differences between the PCL-retained and PCL-resected groups were assessed using a Student's $t$-test.

kneeling averaged 10 mm in the PCL-retained group, which was significantly larger ($P = 0.01$) than the average 5 mm in the PCL-resected group. Maximum skeletal flexion for the lunge activity averaged 120° ± 11° and 123° ± 17° for the PCL-retained and PCL-resected groups, respectively. In the PCL-resected group during the lunge, three patients showed slight articular lift-off in the medial compartment at flexion angles greater than 139°, consistent with observations from normal knees in deep flexion [40]. Tibial axial rotation and lateral femoral rollback were statistically similar for both groups, averaging 9° to 11° of rotation and 8 mm to 9 mm of rollback.

## 4. Discussion

Much of the clinical success of TKA is partially dependent upon using TKA designs with suitable congruity and constraint to provide adequate knee joint stability throughout the full range of motion [3–17]. AP stability during TKA is achieved by proper handling of soft tissues, implanting knee prostheses with suitable thickness, proper alignment, and conforming surfaces, helping to restore tension to the remaining ligament structures [20, 25]. However, it remains unclear precisely how much conformity is required for successful TKA [30]. The current study demonstrated that a TKA articular design with progressive congruency in the lateral compartment (Figures 1 and 2) can provide for femoral condyle rollback in maximal flexion activities and good clinical outcomes at midterm follow-up. Positive clinical and functional performance was achieved in patients whose PCL was either meticulously maintained or summarily excised (Table 1), demonstrating the suitability of using this TKA design with either surgical technique.

Physical examinations and in vivo fluoroscopic analysis showed reasonably consistent flexion kinematics in knees with or without a PCL (Tables 1 and 2). Average passive flexion ranged from 122° to 127° for all TKA in the clinical groups and average flexion during the kneeling and lunge activities ranged from 120° to 131°. This maximum flexion measurement is equivalent to or better than flexion reported

in American patient populations with contemporary TKA including the asymmetrically constrained high-flexion TKA and posterior-stabilized TKA [16, 18, 21, 24]. Our findings also are very comparable to results previously reported for Japanese patients implanted with the same TKA design (3D Knee) using a PCL-preserving surgical technique [41]. In that study [41], patients achieved 127° ± 13° (range, 115° to 160°) of passive flexion during clinical evaluation, 123° ± 13° (rang, 107° to 156°) during kneeling, and 124° ± 15° (range, 107° to 163°) during squatting.

We evaluated TKA performance using clinical outcome scores, in which stability was assessed using the KSS knee score (25 points are assessed for stability), and functional fluoroscopic assessments during deep flexion activities. This combination was selected because previous studies have been unable to differentiate the performance of different TKA designs using only clinical outcomes or gait analysis, even when comparing vastly different articular geometries such as cruciate-retaining or posterior-stabilized TKA [15, 23, 42–45]. In a large randomized controlled study designed with sufficient statistical power to assess TKA performance in bilateral TKA patients, Kim et al. [23] were unable to detect differences between cruciate-retaining TKA and posterior-stabilized TKA using clinical outcome scores and goniometric measurements of the range of motion. Other studies have used combined clinical outcome scores and fluoroscopic assessment of knee flexion kinematics to detect inferior functional performance of TKA designs [14, 39, 40, 46]. In a randomized controlled study of PCL-retaining mobile-bearing TKA assessed using fluoroscopy, Lützner et al. [46] reported lack of functional improvement in some patients supported by significantly lower KSS function scores and axial rotation biased toward femoral internal rotation during nonweight bearing passive knee flexion. Ploegmakers et al. [39] compared two PCL-retaining TKA designs using fluoroscopy during deep knee flexion and reported inferior functional performance for one design supported by greater anterior condylar translation and corresponding greater joint stiffness and disability WOMAC scores. In a randomized controlled fluoroscopy study, Victor et al. [40] reported more stable function of the femoral medial condyle during a deep flexion lunge in posterior-stabilized TKA compared to cruciate-retaining TKA.

A critical question for TKA designs intended for use with or without the PCL is whether the tibiofemoral articulation provides adequate knee stability to eliminate or reduce unproductive AP sliding during dynamic activities like gait and stair climbing. The larger condylar translations (approximately 10 mm) recorded during the deep flexion activities in the current study are consistent with the TKA achieving femoral rollback essential for accomplishing deep flexion kneeling, lunge, and step up/down activities [39, 40]. The approximately 10° of tibial internal rotation (femoral external rotation) similar to healthy normal knee kinematics is known to aid patellar tracking and enhance the quadriceps function during knee flexion [47]. Similar magnitudes of axial rotation during gait and stair activities have been reported for successful TKA cruciate-retaining and posterior-stabilized designs [14, 15]. The articular constraint provided by the TKA design in the current study provided adequate femoral rollback and intrinsic stability to control tibiofemoral motions during deep flexion activities, which may help to avoid developing compensatory hamstrings cocontraction patterns that can limit functional strength [3].

This new TKA design concept was originally introduced in 2001 and was based on new knowledge from studies of in vivo kinematics and retrieved implant analysis [16]. Based on the current study's midterm clinical and functional outcomes, there were few differences between the PCL-retained and PCL-resected groups. Stability scores recorded within the KSS were perfect for 150 (94%) of these TKA. We conclude that this design is beneficial for addressing the wide range of joint laxity that can occur with patient variation and the PCL-retaining and PCL-resecting surgical techniques. Longer duration clinical follow-up and tracking of the polyethylene wear that occurs with in vivo function are ongoing to fully characterize the longevity of this design as related to the highly congruent lateral femoral condyle and widened medial condyle design features (Figures 1 and 2).

The most widely used design concept for providing AP stability after resection of both cruciate ligaments is to incorporate a femoral cam and tibial post articulation [30]. However, several complications associated with wear of the tibial post and increased strain at the prosthesis-bone interface have emerged with those designs [31, 32, 48–50]. O'Rourke et al. [48] reported osteolysis in 16% of cemented IB-II posterior-stabilized TKA at 5 to 8 years follow-up. Similarly, Mikulak et al. [49] reported osteolysis and a 3% rate of revision for loosening associated with high rotational constraint in TKA with a cam and post articulation. Femoral component loosening associated with weight bearing maximum flexion also has been reported for more modern high-flexion TKA designs having a cam and post articulation, with Han et al. [50] reporting a 38% loosening rate in Legacy PS-Flex TKA at 2 to 4 years follow-up. In the current study, there was a notable absence of progressive radiolucent lines at five to ten years of follow-up, suggesting that the forces developed by articular constraints are well-tolerated throughout the midterm duration. Therefore, the stability provided by the TKA design in the current study, which does not depend on a cam and post mechanism, appears to provide a considerable advantage for avoiding such documented complications with cam and post designs.

Several limitations are recognized. Outcomes were assessed solely using KSS knee and function scores, as was the clinical standard for the involved clinics at the start of this study. KSS are known to be weak predictors of differences between patients. While other clinical outcome measures may have detected outcome differences between the study groups, the current study incorporated quantitative radiographic assessments and functional fluoroscopic analysis to supplement the KSS. Regarding surgical technique, one of the known differences between PCL-retaining and PCL-sacrificing surgical techniques is the potential for an increased flexion gap in the latter case. When noted intraoperatively, this was accommodated through the use of thicker tibial inserts in the latter case. The proportion of TKA having nonprogressive radiolucent lines was greater for the PCL-retained group than for the PCL-resected group. This is likely due to technicians who were more demanding in aligning the beam with the prostheses and newer radiography equipment in use at the clinic where the PCL-retained group were followed up. These factors combined to produce better views of the interface between the bone and cement on higher resolution images, aiding detection and follow-up of any progression of observed radiolucent lines at that clinical site.

Limitations related to the limited size of patient cohorts are noted. Dissimilar surgical volume at the two involved clinical sites led to unequally sized patient cohorts with suitable follow-up data acquired within the timeframe of this study. While such dissimilarity can lead to overly broad population variance, and contributed to the differences in patient ages for each group, the authors chose to err on inclusion rather than reduce the PCL-retaining group from 116 TKA down to 43 TKA. The follow-up rate was less than 75% because of the decision to capture an initial group of 150 TKA in patients who met the inclusion criteria and were willing to come to the clinic for follow-up, rather than trying to follow up all patients, many of whom maintain only seasonal residency in the geographic regions surrounding the clinical sites. Studies involving a sequential series of TKA patients operated with this TKA are needed to fully characterize outcomes from patients who are not motivated to return for follow-up or have reduced willingness to participate in clinical studies. The fluoroscopic analysis included only 33 patients who all had high outcome scores. Such selection criteria have been used in many previously published fluoroscopic studies and have proven to yield significant results [4, 5, 14–16, 38–40].

## 5. Conclusion

This novel TKA design showed excellent functional performance with or without the posterior cruciate ligament over the intermediate time period of five to ten years. The standard implantation technique provided surgeons with the option of using one implant solution when dealing with variable posterior cruciate ligament integrity. The 3D Knee provided the required stability to achieve excellent clinical and radiographic outcomes and consistent kinematic results in both the PCL-retained and PCL-resected patient cohorts. Continued multicentered studies of this TKA design will be necessary to produce the evidence-based data to ultimately prove long-term clinical success.

## Conflict of Interests

The authors disclose institutional support from DJO Surgical (MK Harman, SA Banks, WA Hodge), including funding for the project; royalties from DJO Surgical (CJ Leslie, SA Banks, WA Hodge); and payment for lectures and consultant activities from DJO Surgical (MK Harman, CJ Leslie, SA Banks, WA Hodge).

## Acknowledgments

The authors acknowledge assistance from our clinical (Lewjack Dorrance, PA and David Rondon, MD) and technical (Akiko Mori, James Coburn, and Kim Mitchell) collaborators, as well as numerous student interns employed by The BioMotion Foundation. This research was sponsored by The Institute of Mobility and Longevity, with funding obtained through an institutional research grant provided by DJO Global, L.P., Austin, Texas.

## References

[1] M. Manley, K. Ong, E. Lau, and S. M. Kurtz, "Total knee arthroplasty survivorship in the United States Medicare population: effect of hospital and surgeon procedure volume," *Journal of Arthroplasty*, vol. 24, no. 7, pp. 1061–1067, 2009.

[2] E. W. Paxton, O. Furnes, R. S. Namba, M. C. S. Inacio, A. M. Fenstad, and L. I. Havelin, "Comparison of the Norwegian knee arthroplasty register and a United States arthroplasty registry," *The Journal of Bone and Joint Surgery. American*, vol. 93, supplement 3, pp. 20–30, 2011.

[3] T. P. Andriacchi, J. O. Galante, and R. W. Fermier, "The influence of total knee-replacement design on walking and stair-climbing," *Journal of Bone and Joint Surgery A*, vol. 64, no. 9, pp. 1328–1335, 1982.

[4] S. A. Banks, G. D. Markovich, and W. A. Hodge, "In vivo kinematics of cruciate-retaining and -substituting knee arthroplasties," *Journal of Arthroplasty*, vol. 12, no. 3, pp. 297–304, 1997.

[5] S. A. Banks, J. Bellemans, H. Nozaki, L. A. Whiteside, M. Harman, and W. A. Hodge, "Knee motions during maximum flexion in fixed and mobile-bearing arthroplasties," *Clinical Orthopaedics and Related Research*, no. 410, pp. 131–138, 2003.

[6] J. D. Blaha, "The rationale for a total knee implant that confers anteroposterior stability throughout range of motion," *Journal of Arthroplasty*, vol. 19, supplement 1, no. 4, pp. 22–26, 2004.

[7] L. F. Draganich, G. A. Piotrowski, J. Martell, and L. A. Pottenger, "The effects of early rollback in total knee arthroplasty on stair stepping," *Journal of Arthroplasty*, vol. 17, no. 6, pp. 723–730, 2002.

[8] O. M. Mahoney, C. D. McClung, M. A. Dela Rosa, and T. P. Schmalzried, "The effect of total knee arthroplasty design on extensor mechanism function," *Journal of Arthroplasty*, vol. 17, no. 4, pp. 416–421, 2002.

[9] J. B. Stiehl, R. D. Komistek, D. A. Dennis, R. D. Paxson, and W. A. Hoff, "Fluroscopic analysis of kinematics after posterior-cruciate-retaining knee arthroplasty," *Journal of Bone and Joint Surgery B*, vol. 77, no. 6, pp. 884–889, 1995.

[10] J. B. Stiehl, R. D. Komistek, and D. A. Dennis, "Detrimental kinematics of a flat on flat total condylar knee arthroplasty," *Clinical Orthopaedics and Related Research*, no. 365, pp. 139–148, 1999.

[11] H. Wang, K. J. Simpson, S. Chamnongkich, T. Kinsey, and O. M. Mahoney, "A biomechanical comparison between the single-axis and multi-axis total knee arthroplasty systems for the stand-to-sit movement," *Clinical Biomechanics*, vol. 20, no. 4, pp. 428–433, 2005.

[12] P. J. Warren, T. K. Olanlokun, A. G. Cobb, P. S. Walker, and B. F. Iverson, "Laxity and function in knee replacements: a comparative study of three prosthetic designs," *Clinical Orthopaedics and Related Research*, no. 305, pp. 200–208, 1994.

[13] J. D. DesJardins, S. A. Banks, L. C. Benson, T. Pace, and M. LaBerge, "A direct comparison of patient and force-controlled simulator total knee replacement kinematics," *Journal of Biomechanics*, vol. 40, no. 15, pp. 3458–3466, 2007.

[14] S. A. Banks and W. A. Hodge, "Implant design affects knee arthroplasty kinematics during stair-stepping," *Clinical Orthopaedics and Related Research*, no. 426, pp. 187–193, 2004.

[15] S. A. Banks and W. A. Hodge, "2003 Hap Paul Award Paper of the International Society for Technology in Arthroplasty: Design and activity dependence of kinematics in fixed and mobile-bearing knee arthroplasties," *Journal of Arthroplasty*, vol. 19, no. 7, pp. 809–816, 2004.

[16] S. A. Banks, M. K. Harman, J. Bellemans, and W. A. Hodge, "Making sense of knee arthroplasty kinematics: news you can use," *Journal of Bone and Joint Surgery. American*, vol. 85-A, supplement 4, pp. 64–72, 2003.

[17] B. Yue, K. M. Varadarajan, A. L. Moynihan, F. Liu, H. E. Rubash, and G. Li, "Kinematics of medial osteoarthritic knees before and after posterior cruciate ligament retaining total knee arthroplasty," *Journal of Orthopaedic Research*, vol. 29, no. 1, pp. 40–46, 2011.

[18] M. J. Anderson, R. L. Kruse, C. Leslie, L. J. Levy Jr., J. W. Pritchett, and J. Hodge, "Medium-term results of total knee arthroplasty using a medially pivoting implant: a multicenter study," *Journal of surgical orthopaedic advances*, vol. 19, no. 4, pp. 191–195, 2010.

[19] M. Arabori, N. Matsui, R. Kuroda et al., "Posterior condylar offset and flexion in posterior cruciate-retaining and posterior stabilized TKA," *Journal of Orthopaedic Science*, vol. 13, no. 1, pp. 46–50, 2008.

[20] J. Bellemans, M. D. Ries, and J. Victor, *Total Knee Arthroplasty: A Guide to Get Better Performance*, Springer, Heidelberg, Germany, 2005.

[21] W. G. Hamilton, S. Sritulanondha, and C. A. Engh Jr., "Results of prospective, randomized clinical trials comparing standard and high-flexion posterior-stabilized TKA: a focused review," *Orthopedics*, vol. 34, no. 9, pp. e500–e503, 2011.

[22] K. Harato, R. B. Bourne, J. Victor, M. Snyder, J. Hart, and M. D. Ries, "Midterm comparison of posterior cruciate-retaining versus -substituting total knee arthroplasty using the Genesis II prosthesis. A multicenter prospective randomized clinical trial," *Knee*, vol. 15, no. 3, pp. 217–221, 2008.

[23] Y.-H. Kim, Y. Choi, O.-R. Kwon, and J.-S. Kim, "Functional outcome and range of motion of high-flexion posterior cruciate-retaining and high-flexion posterior cruciate-substituting total knee prostheses: a prospective, randomized study," *Journal of Bone and Joint Surgery A*, vol. 91, no. 4, pp. 753–760, 2009.

[24] R. Schmidt, R. D. Komistek, J. D. Blaha, B. L. Penenberg, and W. J. Maloney, "Fluoroscopic analyses of cruciate-retaining and Medial Pivot knee implants," *Clinical Orthopaedics and Related Research*, no. 410, pp. 139–147, 2003.

[25] J. Victor and J. Bellemans, "Physiologic kinematics as a concept for better flexion in TKA," *Clinical Orthopaedics and Related Research*, no. 452, pp. 53–58, 2006.

[26] J. Victor, J. K. P. Mueller, R. D. Komistek, A. Sharma, M. C. Nadaud, and J. Bellemans, "In vivo kinematics after a cruciate-substituting TKA," *Clinical Orthopaedics and Related Research*, vol. 468, no. 3, pp. 807–814, 2010.

[27] H. Morgan, V. Battista, and S. S. Leopold, "Constraint in primary total knee arthroplasty.," *The Journal of the American Academy of Orthopaedic Surgeons.*, vol. 13, no. 8, pp. 515–524, 2005.

[28] W. C. H. Jacobs, D. J. Clement, and A. B. Wymenga, "Retention versus removal of the posterior cruciate ligament in total knee replacement: a systematic literature review within the Cochrane framework," *Acta Orthopaedica*, vol. 76, no. 6, pp. 757–768, 2005.

[29] G. Matziolis, S. Mehlhorn, N. Schattat et al., "How much of the PCL is really preserved during the tibial cut?" *Knee Surgery, Sports Traumatology, Arthroscopy*, vol. 20, no. 6, pp. 1083–1086, 2012.

[30] H. Shoji, A. Wolf, S. Packard, and S. Yoshino, "Cruciate retained and excised total knee arthroplasty: a comparative study in patients with bilateral total knee arthroplasty," *Clinical Orthopaedics and Related Research*, no. 305, pp. 218–222, 1994.

[31] H. Shoji, S. Yoshino, and M. Komagamine, "Improved range of motion with the Y/S total knee arthroplasty system," *Clinical Orthopaedics and Related Research*, vol. 218, pp. 150–163, 1987.

[32] M. M. Dolan, N. H. Kelly, J. T. Nguyen, T. M. Wright, and S. B. Haas, "Implant design influences tibial post wear damage in posterior-stabilized knees," *Clinical Orthopaedics and Related Research*, vol. 469, no. 1, pp. 160–167, 2011.

[33] F. J. Medel, S. M. Kurtz, P. F. Sharkey et al., "Post damage in contemporary posterior-stabilized tibial inserts: Influence of implant design and clinical relevance," *Journal of Arthroplasty*, vol. 26, no. 4, pp. 606–614, 2011.

[34] R. J. Sierra and D. J. Berry, "Surgical technique differences between posterior-substituting and cruciate-retaining total knee arthroplasty," *Journal of Arthroplasty*, vol. 23, no. 7, pp. 20–23, 2008.

[35] M. Barink, M. de Waal Malefijt, P. Celada, P. Vena, A. van Kampen, and N. Verdonschot, "A mechanical comparison of high-flexion and conventional total knee arthroplasty," *Proceedings of the Institution of Mechanical Engineers H: Journal of Engineering in Medicine*, vol. 222, no. 3, pp. 297–307, 2008.

[36] J. N. Insall, L. D. Dorr, R. D. Scott, and W. N. Scott, "Rationale of the knee society clinical rating system," *Clinical Orthopaedics and Related Research*, no. 248, pp. 13–14, 1989.

[37] F. C. Ewald, "The Knee Society total knee arthroplasty roentgenographic evaluation and scoring system," *Clinical Orthopaedics and Related Research*, no. 248, pp. 9–12, 1989.

[38] S. A. Banks and W. A. Hodge, "Accurate measurement of three-dimensional knee replacement kinematics using single-plane fluoroscopy," *IEEE Transactions on Biomedical Engineering*, vol. 43, no. 6, pp. 638–649, 1996.

[39] M. J. M. Ploegmakers, B. Ginsel, H. J. Meijerink et al., "Physical examination and in vivo kinematics in two posterior cruciate ligament retaining total knee arthroplasty designs," *The Knee*, vol. 17, no. 3, pp. 204–209, 2010.

[40] J. Victor, S. Banks, and J. Bellemans, "Kinematics of posterior cruciate ligament-retaining and -substituting total knee arthroplasty. A prospective randomised outcome study," *Journal of Bone and Joint Surgery. British*, vol. 87, no. 5, pp. 646–655, 2005.

[41] S. Nakagawa, Y. Kadoya, S. Todo et al., "Tibiofemoral movement 3: full flexion in the living knee studied by MRI," *Journal of Bone and Joint Surgery*, vol. 82, no. 8, pp. 1199–1200, 2000.

[42] T. Saari, R. Tranberg, R. Zügner, J. Uvehammer, and J. Kärrholm, "Changed gait pattern in patients with total knee arthroplasty but minimal influence of tibial insert design: gait analysis during level walking in 39 TKR patients and 18 healthy controls," *Acta Orthopaedica*, vol. 76, no. 2, pp. 253–260, 2005.

[43] A. Ş. Solak, B. Kentel, and Y. Ateş, "Does bilateral total knee arthroplasty affect gait in women? Comparison of gait analyses before and after total knee arthroplasty compared with normal knees," *Journal of Arthroplasty*, vol. 20, no. 6, pp. 745–750, 2005.

[44] L. G. van den Boom, J. P. Halbertsma, J. J. van Raaij, R. W. Brouwer, S. K. Bulstra, and I. van den Akker-Scheek, "No difference in gait between posterior cruciate retention and the posterior stabilized design after total knee arthroplasty," *Knee Surgery, Sports Traumatology, Arthroscopy*, 2014.

[45] N. Wolterbeek, R. G. H. H. Nelissen, and E. R. Valstar, "No differences in in vivo kinematics between six different types of knee prostheses," *Knee Surgery, Sports Traumatology, Arthroscopy*, vol. 20, no. 3, pp. 559–564, 2012.

[46] J. Lützner, S. Kirschner, K.-P. Günther, and M. K. Harman, "Patients with no functional improvement after total knee arthroplasty show different kinematics," *International Orthopaedics*, vol. 36, no. 9, pp. 1841–1847, 2012.

[47] J. T. H. Chew, N. J. Stewart, A. D. Hanssen, Z.-P. Luo, J. A. Rand, and K.-N. An, "Differences in patellar tracking and knee kinematics among three different total knee designs," *Clinical Orthopaedics and Related Research*, no. 345, pp. 87–98, 1997.

[48] M. R. O'Rourke, J. J. Callaghan, D. D. Goetz, P. M. Sullivan, and R. C. Johnston, "Osteolysis associated with a cemented modular posterior-cruciate-substituting total knee design: five to eight-year follow-up," *Journal of Bone and Joint Surgery—Series A*, vol. 84, no. 8, pp. 1362–1371, 2002.

[49] S. A. Mikulak, O. M. Mahoney, M. A. Dela Rosa, and T. P. Schmalzried, "Loosening and osteolysis with the press-fit condylar posterior-cruciate-substituting total knee replacement," *Journal of Bone and Joint Surgery A*, vol. 83, no. 3, pp. 398–403, 2001.

[50] H. S. Han, S.-B. Kang, and K. S. Yoon, "High incidence of loosening of the femoral component in legacy posterior stabilised-flex total knee replacement," *Journal of Bone and Joint Surgery B*, vol. 89, no. 11, pp. 1457–1461, 2007.

# 3

# Cemented versus Uncemented Oxford Unicompartmental Knee Arthroplasty: Is There a Difference?

**Burak Akan,**[1,2] **Dogac Karaguven,**[1] **Berk Guclu,**[1] **Tugrul Yildirim,**[1] **Alper Kaya,**[1] **Mehmet Armangil,**[3] **and Ilker Cetin**[1]

[1] *Department of Orthopedics and Traumatology, Ufuk University Faculty of Medicine, Ankara, Turkey*
[2] *Dikmen C Parkpinar Evleri, 9/B No 28 Keklikpinari Cankaya, 06420 Ankara, Turkey*
[3] *Department of Orthopedics and Traumatology, Ankara University Faculty of Medicine, Ankara, Turkey*

Correspondence should be addressed to Burak Akan; drburakakan@hotmail.com

Academic Editor: Bach Christian

*Purpose.* The use of uncemented unicompartmental knee prostheses has recently increased. However, few studies on the outcomes of uncemented unicompartmental knee prostheses have been performed. The purpose of this study was to compare the outcomes of cemented and uncemented Oxford unicompartmental knee arthroplasty. *Materials and Methods.* This retrospective observational study evaluated the clinical and radiological outcomes of 263 medial Oxford unicompartmental prostheses (141 cemented, 122 uncemented) implanted in 235 patients. The mean follow-up was 42 months in the cemented group and 30 months in the uncemented group. *Results.* At the last follow-up, there were no significant differences in the clinical results or survival rates between the two groups. However, the operation time in the uncemented unicompartmental knee arthroplasty group was shorter than that in the cemented unicompartmental knee arthroplasty group. In addition, the cost of uncemented arthroplasty was greater. *Conclusion.* Despite the successful midterm results in the uncemented unicompartmental knee arthroplasty group, a longer follow-up period is required to determine the best fixation mode.

## 1. Introduction

Unicompartmental knee replacement arthroplasty (UKA) has been a popular treatment of osteoarthritis since the 1970s. Initial reports showed high failure rates in short-term follow-ups [1]. Because of these high failure rates and instrumentation problems, the use of these implants decreased in the 1990s. However, during the last 20 years, UKA has become a well-established treatment method for unicompartmental osteoarthritis of the knee. Recent reports have described success rates of 90% or higher at a minimum 10-year follow-up [2, 3]. These higher success rates have been attributed to better surgical techniques, new implant designs, improved instrumentation, and careful patient selection [4]. With the improvements in surgical techniques and instruments, this procedure has many advantages over total knee replacement such as a smaller incision, less soft tissue injury, preservation of bone stock, preservation of normal knee kinematics, less morbidity because of minimal postoperative blood loss, lower

infection rate, shortened hospital stay, and rapid recovery [5]. However, controversy on the validity and durability of UKA remains. Although UKA is associated with better clinical results than total knee replacement arthroplasty (TKA), registry data show higher revision rates [6]. On the other hand, Goodfellow et al. reported that the revision rate is a poor and misleading outcome and questioned its use in comparing UKA and TKA [7].

Most UKA designs use cement to fix the components to the bone. Disadvantages of cemented UKA prostheses are aseptic loosening, third-body particles in the joints, and extended surgical times. A porous-coated UKA design is an alternative to cemented fixation [8]. In addition to inducing bone growth, it also provides more reliable fixation, especially in younger patients. Some studies have reported excellent results of uncemented TKA, and these results were similar to those of cemented TKA [9, 10]. However, registry data and meta-analyses show superior results and durability in cemented TKA over uncemented TKA [11]. The efficacy of the uncemented design in UKA remains unclear. A few encouraging reports of cemented and uncemented UKAs have been published, but few direct comparisons of these two methods have been made [12]. In this study, we retrospectively evaluated the early clinical and functional outcomes of cemented and uncemented Oxford Phase 3 UKAs.

## 2. Materials and Methods

From August 2008 to May 2011, a total of 235 patients (263 knees) underwent UKAs with mobile-bearing Oxford unicompartmental knee prostheses (Biomet UK Ltd., Bridgend, UK). There were 141 cemented and 122 uncemented UKAs. All patients had anteromedial osteoarthritis and conformed to the indications described by Goodfellow et al.: patients with medial osteoarthritis, a correctable varus deformity, an intact anterior cruciate ligament and collateral ligaments, absence of degenerative findings in the lateral compartment of the knee on standing radiographs, and femoral flexion deformity of less than 15° [13]. Osteoarthritis of the patellofemoral joint, obesity, old age, and high activity level were not considered to be contraindications to this procedure, unlike the Kozinn and Scott criteria [14, 15]. The final decision to proceed with unicompartmental arthroplasty was made at the time of surgery. If arthritis was found in the lateral compartment or if there was no anterior cruciate ligament, then the operation was converted to total knee arthroplasty. One patient in the uncemented group had undergone arthroscopic anterior cruciate ligament reconstruction 1 year before the index surgery.

The two groups were well matched for age. The mean age was 64.2 years in the cemented group (range, 42–84 years) and 64.9 years in the uncemented group (range, 35–79 years). There were 20 male and 100 female patients in the cemented group and 11 male and 104 female patients in the uncemented group. The mean body mass index was 29.8 (range, 18.5–41.8) in the cemented group and 28.6 (range, 18.8–38.8) in the uncemented group.

The use of cementless components began in 2009; previous to this time, they were not available in the market. Because the manufacturers introduced cementless components during the study period, all surgeons started to perform cementless UKA. In contrast to cemented prostheses, the cementless UKA has a layer of porous titanium with calcium hydroxyapatite under its components and some mechanical modifications to allow for cementless fixation.

All of the surgical procedures were performed by four surgeons (Ilker Cetin, Alper Kaya, Berk Guclu, and Burak Akan) or under their supervision. All operations were performed under tourniquet control, via a short paramedian skin incision, following a medial parapatellar arthrotomy. The cemented and uncemented surgical techniques were identical with the exception of application of the last components.

Early active movement and full weight-bearing were allowed postoperatively, and thromboprophylaxis was prescribed for all patients. All patients were routinely followed up at 6 weeks, 3 months, 6 months, and 1 year postoperatively. The Knee Society objective and functional scores and the Oxford Knee score were used to assess the clinical outcomes.

SSPS ver. 15.0 (SPSS Inc., Chicago, IL, USA) was used for the statistical analyses. Quantitative variables are shown as means, standard deviations, medians, numbers, and percentages. Normality of continuous variables was evaluated by the Kolmogorov-Smirnov test. An independent-samples $t$-test was used to determine the difference between the two groups when parametric test assumptions were satisfied. The groups were compared by the Mann-Whitney $U$ test when parametric test assumptions were not satisfied. The chi-square test was used to compare qualitative variables. Differences between the preoperative and postoperative values were evaluated within each group and between the two groups using a variance analysis in repeated measurements. The level of statistical significance was set at $P = 0.05$.

## 3. Results

A total of 235 patients (263 knees) were included in the study. The mean follow-up was 42 months (range, 24–52 months) in the cemented group and 30 months (range, 24–36 months) in the uncemented group. The mean preoperative and postoperative range of motion of the cemented cases were 114° (range, 100°–130°) and 128° (range, 115°–145°), respectively. The mean preoperative and postoperative range of motion of the uncemented cases were 119° (range, 105°–132°) and 133° (range, 120°–150°), respectively. There were no statistically significant differences in the demographic data (Table 1).

The mean preoperative Oxford Knee score in the cemented group was 15.4 points (range, 9–23 points), and that in the uncemented group was 20.9 points (range, 12–29 points). The mean postoperative Oxford knee score in the cemented group was 39.3 points (range, 29–47 points), and that in the uncemented group was 41.1 points (range, 34–47 points). There were no statistically significant differences in the outcomes between the groups ($P = 0.452$). The mean preoperative Knee Society score for cemented UKA improved from 43.7 points (range, 32–55 points) to 87.7 points (range, 71–100 points) at the last follow-up. The mean preoperative Knee Society score for uncemented UKA increased from 43.8 points (range, 32–57 points) to 87.6 points (range, 72–100 points) at the last follow-up. There were no significant intergroup differences in the knee scores ($P = 0.897$, $P = 0.721$). The mean preoperative functional score for cemented UKA increased from 58.4 points (range, 42–69 points) to 88.2 points (range, 72–100 points). The mean preoperative and postoperative functional scores for uncemented UKA were 59.0 points (range, 40–76 points) and 90.2 points (range, 68–100 points), respectively. There were no significant intergroup differences in the functional scores ($P = 0.841$, $P = 0.624$).

The revision rate was 7.09% (10 knees) in the cemented group and 4.91% (6 knees) in the uncemented group (Table 2). There was no statistically significant difference in the revision rate ($P = 0.155$). Mobile-bearing dislocation occurred in four patients in the cemented group and three patients in the uncemented group. One patient was revised to a mobile bearing that was one size thicker; the other patients were converted to TKA. Four patients in the cemented group and three patients in the uncemented group underwent

TABLE 1: Demographical data.

| | Cemented group ($n = 141$) | Uncemented group ($n = 122$) | $P$ value |
|---|---|---|---|
| Age (years) | 64.2 | 64.9 | $P = 0.746$ |
| Weight (kg) | 74 ± 4.2 | 77 ± 5.5 | $P = 0.731$ |
| Height (cm) | 158 ± 9.2 | 166 ± 10.0 | $P = 0.294$ |
| Body mass index (kg/cm$^2$) | 29.8 ± 11.2 | 28.6 ± 9.7 | $P = 0.771$ |
| Gender (female/male) | 100/20 | 104/11 | $P = 0.213$ |
| Duration of surgery (min) | 45.3 ± 12.1 | 36.1 ± 11.4 | $P < 0.001$ |
| Revision rate (%) | 7.09% | 4.91% | $P = 0.153$ |
| Preoperative Oxford Knee score | 15.4 ± 5.8 | 20.9 ± 6.2 | $P = 0.614$ |
| Postoperative Oxford Knee score | 39.3 ± 7.6 | 41.1 ± 6.0 | $P = 0.452$ |
| Preoperative Knee Society score | 43.7 ± 8.9 | 43.8 ± 9.2 | $P = 0.897$ |
| Postoperative Knee Society score | 87.7 ± 10.5 | 87.6 ± 10.2 | $P = 0.721$ |
| Preoperative functional score | 58.4 ± 7.8 | 59.0 ± 11.6 | $P = 0.841$ |
| Postoperative functional score | 88.2 ± 8.1 | 90.2 ± 6.5 | $P = 0.624$ |

TABLE 2: Reasons for revision.

| | Cemented Oxford unicompartmental | Uncemented Oxford unicompartmental |
|---|---|---|
| Unexplained pain | 4 | 2 |
| Mobile-bearing dislocation | 4 | 3 |
| Lateral osteoarthritis | 1 | 0 |
| Tibial plateau fracture | 1 | 1 |
| Total | 10 | 6 |

TKA because of persistent unexplained pain. Lateral arthritis occurred in one patient in the cemented group. This patient underwent TKA. In the uncemented group, one medial tibial plateau fracture and one medial femoral condyle fracture occurred. There was one medial tibial plateau fracture in the cemented group. The tibial plateau fractures were treated with TKA, and the femoral condyle fracture was treated with percutaneous cannulated screws.

The mean operation time of cemented UKA was 45.3 minutes (range, 30–58 minutes), and the mean operation time of uncemented UKA was 36.1 minutes (range, 27–47 minutes). There was a significant difference between these operation times ($P < 0.001$). The mean follow-up was 42 months in the cemented group and 30 months in the uncemented group. There is a significant statistical difference in the follow-up period between the two groups ($P < 0.001$).

## 4. Discussion

The most important finding of the present study was that uncemented Oxford UKA provided good clinical and functional patient outcomes similar to those obtained with cemented prostheses. The medial tibiofemoral compartment is the most common of the three knee compartments affected by degenerative joint disease [16]. The predictable advantages of UKA over proximal tibial osteotomy are quicker recovery, relief of pain, and much better long-term results. In appropriately selected patients described by designers, UKA has many advantages over total arthroplasty including more satisfactory physiological functions, quicker recovery, and easier revision in cases of failure [5, 17]. Although unicompartmental knee arthroplasty is not a new procedure, the use of and interest in this technique have increased in Turkey during the last 5 years. The main reasons for the increased popularity of unicompartmental knee arthroplasty are the introduction of minimally invasive surgical techniques with modified surgical equipment and the publication of excellent mid- and long-term results [16, 18]. Among the many controversies concerning UKA is the question of which design concept is associated with the most simple, reproducible surgical technique and optimal long-term results. Other specific controversies include fixed-bearing versus mobile-bearing designs, onlay versus inlay designs, the use of robotics and customization, and whether total knee arthroplasty represents a better treatment solution. However, there is no controversy between cemented and uncemented fixation.

The results of cemented and uncemented total knee replacements have been examined in many previous studies, but ongoing debate about the fixation type remains. The Oxford UKA prosthesis (Biomet UK Ltd., Bridgend, UK), which has been used as a cemented implant for many years, required relatively few modifications of its components to satisfy the perceived requirements for uncemented fixation (Figures 1 and 2). Many surgeons prefer using cemented knee prostheses, although there is a considerable debate regarding the possible benefits of using cementless fixation in joint replacement surgery. These debates include bone stock preservation, avoidance of cementation complications, ease of revision surgery, and improved long-term survival of the implant. Cementation errors and third bodies can cause pain, impingement, dislocation and wear of the bearing, and unnecessary revision because of misunderstandings of the significance of radiolucency, as in aseptic loosening. In minimally invasive surgical techniques, it is difficult to clean the cementation residuals from the posterior aspect, and it is possible that these residuals can prevent mobility of the bearings.

Another benefit of using an uncemented prosthesis is the shortened operation time. In our study, the operation time was significantly shorter in the uncemented group. Shortening the operation time reduces the infection rate

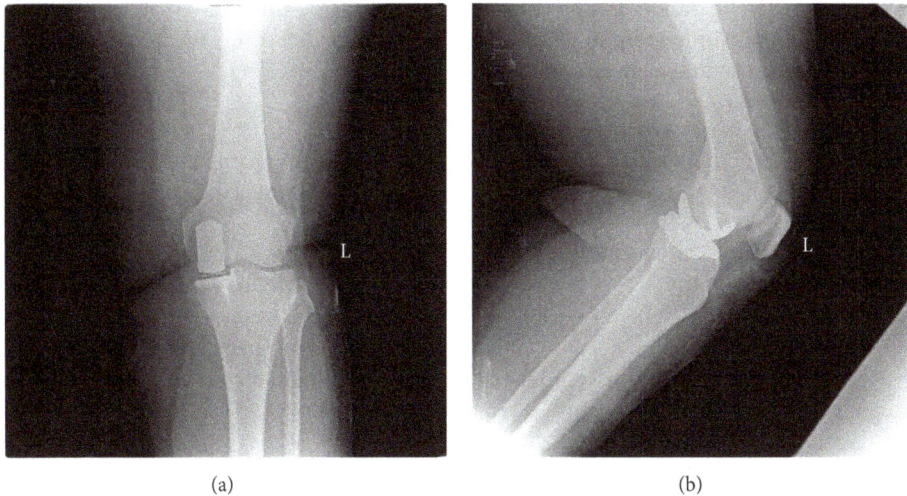

(a)                                                                    (b)

FIGURE 1: (a) A 56-year-old female patient that underwent cemented Oxford UKA, anterior-posterior view. (b) Lateral view.

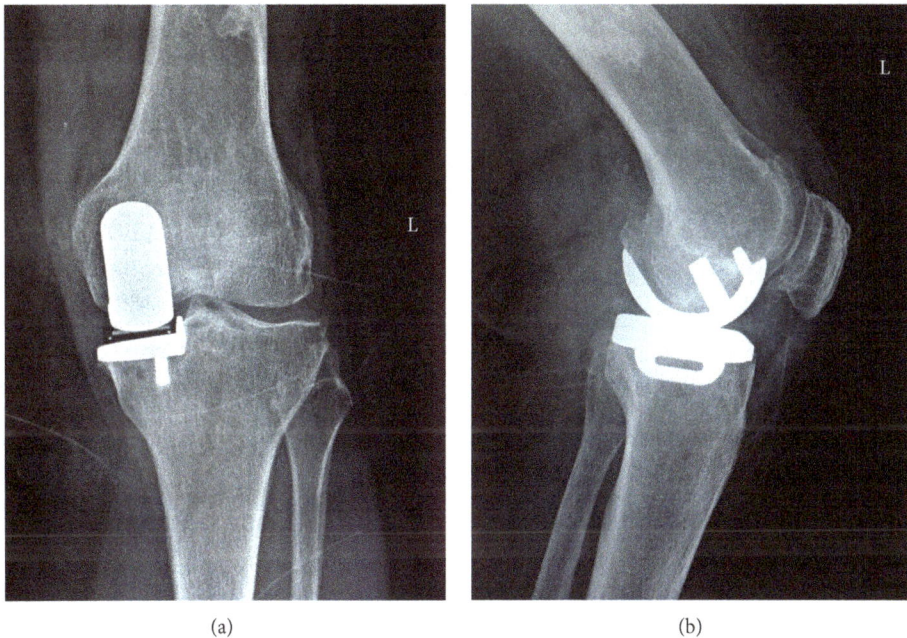

(a)                                                                    (b)

FIGURE 2: (a) A 51-year-old female patient that underwent uncemented Oxford UKA, anterior-posterior view. (b) Lateral view.

and tourniquet side effects and improves operation room productivity [19].

However, whether cementless implants improve long-term patient survival is unclear. Few studies have researched uncemented unicompartmental knee arthroplasty. Pandit et al. reported no differences in patient outcomes between cemented and uncemented fixation, and uncemented fixation was associated with reduced radiolucency after 1 year [8]. This radiolucency has been implicated in aseptic failure, particularly with persistent unexplained pain in surgeries performed by inexperienced surgeons. Using an uncemented prosthesis may help to avoid unnecessary revision surgeries. On the other hand, the cost of uncemented UKA is approximately 450 Euros more than the cost of cemented UKA in

the UK market, and this may be a disadvantage of uncemented arthroplasty because no differences were noted in the clinical and functional results between the groups. The costs of uncemented and cemented UKA are very similar in Turkey; thus, we have improved accessibility to uncemented designs compared with other countries.

The rate of revision to TKA was not significantly different between the cemented and uncemented UKA groups in our study. The most common reasons for revision were unexplained pain and insert dislocation. These failures appeared more often than in independent series, but their incidence was similar to that in designer series [20, 21]. Some of our cases showing physiological radiolucency without pain were not considered to involve component loosening, and they were not revised to UKA. According to designers, physiological radiolucencies are generally 1 mm or less, are surrounded by a sclerotic margin, develop in the first year, and remain static; however, pathologic radiolucencies are wide and do not have a sclerotic margin [22]. It was reported that the incidence of radiolucent lines associated with uncemented Oxford medial unicompartmental knee replacements was significantly lower than that associated with cemented UKA [23]. We found no pathologic radiolucencies in either the cemented or uncemented UKA group.

Many surgeons tend to believe that UKA revision is more beneficial for patients with unexplained pain. Unicompartmental implants are reportedly more susceptible to revision, especially in patients with unexplained pain [7]. We experienced six patients with unexplained pain for whom initial UKA was converted to TKA. Causes of pain such as component loosening, periprosthetic infection, component malpositioning, and spine and hip diseases were all excluded before the revision surgery. The average interval from the primary UKA to the revision TKA for patients with unexplained pain was 15 months (range, 9–22 months). It is recommended to wait at least 2 years after surgery for pain relief because of bone remodeling [24].

We experienced both anterior and posterior mobile-bearing dislocations caused by retained osteophytes or imbalanced flexion-extension gaps. Individuals in Turkey require high degrees of knee flexion for religious and social reasons. Lim et al. reported that bearing dislocations occur more commonly in Asian than in Western cultures because of these demands [25]. Another cause of failure, lateral osteoarthritis, appeared in the early period in one patient.

There were two tibial periprosthetic fractures in cemented and uncemented UKA that were recognized during the postoperative follow-up period. These fractures occurred during daily life weight-bearing activities with minor trauma. Both were treated with standard TKA. Periprosthetic tibial fracture is an uncommon complication of cemented UKA and is related to technical errors. Seeger et al. reported that patients with an extended sagittal bone cut, especially those treated with cementless UKA, are at higher risk for periprosthetic tibial fracture [26]. Although a greater impaction force was applied to uncemented tibial components, there were no differences in the tibial periprosthetic fracture rates among our cases. There was one femoral condyle fracture in the uncemented UKA group that was treated with closed reduction and percutaneous fixation [27].

Our study shows that uncemented UKA provides good clinical and functional outcomes similar to those of cemented UKA. It has a similar complication rate and shorter operation time than cemented UKA. Unlike uncemented TKA, in countries where uncemented UKA prosthesis costs are similar to those of cemented prostheses, we suggest the use of uncemented UKA.

## 5. Conclusions

No clinical difference was observed between cemented and uncemented unicondylar knee prostheses. Uncemented UKA is as safe as cemented UKA. A longer follow-up period is required to determine the best fixation mode.

## Abbreviations

UKA: Unicompartmental knee arthroplasty
TKA: Total knee arthoplasty.

## Disclosure

No funds were received in support of this study. No benefits in any form have been or will be received from a commercial party related directly or indirectly to the subject of this paper. Level of evidence: III.

## References

[1] R. S. Laskin, "Unicompartmental tibiofemoral resurfacing arthroplasty," *The Journal of Bone & Joint Surgery A*, vol. 60, no. 2, pp. 182–185, 1978.

[2] D. W. Murray, J. W. Goodfellow, and J. J. O'Connor, "The oxford medial unicompartmental arthroplasty. A ten-year survival study," *The Journal of Bone & Joint Surgery B*, vol. 80, no. 6, pp. 983–989, 1998.

[3] M. W. Squire, J. J. Callaghan, D. D. Goetz, P. M. Sullivan, and R. C. Johnston, "Unicompartmental knee replacement: a minimum 15 year followup study," *Clinical Orthopaedics and Related Research*, no. 367, pp. 61–72, 1999.

[4] C. L. Saenz, M. S. McGrath, D. R. Marker, T. M. Seyler, M. A. Mont, and P. M. Bonutti, "Early failure of a unicompartmental knee arthroplasty design with an all-polyethylene tibial component," *Knee*, vol. 17, no. 1, pp. 53–56, 2010.

[5] J. H. Newman, C. E. Ackroyd, and N. A. Shah, "Unicompartmental or total knee replacement: the 15-year results of a prospective randomised controlled trial," *The Journal of Bone & Joint Surgery B*, vol. 80, no. 5, pp. 862–865, 1998.

[6] O. Furnes, B. Espehaug, S. A. Lie, S. E. Vollset, L. B. Engesæter, and L. I. Havelin, "Failure mechanisms after unicompartmental and tricompartmental primary knee replacement with cement," *The Journal of Bone & Joint Surgery A*, vol. 89, no. 3, pp. 519–525, 2007.

[7] J. W. Goodfellow, J. J. O'Connor, and D. W. Murray, "A critique of revision rate as an outcome measure: re-interpretation of knee joint registry data," *The Journal of Bone & Joint Surgery B*, vol. 92, no. 12, pp. 1628–1631, 2010.

[8] H. Pandit, C. Jenkins, D. J. Beard et al., "Cementless Oxford unicompartmental knee replacement shows reduced radiolucency at one year," *The Journal of Bone & Joint Surgery B*, vol. 91, no. 2, pp. 185–189, 2009.

[9] Å. Carlsson, A. Björkman, J. Besjakov, and I. Önsten, "Cemented tibial component fixation performs better than cementless fixation: a randomized radiostereometric study comparing porous-coated, hydroxyapatite-coated and cemented tibial components over 5 years," *Acta Orthopaedica*, vol. 76, no. 3, pp. 362–369, 2005.

[10] M. A. Ritter and R. M. Meneghini, "Twenty-year survivorship of cementless anatomic graduated component total knee arthroplasty," *Journal of Arthroplasty*, vol. 25, no. 4, pp. 507–513, 2010.

[11] C. S. Ranawat, M. Meftah, E. N. Windsor, and A. S. Ranawat, "Cementless fixation in total knee arthroplasty: down

the boulevard of broken dreams—affirms," *The Journal of Bone & Joint Surgery B*, vol. 94, pp. 82–84, 2012.

[12] K. Daniilidis, A. Skwara, A. Skuginna, F. Fischer, and C. O. Tibesku, "Comparison of medium-term clinical and radiological outcome between cemented and cementless medial unicompartmental knee arthroplasty," *Zeitschrift für Orthopädie und Unfallchirurgie*, vol. 147, no. 2, pp. 188–193, 2009.

[13] J. W. Goodfellow, C. J. Kershaw, M. K. D'A Benson, and J. J. O'Connor, "The Oxford knee for unicompartmental osteoarthritis. The first 103 cases," *The Journal of Bone & Joint Surgery B*, vol. 70, no. 5, pp. 692–701, 1988.

[14] H. Pandit, C. Jenkins, H. S. Gill et al., "Unnecessary contraindications for mobile-bearing unicompartmental knee replacement," *The Journal of Bone & Joint Surgery B*, vol. 93, no. 5, pp. 622–628, 2011.

[15] S. C. Kozinn and R. Scott, "Current concepts review unicondylar knee arthroplasty," *The Journal of Bone & Joint Surgery A*, vol. 71, no. 1, pp. 145–150, 1989.

[16] J. Goodfellow, J. O'Connor, and D. W. Murray, "The Oxford meniscal unicompartmental knee," *The Journal of Knee Surgery*, vol. 15, no. 4, pp. 240–246, 2002.

[17] W. P. Barrett and R. D. Scott, "Revision of failed unicondylar unicompartmental knee arthroplasty," *The Journal of Bone & Joint Surgery A*, vol. 69, no. 9, pp. 1328–1335, 1987.

[18] P. Vorlat, R. Verdonk, and H. Schauvlieghe, "The Oxford unicompartmental knee prosthesis: a 5-year follow-up," *Knee Surgery, Sports Traumatology, Arthroscopy*, vol. 8, no. 3, pp. 154–158, 2000.

[19] F. M. Khaw, L. M. G. Kirk, R. W. Morris, and P. J. Gregg, "A randomised, controlled trial of cemented versus cementless press-fit condylar total knee replacement. Ten-year survival analysis," *The Journal of Bone & Joint Surgery B*, vol. 84, no. 5, pp. 658–666, 2002.

[20] A. J. Price and U. Svard, "A second decade lifetable survival analysis of the oxford unicompartmental knee arthroplasty," *Clinical Orthopaedics and Related Research*, vol. 469, no. 1, pp. 174–179, 2011.

[21] H. Pandit, C. Jenkins, H. S. Gill, K. Barker, C. A. F. Dodd, and D. W. Murray, "Minimally invasive Oxford phase 3 unicompartmental knee replacement: results of 1000 cases," *The Journal of Bone & Joint Surgery B*, vol. 93, no. 2, pp. 198–204, 2011.

[22] J. W. Goodfellow, J. J. O'Connor, C. Dodd, and D. W. Murray, *Unicompartmental Arthroplasty with the Oxford Knee*, Goodfellow Publishers, Oxford, UK, 1st edition, 2006.

[23] G. J. Hooper, A. R. Maxwell, B. Wilkinson et al., "The early radiological results of the uncemented Oxford medial compartment knee replacement," *The Journal of Bone & Joint Surgery B*, vol. 94, no. 3, pp. 334–338, 2012.

[24] M. Clarius, D. Haas, P. R. Aldinger, S. Jaeger, E. Jakubowitz, and J. B. Seeger, "Periprosthetic tibial fractures in unicompartmental knee arthroplasty as a function of extended sagittal saw cuts: an experimental study," *Knee*, vol. 17, no. 1, pp. 57–60, 2010.

[25] H. C. Lim, J. H. Bae, S. H. Song, and S. J. Kim, "Oxford phase 3 unicompartmental knee replacement in Korean patients," *The Journal of Bone & Joint Surgery B*, vol. 94, pp. 1071–1076, 2012.

[26] J. B. Seeger, D. Haas, S. Jäger, E. Röhner, S. Tohtz, and M. Clarius, "Extended sagittal saw cut significantly reduces fracture load in cementless unicompartmental knee arthroplasty compared to cemented tibia plateaus: an experimental cadaver study," *Knee Surgery, Sports Traumatology, Arthroscopy*, vol. 20, no. 6, pp. 1087–1091, 2012.

[27] B. Akan, T. Yildirim, and D. Karaguven, "Medial femoral condyle fracture after cementless unicompartmental knee replacement: a rare complication," *Knee*, vol. 20, pp. 295–297, 2013.

# 4

# Utility of Intraoperative Neuromonitoring during Minimally Invasive Fusion of the Sacroiliac Joint

Michael Woods,[1] Denise Birkholz,[2] Regina MacBarb,[3] Robyn Capobianco,[3] and Adam Woods[2]

[1]Missoula Bone and Joint, 2360 Mullan Road, Suite C, Missoula, MT 59808, USA
[2]Pronerve, 7600 East Orchard Road, Suite 200, Greenwood Village, CO 80111, USA
[3]SI-BONE, Inc., 3055 Olin Avenue, Suite 2200, San Jose, CA 95128, USA

Correspondence should be addressed to Robyn Capobianco; rcapobianco@si-bone.com

Academic Editor: Allen L. Carl

*Study Design.* Retrospective case series. *Objective.* To document the clinical utility of intraoperative neuromonitoring during minimally invasive surgical sacroiliac joint fusion for patients diagnosed with sacroiliac joint dysfunction (as a direct result of sacroiliac joint disruptions or degenerative sacroiliitis) and determine stimulated electromyography thresholds reflective of favorable implant position. *Summary of Background Data.* Intraoperative neuromonitoring is a well-accepted adjunct to minimally invasive pedicle screw placement. The utility of intraoperative neuromonitoring during minimally invasive surgical sacroiliac joint fusion using a series of triangular, titanium porous plasma coated implants has not been evaluated. *Methods.* A medical chart review of consecutive patients treated with minimally invasive surgical sacroiliac joint fusion was undertaken at a single center. Baseline patient demographics and medical history, intraoperative electromyography thresholds, and perioperative adverse events were collected after obtaining IRB approval. *Results.* 111 implants were placed in 37 patients. Sensitivity of EMG was 80% and specificity was 97%. Intraoperative neuromonitoring potentially avoided neurologic sequelae as a result of improper positioning in 7% of implants. *Conclusions.* The results of this study suggest that intraoperative neuromonitoring may be a useful adjunct to minimally invasive surgical sacroiliac joint fusion in avoiding nerve injury during implant placement.

## 1. Introduction

Minimally invasive (MIS) sacroiliac (SI) joint fusion has gained popularity as a safe and effective treatment option for patients with recalcitrant symptoms of SI joint degeneration or disruption (based on joint asymmetry via radiographic imaging or contrast leakage during diagnostic joint block) [1, 2]. A common method uses a series of triangular, titanium porous plasma spray (TPS) coated implants (iFuse Implant System, SI-BONE, Inc; San Jose, CA) [3].

Similar to MIS pedicle screw procedures, surgery is performed under indirect visualization using fluoroscopic guidance and the implants are placed in bone adjacent to several neural structures. Achieving clear visualization can be difficult as the trajectory is much more anatomically complex than in lumbar spinal procedures (Figure 1). Bony landmarks are often obscured and can therefore be misinterpreted [4].

Thus, there is a potential risk for neural encroachment due to improper implant placement with possible neurologic sequelae. Given the consequences of iatrogenic nerve injury, it is advisable to employ neurologic structure localization techniques.

Intraoperative neuromonitoring (IOM) is a well-documented technique used to decrease the risk of iatrogenic nerve injury during MIS spinal procedures performed under limited visualization [5, 6]. This technology is dependent upon the greater electrical resistance of bone compared to the surrounding fluid and soft tissue. As a result, an implant that is entirely embedded in bone will be electrically shielded within certain limits from adjacent neural structures [7]. Should the implant come within close proximity to a nerve, the implant will no longer be electrically shielded, resulting in neural stimulation upon passage of current through

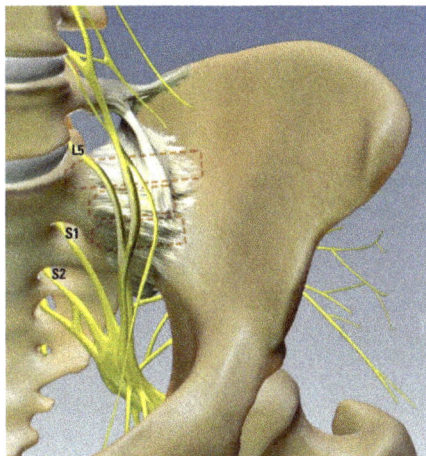

FIGURE 1: A three-dimensional representation of the lumbar spine, sacrum, and ilium. Red dashed outlines depict common positioning of three iFuse implants across the sacroiliac joint. Of the neural structures shown, the L5, S1, and S2 nerves (labeled in the figure) are at greatest risk of injury during such procedures.

the implant. The resultant response of the muscle that is being monitored alerts the surgeon to possible implant misplacement so that action may be taken to avoid potential neurologic sequelae.

Several methods of neuromonitoring have been utilized in spinal procedures, including electromyography (EMG) recordings, somatosensory evoked potentials, and motor-evoked potentials [8–10]. In comparison to EMG monitoring, the latter methods monitor the ascending and descending pathways of the spinal cord, which are not considered to be at risk during SI joint fusion surgery. Conversely, intraoperative EMG monitoring provides the surgeon with real-time neurophysiological feedback from the individual nerve roots at risk, enabling a rapid response if unfavorable readings are obtained. Intraoperative EMG has a high documented success rate for detecting the proximity of an implant or instrument to neural structures during spinal procedures [7, 11, 12]. Given the potential benefits of EMG monitoring, the purpose of the present study is to document its clinical utility during MIS SI joint fusion and determine stimulated EMG thresholds reflective of favorable implant position.

## 2. Materials and Methods

After IRB approval was obtained, a medical chart review was undertaken for consecutive patients operated on by a single orthopedic surgeon (MW). Thirty-seven consecutive patients, treated with MIS SI joint fusion using IOM between November 2012 and January 2014, were identified. Data extracted from the medical chart included demographics, comorbidities, neurological status, pertinent medical history related to the lumbopelvic hip complex, relevant imaging studies, estimated blood loss, and perioperative and postoperative complications. Stimulated EMG thresholds during surgery were obtained directly from the neuromonitoring technologist's records.

The primary endpoint of this study was the relationship of EMG threshold values to device reposition and overall success of the surgery defined by lack of reoperation within 30 days and absence of postoperative neurological impairment.

*2.1. Procedure Description.* Prior to surgery, a computed tomography (CT) scan was obtained to determine the presence of anomalous sacral anatomy. MIS SI joint fusion surgery using a series of triangular, titanium porous plasma (TPS) coated titanium implants was performed with the patient on a radiolucent table to facilitate the use of intraoperative fluoroscopy. After general endotracheal anesthesia was administered, the patient was connected via subdermal needle electrodes to a standard neuromonitoring system (NIM-ECLIPSE, Medtronic, Memphis, TN). Continuous free-running EMG monitoring of selected muscle groups innervated by nerves at risk was employed throughout the surgery (IOM procedure description below). The patient was then carefully positioned prone, padded appropriately, and prepped in the normal sterile fashion. A lateral incision (3 cm) was made parallel to the sacral body as viewed on a lateral fluoroscopic image. The gluteal fascia was then incised in line with the incision and the gluteal musculature was bluntly dissected to reach the outer table of the ilium. A 3.2 mm guide pin was passed through the ilium, across the SI joint, and into the sacrum lateral to the neural foramen using an insulated soft tissue retractor. The pin was intermittently stimulated at 8 milliamperes (mA) during advancement to ensure that no neurologic structures were encountered. After the first pin was in an acceptable position, two additional pins were sequentially placed caudally in a triangular pattern to reflect the anatomy of the joint and ensure optimal bony purchase (Figure 2). Pin length was measured to determine implant length. A larger soft tissue protector was then passed over the first pin and a center channel was drilled from the ilium, across the SI joint, and into the sacrum. Drill progression was monitored under fluoroscopy to prevent medial migration of the pin. A cannulated broach was used to prepare a triangular channel and the implant was then delivered into its final position. The guide pin was then removed. A standard ball-tip probe was passed through the center channel of the implant and was progressively stimulated up to a maximum of 20 mA. The implant was considered to be in a safe position if no distal muscle activity was detected at or below 16 mA. If activity was detected, a "search" technique was used, where the probe was set to a constant current of 8 mA and slowly advanced out of the distal end of the implant under fluoroscopic guidance in an effort to identify the location of the adjacent neurologic structure (Figure 3). Based on this information, the implant position was modified if necessary, typically by retracting its position a few millimeters laterally. If the implant was adjusted, stimulation was repeated (as previously described) to ensure proper positioning. This technique was repeated for the remaining 2 guide pins; all 37 patients received 3 implants (Figure 4). Following placement of all implants, the wound was irrigated, final hemostasis was achieved, tissue layers were closed, and local anesthetic was injected. A postoperative CT scan to evaluate final implant position

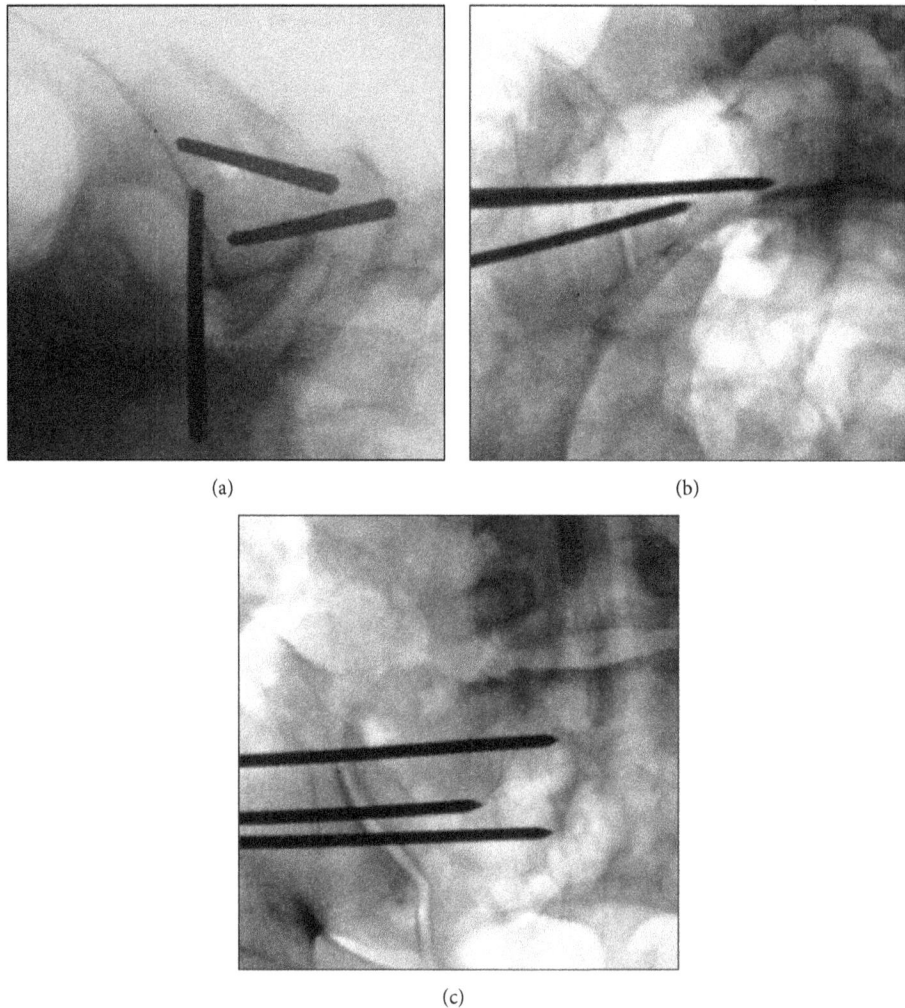

(a)

(b)

(c)

FIGURE 2: Lateral (a), inlet (b), and outlet (c) views of guide wire placement through the ilium, across the sacroiliac joint, and into the sacrum. Note the difficulty in visualizing the sacral foramen in (c).

was obtained if clinically indicated but was not performed routinely to avoid excessive patient radiation exposure.

A program of gradual return to full weight bearing was prescribed for all patients. In general, patients were instructed to ambulate 50% weight bearing with the assistance of crutches or walker for the first 3 weeks; after which time a regimen of gradual return to full weight bearing was recommended. Postoperative physical therapy was tailored to individualized clinical need. Patients were followed up in the office at 2, 6, and 12 weeks postoperatively.

*2.2. Intraoperative Neuromonitoring Protocol.* Both free-running and stimulated-EMG are used during the procedure to detect any nerve irritation. Subdermal needles are placed to monitor muscle activity triggered by the corresponding nerve roots as follows: tibialis anterior for L4-5, extensor hallucis longus for L5-S1, and gastrocnemius, abductor hallucis brevis, and flexor digitorum brevis for S1-2. Once all 3 guide pins are placed, a current of 8 mA is applied to each pin, utilizing an insulated pin guide to prevent shunting. Lack of

response at this threshold is used as an additional guideline to determine correct depth of penetration, in addition to fluoroscopic imaging. Once the first implant is sited and the guide pin is removed, a ball tip probe is passed into the cannulated implant. Current is gradually applied until a response is noted or the current reaches 20 mA. Any response noted at 16 mA or lower warrants close implant reevaluation. To assess implant proximity to the adjacent nerve structure(s), a "search" technique is also used. The ball tip probe is inserted through the cannulated implant and advanced past the distal end using a constant current of 8 mA (Figure 3). The probe is slowly advanced under fluoroscopic guidance until a response is noted.

## 3. Results

A total of 111 implants were placed in 37 patients. Eight (8/111) implants were repositioned in response to EMG thresholds of ≤16 mA.

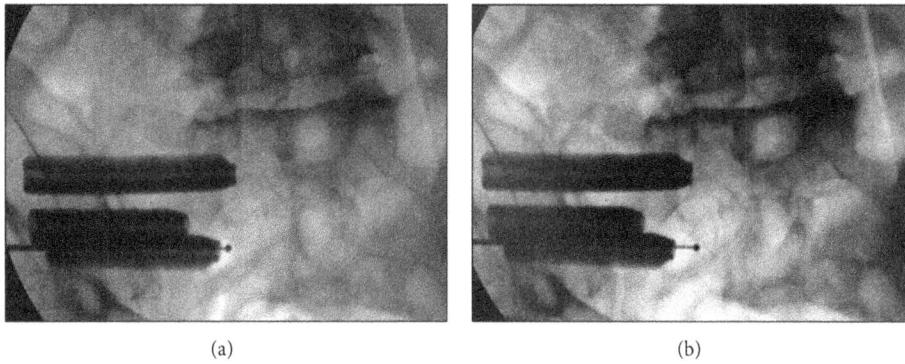

(a)          (b)

FIGURE 3: Following implant placement, the neuromonitoring probe is placed through the cannula of the implant and set to "searching" mode at 8 mA. In (a), monitoring of the probe past the distal end of the implant reveals a safe response, while further advancement of the probe to the position shown in (b) results in a positive EMG response, indicating that the probe has come within close proximity to a neural structure.

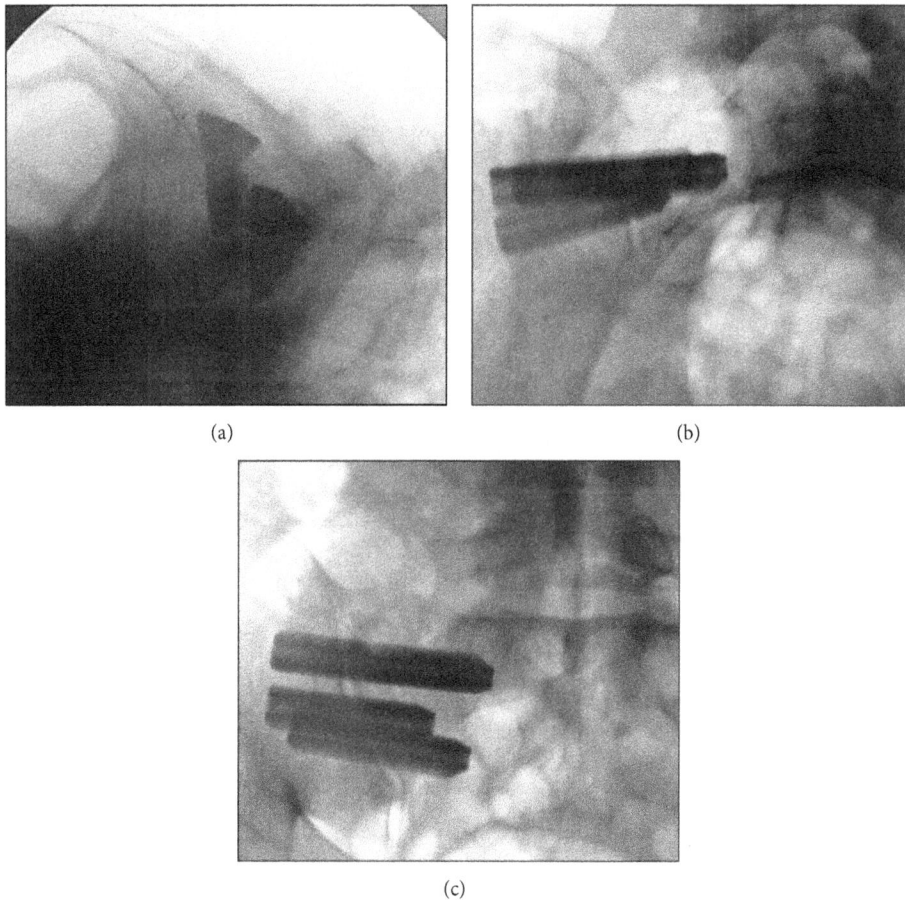

(a)          (b)

(c)

FIGURE 4: Lateral (a), inlet (b), and outlet (c) views of final implant placement through the ilium, across the sacroiliac joint, and into the sacrum, representing safe implant placement as measured via continuous passive EMG monitoring and fluoroscopy.

Two false negative results were noted. One patient had an immediate repositioning of an implant based on a search mode reading that suggested close neural proximity. The second patient recorded a final EMG threshold of 17 mA, with good implant placement noted on intraoperative fluoroscopy. The patient reported new neurologic symptoms postoperatively. A CT scan done immediately postoperatively revealed the caudal implant in close proximity to, but not impinging on, a nerve root. The patient elected not to reposition immediately, but, after thirty days, the patient was returned to the operating room to revise the implant. Postoperatively, the patient's symptoms were somewhat improved but not resolved. Further evaluation revealed additional pathology unrelated to the SI joint (lumbar spinal stenosis and piriformis syndrome) requiring surgical intervention.

Three false positive results were obtained in one patient. Readings of 10 mA were obtained for all three implants in final position. Using intraoperative imaging and search mode techniques, all three implants were determined to be in an acceptable position. This was confirmed on postoperative CT imaging. Postoperatively, the patient experienced satisfactory relief of SI joint symptoms and no postoperative issues. The relationship between anatomy and the potential for false positives is discussed below.

EMG readings obtained for 111 implants resulted in 8 true positives, 3 false positives, 2 false negatives, and 98 true negatives. These results provide sensitivity and specificity rates of 80% and 97%, respectively.

## 4. Discussion

To our knowledge, this is the first assessment of the utility of intraoperative neuromonitoring during MIS SI joint fusion using a series of triangular, TPS-coated implants. In spine surgery, iatrogenic nerve injury most commonly occurs directly via mechanical compression, stretching, or laceration or indirectly via ischemia [13]. The extent of neural injury is further dependent on the magnitude, degree, and duration of compression or laceration [14, 15]. Depending on the severity of the initial insult, the resulting injury can range anywhere from recoverable neurapraxia to the irreversible axonotmesis [16]. The current study shows that intraoperative EMG monitoring may be useful in decreasing the potential risk of neural injury utilizing a relatively simple and reproducible technique.

Intraoperative neuromonitoring was first used in 1898 during operations where the facial and trigeminal nerves were at high risk [17]. Advancements in the technique and science of neuromonitoring over the last century have led to its widespread acceptance in several areas of medicine, particularly spinal surgery. One of the earliest applications of IOM in MIS spine surgery was for detecting pedicle wall breaches during pedicle screw placement [18]. Of the various types of IOM, EMG has been highly regarded and well-documented for its ease of use and clinical utility in improving the safety and accuracy of pedicle screw procedures under limited visualization [18–24].

EMG monitoring may likewise prove useful as an adjunct to MIS SI joint fusion surgery as several neural structures, including the cauda equina, L5, S1, and S2 exiting nerves, lie within close proximity to implant trajectory (Figure 1) [25]. Specifically, the trajectory of the most cephalad implant passes in close proximity to the fifth lumbar nerve root [26], while the trajectories of the more caudal implants come close to the first and second sacral foramina, respectively (Figure 1). Not only bony landmarks for placing the implants are often obscured and difficult to visualize on fluoroscopy, but also the anatomy of the sacrum can be highly variable and dysplastic [27]. Safe instrument and implant positioning minimize the potential for neurologic injury [11]. Use of

IOM decreases this possibility by providing additional data to assist intraoperative maneuvering during instrumentation and implantation.

Threshold response ranges that indicate a "positive," or possibly injurious, versus a "negative," or safe, distance from a nerve must be identified before EMG can be used successfully. Moed et al. studied the correlation of EMG with CT for guide pin placement in the sacrum of a canine animal model [13]. Stimulus-evoked EMG monitoring was used in conjunction with high speed CT imaging to correlate pin tip location within the sacral body to determine a neural proximity EMG response range. A current threshold of 6.3 mA showed the guide pin 1 mm lateral to the sacral canal, while a response ≤5.9 mA resulted in compression or penetration of the L5 nerve root [26]. The authors reported a 0.801 correlation coefficient between recorded thresholds and pin location with respect to the adjacent nerve. Pedicle screw studies in the lower thoracic and lumbosacral spine correlated a threshold range of 8–15 mA as reliable for detecting nerve root proximity [13, 21] and currents of ≤6–10 mA as indicative of possible neural injury [28–30]. A study of 512 lumbar pedicle screw cases determined a threshold response of ≥15 mA to coincide with a 98% confidence that the screw was within the pedicle (as verified via CT), while thresholds between 10 and 15 mA provided an 87% confidence [21].

In the current study, a stimulus of 8 mA was chosen as an upper limit response for initial guide pin placement and 16 mA as the lower limit for implant placement. The lower threshold of 8 mA necessitates a closer proximity to the neural structure to elicit a signal, aiding the surgeon in more accurately determining distance from the nerve. An implant response of 16 mA was chosen based on a combination of literature reports and careful consideration after studying many patients during the SI joint fusion procedure. In the present study, 8 of 111 implants were repositioned following a recording of ≤16 mA. These findings suggest that a neuromonitoring threshold of 16 mA potentially avoided nerve irritation or injury in 7% of device implantations, leading to successful outcomes. These results are similar to those reported in pedicle screw literature, as indicated in the above paragraph [21–23, 28–30].

While intraoperative EMG monitoring adds an element of safety, it is important to note that it is not 100% sensitive and specific. In the current cohort, EMG sensitivity (true positive) was 80% and specificity (true negative) was 97%. The reported average rate of false-negative EMG responses during lumbar surgery is 23% [24]. In a separate study, 2 out of 32 patients were found to develop nerve root irritation in the absence of irregular EMG activity during pedicle screw placement [31]. In the current cohort, two false-negative results were noted. It is worth noting that we never encountered abnormal readings on spontaneous EMG monitoring alone. Only with active stimulation protocols were we able to elicit positive responses. This study emphasizes the need to not rely only on "passive monitoring" or a false sense of security will potentially exist.

In regards to our false positive findings, the patient we brought back to the OR had a superior and lateral sacral deficiency, which is not uncommon. This resulted in an unusually wide SI joint superiorly that was traversed by the implants, especially the superior implant. Our hypothesis is that even though the implants in this case were safely positioned as confirmed by CT, the superior edge of the implant was effectively uncovered for a variable distance by the lack of a bony "roof" due to the dysplasia and, therefore, not as well insulated. This could have contributed to the lower threshold readings.

Such situations demonstrate the technical limitations of neuromonitoring. Specifically, it is imperative that surgeons and neurophysiologists are aware that a negative neuromonitoring reading cannot determine safe implant position with 100% certainty. The benefits of neuromonitoring, when used in conjunction with preoperative CT imaging, fluoroscopy, and meticulous surgical technique, merit its use in MIS SI joint implantation. This surgical adjunctive technique has the potential to optimize positive patient outcomes when implanting medical devices in close proximity to neural structures. However, there is no substitute for experience and sound surgical judgment in each specific case.

Limitations of this study include small sample size, single surgeon experience, and absence of a control group. The small patient size was reflective of the number of patients available in the private practice office. All patients included in this study were followed postoperatively for a minimum of 3 months. The benefits of evaluating patients from a single center include a consistent diagnostic and therapeutic approach. Hopefully, in the near future, other surgeons will add to this body of knowledge and help validate the outcomes of this limited study.

## 5. Conclusions

This study provides insight into the potential benefit of IOM for MIS SI joint fusion. Specifically, results suggest that a stimulation threshold of ≤16 mA may indicate a potentially hazardous implant placement. In addition, the use of an 8 mA search mode technique for initial guide pin placement and final implant position allows the surgeon to determine proximity to adjacent neural structures. Given the potential of these thresholds to decrease the risk of iatrogenic nerve injury, IOM may be a useful adjunct to MIS SI joint fusion surgery.

## Conflict of Interests

This study was performed at Missoula Bone & Joint, LLC and was sponsored by SI-BONE, Inc. No funds were received by Michael Woods, Denise Birkholz, Adam Woods or Missoula Bone & Joint LL in support of this work. Michael Woods is a paid consultant for SI-BONE, Inc. Robyn Capobianco and Regina MacBarb are employees of SI-BONE, Inc.

## Acknowledgments

The authors wish to thank Kristen Munk for her assistance with chart preparation.

## References

[1] A. G. Smith, R. Capobianco, D. Cher et al., "Open versus minimally invasive sacroiliac joint fusion: a multi-center comparison of perioperative measures and clinical outcomes," *Annals of Surgical Innovation and Research*, vol. 7, no. 1, article 14, 2013.

[2] L. Rudolf, "Sacroiliac joint arthrodesis-MIS technique with titanium implants: report of the first 50 patients and outcomes," *The Open Orthopaedics Journal*, vol. 6, no. 1, pp. 495–502, 2012.

[3] M. P. Lorio, D. W. Polly Jr., I. Ninkovic et al., "Utilization of minimally invasive surgical approach for sacroiliac joint fusion in surgeon population of ISASS and SMISS membership," *The Open Orthopaedics Journal*, vol. 8, pp. 1–6, 2014.

[4] M. L. C. Routt Jr., P. T. Simonian, S. G. Agnew, and F. A. Mann, "Radiographic recognition of the sacral alar slope for optimal placement of iliosacral screws: a cadaveric and clinical study," *Journal of Orthopaedic Trauma*, vol. 10, no. 3, pp. 171–177, 1996.

[5] M. G. Fehlings, D. S. Brodke, D. C. Norvell, and J. R. Dettori, "The evidence for intraoperative neurophysiological monitoring in spine surgery: does it make a difference?" *Spine*, vol. 35, no. 9S, pp. S37–S46, 2010.

[6] R. R. Lall, J. S. Hauptman, C. Munoz et al., "Intraoperative neurophysiological monitoring in spine surgery: indications, efficacy, and role of the preoperative checklist," *Neurosurgical Focus*, vol. 33, no. 5, article E10, 2012.

[7] B. Bose, L. R. Wierzbowski, and A. K. Sestokas, "Neurophysiologic monitoring of spinal nerve root function during instrumented posterior lumbar spine surgery," *Spine*, vol. 27, no. 13, pp. 1444–1450, 2002.

[8] D. S. Dinner, H. Luders, R. P. Lesser, and H. H. Morris, "Invasive methods of somatosensory evoked potential monitoring," *Journal of Clinical Neurophysiology*, vol. 3, no. 2, pp. 113–130, 1986.

[9] D. H. York, R. J. Chabot, and R. W. Gaines, "Response variability of somatosensory evoked potentials during scoliosis surgery," *Spine*, vol. 12, no. 9, pp. 864–876, 1987.

[10] D. L. Helfet, E. A. Hissa, S. Sergay, and J. W. Mast, "Somatosensory evoked potential monitoring in the surgical management of acute acetabular fractures," *Journal of orthopaedic trauma*, vol. 5, no. 2, pp. 161–166, 1991.

[11] B. R. Moed, B. K. Ahmad, J. G. Craig, G. P. Jacobson, and M. J. Anders, "Intraoperative monitoring with stimulus-evoked electromyography during placement of iliosacral screws: an initial clinical study," *Journal of Bone and Joint Surgery*, vol. 80, no. 4, pp. 537–546, 1998.

[12] L. X. Webb, W. de Araujo, P. Donofrio et al., "Electromyography monitoring for percutaneous placement of iliosacral screws," *Journal of Orthopaedic Trauma*, vol. 14, no. 4, pp. 245–254, 2000.

[13] B. R. Moed, J. W. Maxey, and G. J. Minster, "Intraoperative somatosensory evoked potential monitoring of the sciatic nerve: an animal model," *Journal of Orthopaedic Trauma*, vol. 6, no. 1, pp. 59–65, 1992.

[14] S. Sunderland, "A classification of peripheral nerve injuries producing loss of function," *Brain*, vol. 74, no. 4, pp. 491–516, 1951.

[15] M. G. Burnett and E. L. Zager, "Pathophysiology of peripheral nerve injury: a brief review," *Neurosurg Focus*, vol. 16, no. 5, article E1, 2004.

[16] A. Ahmadian, A. R. Deukmedjian, N. Abel, E. Dakwar, and J. S. Uribe, "Analysis of lumbar plexopathies and nerve injury after lateral retroperitoneal transpsoas approach: diagnostic standardization," *Journal of Neurosurgery: Spine*, vol. 18, no. 3, pp. 289–297, 2013.

[17] R. E. Minahan and A. S. Mandir, "Neurophysiologic intraoperative monitoring of trigeminal and facial nerves," *Journal of Clinical Neurophysiology*, vol. 28, no. 6, pp. 551–565, 2011.

[18] M. R. Isley, X.-F. Zhang, J. R. Balzer, and R. E. Leppanen, "Current trends in pedicle screw stimulation techniques: lumbosacral, thoracic, and cervical levels," *Neurodiagnostic Journal*, vol. 52, no. 2, pp. 100–175, 2012.

[19] J. C. Rodriguez-Olaverri, N. C. Zimick, A. Merola et al., "Using triggered electromyographic threshold in the intercostal muscles to evaluate the accuracy of upper thoracic pedicle screw placement (T3-T6)," *Spine*, vol. 33, no. 7, pp. E194–E197, 2008.

[20] B. Calancie, N. Lebwohl, P. Madsen, and K. J. Klose, "Intraoperative evoked EMG monitoring in an animal model: a new technique for evaluating pedicle screw placement," *Spine*, vol. 17, no. 10, pp. 1229–1235, 1992.

[21] S. D. Glassman, J. R. Dimar, R. M. Puno, J. R. Johnson, C. B. Shields, and R. D. Linden, "A prospective analysis of intraoperative electromyographic monitoring of pedicle screw placement with computed tomographic scan confirmation," *Spine*, vol. 20, no. 12, pp. 1375–1379, 1995.

[22] D. H. Clements, D. E. Morledge, W. H. Martin, and R. R. Betz, "Evoked and spontaneous electromyography to evaluate lumbosacral pedicle screw placement," *Spine*, vol. 21, no. 5, pp. 600–604, 1996.

[23] B. L. Raynor, L. G. Lenke, K. H. Bridwell, B. A. Taylor, and A. M. Padberg, "Correlation between low triggered electromyographic thresholds and lumbar pedicle screw malposition: analysis of 4857 screws," *Spine*, vol. 32, no. 24, pp. 2673–2678, 2007.

[24] R. M. Beatty, P. McGuire, J. M. Moroney, and F. P. Holladay, "Continuous intraoperative electromyographic recording during spinal surgery," *Journal of Neurosurgery*, vol. 82, no. 3, pp. 401–405, 1995.

[25] S. Mirkovic, J. J. Abitbol, J. Steinman et al., "Anatomic consideration for sacral screw placement," *Spine*, vol. 16, no. 6, pp. S289–S294, 1991.

[26] B. R. Moed, M. J. Hartman, B. K. Ahmad, D. D. Cody, and J. G. Craig, "Evaluation of intraoperative nerve-monitoring during insertion of an iliosacral implant in an animal model," *Journal of Bone and Joint Surgery—American Volume*, vol. 81, no. 11, pp. 1529–1537, 1999.

[27] A. N. Miller and M. L. C. Routt Jr., "Variations in sacral morphology and implications for iliosacral screw fixation," *Journal of the American Academy of Orthopaedic Surgeons*, vol. 20, no. 1, pp. 8–16, 2012.

[28] B. Calancie, P. Madsen, N. Lebwohl, and J. H. Owen, "Stimulus-evoked EMG monitoring during transpedicular lumbosacral spine instrumentation: initial clinical results," *Spine*, vol. 19, no. 24, pp. 2780–2786, 1994.

[29] L. G. Lenke, A. M. Padberg, M. H. Russo, K. H. Bridwell, and D. E. Gelb, "Triggered electromyographic threshold for accuracy of pedicle screw placement: an animal model and clinical correlation," *Spine*, vol. 20, no. 14, pp. 1585–1591, 1995.

[30] J. Maguire, S. Wallace, R. Madiga, R. Leppanen, and V. Draper, "Evaluation of intrapedicular screw position using intraoperative evoked electromyography," *Spine*, vol. 20, no. 9, pp. 1068–1074, 1995.

[31] W. C. Welch, R. D. Rose, J. R. Balzer, and G. B. Jacobs, "Evaluation with evoked and spontaneous electromyography during lumbar instrumentation: a prospective study," *Journal of Neurosurgery*, vol. 87, no. 3, pp. 397–402, 1997.

# 5

# Obtaining Glenoid Positioning Data from Scapular Palpable Points In Vitro

## Jordan H. Trafimow and Alexander S. Aruin

*Department of Physical Therapy (MC 898), University of Illinois at Chicago, 1919 W. Taylor Street, Chicago, IL 60612, USA*

Correspondence should be addressed to Alexander S. Aruin; aaruin@uic.edu

Academic Editor: Christian Bach

Both clinical and biomechanical problems affecting the shoulder joint suggest that investigators should study force transmission into and out from the scapula. To analyze force transmission between the humeral head and the glenoid, one must know the position of the glenoid. Studies have analyzed the position of the scapula from the positions of three palpable points, but the position of the glenoid relative to three palpable points has not been studied. Dry scapulae ($N = 13$) were subjected to X-rays and a critical angle, $\Theta$ (which relates the plane determined by the three palpable points on the scapula to a plane containing the glenoid center and the first two palpable points) was calculated. The mean value for $\Theta$ was $28.5 \pm 5.60$ degrees. The obtained $\Theta$ allows us to determine the position of the glenoid from three palpable points. This information could be used in calculation of forces across the shoulder joint, which in turn would allow optimizing the choice of strengthening exercises.

## 1. Introduction

Both clinical and biomechanical problems affecting the shoulder joint suggest that investigators should study force transmission into and out from the scapula [1]. One clinical problem is the wearing away of the posterior part of the glenoid in patients who need total shoulder replacement [2]. Another problem is dyskinesis, (e.g., abnormal scapular motion) due to various clinical entities such as internal derangement of the shoulder, acromioclavicular instability, and fractured clavicle [1, 3]. In addition, movements of the scapula are subjected to extensive variations, which in itself influence the interaction of glenoid and humeral head [4]. Some authors postulate that dyskinesis causes swimmer's shoulder and impingement syndrome [5, 6].

The biomechanical problem is finding the location of the glenoid. Since the glenoid is always centered about the humeral head [7], the problem becomes finding two coordinates of the glenoid, for example, Euler angles. To the best of our knowledge, there are no studies dealing with this problem. This is mainly because current techniques lack the ability to locate, in three dimensions, the angle between glenoid center and the force vector from the humeral head.

This angle is needed in the calculation of force transmission across the shoulder and to make more definite the diagnosis of dyskinesia.

To solve these problems there is a need to define the position of the glenoid. We define the center line as a line running from the point at which the spine and medial border meet (O) through the center of the glenoid (G) to a point midway between the most anterior and the most posterior points on the glenoid rim [8, 9]. Since the scapula rotates around the humeral head [7], the center of the humeral head is also on the center line. Thus, the location of the glenoid could be determined using the center line.

There is also a need to obtain three points to determine the location of the scapula. Most of the studies on the scapula in the past have used the vertex of the inferior angle of the scapula (Q) and junction (O) of the scapular spine and the medial border (e.g., [10]) providing two points. The third point is one of various points on the acromion [11]. All the previous points are palpable. However, there is no literature data linking the position of the glenoid to the positions of the three palpable points mentioned previously. A possible way of solving such a problem would be obtaining MRIs with the arm in various positions [4]. The problem is getting

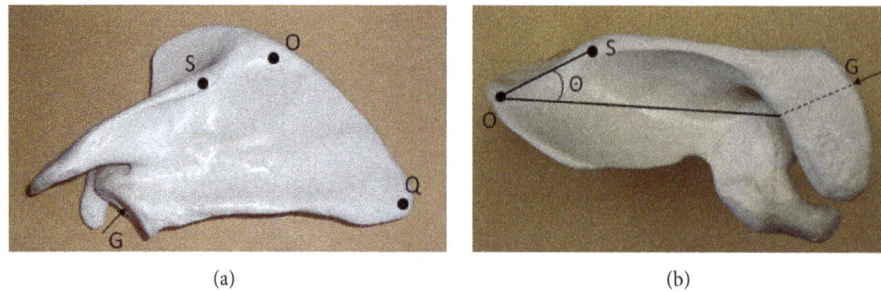

(a)                                                                    (b)

FIGURE 1: (a) Posterior view of the scapula. The following points are shown: G: center of the glenoid, Q: vertex of the inferior angle of the scapula, O: junction of the medial border of the scapula with the medial border of the scapular spine, S: is the point where the medial and lateral parts of the edge of the scapular spine meet. (b) Superior view of the scapula. Points O, S, and G are shown (G is covered by the acromion); Θ is defined as the angle between OS and OG.

the central ray parallel to OQ, the line between the inferior angle (Q) and the junction (O). If the central ray is not perpendicular the angle (our Θ) will be incorrect.

The aim of the study was to introduce a method of locating the glenoid given three palpable points on the scapula.

## 2. Methods

*2.1. Materials and Technique.* The study was conducted on 13 dry, intact adult scapulae (7 from the right and 6 from the left side of the body) of unknown sex procured from the University of Illinois at Chicago Anatomy Department collection. No existing pathologies or abnormalities of the scapulae were found except differences in size and the specimens were random. X-ray opaque lead balls 4 mm in diameter were mounted on each specimen with glue on points O, Q, and G. In addition a lead ball was placed on point S, which is the point where the medial and lateral parts of the edge of the scapular spine meet (Figure 1). This point is described in the literature [12] but is not named. The scapulae were then mounted in metal cages, using glue and plastic strings. The line OQ was kept vertical. The cages were numbered.

An X-ray was taken of each specimen. The central ray went through the scapula from superior to inferior. A film in a 2 cm thick cassette was placed under the cage. The central ray of the X-ray ran vertically downward from a source 183 cm above the floor, passing through the specimen from superior to inferior. All X-rays were taken by an experienced technician.

The positions of the lead balls were identified on the X-rays. The lead ball at point Q was easily identified because on the X-ray its image was smaller than the images of the other balls; Q was roughly 10 cm. closer to the X-ray cassette than the other points, so its image was smaller.

*2.2. Rationale.* The data are often obtained from recording devices that use vertical and horizontal coordinates. We first convert the coordinates to their equivalents based on the scapula.

Secondly we rotate the coordinate axes to positions OQ and the center line. Using cylindrical coordinates, we choose the third coordinate as the angle Θ between the center line (OG) and OS. In our study we measure this angle on the X-ray. In biomechanical studies we use the value of Θ determined by this and subsequent studies. We are interested only in the angle of the center line and we do not need the length of the center line as it runs to the humeral head.

In summary, these points, O, Q, and S, are palpable, so their location can be established by light emitting diodes or other instruments. With Θ known, we can calculate the location of the center line; OG is perpendicular to OQ [3, 13].

*2.3. Calculations.* We defined the point P as the point on the X-ray at which the perpendicular from S to line OG met line OG (Figure 1). PS and OP were measured on the X-ray 3 times and the means were obtained. Θ was obtained from the equation PS/OP = tan Θ.

## 3. Results

Means measured for each specimen, OP and PS lengths, and Θ are shown in Table 1. The obtained Θ for the group was $28.74 \pm 5.60°$.

## 4. Discussion

Knowing the position of glenoid is essential in analyzing force transmission from the humerus to the glenoid. However, to date we could find no study which determines the position of the glenoid from palpable points on the scapula. To obtain the glenoid position one must start with points on the scapula that are palpable. However, what we need is the position of the glenoid. Obtaining Θ would allow us to determine this position.

The study was conducted to test a method of finding the location of the glenoid using three palpable points on the scapula (O, Q, S). The Θ magnitude obtained in the current study allows calculation of the position of the glenoid using three palpable points (the inferior angle of the scapula (Q) and the junction between the scapular spine and the

TABLE 1: Values of $\Theta$ and the means of OP and PS.

| Specimen # | OP (cm) | PS (cm) | $\Theta$ (deg) |
|---|---|---|---|
| 5 | 2.7 | 1.4 | 1.3 |
| 6 | 3.0 | 2.0 | 1.9 |
| 7 | 3.43 | 1.59 | 0.18 |
| 8 | 4.36 | 2.02 | 0.63 |
| 9 | 3.78 | 2.13 | 1.48 |
| 10 | 5.64 | 2.44 | 0.83 |
| 11 | 4.19 | 1.81 | 2.18 |
| 12 | 4.69 | 3.19 | 0 |
| 13 | 2.67 | 1.47 | 1.4 |
| 14 | 10.94 | 4.67 | 2.2 |
| 15 | 4.87 | 2.78 | 1.38 |
| 17 | 3.81 | 3.42 | 2.33 |

medial border of the scapula (O)) and the angle $\Theta$ between the OS line and the center line (that are obtained from X-rays).

The obtained data on the position of glenoid could be used in calculation of forces across the shoulder joint. For example, to calculate the force vector from the humeral head across the shoulder, one can use a linked rigid body model. The obtained force and the angle of the glenoid and a critical angle, $\Theta$, would allow calculating the amount of force transferred from the humeral head to the glenoid.

There are some limitations that should be taken into consideration. First, following the literature [14, 15], we assumed that the body of the scapula is a plane, our plane OQG which might not be always true [16]. Second, we used the lead balls (4 mm in diameter); using smaller balls would allow more accurate measurements. The small number of specimens used in the current study allows us to obtain preliminary data only. Finally, the number of specimens needs to be larger to be able to apply the study outcome to individuals of different genders and ages.

Nevertheless, the study outcome allows investigators to obtain the center line (OG-Figure 1(b)) from 3 palpable points. Furthermore, the direction of force from the humeral head can be compared with the direction of the center line in various positions, and normal positioning of the scapula and glenoid could be established. This could be applied to patients with certain conditions. Thus, in patients with dyskinesis, force direction from the humerus and glenoid could be found. Based on the obtained force direction, strengthening exercises could be prescribed so that normal force transmission can be restored. Also, in patients who need total shoulder replacement, the posterior part of the humeral head is very often worn away [2]. Appropriate exercises could be prescribed in the early stages of this condition, to redirect the force away from the abnormal part of the humeral head. It is also reported in the literature that overhead athletes (swimmers and pitcher in baseball) frequently develop shoulder problems. It is quite possible that these individuals develop dyskinesis and thus would benefit from appropriately designed physical therapy [5, 6].

## 5. Conclusions

The study outcome allows obtaining the position of the center line and as such the position of the glenoid from the positions of three palpable points on the scapula. This information could be used in calculation of forces across the shoulder joint, which in turn would allow optimizing the choice of strengthening exercises in patients with dyskinesis.

## Acknowledgment

The authors would like to thank Hazel L. Radloff for the help in obtaining the X-rays.

## References

[1] P. W. McClure, L. A. Michener, B. J. Sennett, and A. R. Karduna, "Direct 3-dimensional measurement of scapular kinematics during dynamic movements *in vivo*," *Journal of Shoulder and Elbow Surgery*, vol. 10, no. 3, pp. 269–277, 2001.

[2] R. J. Friedman, K. B. Hawthorne, and B. M. Genez, "The use of computerized tomography in the measurement of glenoid version," *Journal of Bone and Joint Surgery A*, vol. 74, no. 7, pp. 1032–1037, 1992.

[3] W. B. Kibler, A. Sciascia, and T. Wilkes, "Scapular dyskinesis and its relation to shoulder injury," *Journal of the American Academy of Orthopaedic Surgeons*, vol. 20, no. 6, pp. 364–372, 2012.

[4] R. von Eisenhart-Rothe, S. Hinterwimmer, C. Braune et al., "MR-based 3D-analysis of the pathomechanics of traumatic and atraumatic shoulder instability," *Zeitschrift fur Orthopadie und Ihre Grenzgebiete*, vol. 143, no. 4, pp. 461–467, 2005.

[5] K. Bak, "Nontraumatic glenohumeral instability and cora-coacromial impingement in swimmers," *Scandinavian Journal of Medicine and Science in Sports*, vol. 6, no. 3, pp. 132–144, 1996.

[6] P. Page, "Shoulder muscle imbalance and subacromial impingement syndrome in overhead athletes," *International Journal of Sports Physical Therapy*, vol. 6, no. 1, pp. 51–58, 2011.

[7] C. F. Beaulieu, D. K. Hodge, A. G. Bergman et al., "Glenohumeral relationships during physiologic shoulder motion and stress testing: initial experience with open MR imaging and active imaging-plane registration," *Radiology*, vol. 212, no. 3, pp. 699–705, 1999.

[8] G. S. Lewis, C. D. Bryce, A. C. Davison, C. S. Hollenbeak, S. J. Piazza, and A. D. Armstrong, "Location of the optimized centerline of the glenoid vault: a comparison of two operative techniques with use of three-dimensional computer modeling," *Journal of Bone and Joint Surgery A*, vol. 92, no. 5, pp. 1188–1194, 2010.

[9] A. K. Saha, "Dynamic stability of the glenohumeral joint," *Acta Orthopaedica Scandinavica*, vol. 42, no. 6, pp. 491–505, 1971.

[10] P. M. Ludewig, D. R. Hassett, R. F. Laprade, P. R. Camargo, and J. P. Braman, "Comparison of scapular local coordinate systems," *Clinical Biomechanics*, vol. 25, no. 5, pp. 415–421, 2010.

[11] S. Oyama, J. B. Myers, C. A. Wassinger, R. D. Ricci, and S. M. Lephart, "Asymmetric resting scapular posture in healthy overhead athletes," *Journal of Athletic Training*, vol. 43, no. 6, pp. 565–570, 2008.

[12] H. Gray and C. M. Goss, *Anatomy of the Human Body*, Lea & Febiger, Philadelphia, Pa, USA, 26th edition, 1954.

[13] J. Sobotta, *Atlas of Descriptive Human Anatomy*, vol. 1, Hafner Publishing, New York, NY, USA, 6th edition, 1954, edited by E. Uhlenhuth.

[14] P. A. Borsa, M. K. Timmons, and E. L. Sauers, "Scapular-positioning patterns during humeral elevation in unimpaired shoulders," *Journal of Athletic Training*, vol. 38, no. 1, pp. 12–17, 2003.

[15] N. K. Poppen and P. S. Walker, "Normal and abnormal motion of the shoulder," *Journal of Bone and Joint Surgery A*, vol. 58, no. 2, pp. 195–201, 1976.

[16] W. Hollinshead, *Anatomy for Surgeons: The Back and Limbs*, vol. 3, Hoeber-Harper, New York, NY, USA, 1958.

# 6

# Cement Removal from the Femur Using the ROBODOC System in Revision Total Hip Arthroplasty

**Mitsuyoshi Yamamura,**[1] **Nobuo Nakamura,**[1] **Hidenobu Miki,**[2]
**Takashi Nishii,**[2] **and Nobuhiko Sugano**[2,3]

[1] Center of Arthroplasty, Kyowakai Hospital, 1-24-1 Kishibekita, Suita, Osaka 564-0001, Japan
[2] Department of Orthopaedic Surgery, Osaka University Graduate School of Medicine, 2-2 Yamadaoka, Suita, Osaka 565-0871, Japan
[3] Department of Orthopaedic Medical Engineering, Osaka University Graduate School of Medicine, 2-2 Yamadaoka, Suita,
  Osaka 565-0871, Japan

Correspondence should be addressed to Nobuhiko Sugano; n-sugano@umin.net

Academic Editor: Michael A. Conditt

*Introduction.* The perforation and fracture of the femur during the removal of bone cement in revision total hip arthroplasty (THA) are serious complications. The ROBODOC system has been designed to selectively remove bone cement from the femoral canal, but results have not been reported yet. The purpose of our study was to evaluate the clinical and radiographic results of revision THA using the ROBODOC system for cement removal. *Materials and Methods.* The subjects comprised 19 patients who underwent revision THA using the ROBODOC system. The minimum duration of follow-up was 76 months (median, 109 months; range, 76–150 months). The extent of remaining bone cement on postoperative radiography, timing of weight bearing, and the complications were evaluated. *Results.* The mean Merle d'Aubigne and Postel score increased from 10 points preoperatively to 14 points by final follow-up. Bone cement was completely removed in all cases. Full weight bearing was possible within 1 week after surgery in 9 of the 19 cases and within 2 months in all remaining cases. No instances of perforation or fracture of the femur were encountered. *Conclusions.* Bone cement could be safely removed using the ROBODOC system, and no serious complications occurred. Full weight bearing was achieved early in the postoperative course because of circumferential preservation of the femoral cortex.

## 1. Introduction

The perforation and fracture of the femur during the removal of bone cement in revision total hip arthroplasty (THA) are serious complications that considerably affect the postoperative protocols and clinical results [1]. With the increasing frequency of revision THA, the incidence of intraoperative femoral fracture has increased recently [2, 3]. To prevent the perforation and fracture of the femur, several instruments and procedures have been developed especially for bone cement removal. However, sufficient results have not been achieved yet in the clinical setting [4–7]. Extended trochanteric osteotomy was introduced for difficult situations in revision THA [8–11], but good results have not necessarily been obtained with the procedure in terms of intraoperative femoral fracture [8, 10, 12].

Since 1992, a computer-assisted surgical system called ROBODOC (Integrated Surgical Systems, Davis, CA) has been used in clinical settings and is highly regarded for the accuracy of the surgical process [13–15]. After making system improvements, the ROBODOC system received 510(k) clearance from the US Food and Drug Administration in 2008. Using ROBODOC, the rate of intraoperative femoral fissures was significantly lower than that of the hand rasping conventional THA [16]. This system can also selectively remove bone cement from the femoral canal in revision THA [13]. However, results have not been reported yet.

The purpose of our study was to evaluate the clinical and radiographic results of revision THA using the ROBODOC system. Our research questions were as follows: (1) Did the system contribute to a reduced rate of intraoperative complications such as femoral fracture? (2) Did the use of the system

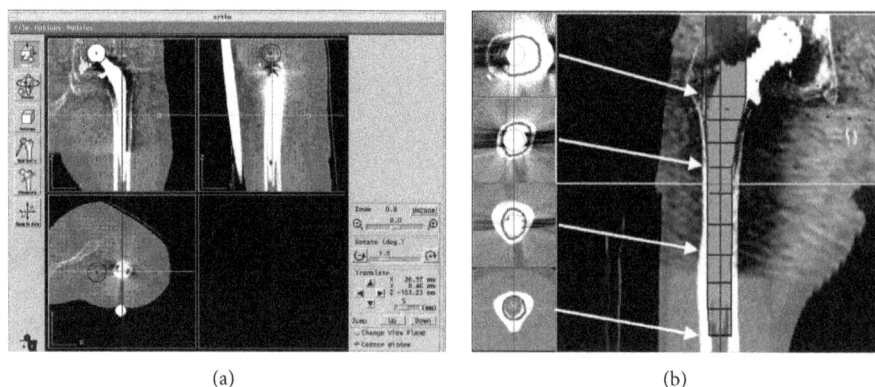

|            (a)            |            (b)            |

FIGURE 1: (a) Multiplanar reconstruction of the proximal femur on ORTHODOC. A minimum of 8 cross sections are defined on a coronal view. A perimeter around the bone is demarcated on each section. (b) A cutting path (hatched area) is automatically created.

affect the postoperative rehabilitation protocol with regard to weight bearing? (3) Was bone cement completely removed from the femur?

## 2. Materials and Methods

We reviewed the medical records and radiographs of the studied subjects after the approval of this study by the institutional review board committee. The subjects comprised 19 patients (17 women, 2 men) for whom bone cement of the femoral canal was removed using the ROBODOC system in revision THA, between 2000 and 2006. All patients provided informed consent for participation before surgery, and the procedure was approved by the institutional review board committee. The mean patient age at the time of surgery was 70 years (range, 51–85 years). Cemented femoral component had been implanted in all patients. The primary diagnosis was osteoarthritis in 14 hips, femoral neck fracture in 4 hips, and rheumatoid arthritis in 1 hip. The reason for revision was aseptic loosening in 17 hips, septic loosening in 1 hip (infection was completely cleared up at the time of surgery), and central migration of the bipolar head in 1 hip. The minimum duration of follow-up was 76 months (median, 109 months; range, 76–150 months).

Prior to the index surgery, 2 locater pins were implanted into the greater trochanter and lateral condyle of the affected femur under local anesthesia. Computed tomography (CT) (General Electric, Waukesha, WI) was then performed in accordance with the protocol specified by the manufacturer (slice thickness, 1 mm; scan interval, 1–6 mm; field of view, 200 mm; total slices, <200). CT data were imported into a preoperative planning workstation (ORTHODOC; Integrated Surgical Systems, Davis, CA) that displayed a 3-dimensional image of the femur (Figure 1(a)). The long axis of the femur was aligned. At least 8 cross sections were defined, and the surgeon demarcated a perimeter around the bone cement in the axial views of the femur. From these data, the ORTHODOC program automatically created a 3-dimensional cutting path for cement removal (Figure 1(b)). At this time, the surgeon could check and modify the cutting path. These preoperative planning data were recorded on

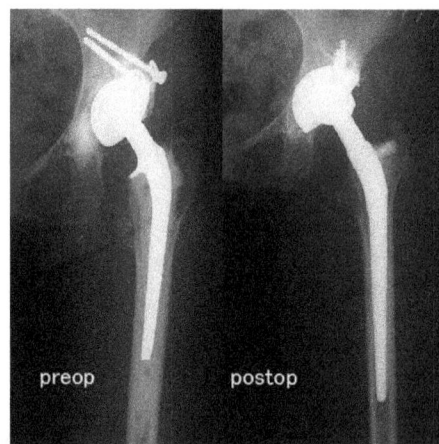

FIGURE 2: A 54-year-old woman underwent primary THA for osteoarthritis of the hip. Eleven years later, revision THA was performed using the ROBODOC system due to aseptic loosening. Full weight bearing was possible within 1 week after surgery. At the latest follow-up, 9 years postoperatively, no clinical or radiographic problems were identified.

a compact disc (CD). Before each surgical procedure, the surgeon loaded the data for that patient from this CD into the ROBODOC system and performed a startup self-diagnosis of the robot.

During the operation, the femur was exposed through a posterolateral approach in all cases, and the femoral component was removed using a conventional procedure. After the patient's leg was fixed to ROBODOC and to the surgical table, registration was performed using the 2 locater pins. After the gluteus medius muscle was firmly retracted, ROBODOC milled the femoral canal to remove the bone cement. Finally, the surgeon performed manual reaming of the femoral canal and a long-straight-tapered cementless stem (Wagner, Zimmer, Warsaw, USA) was inserted (Figure 2).

Clinical and radiographic evaluations were performed on the day of operation and 6 weeks and 3, 6, and 12 months postoperatively, then annually thereafter. No patients were excluded or lost to followup. Clinical results were measured

TABLE 1: The patients demographic and operative data.

| Case | Age (years) | Sex | Primary diagnosis | Reason for revision | Operation time (min) | Blood loss (g) | FWB (weeks) | Stem subsidence |
|------|------|-----|------|------|------|------|------|------|
| 1 | 76 | M | FNF | Aseptic loosening | 210 | 600 | 9 | – |
| 2 | 72 | F | OA | Aseptic loosening | 225 | 1600 | 1 | – |
| 3 | 69 | F | OA | Aseptic loosening | 250 | 450 | 5 | – |
| 4 | 63 | F | RA | Aseptic loosening | 215 | 1100 | 1 | – |
| 5 | 51 | F | OA | Aseptic loosening | 180 | 960 | 4 | + |
| 6 | 70 | F | OA | Aseptic loosening | 225 | 550 | 5 | – |
| 7 | 78 | F | OA | Aseptic loosening | 258 | 1000 | 1 | – |
| 8 | 73 | F | OA | Aseptic loosening | 285 | 1100 | 9 | – |
| 9 | 71 | M | FNF | Septic loosening | 251 | 3000 | 1 | + |
| 10 | 74 | F | OA | Aseptic loosening | 420 | 1350 | 9 | – |
| 11 | 77 | F | FNF | Aseptic loosening | 300 | 700 | 8 | – |
| 12 | 54 | F | OA | Aseptic loosening | 285 | 570 | 1 | – |
| 13 | 64 | F | OA | Aseptic loosening | 405 | 1450 | 9 | – |
| 14 | 75 | F | OA | Aseptic loosening | 335 | 1750 | 1 | – |
| 15 | 82 | F | OA | Aseptic loosening | 205 | 1100 | 1 | – |
| 16 | 59 | F | OA | Aseptic loosening | 275 | 2100 | 1 | – |
| 17 | 80 | F | OA | Aseptic loosening | 212 | 1500 | 1 | – |
| 18 | 75 | F | OA | Aseptic loosening | 260 | 1000 | 1 | – |
| 19 | 72 | F | FNF | Bipolar head migration | 290 | 1600 | 1 | – |

Abbreviations: FWB: full weight bearing; FNF: femoral neck fracture; OA: osteoarthritis; RA: rheumatoid arthritis.

using Merle d'Aubigne and Postel score [17]. Each patient was questioned on each visit, regarding the presence of thigh pain, which was considered as a complication related to the femoral component. The time at which full weight bearing was resumed was recorded. The extent of remaining bone cement was assessed on postoperative anteroposterior and lateral radiographs of the femur, taken immediately after surgery. A stem was considered unstable when progressive subsidence >3 mm, any change in position, or a continuous radiolucent line wider than 2 mm was seen [18].

## 3. Results

The patients' demographic and operative data are provided in Table 1. The mean operation time was 267 min (range, 180–420 min). The mean robotic milling time was 34 min (range, 17–51 min). The mean blood loss was 1236 g (range, 450–3000 g). The mean clinical score increased from 10 points (range, 6–12 points) preoperatively to 14 points (range, 9–17 points) at final follow-up. No instances of the perforation or fracture of the femur were seen during surgery or follow-up. No patients in this series displayed nerve palsy or infection, including locater pin cite. The only patient who complained of thigh pain displayed 3 mm of stem subsidence immediately after surgery. However, symptoms disappeared when subsidence stopped 6 months after surgery. Further revision was required in 2 cases for acetabular loosening.

Of the 19 cases, full weight bearing was possible within 1 week in 9 cases. In other 9 cases, because bone grafting was performed to correct an acetabular bone defect, the patients

were forced to delay full weight bearing due to the unreliable stability of the acetabular cup. The remaining patient was the first case in this study, and we were overly careful not to allow full weight bearing too early. However, full weight-bearing was achieved by all 19 patients within 2 months postoperatively, and they all became able to walk with a single cane.

Radiographically, bone cement was completely removed in all cases. Stem subsidence was seen in 2 cases, including the one mentioned previously. In the other case, subsidence progressed to 2 cm because of an undersized stem. Dislocation was seen only in this patient and was successfully treated using an abduction brace for three months after close reduction. As of final follow-up, all stems were considered to be bone stable.

## 4. Discussion

The results of revision THA using the ROBODOC system have not previously been reported. The purpose of this study was to evaluate the clinical and radiographic results for the ROBODOC system. In particular, we focused on the presence of intraoperative femoral fracture, the timing of full weight bearing, and the extent of remaining bone cement.

Several limitations in this study warrant consideration. First, the study design was retrospective, and we had no control group. Second, the number of cases was small, so the efficacy of this system needs to be confirmed in a larger number of cases. In addition, this system is strictly designed for the removal of bone cement and cannot be used for the removal of the stem itself. The primary disadvantages of this system are the need to implant locater pins before the revision surgery and the cost of the equipment.

The rate of the intraoperative fractures of the femur in revision THA ranges widely from 2.3% to 50% [19–23]. To remove the intramedullary bone cement safely, many new instruments and procedures, such as a ballistically driven chiseling system [7], a water jet [6], and high-energy shock waves [24], have been introduced, but clinical results have not yet been reported. Although an ultrasonic device presented some good clinical results [4, 5], Gardiner et al. reported complications related to the use of the device, such as superficial bone burns (9%) and bone perforation (3.3%) [5]. In addition, cases of radial nerve palsy and pathological humeral fracture reportedly developed after ultrasonic cement removal from the humerus [25]. Extended trochanteric osteotomies have been recommended to facilitate femoral component removal, femoral cement removal, and acetabular exposure in cases of difficult revision THA [8–11]. However, Noble et al. reported in an in vitro cadaveric study that extended trochanteric osteotomy reduced the torsional strength of the femur by 73%, even when the osteotomy fragment was repaired [26]. Moreover, Busch et al. postulated in a series of 219 revision procedures that the use of extended trochanteric osteotomy would represent a risk factor for stem fracture after revision surgery due to the poor proximal femoral bone support [19]. Cement-in-cement techniques have been introduced to reduce intraoperative complications in cases of well-fixed cemented stem revisions. Some good midterm results have been reported, but the perforation and fracture of the femur could not be completely avoided (1.5–20.4%) [27–29]. The ROBODOC system has been used without femoral fracture in a total of 900 cases of primary THA, clearly establishing the safety of this method [13]. Of note is the fact that no perforations or fractures of the femur occurred in our series. The ROBODOC system has an advantage over other new procedures, because the cutting area can be assessed 3-dimensionally before surgery and reproduced reliably during the operation.

The ROBODOC system allows early full weight bearing because of the circumferential preservation of the femoral cortex, which may help reduce the hospital stay and expenses. Among our 19 cases, full weight bearing was possible within 1 week after surgery in 9 cases and in all remaining patients within 2 months. The use of the extended trochanteric osteotomy reduces the rates of nonunion and migration of the osteotomy site (0–2%) [9–11]. However, to prevent these events, postoperative rehabilitation protocols must be restrictive. Brace wear and partial weight bearing may be continued for about 8–12 weeks before full weight bearing is allowed [9, 11].

Removing all cement from the femoral canal without using a cortical window or osteotomy is challenging. Schurman reported that in 12 of 15 cases, cement mantles were completely removed using the segmental cement extraction system. However, 2 cases showed retained cement along the medial wall of the femur, and the plug could not be extracted using this system in 1 case [30]. Jingushi et al. reported remaining parts of cement in the canal in postoperative radiography in 65% patients (13/20) using standard instruments for revision arthroplasty [31]. The clinical reports of the ultrasonic device did not refer to whether bone cement was completely removed [4, 5]. In our study, bone cement was completely removed without osteotomy in all 19 cases, thanks to the 3-dimensional assessment of the cutting area and the reproducibility of the ROBODOC system.

Nogler et al. pointed out the risk of heat injury during the ROBODOC milling process of cement removal, if cooling facilities were insufficient [32]. Although heat generation may cause soft tissue damage and bone necrosis, no nerve palsy or pathological fracture was encountered in our series, and bone ongrowth fixation between stem and femur was achieved in all cases. This result indicates that the intramedullary irrigation system functioned well for cooling, and bone around the stem remained viable.

In revision THA using the ROBODOC system, bone cement could be safely removed without the perforation or fracture of the femur, and full weight bearing was achieved early in the postoperative course due to the circumferential preservation of the femoral cortex.

## Conflict of Interests

The authors report no conflict of interests.

## References

[1] S.-R. Lee and M. P. G. Bostrom, "Periprosthetic fractures of the femur after total hip arthroplasty," *Instructional Course Lectures*, vol. 53, pp. 111–118, 2004.

[2] D. J. Berry, "Epidemiology: hip and knee," *Orthopedic Clinics of North America*, vol. 30, no. 2, pp. 183–190, 1999.

[3] S. Terzi, A. Toni, M. C. Zanotlí Russo, D. Nardi, A. Sudanese, and A. Giunti, "Intraoperative fractures of the femur in prosthetic hip reimplantations," *La Chirurgia Degli Organi di Movimento*, vol. 82, no. 3, pp. 221–230, 1997.

[4] R. C. Klapper, J. T. Caillouette, J. J. Callaghan, and W. J. Hozack, "Ultrasonic technology in revision joint arthroplasty," *Clinical Orthopaedics and Related Research*, no. 285, pp. 147–154, 1992.

[5] R. Gardiner, W. J. Hozack, C. Nelson, and E. M. Keating, "Revision total hip arthroplasty using ultrasonically driven tools: a clinical evaluation," *Journal of Arthroplasty*, vol. 8, no. 5, pp. 517–521, 1993.

[6] M. Honl, R. Rentzsch, K. Schwieger et al., "The water jet as a new tool for endoprosthesis revision surgery—an in vitro study on human bone and bone cement," *Bio-Medical Materials and Engineering*, vol. 13, no. 4, pp. 317–325, 2003.

[7] M. Porsch and J. Schmidt, "Histological findings of the femoral bone after cement removal in hip revision. An experimental study of cadaver femurs with two different cement removal procedures," *Archives of Orthopaedic and Trauma Surgery*, vol. 123, no. 5, pp. 199–202, 2003.

[8] R. Aribindi, W. Paprosky, P. Nourbash, J. Kronick, and M. Barba, "Extended proximal femoral osteotomy," *Instructional Course Lectures*, vol. 48, pp. 19–26, 1999.

[9] W.-M. Chen, J. P. McAuley, J. Engh C.A., J. Hopper R.H., and C. A. Engh, "Extended slide trochanteric osteotomy for revision total hip arthroplasty," *The Journal of Bone and Joint Surgery. American*, vol. 82, no. 9, pp. 1215–1219, 2000.

[10] T. M. Miner, N. G. Momberger, D. Chong, and W. L. Paprosky, "The extended trochanteric osteotomy in revision hip arthroplasty: a critical review of 166 cases at mean 3-year, 9-month follow-up," *Journal of Arthroplasty*, vol. 16, no. 8, pp. 188–194, 2001.

[11] T. I. Younger, M. S. Bradford, R. E. Magnus, and W. G. Paprosky, "Extended proximal femoral osteotomy: a new technique for femoral revision arthroplasty," *Journal of Arthroplasty*, vol. 10, no. 3, pp. 329–338, 1995.

[12] G. R. Huffman and M. D. Ries, "Combined vertical and horizontal cable fixation of an extended trochanteric osteotomy site," *The Journal of Bone and Joint Surgery. American*, vol. 85, no. 2, pp. 273–277, 2003.

[13] W. L. Bargar, A. Bauer, and M. Börner, "Primary and revision total hip replacement using the ROBODOC system," *Clinical Orthopaedics and Related Research*, no. 354, pp. 82–91, 1998.

[14] H. A. Paul, W. L. Bargar, B. Mittlestadt et al., "Development of a surgical robot for cementless total hip arthroplasty," *Clinical Orthopaedics and Related Research*, no. 285, pp. 57–66, 1992.

[15] N. Sugano, "Computer-assisted orthopedic surgery," *Journal of Orthopaedic Science*, vol. 8, no. 3, pp. 442–448, 2003.

[16] N. Nakamura, N. Sugano, T. Nishii, A. Kakimoto, and H. Miki, "A comparison between robotic-assisted and manual implantation of cementless total hip arthroplasty," *Clinical Orthopaedics and Related Research*, vol. 468, no. 4, pp. 1072–1081, 2010.

[17] R. M. Melre d'Aubigne and M. Postel, "Function al results of hip arthroplasty with acrylic prosthesis," *The Journal of Bone and Joint Surgery. American*, vol. 36, no. 3, pp. 451–475, 1954.

[18] C. A. Engh, P. Massin, and K. E. Suthers, "Roentgenographic assessment of the biologic fixation of porous-surfaced femoral components," *Clinical Orthopaedics and Related Research*, no. 257, pp. 107–128, 1990.

[19] C. A. Busch, M. N. Charles, C. M. Haydon et al., "Fractures of distally-fixed femoral stems after revision arthroplasty," *The Journal of Bone and Joint Surgery. British*, vol. 87, no. 10, pp. 1333–1336, 2005.

[20] K. J. Egan and P. E. Di Cesare, "Intraoperative complications of revision hip arthroplasty using a fully porous-coated straight cobalt-chrome femoral stem," *Journal of Arthroplasty*, vol. 10, pp. S45–S51, 1995.

[21] J. M. Lawrence, C. A. Engh, G. E. Macalino, and G. R. Lauro, "Outcome of revision hip arthroplasty done without cement," *The Journal of Bone and Joint Surgery. American*, vol. 76, no. 7, pp. 965–973, 1994.

[22] A. L. Malkani, D. G. Lewallen, M. E. Cabanela, and S. L. Wallrichs, "Femoral component revision using an uncemented, proximally coated, long-stem prosthesis," *Journal of Arthroplasty*, vol. 11, no. 4, pp. 411–418, 1996.

[23] B. F. Morrey and B. F. Kavanagh, "Complications with revision of the femoral component of total hip arthroplasty: comparison between cemented and uncemented techniques," *Journal of Arthroplasty*, vol. 7, no. 1, pp. 71–79, 1992.

[24] T. C. May, W. R. Krause, A. J. Preslar, M. J. Vernon Smith, A. J. Beaudoin, and J. A. Cardea, "Use of high-energy shock waves for bone cement removal," *Journal of Arthroplasty*, vol. 5, no. 1, pp. 19–27, 1990.

[25] S. H. Goldberg, M. S. Cohen, M. Young, and B. Bradnock, "Thermal tissue damage caused by ultrasonic cement removal from the humerus," *The Journal of Bone and Joint Surgery. American*, vol. 87, no. 3, pp. 583–591, 2005.

[26] A. R. Noble, D. B. Branham, M. C. Willis et al., "Mechanical effects of the extended trochanteric osteotomy," *The Journal of Bone and Joint Surgery. American*, vol. 87, no. 3, pp. 521–529, 2005.

[27] W. W. Duncan, M. J. W. Hubble, J. R. Howell, S. L. Whitehouse, A. J. Timperley, and G. A. Gie, "Revision of the cemented femoral stem using a cement-in-cement technique: a five- to 15-year review," *The Journal of Bone and Joint Surgery. British*, vol. 91, no. 5, pp. 577–582, 2009.

[28] K. Goto, K. Kawanabe, H. Akiyama, T. Morimoto, and T. Nakamura, "Clinical and radiological evaluation of revision hip arthroplasty using the cement-incement technique," *The Journal of Bone and Joint Surgery. British*, vol. 90, no. 8, pp. 1013–1018, 2008.

[29] P. Keeling, P. J. Prendergast, A. B. Lennon, and P. J. Kenny, "Cement-in-cement revision hip arthroplasty: an analysis of clinical and biomechanical literature," *Archives of Orthopaedic and Trauma Surgery*, vol. 128, no. 10, pp. 1193–1199, 2008.

[30] D. J. Schurman and W. J. Maloney, "Segmental cement extraction at revision total hip arthroplasty," *Clinical Orthopaedics and Related Research*, no. 285, pp. 158–163, 1992.

[31] S. Jingushi, Y. Noguchi, T. Shuto, T. Nakashima, and Y. Iwamoto, "A device for removal of femoral distal cement plug during hip revision arthroplasty: a high-powered drill equipped with a centralizer," *Journal of Arthroplasty*, vol. 15, no. 2, pp. 231–233, 2000.

[32] M. Nogler, M. Krismer, C. Haid, M. Ogon, C. Bach, and C. Wimmer, "Excessive heat generation during cutting of cement in the ROBODOC hip-revision procedure," *Acta Orthopaedica Scandinavica*, vol. 72, no. 6, pp. 595–599, 2001.

# 7

# A Novel Approach to the Surgical Treatment of Lumbar Disc Herniations: Indications of Simple Discectomy and Posterior Transpedicular Dynamic Stabilization Based on Carragee Classification

**A. F. Ozer,[1] F. Keskin,[2] T. Oktenoglu,[3] T. Suzer,[3] Y. Ataker,[4] C. Gomleksiz,[5] and M. Sasani[3]**

[1] *Neurosurgery Department, Koç University School of Medicine, Rumelifeneri Yolu Sarıyer, 34450 Istanbul, Turkey*

[2] *Neurosurgery Department, Necmettin Erbakan University Meram Medical Faculty Hospital, 42080 Konya, Turkey*

[3] *Neurosurgery Department, American Hospital, 34365 Istanbul, Turkey*

[4] *Physical Therapy and Rehabilitation Department, American Hospital, 34365 Istanbul, Turkey*

[5] *Neurosurgery Department, Mengücek Gazi Training and Research Hospital, School of Medicine, Erzincan University, 24100 Erzincan, Turkey*

Correspondence should be addressed to A. F. Ozer; alifahirozer@gmail.com

Academic Editor: Deniz Erbulut

Surgery of lumbar disc herniation is still a problem since Mixter and Barr. Main trouble is dissatisfaction after the operation. Today there is a debate on surgical or conservative treatment despite spending great effort to provide patients with satisfaction. The main problem is segmental instability, and the minimally invasive approach via microscope or endoscope is not necessarily appropriate solution for all cases. Microsurgery or endoscopy would be appropriate for the treatment of Carragee type I and type III herniations. On the other hand in Carragee type II and type IV herniations that are prone to develop recurrent disc herniation and segmental instability, the minimal invasive techniques might be insufficient to achieve satisfactory results. The posterior transpedicular dynamic stabilization method might be a good solution to prevent or diminish the recurrent disc herniation and development of segmental instability. In this study we present our experience in the surgical treatment of disc herniations.

## 1. Introduction

The surgical treatment of lumbar disc herniation is performed when the conservative treatment is recalcitrant and only ten percent of all lumbar disc herniations cases are candidates to surgery [1]. The main problem with the surgery is that the lumbar pain of the patients does not necessarily relieved following surgery and even they might become worse. For this reason, there are serious anxiety and suspicion against the surgical treatment of lumbar disc herniations. This phenomenon is also valid for some spine surgeons who will perform the operation. Even on their own series of Mixter and Barr, who first performed the discectomy of lumbar disc herniations, the success and failure rates compete head to head [2]. Later Caspar and Yasargil introduced

the microscope into the disc surgery and allowed minimal anatomic damage; however, no significant rise was achieved in satisfactory results [3, 4].

Carragee et al. revealed that the occurrence of disc herniation, the type of surgery, and the rates of reherniation are in a close relation with the defect on posterior annulus [5]. Lumbar disc herniation is not a separate illness but a part of a degenerative process, so the treatment should be designed in this manner. It is known that if the defect on the annulus is small, annulus has capacity to repair itself after fragmentectomy with both operative techniques: endoscopy and microdiscectomy. On the other hand, if the defect is large, problem arises at that time [6, 7].

In this paper, we discussed our results in the light of literature. We evaluated the role of load sharing principle with application of posterior transpedicular dynamic stabilization (PTDS) in lumbar disc herniation cases with large annulus defect, instead of performing radical discectomy.

## 2. Materials and Methods

This is a prospective study held between 2008 and 2012. Totally 98 patients were included in the study who did not respond to conservative treatment and minimal invasive pain procedure that was applied at a minimum of 6 weeks. Conservative treatment includes back exercises program and medicine. Epidural steroid injection and anauloplasty with laser were also performed for some of these cases as a minimal invasive pain procedure. Five surgeons performed the operations. The patients included for the study met the following inclusion criteria: (1) the findings of neurologic examination concordant with the patient's sciatica, (2) one level lumbar disc herniation determined with MR, (3) the surgical procedure applied electively, and (4) not having a spine operation before. Additionally, the patients with infection, instability, scoliosis, and malignancy are excluded from the study. The type of the operation to be applied was told to all the patients and the consent of patients was taken. Before the operation, magnetic resonance imaging was done to all cases and the deformation of annulus was evaluated with MR study and under the surgical microscope in operation. Patients were divided into four groups according to the classification of Carragee et al. [5] with a slight modification. In regard to achieving low recurrence notes, we accepted annulus defect as 4 mm difference from Carragee:

(i) Type I: there is no significant defect on annulus (Figure 1),

(ii) Type II: annular defect > 4 mm (Figure 2),

(iii) Type III: annular defect < 4 mm (Figure 3),

(iv) Type IV: massive-large annular defect (Figure 4).

The mean age of the patients was 48.19 (between 16 and 80). We determined the type of surgical intervention in reference to CS based on intraoperative observation and MR study. Clinic results were evaluated with visual analog scale (VAS) and Oswestry Disability Index (ODI) in the 3rd, 12th, and 24th months after the surgery. All patients who developed severe low back pain and/or recurrence sciatica were evaluated with MR for recurrence of disc herniation.

*2.1. Surgical Technique.* The surgical interventions were applied by five surgeons using standard microsurgical techniques at the same hospital. Before the surgical intervention, a single prophylactic antibiotic was given. According to the classification of modified Carragee, only fragmentectomy was applied to the cases of Type I herniation and discectomy was not applied in the course of the operation since annular tear was not observed under the surgical microscope. Limited discectomy was applied to the patients in the other groups. While discectomy was performed through the interlaminar gap in most of the patients, discectomy was applied to some patients following laminotomy with use of high speed drill. In

the course of the operation the types of disc herniation were defined with regard to MCC.

In the cases with MC Type II herniation, fragmentectomy (annular tear > 4 mm), limited discectomy with excision of degenerate nucleus pulposus, and annulus repair were performed. Annulus repair is carried out with bipolar cauterization of damaged outer layers of annulus fibrosus under the surgical microscope. PTDS was applied under C-arm scopy through paravertebral muscles as per Wiltse method, Cosmic (Ulrich GmbH & Co. KG, Ulm, Germany) and Safinaz (Medikon, Ankara, Turkey) screw and rods used for PTDS. In the cases with MC Type III herniations, limited discectomy (annular tear < 4 mm) with excision of degenerate nucleus pulposus and annulus repair were performed and PTDS was applied. In the cases with MC Type IV herniations, limited discectomy (massive annular tear) with excision of degenerate nucleus pulposus and annulus repair were performed. Then PTDS was applied.

In the course of operation, annular structure and the size of the annular defect were evaluated by at least two surgeons.

## 3. Results

Totally 13 out of 98 patients, operated with fragmentectomy, limited discectomy applied to 20 patients, and limited discectomy and PTDS were applied to 65 patients. The frequent type of herniation observed in our study was MCC Type II (47.8%) and the frequency of Type I, Type III, and Type IV was 18.3%, 26.5%, and 7.4%, respectively. Intraoperative complication was not observed. In the course of followup, for patients with Type II herniation, one patient developed a screw break and in one patient we observed screw loosening. It was noticed that these two patients were morbid obese. In the postoperative 8th and 12th month, the instrumentation systems were revised. In Type IV group, in one patient screw break was observed following a severe trauma. The instrumentation system of this patient was revised in 16th postoperative month. Finally a recurrence disc herniation was observed in a patient whose body structure was above the normal standards according to her age. In two patients with Type II and one patient with Type IV, adjacent segment degeneration was monitored. On the other hand, these patients did not complain clinically; therefore an extra surgical intervention was not considered. The follow-up period of cases with Type I group, reherniation, and recurrence herniation were not recorded. In two patients with Type II group reherniation, I in two cases with Type III group reherniation, and in one case with Type IV group, and reherniation as recorded.

## 4. Discussion

Even though it is thought that lumbar disc herniation is a separate disease; in fact, the degenerative change of the vertebrae is a part of the process. Following disc degeneration and before the loss of total disc integrity, the disc becomes clinically problematic due to improvement of painful black

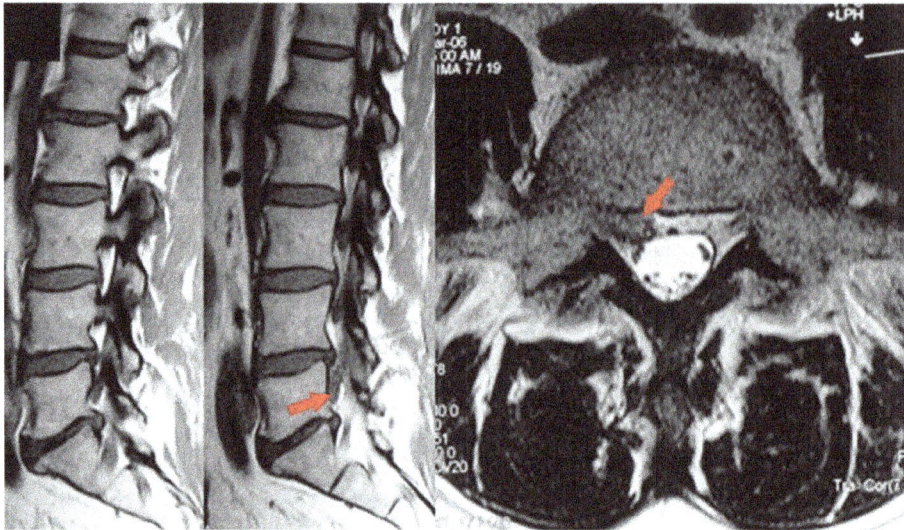

FIGURE 1: A small extruded fragment was observed under the nerve root. Notice that there is no apparent annulus defect (Carragee Type I).

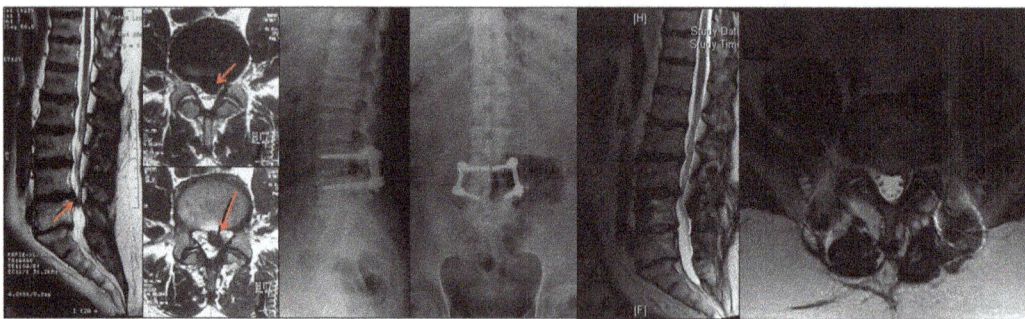

FIGURE 2: A large extruded fragment and noncontained disc herniation compress right S1 nerve root and cauda equina. Integrity of annulus fibrosus completely destroyed (Carragee Type II). The patient was operated on due to severe neurologic deficit and PTDS was applied to the patient after L5-S1 microdiscectomy and annular repair.

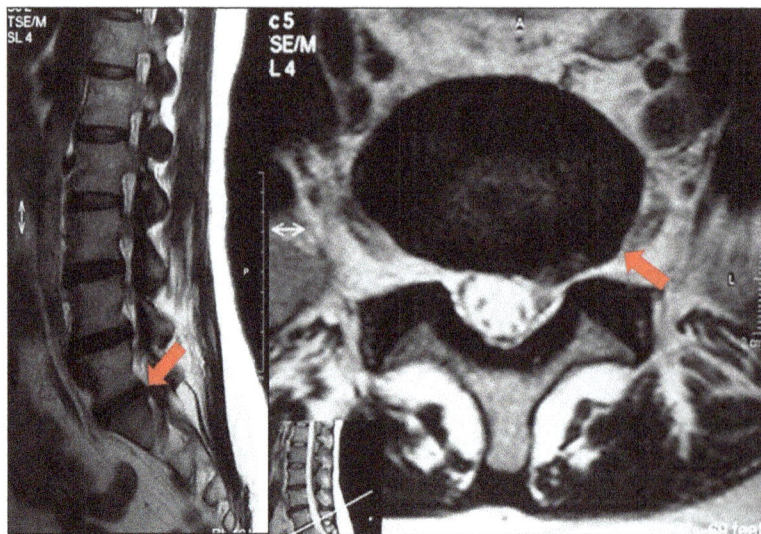

FIGURE 3: A small annulus defect (<4 mm) was observed at the left side just under the S1 nerve root. Integrity of the annulus fibrosus is preserved (Carragee Type III).

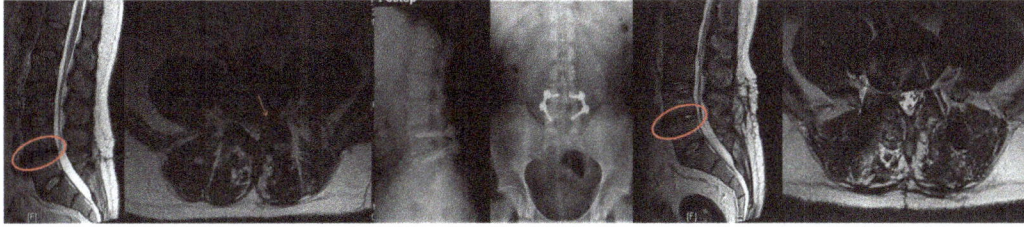

Figure 4: A large annulus defect (>4 mm) was observed at the midline of posterior annulus fibrosus. Integrity of annulus is preserved (Carragee Type IV). The patient is unresponsive to the conservative treatment and PTDS was applied to the patient after L5-S1 microdiscectomy and annular repair.

disc, degenerative spondylolisthesis, or lumbar disc herniation pathologies. That is why its treatment should be with the concepts by which we approach the degenerative process.

Since the beginning of the surgery for the treatment of lumbar disc herniation, the basic aim has been to increase the rate of success of the surgical treatment. Because while in some patients even there was no recurrence or residue herniation radiologically, there is still low back and/or radicular pain and in the other group who had very successful operation, they might have several recurrences on the same level and the same side. It has been thought that the results of the surgery implemented with little anatomic damage by using surgical microscope will affect in a positive way, and some reports supported this method [3, 4]. But the issues occurring after that period. However the later reports showed that the result did not change much in reference to the classic surgery [8, 9]. For a long time period, it is believed that fibrosis is sufical area which is somewhat more in some patients due to an unknown reason, and it is thought that the surgical success would increase if the improvement of fibrosis is prevented and made a big bid for this subject; yet, in the meantime the segmental instability was missed out [10–12]. Following the symptomatic lumbar disc herniation surgery at the height loss on disc space, the relaxation on the facet joint capsule, and ligamentous structures were well-known alternations. After the surgery, the load on the facet joints increases and it may lead to segmental instability [13–15]. For this reason, segmental instability and chronic lumbar pain which improve after the lumbar discectomy cause this type of treatment to which has been used for long years, become disputable [16]. Only the removal of nucleus pulposus is not suitable to stop the segmental degeneration related to the rotational and translational motions [17–19]. Therefore one of the important reasons of the failure of lumbar surgery is segmental instability. Yorimitsu has been following his patients for more than ten years after the disc surgery and concluded that the frequency of the chronic lumbar pain was more in proportion to reherniation based on the height loss on disc space [16].

Segmental instability has been shown with the radiological and clinical findings. These findings may not always support each other [20, 21]. The association of lumbar disc herniation and segmental instability is declared to be 20% in the literature [22]. Kotilainen determined that 22% of the patients developed segmental instability following one level

microlumbar discectomy studies and concluded that 29% of them had chronic lumbar pain [23]. Frymoyer signified that on wide based L4-5 disc hernias, there was severe lumbar pain and it is related to degenerative instability [22].

In the surgical treatment of lumbar disc herniation, it is very obvious that disc tried to be taken out; that is to say, radical discectomy does not solve the problem. Although it was realized, disc should not be completely removed. The more the existing disc structure is kept, the better the patient will become after the operation. That is to say, the theory of being respectful of the integrity became the main topic of the conversation with Spengeler who defined limited discectomy in 1990. This concept was improved more, and it is suggested by Williams that the fragment only should be removed and the integrity of the disc should be protected [24, 25].

Williams reported successful clinic results with minimal disc tissue taken out from the disc while they documented 4–9% recurrence rate and 90% clinic success rate [25, 26].

Afterwards, in the literature the discussions began if fragmentectomy or discectomy would be better. Wera et al. compared subtotal discectomy and sequestrectomy in the cases of herniation in Type II. They found that while in the events made with subtotal discectomy, reoperation rate was 3.4%, in the events made only fragmentectomy reoperation rate was 21.2%. Consequently, they informed that in the herniation events in Type II, subtotal discectomy would be more suitable [6]. Rogers compared massive discectomy with fragmentectomy in the disc herniations which are ruptured and reported that in the events of fragmentectomy the recurrence rate was 21% which is in a high rate [27]. Mochida et al. compared the clinical and radiological results of the patients who were operated on by percutaneous nucleotomy and standard discectomy. They documented that in the younger people below 40, surgery performed by protected nucleus pulposus, there were better radiological and clinic results [28]. Thomé et al. stated that recurrence rate is higher by microdiscectomy compared to sequestrectomy [13]. Barth et al. compared the two year rates of reherniation with microdiscectomy and microscopic sequestrectomy. They observed 10.5% reherniation rate in the microdiscectomy group and 12.5% in the events of fragmentectomy and concluded that there was no significant difference between these two groups [29]. However even the results of the patients who had fragmentectomy are better;

due to high recurrence rates, some surgeons did not give up performing subtotal discectomy [6, 7].

It is Carragee who emphasized that in the treatment of the lumbar disc herniation, the success is related to the defect on the posterior annulus. Carragee et al. reported in their study that for the patients of Type I group (who had small annular defect with fragment), only fragmentectomy was applied. The rate of reherniation and reoperation was 1%. In the group of Type II (fragment defect), the rate of recurrence sciatica was 27.3%, reoperation rate was high like 21.2%. In the group of Type III (fragment-contained), the rate of recurrence was 11.9% and the reoperation rate was 4.8%. In the group of Type IV (non-fragment-contained), reherniation rate was 37.5% and the rate of reoperation was 6.3%. Only fragmentectomy was applied to Type I group; the other groups were operated on by limited discectomy. Although the clinic results in Type I group were satisfactory, for the other groups, it was observed that the rates of reherniation and reoperation were rather high [5].

Therefore, the persistent pain after the operation and the recurrence is related to segmental instability and directly proportional to the integrity of defect in the posterior annulus. In this study, we applied limited discectomy or fragmentectomy to support posterior tension band; appropriate cases are required in respect to the integrity of disc material. We supported the spine with PTDS. The system shares the load applied on to spine thus decreases the load on the anterior column and this might allow disc to repair itself. Despite the fact that for the patients in Type I and Type III, our approach is the same with Carragee, for patients in Type II and Type IV, we used PTDS in addition to decompression. As a result of this, we achieved better VAS and Oswestry results compared to Carragee and Wera. The rates of recurrence for Type II is 5% and in Type IV is 4%. When we review the patients with recurrence, it was determined that one of them had a trauma in earlier time after the operation and the rest of them were those whose height and weight standards were really high according to the standards of society.

Practically if we exclude the patients who are overweight and had trauma, the rate of recurrence will be lower. It is a necessity that for the overweight people in reference to standards, dynamic systems should be designed restoratively.

In conclusion, the concept of the stabilisation of the spine in motion has been developed lately.

There are still many dark spots such as how much it keeps the motion, long term clinic results are unknown; the effect of it on the adjacent segments are unknown. On the other hand, it has an undeniable reality in its clinical success. Dynamic system technology is open to improvement and it is very certain that we will see the breakthroughs. By time, the dynamic screws, dynamic rods, and even those screws will have the flexibility of their body in the course of adaptation to the bone, will be developed. The rigid systems will leave their places to the systems which will be close to the structure of ligaments. Thus, the use of dynamic systems in the treatment of the cases with Type II and Type IV disc herniations would not be an overtreated approach but it is a step directed to the protection of the disc space following discectomy in more physiological conditionsç.

# References

[1] S. S. Hu, "Lumbar disc herniation section of disorders, diseases, and injuries of the spine," in *Current Diagnosis and Treatment in Orthopedics*, H. B. Skinner, Ed., pp. 246–249, McGraw-Hill, New York, NY, USA, 4th edition, 2006.

[2] W. J. Mixter and J. S. Barr, "Rupture of intervertebral disc with involvement of spinal canal," *New England Journal of Medicine*, vol. 211, pp. 210–215, 1934.

[3] W. Caspar, "A new surgical procedure for lumbar disc herniation causing less tissue damage through a microsurgical approach," *Lumbar Disc Adult Hydrocephalus*, vol. 4, pp. 74–80, 1977.

[4] M. G. Yasargil, "Microsurgical operation of herniated lumbar disc," *Advances in Neurosurgery*, vol. 4, p. 81, 1977.

[5] E. J. Carragee, M. Y. Han, P. W. Suen, and D. Kim, "Clinical outcomes after lumbar discectomy for sciatica: the effects of fragment type and anular competence," *Journal of Bone and Joint Surgery A*, vol. 85, no. 1, pp. 102–108, 2003.

[6] G. D. Wera, C. L. Dean, U. M. Ahn et al., "Reherniation and failure after lumbar discectomy: a comparison of fragment excision alone versus subtotal discectomy," *Journal of Spinal Disorders and Techniques*, vol. 21, no. 5, pp. 316–319, 2008.

[7] E. J. Carragee, A. O. Spinnickie, T. F. Alamin, and S. Paragioudakis, "A prospective controlled study of limited Versus subtotal posterior discectomy: short-term outcomes in patients with herniated lumbar intervertebral discs and large posterior anular defect," *Spine*, vol. 31, no. 6, pp. 653–657, 2006.

[8] Y. Katayama, Y. Matsuyama, H. Yoshihara ct al., "Comparison of surgical outcomes between macro discectomy and micro discectomy for lumbar disc herniation: a prospective randomized study with surgery performed by the same spine surgeon," *Journal of Spinal Disorders and Techniques*, vol. 19, no. 5, pp. 344–347, 2006.

[9] K. Türeyen, "One-level one-sided lumbar disc surgery with and without microscopic assistance: 1-year outcome in 114 consecutive patients," *Journal of neurosurgery*, vol. 99, no. 3, pp. 247–250, 2003.

[10] A. F. Ozer, T. Oktenoglu, M. Sasani et al., "Preserving the ligamentum flavum in lumbar discectomy: a new technique that prevents scar tissue formation in the first 6 months postsurgery," *Neurosurgery*, vol. 59, supplement 1, pp. S126–S133, 2006.

[11] J. Brotchi, B. Pirotte, O. De Witte, and M. Levivier, "Prevention of epidural fibrosis in a prospective series of 100 primary lumbosacral discectomy patients: follow-up and assessment at reoperation," *Neurological Research*, vol. 21, supplement 1, pp. S47–S50, 1999.

[12] R. N. Alkalay, D. H. Kim, D. W. Urry, J. Xu, T. M. Parker, and P. A. Glazer, "Prevention of postlaminectomy epidural fibrosis using bioelastic materials," *Spine*, vol. 28, no. 15, pp. 1659–1665, 2003.

[13] C. Thomé, M. Barth, J. Scharf, and P. Schmiedek, "Outcome after lumbar sequestrectomy compared with microdiscectomy: a prospective randomized study," *Journal of Neurosurgery*, vol. 2, no. 3, pp. 271–278, 2005.

[14] C. Cinotti and F. Postacchini, "Biomechanics," in *Lumbar Disc Herniation*, F. Postacchini, Ed., pp. 81–93, Springer-Verlag, Wien, Austria, 1999.

[15] M. Wenger, L. Mariani, A. Kalbarczyk, and U. Gröger, "Long-term outcome of 104 patients after lumbar sequestrectomy according to Williams," *Neurosurgery*, vol. 49, no. 2, pp. 329–335, 2001.

[16] E. Yorimitsu, K. Chiba, Y. Toyama, and K. Hirabayashi, "Long-term outcomes of standard discectomy for lumbar disc herniation: a follow-up study of more than 10 years," *Spine*, vol. 26, no. 6, pp. 652–657, 2001.

[17] A. Fujiwara, K. Tamai, M. Yamato et al., "The relationship between facet joint osteoarthritis and disc degeneration of the lumbar spine: an MRI study," *European Spine Journal*, vol. 8, no. 5, pp. 396–401, 1999.

[18] C. A. Niosi, Q. A. Zhu, D. C. Wilson, O. Keynan, D. R. Wilson, and T. R. Oxland, "Biomechanical characterization of the three-dimensional kinematic behaviour of the Dynesys dynamic stabilization system: an in vitro study," *European Spine Journal*, vol. 15, no. 6, pp. 913–922, 2006.

[19] A. Rohlmann, T. Zander, H. Schmidt, H. J. Wilke, and G. Bergmann, "Analysis of the influence of disc degeneration on the mechanical behaviour of a lumbar motion segment using the finite element method," *Journal of Biomechanics*, vol. 39, no. 13, pp. 2484–2490, 2006.

[20] J. W. Frymoyer, E. N. Hanley, and J. Howe, "A comparison of radiographic findings in fusion and nonfusion patients ten or more years following lumbar disc surgery," *Spine*, vol. 4, no. 5, pp. 435–440, 1979.

[21] S. Sano, S. Yokokura, Y. Nagata, and Seong Zeon Young, "Unstable lumbar spine without hypermobility in postlaminectomy cases: mechanism of symptoms and effect of spinal fusion with and without spinal instrumentation," *Spine*, vol. 15, no. 11, pp. 1190–1197, 1990.

[22] J. W. Frymoyer and D. K. Selby, "Segmental instability: rationale for treatment," *Spine*, vol. 10, no. 3, pp. 280–286, 1985.

[23] E. Kotilainen and S. Valtonen, "Clinical instability of the lumbar spine after microdiscectomy," *Acta Neurochirurgica*, vol. 125, no. 1–4, pp. 120–126, 1993.

[24] D. M. Spengler, E. A. Ouellette, M. Battie, and J. Zeh, "Elective discectomy for herniation of a lumbar disc. Additional experience with an objective method," *Journal of Bone and Joint Surgery A*, vol. 72, no. 2, pp. 230–237, 1990.

[25] R. W. Williams, "Microlumbar discectomy. A conservative surgical approach to the virgin herniated lumbar disc," *Spine*, vol. 3, no. 2, pp. 175–182, 1978.

[26] R. W. Williams, "Microlumbar discectomy. A 12-year statistical review," *Spine*, vol. 11, no. 8, pp. 851–852, 1986.

[27] L. A. Rogers, "Experience with limited versus extensive disc removal in patients undergoing microsurgical operations for ruptured lumbar discs," *Neurosurgery*, vol. 22, no. 1, pp. 82–85, 1988.

[28] J. Mochida, K. Nishimura, T. Nomura, E. Toh, and M. Chiba, "The importance of preserving disc structure in surgical approaches to lumbar disc herniation," *Spine*, vol. 21, no. 13, pp. 1556–1564, 1996.

[29] M. Barth, C. Weiss, and C. Thomé, "Two-year outcome after lumbar microdiscectomy versus microscopic sequestrectomy-part 1: evaluation of clinical outcome," *Spine*, vol. 33, no. 3, pp. 265–272, 2008.

# 8

# Vacuum Assisted Closure Therapy versus Standard Wound Therapy for Open Musculoskeletal Injuries

**Kushagra Sinha,[1] Vijendra D. Chauhan,[2] Rajesh Maheshwari,[1] Neena Chauhan,[3] Manu Rajan,[4] and Atul Agrawal[1]**

[1] Department of Orthopaedics, Himalayan Institute of Medical Sciences, Dehradun, Uttarakhand 248140, India
[2] Himalayan Institute of Medical Sciences, Dehradun, Uttarakhand 248140, India
[3] Department of Pathology, Himalayan Institute of Medical Sciences, Dehradun, Uttarakhand 248140, India
[4] Department of Plastic Surgery, Himalayan Institute of Medical Sciences, Dehradun, Uttarakhand 248140, India

Correspondence should be addressed to Vijendra D. Chauhan; vchauhan16@yahoo.co.in

Academic Editor: Hiroshi Hashizume

*Background.* This study was performed to evaluate the results of vacuum assisted wound therapy in patients with open musculoskeletal injuries. *Study Design and Setting.* Prospective, randomized, and interventional at tertiary care hospital, from 2011 to 2012. *Materials and Methods.* 30 patients of open musculoskeletal injuries underwent randomized trial of vacuum assisted closure therapy versus standard wound therapy around the upper limb and lower limb. Mean patient age was $39 \pm 18$ years (range, 18 to 76 years). Necrotic tissues were debrided before applying VAC therapy. Dressings were changed every 3 or 4 days. For standard wound therapy, debridement followed by daily dressings was done. *Data Management and Statistical Analysis.* The results obtained were subjected to statistical analysis. *Results.* The size of soft tissue defects reduced more than 5 mm to 25 mm after VAC (mean decrease of 26.66%), whereas in standard wound therapy, reduction in wound size was less than 5 mm. A free flap was needed to cover exposed bone and tendon in one case in standard wound therapy group. No major complication occurred that was directly attributable to treatment. *Conclusion.* Vacuum assisted wound therapy was found to facilitate the rapid formation of healthy granulation tissue on open wounds in the upper limb and lower limb, thus to shorten healing time and minimize secondary soft tissue defect coverage procedures.

## 1. Introduction

Wound healing is a complex and dynamic process that includes an immediate sequence of cell migration leading to repair and closure. This sequence begins with removal of debris, control of infection, clearance of inflammation, angiogenesis, deposition of granulation tissue, contraction, remodelling of the connective tissue matrix, and maturation. When wound fails to undergo this sequence of events, a chronic open wound without anatomical or functional integrity results [1].

High-energy open fractures require both skeletal stability and adequate soft tissue coverage. In such injuries, debridement of all nonviable tissue can produce significant soft-tissue defects precluding healing through primary closures, delayed primary closures, or secondary intention [2]. Various

surgical methods have been developed to obtain coverage in these difficult situations. These include skin grafts, local rotation flaps, and myocutaneous or fasciocutaneous tissue transfers. Although skin grafts are readily obtainable, they are dependent on the vascularity of its recipient bed and may be contraindicated when exposed bone, cartilage, tendons, or surgical implants exist [3]. In such situation, a local rotation flap may be needed. When the soft tissue defect prevents local coverage [4], free tissue transfers are usually required, but the transfer may produce donor site morbidity and require late revisions due to the size of the muscle flap [5].

Although nonoperative modalities, such as hyperbaric oxygen, have been used to enhance wound coverage, these devices may not be available to all patients and may not be adequate for use in patients presenting with high-energy injuries due to edema, retraction of the skin and soft tissue, wound size, or loss of available local coverage [6]. Attempts have been made to identify an alternative treatment of wound management in these patients.

Clinically, chronic wounds may be associated with pressure sore, trauma, venous insufficiency, diabetes, vascular disease, or prolonged immobilization. The treatment of chronic, open wounds is variable and costly, demanding lengthy hospital stays or specialized home care requiring skilled nursing and costly supplies. Rapid healing of chronic wounds could result in decreased hospitalization and an earlier return of function. A method that improves the healing process could greatly decrease the risk of infection, amputation, and length of hospital stay and result in an estimated potential annual savings of billions of rupees of healthcare cost [1].

Initially developed in the early 1990s, for the management of large, chronically infected wounds that could not be closed in extremely debilitated patients, the use of vacuum-assisted closure (VAC) has been more recently used in the treatment of traumatic wounds [7].

The purpose of this study is to evaluate the results of this therapy for the management of patients presenting with open musculoskeletal injuries.

## 2. Materials and Methods

The study was conducted on 30 patients in the Department of Orthopaedics, Himalayan Institute of Medical Sciences, over a period of 12 months, after obtaining the permission from institutional ethical committee and taking informed and written consents from the patients.

All patients above 18 years of age with open musculoskeletal injuries in extremities that required coverage procedures were included in the study. However, patients with preexisting osteomyelitis in the wounds, neurovascular deficit in the injured limb, diabetics, malignancy, and peripheral vascular disease were excluded from the study.

The patients were prospectively randomized into one of the two treatment groups receiving either the vacuum assisted closure therapy or standard saline-wet-to-moist wound care. Files were marked with red (vacuum assisted closure therapy) or yellow (saline-wet-to-moist dressings) labels on the inside panel and were randomly organized. A file was randomly picked for each wound with the treatment determined by the label colour.

Participation in the study did not deviate from the standard care of the acute wound. All patients for wound management were subjected to

(1) standard radiological assessment of the injured wound,

(2) routine haematological investigation, for example, complete blood count, ESR, blood sugar, HIV and HbsAg, gram stain and culture,

(3) all patients were supplemented with standard nutritional supplements, including zinc and multivitamin daily.

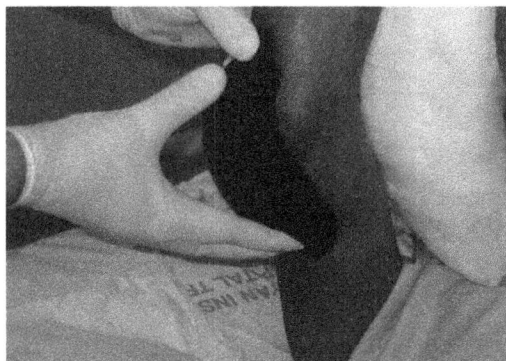

FIGURE 1: Foam was cut according to wound size.

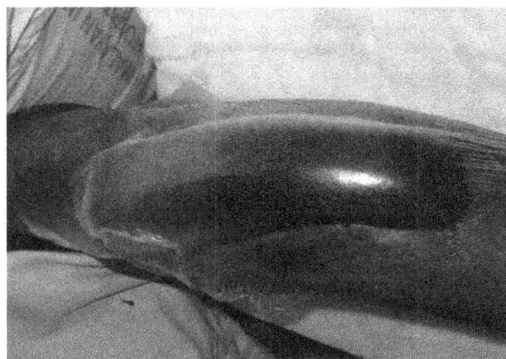

FIGURE 2: Sterile drape was applied covering the foam and 2-3 cm of the surrounding skin.

### 2.1. Vacuum Assisted Wound Therapy Procedure

*2.1.1. Wound Preparation.* Any dressings from the wound were removed and discarded. A culture swab for microbiology was taken before wound irrigation with normal saline. Necrotic tissues were surgically removed (surgical debridement), and adequate haemostasis was achieved. Prior to application of the drape, it was essential to prepare the peri-wound skin and ensure that it was dry.

*2.1.2. Placement of Foam.* Sterile, open-pore foam (35 ppi density and 33 mm thick) dressing was gently placed into the wound cavity. Open-pore foams are polyurethane with 400–600 microns size having hydrophobic open cell structured network. Such sizes of pores are most effective at transmitting mechanical forces across the wound and provide an even distribution of negative pressure over the entire wound bed to aid in wound healing (Figure 1).

*2.1.3. Sealing with Drapes.* The site was then sealed with an adhesive drape covering the foam and tubing and at least three to five centimetres of surrounding healthy tissue to ensure a seal (Figures 2 and 3).

*2.1.4. The Application of Negative Pressure.* Controlled pressure was uniformly applied to all tissues on the inner surface of the wound. The pump delivered an intermittent negative pressure of −125 mmHg. The cycle was of seven minutes in

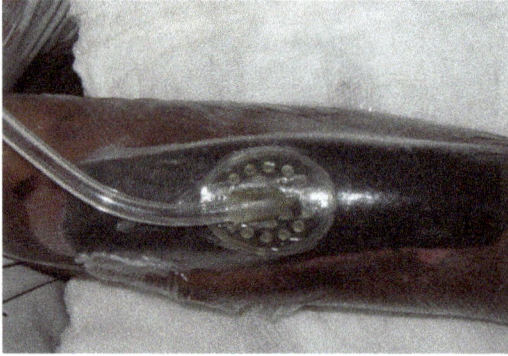

FIGURE 3: The connecting tube was applied after making a small opening (3-4 mm) on the drape.

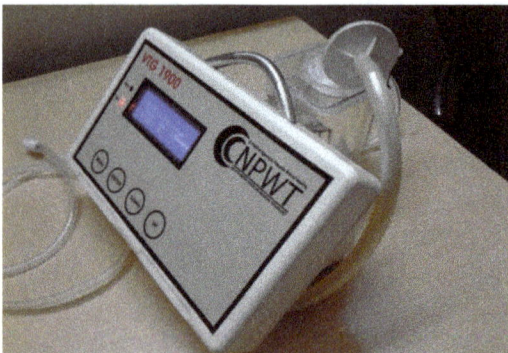

FIGURE 4: The connecting tube was connected to the negative pressure wound therapy.

which pump was on for five minutes and off for two minutes (Figure 4).

The dressings were changed on the fourth day.

*2.2. Saline-Wet-to-Moist Group Procedure.* Wound preparation—any dressings from the wound was removed and discarded. A culture swab for microbiology was taken before wound irrigation with normal saline. Surface slough or necrotic tissue was surgically removed (surgical debridement), and adequate haemostasis was achieved.

Daily dressings by conventional methods, that is, cleaning with hydrogen peroxide and normal saline and dressing the wound with povidone iodine (5%) and saline-soaked gauze was done and wound examined daily.

Resident who had measured the wounds was not involved in the daily care of the study patients. It was not mentioned to which treatment group the patient was assigned. This blinding arrangement ensured that the person evaluating the wound and collecting data initially at day zero and whenever dressings were subsequently changed had seen the wound only after all dressings, supplies, and equipment were removed from the patient and the room. He took photographs and measured the wound by Vernier Caliper and transparent O.H.P sheets (overhead projector sheet).

The resident doctor also clinically assessed the wounds for signs of infection and obtained 4–6 mm punch biopsy

TABLE 1: Decrease in wound size from day 0 to day 8.

| Measurements (mm) | VAC ($n = 15$) | Saline-wet-to-moist ($n = 15$) |
|---|---|---|
| 1–4.9 | 4 (26.66%) | 14 (93.33%) |
| 5–9.9 | 1 (6.66%) | 0 |
| 10–14.9 | 4 (26.66%) | 1 (6.66%) |
| 15–19.9 | 3 (20%) | 0 |
| 20–24.9 | 1 (6.66%) | 0 |
| >25 | 2 (13.33%) | 0 |

Chi Square = 14.4, d.f = 5, $P = 0.013$.

samples for histology and culture. Biopsies were obtained from the four corners and the most "healthy" portion of the wound bed. Samples were taken on day zero, day four, and day eight. The presence of drainage, edema, erythema, exposed bone, or exposed tendon wasdocumented. Any complications associated with vacuum assisted closure therapy were also documented. Such measurements and findings were recorded on day zero, day four, and day eight in both the groups.

The wounds were also evaluated by plastic surgeon on day one and on day eight to assess the nature of surgical procedure to be adopted to cover the wound.

The pathologist noted and quantified the presence of inflammatory cells, bacteria, arterioles, proliferative fibroblasts, excessive collagen formation, and fibrosis in the biopsy samples.

*2.3. Data Management and Statistical Analysis.* The results obtained were subjected to statistical analysis which was done by using statistical software SPSS-version 19. Normality of data was checked by Kolmogorov-Smirnov test for unpaired $t$-test. Quantitative data was expressed in terms of mean ± SD. Categorical data was analysed by Chi-square and Wilcoxon signed ranks test.

For Wilcoxon signed ranks test, the evaluation of histological parameters (Inflammatory cells, proliferative fibroblasts, collagen formation, and fibrosis) was ranked as absent—0, mild—1, moderate—2, and severe—3.

## 3. Results

Mean patient age was 39 ± 18 years (range, 18 to 76 years). All patients had suffered an acute trauma. Road traffic accident was found to be most common cause with 22 (73.33%) patients, followed by machinery injury in 5 (16.66%) patients and 3 (10%) patients had a fall from height. According to Gustilo Anderson classification, out of 30 patients, 16 patients had grade IIIb injury, 7 had grade IIIc injury, 3 had IIIa injury, and 4 had grade II injury.

*Decrease in Wound Size.* There was significant decrease in wound size from day zero to day eight in VAC group in comparison to saline-wet-to-moist group as shown in Tables 1 and 2.

TABLE 2: Mean wound size difference between VAC and saline wet to moist on day 8.

| | VAC ($n = 15$) | Saline wet to moist ($n = 15$) | P value | 95% CI |
|---|---|---|---|---|
| Mean difference (mm) | $13.24 \pm 8.48$ | $3.02 \pm 2.90$ | 0.0001 | 11.053 to 15.327 |

TABLE 3: Bacterial growth ($n = 30$).

| Bacterial growth | VAC patients ($n = 15$) | | | Saline wet to moist ($n = 15$) | | |
|---|---|---|---|---|---|---|
| | Day 0 | Day 4 | Day 8 | Day 0 | Day 4 | Day 8 |
| Present | 15 (100%) | 12 (80%) | 6 (40%) | 15 (100%) | 15 (100%) | 12 (80%) |
| Absent | 0 | 3 (20%) | 9 (60%) | 0 | 0 | 3 (20%) |

TABLE 4: Comparison of histological parameters from day 0 to day 8 by Wilcoxon signed ranks test.

| Stages of wound healing | Saline wet to moist | | | | VAC | | | |
|---|---|---|---|---|---|---|---|---|
| | Positive | Negative | Equal | P value | Positive | Negative | Equal | P value |
| Inflammatory cells | 1 | 10 | 4 | 0.001 | 1 | 12 | 2 | 0.003 |
| Proliferative fibroblasts | 13 | 0 | 2 | 0.001 | 15 | 0 | 0 | 0.001 |
| Collagen formation | 14 | 0 | 1 | 0.001 | 15 | 0 | 0 | 0.001 |
| Fibrosis | 6 | 0 | 9 | 0.03 | 15 | 0 | 0 | 0.001 |

P value < 0.05.
Positive: ranks of day 8 > ranks of day 0.
Negative: ranks of day 8 < ranks of day 0.
Equal: ranks of day 8 is equal to ranks of day 0.

*Bacterial Growth.* There was significant decrease in the bacterial growth in the VAC group as compared to saline-wet-to-moist group, as shown in Table 3.

On histological comparison too, there was a statistical difference between the VAC group and saline-wet-to-moist group, P value being less than 0.05 by using Wilcoxon signed rank test between the findings from day zero to day eighth as shown in Table 4.

*Case No. 1.* In an 18-year-male old a case of open grade IIIb fracture both bone right forearm (middle 3rd), wound was present over anterior aspect of forearm. After thorough debridement and fracture fixation VAC was applied (see Figure 5).

*Case No. 2.* In a 57-year-male old sustained injury open grade IIIa olecranon, debridement was done, and VAC was applied (see Figure 6).

## 4. Discussion

Healing is an intricate, interdependent process that involves complex interactions between cells, the cellular microenvironment, biochemical mediators, and extracellular matrix molecules that usually results in a functional restoration of the injured tissue [8, 9]. The goals of wound healing are to minimize blood loss, replace any defect with new tissue (granulation tissue followed by scar tissue), and restore an intact epithelial barrier as rapidly as possible.

The rate of wound healing is limited by the available vascular supply and the rate of formation of new capillaries and matrix molecules [10]. These events are heavily influenced by locally acting growth factors that affect various processes including proliferation, angiogenesis, chemotaxis and migration, gene expression, proteinases, and protein production [8, 11–14]. Disruption of any of these factors may adversely affect the healing process, resulting in a chronic or nonhealing wound.

Blood flow increases and bacterial colonization of wound tissues decreases following the application of subatmospheric pressure to wounds [7]. Any increase in circulation and oxygenation to compromised or damaged tissue enhances the resistance to infection [15]. Successful, spontaneous healing and healing following surgical intervention are correlated with tissue bacterial counts of less than $10^5$ organisms per gram of tissue [16]. Higher levels uniformly interfere in wound healing. Increase in local tissue oxygen levels reduce or eliminate the growth of anaerobic organisms, which have been correlated to decreased healing rates [17, 18]. Additionally, the increased flow should make greater amounts of oxygen available to neutrophils for the oxidative bursts that kill bacteria [19].

Our study showed that in VAC group after day 4, there were 20% of patients who had no bacterial growth, and on day 8 there were 60% of patients who had no bacterial growth, whereas in saline-wet-to-moist patients only 20% of patients had no bacterial growth on the 8th day. There have been similar studies by Morykwas and Argenta [7], Banwell et al. [20], and Morykwas et al. [21] which showed clearance of bacteria from infected wounds using VAC therapy.

On the other hand, Weed et al. while quantifying bacterial bioburden during negative pressure wound therapy concluded with serial quantitative cultures that there is no

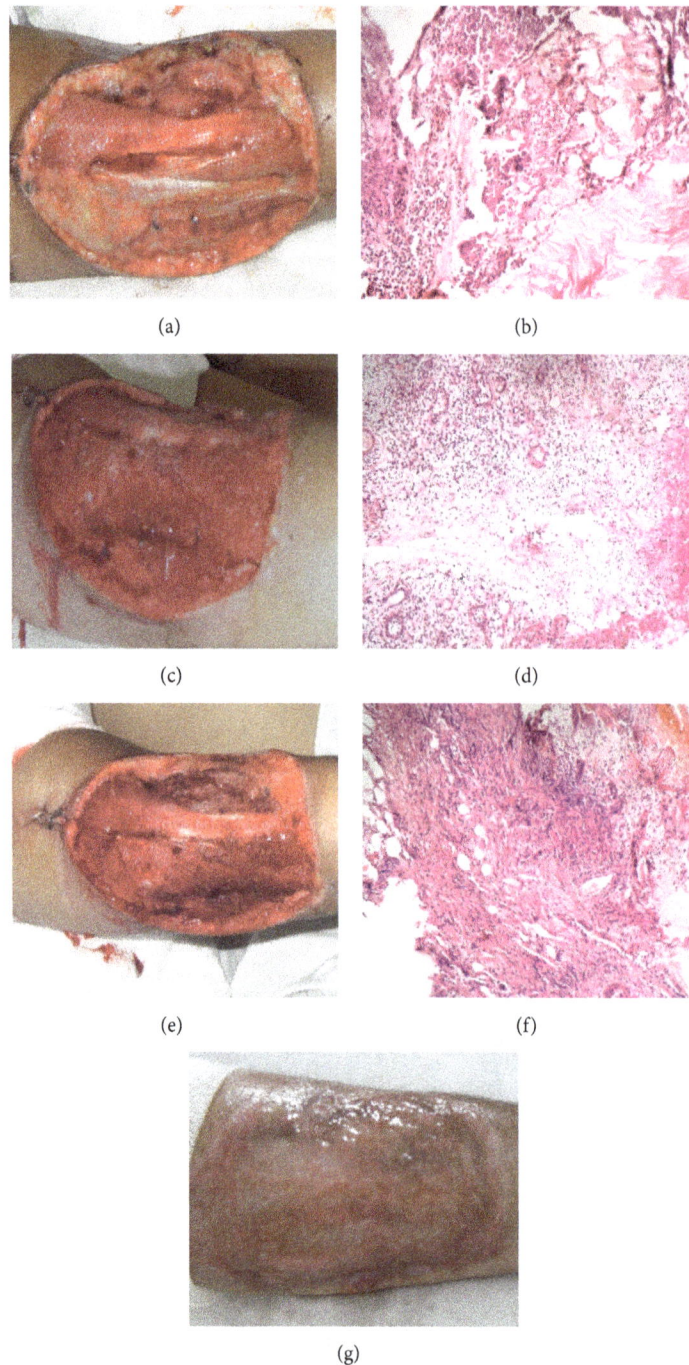

FIGURE 5: (a) Day 0: wound size, $146 \times 135$ mm. (b) Day 0: photomicrograph number 1-H and E stained section (100x) shows: dense neutrophilic exudates on the surface of wound. (c) Day 4: wound size, $130 \times 120$ mm. (d) Day 4: photomicrograph number 2-H and E stained section (100x) shows: fibrinous exhudate on the surface and base of ulcer is formed by moderately inflamed granulation tissue. (e) Day 8: wound size, $130 \times 117$ mm. (f) Day 8: photomicrograph number 3-H and E stained section (100x) shows: many newly formed blood vessels and dense fibro collagenous tissue. (g) SSG uptake seen.

consistent bacterial clearance with the VAC therapy, and the bacterial growth remained in the range of $10^4$–$10^6$ [22].

Thomas first postulated that application of mechanical stress would result in angiogenesis and tissue growth. Unlike sutures or tension devices, the VAC can exert a uniform force at each individual point on the edge of the wound drawing it toward the centre of the defect by mechanically stretching

the cells when negative pressure is applied [23]. This allows the VAC to move distensible soft tissue, similar to expanders, towards the centre of the wound, thereby decreasing the actual size of the wound [24].

Our study showed a decrease in size of 1 to 4.9 mm in 26.66% of patients in VAC group whereas 93.33% in control group from day 0 to day 8. A decrease in size of 10 to 19.9 mm

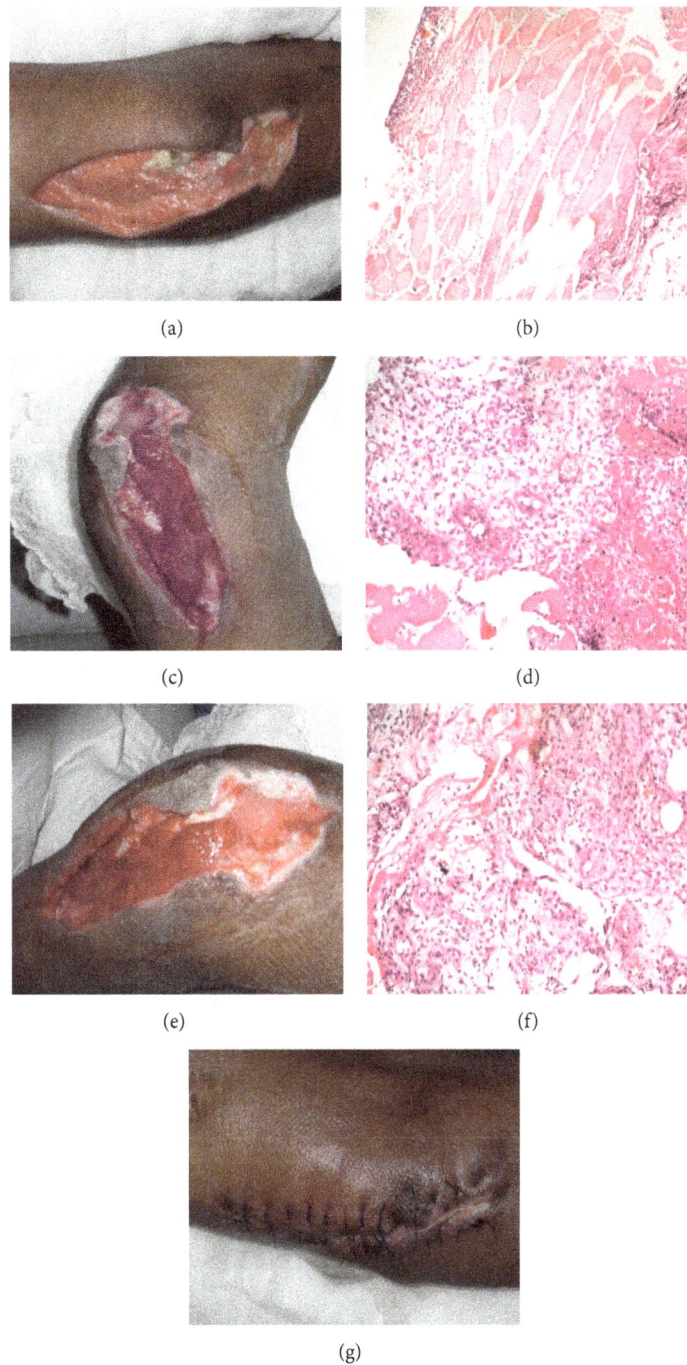

(a)

(b)

(c)

(d)

(e)

(f)

(g)

FIGURE 6: (a) Day 0: wound size, 146 × 61 mm. (b) Day 0: photomicrograph number 1-H and E stained section (100x) shows: thick neutrophillic exhudate on the surface and skeletal muscle bundles. (c) Day 4: wound size, 141 × 51 mm. (d) Day 4: photomicrograph number 2-H and E stained section (100x) shows: Inflammed granulation tissue with little exhudate on the surface. (e) Day 8: Wound size, 135 × 51 mm. (f) Day 8: photomicrograph number 3-H and E stained section (100x) shows: healthy granulation tissue without any exhudate. (g) Secondary closure done.

was seen in 46.66% of patients of VAC group and only 6.66% in control group. A decrease in size of more than 25 mm was seen in 13.33% in VAC group.

There have been similar studies by Joseph et al. [1], Morykwas and Argenta [7], and Morykwas et al. [21] which showed that VAC proved effective in shrinking the widths of wound over time compared to standard wound dressings.

Our study showed that VAC increases the vascularity and the increase in rate of granulation tissue formation compared to standard wound dressing. Histologically, VAC patients showed angiogenesis and healthy tissue growth as compared to the inflammation and fibrosis seen in standard wound dressing. Inflammation had increased in those treated with standard wound therapy and decreased in those patients treated with VAC.

The highly significant increase in the rate of granulation tissue formation of subatmospheric pressure-treated wound is postulated to be due to transmission of the uniformly applied force to the tissues on the periphery of the wound. These forces both recruit tissues through viscoelastic flow and promote granulation tissue formation. Currently, the Ilizarov technique and soft tissue expanders both apply mechanical stress to tissues to increase mitotic rates [25, 26].

Standard wound dressings adhere to devitalized tissue and within four to six hours the gauze can be removed, along with the tissue, as a form of mechanical debridement. This method of wound care has been criticized for removing viable tissue as well as nonviable tissue and being traumatic to granulation tissue and to new epithelial cells [27].

There is very little literature available especially on compound injuries using VAC. Open musculoskeletal injuries have very high incidences of nonunion and infection [28]; they require urgent irrigation and debridement. As wounds are frequently left open and require repeated debridement, resulting in large soft tissue defects, early coverage of exposed bone, tendons, and neurovascular structures is crucial. This is to decrease the risk of infection, nonunion, and further tissue loss. We believe that VAC therapy can be effective to overcome all the aforementioned problems.

The daily rental charges for a VAC machine and consumables are significant. This has discouraged many from using the system. However, there have been some reports showing that the increased healing times and downgrading of required operations correlate to decreased overall costs of care. The dressing should also enable larger wounds to be treated in the community with minimal nursing care impact. This would free up hospital beds permitting faster healing of operative patients and preventing waiting list buildup [29].

VAC therapy can be regarded as a method that combines the benefit of both open and closed treatment and adheres to DeBakey's principles of being short, safe, and simple. It has been shown to work and be beneficial to wound healing. VAC therapy is not the answer for all wounds; however, it can make a significant difference in many cases. VAC is most useful in difficult cavity or highly exudative wounds. VAC is a useful tool in moving a wound to a point where more traditional dressings or more simple surgical reconstructive methods can be used. As such it is a well deserved, although at present pragmatic addition to the wound healing armamentarium and the reconstructive ladder [30].

## 5. Conclusion

Vacuum assisted closure therapy appears to be a viable adjunct for the treatment of open musculoskeletal injuries. Application of subatmospheric pressure after the initial debridement to the wounds results in an increase in local functional blood perfusion, an accelerated rate of granulation tissue formation, and decrease in tissue bacterial levels. Although traditional soft tissue reconstruction may still be required to obtain adequate coverage, the use of this device appears to decrease their need overall.

## Disclosure

Regarding your statistical software SPSS-version 19, Himalayan Institute of Medical Sciences had purchased the software for data analysis for all its ongoing projects. So, even our clinical trial was analyzed with the same software.

## Conflict of Interests

There is no conflict of interests of any sort regarding the software.

## References

[1] E. Joseph, C. A. Hamori, S. Bergman, E. Roaf, N. F. Swann, and G. W. Anastasi, "A prospective randomized trial of vacuum-assisted closure versus standard therapy of chronic nonhealing wounds," *Wounds*, vol. 12, no. 3, pp. 60–67, 2000.

[2] M. J. Yaremchuk, "Concepts in soft tissue management," in *Lower Extremity Salvage and Reconstruction. Orthopaedic and Plastic Surgical Management*, M. J. Yaremchuk, A. R. Burgess, and R. J. Brumback, Eds., pp. 95–106, Elsevier Science, New York, NY, USA, 1989.

[3] J. A. Haller and R. E. Billingham, "Studies of the origin of the vasculature in free skin grafts," *Annals of Surgery*, vol. 166, no. 6, pp. 896–901, 1967.

[4] M. Geishauser, R. W. Staudenmaier, and E. Biemer, "Donor-site morbidity of the segmental rectus abdominis muscle flap," *British Journal of Plastic Surgery*, vol. 51, no. 8, pp. 603–607, 1998.

[5] M. B. Kelly and A. Searle, "Improving the donor site cosmesis of the latissimus dorsi flap," *Annals of Plastic Surgery*, vol. 41, no. 6, pp. 629–632, 1998.

[6] M. C. Y. Heng, "Topical hyperbaric therapy for problem skin wounds," *Journal of Dermatologic Surgery and Oncology*, vol. 19, no. 8, pp. 784–793, 1993.

[7] M. J. Morykwas and L. C. Argenta, "Vacuum-assisted closure: a new method for wound control and treatment: clinical experience," *Annals of Plastic Surgery*, vol. 38, no. 6, pp. 563–577, 1997.

[8] R. A. F. Clarke and P. M. Henson, Eds., *The Molecular and Cellular Biology of Wound Repair*, Plenum Press, New York, NY, USA, 1988.

[9] I. K. Cohen, R. F. Diegelmann, and W. J. Lindblad, *Wound Healing: Biochemical and Clinical Aspects*, WB Saunders, Philadelphia, Pa, USA, 1992.

[10] T. K. Hunt, "Vascular factors govern healing in chronic wounds," in *Clinical and Experimental Approach to Dermal and Epidermal Repair: Normal and Chronic Wounds*, A. Barbul, M. D. Caldwell, W. H. Eaglstein et al., Eds., pp. 1–17, Wiley & Leiss, New York, NY, USA, 1991.

[11] G. F. Pierce, J. Vande Berg, R. Rudolph, J. Tarpley, and T. A. Mustoe, "Platelet-derived growth factor-BB and transforming growth factor beta1 selectively modulate glycosaminoglycans, collagen, and myofibroblasts in excisional wounds," *American Journal of Pathology*, vol. 138, no. 3, pp. 629–646, 1991.

[12] M. Laiho and O. J. Keski, "Growth factors in the regulation of pericellular proteolysis: a review," *Cancer Research*, vol. 49, no. 10, pp. 2533–2553, 1989.

[13] M. Laiho and O. J. Keski, "Growth factors in the regulation of pericellular proteolysis: a review," *Cancer Research*, vol. 49, no. 10, pp. 2533–2553, 1989.

[14] D. J. Whitby and M. W. J. Ferguson, "Immunohistological studies of the extracellular matrix and soluble growth factors in fetal and adult wound healing," in *Fetal Wound Healing*, N. S. Adzick and M. T. Longaker, Eds., pp. 161–177, Elsevier Science, New York, NY, USA, 1992.

[15] T. K. Hunt, "The physiology of wound healing," *Annals of Emergency Medicine*, vol. 17, no. 12, pp. 1265–1273, 1988.

[16] J. O. Kucan, M. C. Robson, and J. P. Heggers, "Comparison of silver sulfadiazine, povidone-iodine and physiologic saline in the treatment of chronic pressure ulcers," *Journal of the American Geriatrics Society*, vol. 29, no. 5, pp. 232–235, 1981.

[17] W. O. Seiler, H. B. Stahelin, and W. Sonabend, "Einflus aerobe und anaerober keime auf den heilungsverlauf von dekubitalulzera," *Schweizerische Medizinische Wochenschrift*, vol. 109, pp. 1595–1599, 1979.

[18] D. C. Daltrey, B. Rhodes, and J. G. Chattwood, "Investigation into the microbial flora of healing and non-healing decubitus ulcers," *Journal of Clinical Pathology*, vol. 34, no. 7, pp. 701–705, 1981.

[19] T. J. Ryan, "Microcirculation in psoriasis: blood vessels, lymphatics and tissue fluid," *Pharmacology and Therapeutics*, vol. 10, no. 1, pp. 27–64, 1980.

[20] P. Banwell, S. Withey, and I. Holten, "The use of negative pressure to promote healing," *British Journal of Plastic Surgery*, vol. 51, no. 1, pp. 79–82, 1998.

[21] M. J. Morykwas, L. C. Argenta, E. I. Shelton-Brown, and W. McGuirt, "Vacuum-assisted closure: a new method for wound control and treatment: animal studies and basic foundation," *Annals of Plastic Surgery*, vol. 38, no. 6, pp. 553–562, 1997.

[22] T. Weed, C. Ratliff, D. B. Drake et al., "Quantifying bacterial bioburden during negative pressure wound therapy: does the wound VAC enhance bacterial clearance?" *Annals of Plastic Surgery*, vol. 52, no. 3, pp. 276–280, 2004.

[23] R. Thoma, "Ueber die histomechanik des gefasssystems und die pathogens der angioskeleroose," *Virchows Archiv für Pathologische Anatomie und Physiologie und für Klinische Medizin*, vol. 204, no. 1, pp. 1–74, 1911.

[24] T. E. Philbeck, K. T. Whittington, M. H. Millsap, R. B. Briones, D. G. Wight, and W. J. Schroeder, "The clinical and cost effectiveness of externally applied negative pressure wound therapy in the treatment of wounds in home healthcare Medicare patients," *Ostomy/Wound Management*, vol. 45, no. 11, pp. 41–50, 1999.

[25] G. A. Ilizarov, "The tension-stress effect on the genesis and growth of tissues. Part I. The influence of stability of fixation and soft-tissue preservation," *Clinical Orthopaedics and Related Research*, no. 238, pp. 249–281, 1989.

[26] G. D. Hall, C. W. Van Way, F. T. K. Fei' Tau Kung, and M. Compton-Allen, "Peripheral nerve elongation with tissue expansion techniques," *Journal of Trauma*, vol. 34, no. 3, pp. 401–405, 1993.

[27] O. M. Alvarez, P. M. Mertz, and W. H. Eaglstein, "The effect of occlusive dressings on collagen synthesis and re-epithelialization in superficial wounds," *Journal of Surgical Research*, vol. 35, no. 2, pp. 142–148, 1983.

[28] A. L. Akin Yoola, A. K. Ako-Nai, O. Dosumu, A. O. Aboderin, and O. O. Kassim, "Microbial isolates in early swabs of open musculoskeletal injuries," *The Nigerian Oostgraduate Medical Journal*, vol. 13, no. 3, pp. 176–181, 2006.

[29] W. Fleischmann, W. Strecker, M. Bombelli, and L. Kinzl, "Vacuum sealing for treatment of soft tissue injury in open fractures," *Unfallchirurg*, vol. 96, no. 9, pp. 488–492, 1993.

[30] S. M. Jones, P. E. Banwell, and P. G. Shakespeare, "Advances in wound healing: topical negative pressure therapy," *Postgraduate Medical Journal*, vol. 81, no. 956, pp. 353–357, 2005.

# 9

# Distal Femur Allograft Prosthetic Composite Reconstruction for Short Proximal Femur Segments following Tumor Resection

**Bryan S. Moon,[1] Nathan F. Gilbert,[2] Christopher P. Cannon,[3] Patrick P. Lin,[1] and Valerae O. Lewis[1]**

[1] *MD Anderson Cancer Center, Department of Orthopaedic Oncology, P.O. Box 301402, Houston, TX 77230-1402, USA*
[2] *Greater Dallas Orthopaedics, 12230 Coit Road, Suite 100, Dallas, TX 75251, USA*
[3] *Polyclinic Department of Orthopaedic Surgery, 1001 Broadway, Suite 109, Seattle, WA 98122, USA*

Correspondence should be addressed to Bryan S. Moon; bsmoon@mdanderson.org

Academic Editor: Allen L. Carl

Short metaphyseal segments remaining after distal femoral tumor resection pose a unique challenge. Limb sparing options include a short stemmed modular prosthesis, total endoprosthetic replacement, cross-pin fixation to a custom implant, and allograft prosthetic composite reconstruction (APC). A series of patients with APC reconstruction were evaluated to determine functional and radiologic outcome and complication rates. Twelve patients were retrospectively identified who had a distal femoral APC reconstruction between 1994 and 2007 to salvage an extremity with a segment of remaining bone that was less than 20 centimeters in length. Seventeen APC reconstructions were performed in twelve patients. Eight were primary procedures and nine were revision procedures. Average f/u was 89 months. Twelve APC reconstructions (71%) united and five (29%) were persistent nonunions. At most recent followup 10 patients (83%) had a healed APC which allowed WBAT. One pt (8%) had an amputation and one pt (8%) died prior to union. Average time to union was 19 months. Four pts (33%) or five APC reconstructions (29%) required further surgery to obtain a united reconstruction. Although Distal Femoral APC reconstruction has a high complication rate, a stable reconstruction was obtained in 83% of patients.

## 1. Introduction

Resection of large skeletal tumors can result in short metaphyseal juxtaarticular segments of host bone which can pose a reconstructive challenge to the musculoskeletal tumor surgeon. In addition, aseptic loosening or fracture around a standard reconstruction can lead to loss of bone stock so that only a short metaphyseal segment of host bone remains for fixation in revision surgery. Limb salvage reconstructive options in this scenario include the use of a standard endoprosthesis with fixation of the stem into the short segment of host bone, use of custom implants allowing for cross-pin fixation of the endoprosthesis to the host bone, use of an endoprosthesis to replace the entire bone, and use of a composite of an allograft and an endoprosthesis [1–3].

Use of a standard, modular endoprosthesis with cement or press fit fixation in this setting has not been directly investigated to our knowledge; however, the use of a short stem cemented into the metaphyseal segment would be expected to have a high rate of aseptic loosening due to the high stress imparted on the relatively short interface between host bone and cement [2] (Figure 1). Use of cross-pin fixation of a custom prosthesis to host bone has been described previously with a low rate of aseptic loosening [1] (Figure 2). This technique is limited by decreasing intraoperative flexibility and adding extra time and cost. Replacement of the entire bone with an endoprosthesis is also a described technique that has the advantage of early weight bearing, but it has the disadvantage of increased rehabilitation and higher rates of joint dislocations [3–5] (Figure 3). Allograft prosthetic

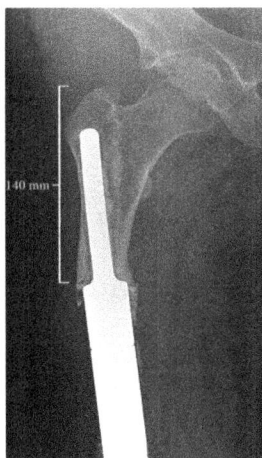

FIGURE 1: Short stemmed cemented endoprosthesis with aseptic loosening.

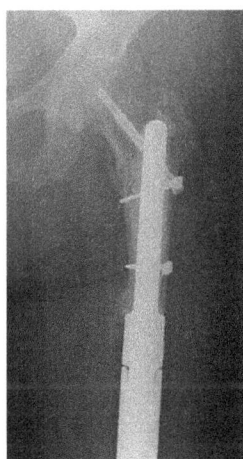

FIGURE 2: Customized cemented stem with screw fixation.

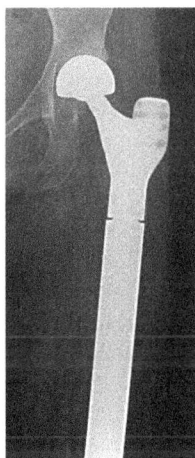

FIGURE 3: Total femur endoprosthesis.

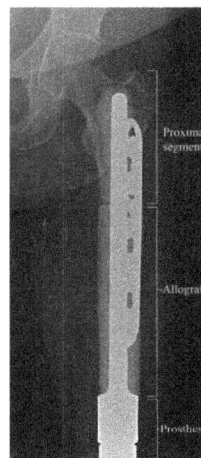

FIGURE 4: Distal femur APC.

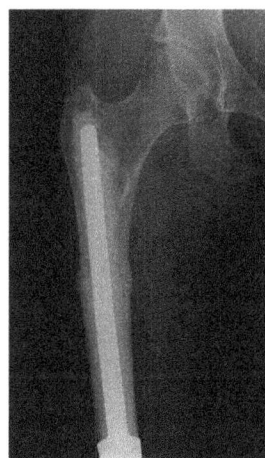

FIGURE 5: Healed distal femur APC.

composite (APC) reconstruction restores bone stock which allows the use of a longer stem, increases intraoperative flexibility, and provides the durability of an endoprosthesis (Figures 4 and 5). Figures 1–4 demonstrate the main types of reconstruction currently used for short juxtaarticular metaphyseal segments. To the best of our knowledge, no series has previously reported on APC reconstruction for short metaphyseal segments of host bone.

Our purposes were to determine (1) the functionality of these patients, union rates, rates of reoperation, and other complications that may occur with this type of reconstruction and (2) if this type of reconstruction is an acceptable alternative to other reconstructive options.

## 2. Methods

We retrospectively reviewed 12 patients who underwent allograft prosthetic composite reconstruction after resection of large skeletal tumors between 1994 and 2007. All patients had 20 cm or less of host bone remaining. Average age of the patients was 19 years (range, 7–56 years). Five males and seven females comprised the study group. Diagnosis was

TABLE 1

| Patient | Age | Diagnosis | Type | Expandable | Residual femur | Union | Followup | Complications |
|---|---|---|---|---|---|---|---|---|
| 1 | 12 | OGS | Primary | Yes | 14 cm | 29 mos | 31 months, death | Death |
| 2 | 15 | OGS | Primary | Yes | 20 cm | No | 133 months, lost | Nonunion |
| | | | Revision | Yes | 16 cm | 12 mos | | Broken stem |
| | | | Revision | Yes | 17 cm | ? mos | | Stem perforation |
| | | | Revision | No | 17 cm | 21 mos | | Bone graft |
| 3 | 25 | OGS | Revision | No | 17 cm | 29 mos | 177 months, lost | Bone graft/plating X2 |
| 4 | 8 | OGS | Primary | Yes | 10 cm | 26 mos | 78 months, lost | Bone graft, stem loosening ? infection |
| 5 | 8 | OGS | Primary | Yes | 7 cm | No | 118 months, current | Nonunion |
| | | | Revision | Yes | 7 cm | No | | Nonunion, infection, amp |
| 6 | 9 | OGS | Primary | Yes | 10 cm | No | 31 months, death | Nonunion, death |
| 7 | 9 | OGS | Revision | No | 17 cm | No | 168 months, current | Fracture, nonunion |
| | | | | No | 17 cm | 12 mos | | None |
| 8 | 7 | OGS | Primary | Yes | 11 cm | 22 mos | 83 months, current | Fungal infection |
| 9 | 31 | OGS | Revision | No | 13 cm | 21 mos | 81 months, current | None |
| 10 | 56 | CHSA | Primary | No | 10 cm | 28 mos | 55 months, current | Bone graft |
| 11 | 35 | GCT | Revision | No | 11 cm | 10 mos | 60 months, current | None |
| 12 | 8 | OGS | Primary | Yes | 10 cm | 4 mos | 52 months, current | Tibia fracture |

osteosarcoma in 10 patients, chondrosarcoma in 1 patient, and giant cell tumor in 1 patient. Location of the tumor was the distal femur in all 12 patients. Six patients received neoadjuvant and adjuvant chemotherapy, one received neoadjuvant chemotherapy, one received adjuvant chemotherapy, and four received no chemotherapy in the perioperative period. No patients received radiation therapy.

A total of seventeen allograft prosthetic reconstructions were performed in these twelve patients. Eight reconstructions were performed as primary limb salvage procedures and nine were performed as revision procedures.

At the time of surgery, all patients had an extensile surgical approach to expose the area of interest. Freeze-dried allografts were used in all cases. The allografts were thawed in antibiotic solution and then prepared on a back table by cutting the allograft to required length and reaming to appropriate diameter. Transverse osteotomies were utilized and were manipulated as needed to maximize allograft-host bone contact. Cement fixation was used in all cases to fix the stem in both the allograft and host bone. A Biomet (Warsaw, IN) custom expandable implant was used in 5 patients, a Biomet long-stem modular rotating hinge total knee replacement was used in 3 patients, a Biomet modular distal femur endoprosthesis was used in one patient, a Stryker (Mahwah, NJ) modular distal femur endoprosthesis was used in one patient, and a Wright Medical (Memphis, TN) noninvasive custom expandable endoprosthesis was used in two patients. Additional plate fixation was used in 7 patients. Supplemental autograft, allograft, or demineralized bone matrix was used at the host-allograft interface in all but one patient. Postoperative rehabilitation involved early range of motion and touchdown weight bearing until there was radiographic evidence of healing.

The radiographs and medical records of these patients were analyzed to determine functional, radiographic, and clinical outcome. The remaining host bone segments were measured from the tip of the greater trochanter to the osteotomy site. Radiographs were also analyzed to determine union, which was defined as osseous bridging of at least 3 of 4 cortices at the osteotomy site.

## 3. Results

Average duration of followup from the date of the original surgery was 89 months (range, 31–177 months). The average length of bone remaining after resection of the tumor was 13 cm (range, 7–20 cm). One patient died of disease prior to union, one died after union occurred, and one patient underwent an amputation. Three patients were lost to followup at 133, 177, and 78 months.

The twelve patients underwent seventeen APC reconstructions (Table 1). The five extra reconstructions in three patients were performed for three nonunions and two prosthesis failures. Primary union was achieved in eight reconstructions (47%), and secondary union was achieved in four reconstructions (24%) via secondary bone grafting. Five reconstructions (29%) were persistent nonunions. Therefore, bony union was achieved in 12 reconstructions (71%) or ten patients (83%) at an average of nineteen months (range, 4–29 months). Of these ten patients, five (50%) required further surgery to obtain union.

Graft related complications including nonunion requiring bone grafting, persistent nonunion requiring APC revision, allograft fracture, infection, and stem perforation occurred in eight patients (67%) (Table 1). Three patients (25%) underwent five complete APC revisions. Three were for persistent nonunions, one was for a broken stem, and one was for stem perforation through the allograft. The average time to revision of the reconstruction in these patients was

29 months (range, 11–48 months). There were two deep infections. One was a fungal infection that was successfully treated with debridement and antifungals. The second was a staph aureus infection that eventually ended in amputation. A third patient made telephone contact 60 months after surgery with concerns of an infection, but the patient did not return for evaluation and was lost to followup.

In terms of functional outcome, all ten patients with united reconstructions were weight bearing as tolerated at their most recent follow-up visit. Two of these patients use assistive devices for ambulation. Current MSTS scores were available for six of the ten patients. The average score was 90%. The average time from surgery to evaluation for scoring was 82 months (range, 52–90 months). The MSTS score for the patient that underwent amputation was 63%.

## 4. Discussion

At first glance, the above results may seem discouraging for the use of APC reconstruction in the setting of short metaphyseal bone segments. Certainly, the complication rate is significant, but it should be noted that the complications were manageable in the majority of patients. It should also be noted that once union was achieved, the reconstruction does appear durable in that there has only been one graft related complication following union. Also, the allograft provided sufficient bone stock for a standard revision in the one case of stem loosening. In the case of the broken stem, it was the surgeon's preference to replant an APC rather than attempting stem extraction from the allograft.

Other limb sparing options are available for this difficult type of reconstruction including cementation of a modular endoprosthesis into the short segment of host bone, resection of the entire bone and replacement with an endoprosthesis, and cross-pin fixation of a custom endoprosthesis to the host bone. All of these approaches have technical challenges, advantages, and disadvantages. Cementing a short stem of a standard modular endoprosthesis into a short metaphyseal segment would be expected to have a high rate of aseptic loosening and implant failure. This has been confirmed in clinical studies that report poor results in lower extremity endoprosthetic reconstruction when addressing bone defects left by larger resections [2, 6]. In addition, biomechanical studies using a canine model have shown that cement fixation of endoprostheses alone leads to a more compliant reconstruction when dealing with large femoral defects [7, 8].

Several techniques have been devised to overcome the limitations of standard modular endoprostheses in this setting, including total replacement endoprostheses, cross-pin fixation of custom endoprostheses, and use of allograft prosthetic composite reconstruction. Total bone endoprostheses are useful reconstructive devices, but their implementation necessitates the removal of two joints. This creates the possibility of complications and wear debris at two articulations [5]. Rehabilitation of two artificial joints is more rigorous and complicated than one, especially if one of the joints has a significant risk of dislocation. There have been techniques described to limit the risk of dislocation in total

femur endoprostheses, but hip joint preservation is favorable for lower extremity function [9]. One advantage of total endoprosthetic replacement is that weightbearing may be allowed right away. In addition, concern for healing the host allograft junction is obviated. Although the numbers of studies on total endoprosthetic replacement are limited, functional outcome has been promising [3, 5].

Cross-pin fixation of a custom prosthesis into the remaining short metaphyseal defect has also been described [1]. Twelve patients with short, metaphyseal segments were included in this study. Cement fixation of the stem into the remaining host bone was used in addition to screws. Only one of the stems used for short metaphyseal articular segments failed, and reconstructive success was achieved with a relatively low complication rate. One drawback to this technique is the fact that all implants must be custom made. Therefore, several weeks of manufacturing time is required and the use of a custom implant diminishes intraoperative flexibility. This may prevent their use in more urgent reconstructive scenarios such as displaced pathologic or periprosthetic fracture.

The use of APCs for reconstruction of short metaphyseal segments has not been examined previously. Allograft prosthetic composite reconstruction has been shown to be a viable reconstructive technique for a variety of reconstruction sites including the proximal femur and tibia [10–13]. The advantage of providing local bone stock is combined with intraoperative flexibility and the durability of an endoprosthesis. Allograft prosthetic composites can be used after primary tumor resection or in revision of a failed reconstruction. The main disadvantage is that weight bearing is usually limited until healing at the host-allograft junction occurs [14]. The use of allograft prosthetic composites used for revision of failed distal femur endoprostheses has been described and it was determined that this was a successful option for revising a failed distal femur endoprosthesis, but the length of remaining bone was not separately analyzed [15]. The results of total femur allograft prosthetic composites have also been previously reported [4]. A total femur allograft with a bipolar hemiarthroplasty and total knee arthroplasty was used. Logistically, this is the same as a total replacement endoprosthesis and different from the technique described in our series.

Limitations of this study include small sample size, retrospective design, and patient heterogeneity. Given that the need for distal femoral APC is an uncommon event, small sample size and retrospective design should not be considered a major weakness. Similarly, since neoplasms of the distal femur affect a wide patient demographic, patient heterogeneity is unavoidable. However, it is reasonable to assume that some aspects of heterogeneity such as the use of chemotherapy, expandable versus unexpandable implants, and primary versus revision reconstructions may have an influence on the rate of union. For example, it is notable that four of the five nonunions occurred in patients with expandable prostheses. Although this may represent an interesting trend, our numbers are too small for any meaningful statistical analysis. Finally, three patients were lost to current followup and MSTS scoring. Given that one of these patients underwent four APC reconstructions and one did not follow up after making contact regarding concerns of infection, it is likely that the MSTS scores are skewed in a positive direction. However, these three patients did have an average followup of 129 months and were all ambulating at their final visits.

Distal femur APC reconstruction can be useful in reconstruction of short metaphyseal segments both after primary tumor resection and for salvage of a failed prior reconstruction. The complication rate was high even in patients who went on to have a durable reconstruction; therefore, patients should be counseled to provide reasonable expectations. As the primary union rate was low, early bone grafting should be considered. It is our current practice to consider bone grafting no earlier than 6 months postoperatively. Autograft, allograft chips, and/or demineralized bone matrix may be used and is determined by patient and surgeon preference. Once union is achieved, the patients can be expected to have an acceptable level of function and a durable reconstruction. Further studies are required to determine optimal reconstructive techniques for this challenging scenario.

## Ethical Approval

This study has received IRB approval.

## Disclosure

Level of Evidence is Level IV, therapeutic study. See guidelines for authors for a complete description of levels of evidence.

## Conflict of Interests

The authors have no conflict of interests to disclose and have full control of all primary data.

## Acknowledgment

The authors work performed at MD Anderson Cancer Center.

## References

[1] C. P. Cannon, J. J. Eckardt, J. M. Kabo et al., "Custom cross-pin fixation of 32 tumor endoprostheses stems," *Clinical Orthopaedics and Related Research*, no. 417, pp. 285–292, 2003.

[2] J. J. Eckardt, F. R. Eilber, G. Rosen et al., "Endoprosthetic replacement for stage IIB osteosarcoma," *Clinical Orthopaedics and Related Research*, no. 270, pp. 202–213, 1991.

[3] H. G. Morris, R. Capanna, D. Campanacci, M. del Ben, and A. Gasbarrini, "Modular endoprosthetic replacement after total resection of the femur for malignant tumour," *International Orthopaedics*, vol. 18, no. 2, pp. 90–95, 1994.

[4] H. J. Mankin, F. J. Hornicek, and M. Harris, "Total femur replacement procedures in tumor treatment," *Clinical Orthopaedics and Related Research*, no. 438, pp. 60–64, 2005.

[5] W. G. Ward, F. Dorey, and J. J. Eckardt, "Total femoral endoprosthetic reconstruction," *Clinical Orthopaedics and Related Research*, no. 316, pp. 195–206, 1995.

[6] P. S. Unwin, S. R. Cannon, R. J. Grimer, H. B. Kemp, R. S. Sneath, and P. S. Walker, "Aseptic loosening in cemented custom-made prosthetic replacements for bone tumours of the lower limb," *Journal of Bone and Joint Surgery B*, vol. 78, no. 1, pp. 5–13, 1996.

[7] S. S. Kohles, M. D. Markel, M. G. Rock, E. Y. Chao, and R. Vanderby Jr., "Mechanical evaluation of six types of reconstruction following 25, 50, and 75% resection of the proximal femur," *Journal of Orthopaedic Research*, vol. 12, no. 6, pp. 834–843, 1994.

[8] M. D. Markel, F. Gottsauner-Wolf, M. G. Rock, F. J. Frassica, and E. Y. S. Chao, "Mechanical characteristics of proximal femoral reconstruction after 50% resection," *Journal of Orthopaedic Research*, vol. 11, no. 3, pp. 339–349, 1993.

[9] J. Bickels, I. Meller, R. M. Henshaw, and M. M. Malawer, "Reconstruction of hip stability after proximal and total femur resections," *Clinical Orthopaedics and Related Research*, no. 375, pp. 218–230, 2000.

[10] Y. Farid, P. P. Lin, V. O. Lewis, and A. W. Yasko, "Endoprosthetic and allograft-prosthetic composite reconstruction of the proximal femur for bone neoplasms," *Clinical Orthopaedics and Related Research*, no. 442, pp. 223–229, 2006.

[11] D. J. Biau, V. Dumaine, A. Babinet, B. Tomeno, and P. Anract, "Allograft-prosthesis composites after bone tumor resection at the proximal tibia," *Clinical Orthopaedics and Related Research*, no. 456, pp. 211–217, 2007.

[12] S. Gitelis and P. Piasecki, "Allograft prosthetic composite arthroplasty for osteosarcoma and other aggressive bone tumors," *Clinical Orthopaedics and Related Research*, no. 270, pp. 197–201, 1991.

[13] M. J. Hejna and S. Gitelis, "Allograft prosthetic composite replacement for bone tumors," *Seminars in Surgical Oncology*, vol. 13, pp. 18–24, 1997.

[14] A. I. Harris, S. Gitelis, M. G. Sheinkop, A. G. Rosenberg, and P. Piasecki, "Allograft prosthetic composite reconstruction for limb salvage and severe deficiency of bone at the knee or hip," *Seminars in Arthroplasty*, vol. 5, no. 2, pp. 85–94, 1994.

[15] R. M. Wilkins and C. M. Kelly, "Revision of the failed distal femoral replacement to allograft prosthetic composite," *Clinical Orthopaedics and Related Research*, no. 397, pp. 114–118, 2002.

# 10

# Adult's Degenerative Scoliosis: Midterm Results of Dynamic Stabilization without Fusion in Elderly Patients—Is It Effective?

**Mario Di Silvestre, Francesco Lolli, Tiziana Greggi,**
**Francesco Vommaro, and Andrea Baioni**

*Spine Surgery Department, Istituti Ortopedici Rizzoli, Via Pupilli 1, 40136 Bologna, Italy*

Correspondence should be addressed to Mario Di Silvestre; mario.disilvestre@ior.it

Academic Editor: Vijay K. Goel

*Study Design.* A retrospective study. *Purpose.* Posterolateral fusion with pedicle screw instrumentation used for degenerative lumbar scoliosis can lead to several complications. In elderly patients without sagittal imbalance, dynamic stabilization could represent an option to avoid these adverse events. *Methods.* 57 patients treated by dynamic stabilization without fusion were included. All patients had degenerative lumbar *de novo* scoliosis (average Cobb angle 17.2°), without sagittal imbalance, associated in 52 cases (91%) with vertebral canal stenosis and in 24 (42%) with degenerative spondylolisthesis. Nineteen patients (33%) had previously undergone lumbar spinal surgery. *Results.* At an average followup of 77 months, clinical results improved with statistical significance. Scoliosis Cobb angle was 17.2° (range, 12° to 38°) before surgery and 11.3° (range, 4° to 26°) at last follow-up. In the patients with associated spondylolisthesis, anterior vertebral translation was 19.5% (range, 12% to 27%) before surgery, 16.7% (range, 0% to 25%) after surgery, and 17.5% (range, 0% to 27%) at followup. Complications incidence was low (14%), and few patients required revision surgery (4%). *Conclusions.* In elderly patients with mild degenerative lumbar scoliosis without sagittal imbalance, pedicle screw-based dynamic stabilization is an effective option, with low complications incidence, granting curve stabilization during time and satisfying clinical results.

## 1. Introduction

Degenerative lumbar scoliosis, also described as *de novo* or "primary degenerative scoliosis" [1] is a frequent disease. Its incidence is reported to be from 6% to 68% [2–5] and increases with age [6]. These curves are located at thoracolumbar or lumbar level and need to be distinguished from degenerated preexisting idiopathic scoliosis; in fact, *de novo* scoliosis is developing after skeletal maturity without previous history of scoliosis. A recent prospective study [3] investigated 60 adults aged 50–84 years, without previous scoliosis. within 12 years, 22 cases (36.7%) developed *de novo* scoliosis with a mean angle of 13°. A previous study reported a similar incidence: Robin et al. [7] followed 160 adults with a straight spine for more than 7 years and found 55 cases of *de novo* scoliosis (34.4%). Decreased bone density was initially considered to be the cause of *de novo* lumbar scoliosis [2]. At present, asymmetric degenerative changes

of the disc, vertebral body wedging, and facet joint arthritis are held to be the predominant causes [1, 3, 7–9], disc degeneration appearing to be the starting point [3, 8]. Lumbar *de novo* scoliosis is frequently associated with degenerative spondylolisthesis and stenosis [6, 10, 11].

The surgical treatment of these deformities included more often a posterolateral fusion with pedicle screw instrumentation in addition to decompression of neural elements [1, 12–15]. In most series, the incidence of complications is high [1, 13–15]. The impact of different factors on the complications rate remains unclear and there are conflicting results in the literature [13–21]. However, older age (over 65 years), medical comorbidities, increased blood loss, and number of levels fused seem to play an important role. Among these, excessive intraoperative blood loss seems to be the most significant risk factor for early perioperative complications [14]. Accordingly, in elderly patients, the surgery should be the least aggressive possible, and the length of the surgical procedure should be considered very carefully [20]. A surgical treatment based on decompression alone presented poor results, related to progression of symptoms and deformity [22]. At the same time, adding an arthrodesis to the decompression procedure increases the operative time and blood loss and consequently can increase the complications rate [13, 16, 21].

The use of dynamic stabilization without fusion can represent an option for treatment of mild degenerative lumbar scoliosis without sagittal imbalance. In a previous study [23], we analyzed the outcomes of dynamic stabilization for these deformities, using Dynesys implants (Zimmer Spine, Minneapolis, MN) as an alternative to fusion in elderly patients. The purpose of the present paper is to assess the midterm results of a larger series of patients over 65 years, in order to determine complications and to evaluate clinical outcomes.

## 2. Materials and Methods

A retrospective data base review was performed to identify all patients affected by degenerative lumbar "*de novo*" scoliosis (Aebi's classification type I [1]), who had been surgically treated by dynamic fixation (Dynesys system) without fusion at our department between January 2002 and December 2006.

Inclusion criteria were (1) minimum age at surgery of 65 years; (2) Cobb angle more than 10° before surgery; (3) no improvement after conservative treatment; (4) minimum-5-year followup.

Exclusion criteria were (1) fixed sagittal imbalance; (2) scoliosis Cobb angle more than 40° before surgery; (3) previous lumbar fusion or stabilization surgery.

An independent spine surgeon reviewed all the selected patients' medical records and X-rays. Inpatient and outpatient charts were used for collecting demographic data, preoperative data (location of pain, neurologic symptoms, and previous surgeries), perioperative data (blood loss, surgical duration, hospital stay, and any medical and surgical-related complication), and postoperative data, including revision surgeries.

*2.1. Questionnaires.* Clinical outcome was assessed by means of the Oswestry Disability Index (ODI), Roland Morris Disability Questionnaire (RMDQ), and separate visual analog scales (VAS) for back and leg pain, completed by patients preoperatively, in the early postoperative period and at last followup. Radiographic evaluation included preoperative CT and MRI of the lumbar spine, as well as pre-operative, postoperative and followup standing plain radiographs. Overall measures from the radiographs included Cobb angle of the lumbar curve, lumbar lordosis (T12-S1) and thoracolumbar junction alignment (T10-L2), apical vertebral lateral displacement, and anterior vertebral translation measurements for spondylolisthesis. Instrumentation loosening or breakage and degenerative alterations of adjacent levels were also investigated.

*2.2. Statistical Evaluation.* The clinical and radiologic results were analyzed using *t*-test. Results are expressed as the mean

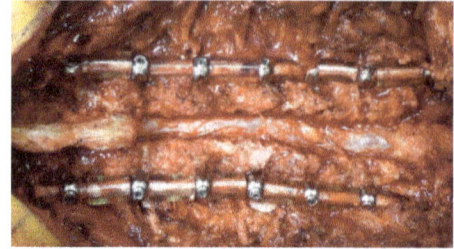

FIGURE 1: Multisegmental dynamic stabilization with decompressive laminectomy.

(range), with a *P* value < 0.05 considered as being statistically significant.

*2.3. Surgical Treatment.* All surgeries were performed by four experienced spine surgeons of our department. Preventive antibiotics were routinely started 12 hours before surgery and continued for an average of 9 days (range, 8 to 11 days). The patients were treated under general anesthesia in the prone position.

Initially, in cases with associated stenosis of the vertebral canal, patients' hips were flexed at an angle of 90° to facilitate decompression of the stenotic levels. Stenosis was treated by laminectomy: the decompression was extended to the lateral recess, and foraminotomy was performed without interrupting the isthmus.

After decompression, the patients' position was modified to obtain the maximum lumbar lordosis, and stabilization was performed.

Dynesys implants were used for dynamic fixation. Dynesys implants consist of titanium alloy pedicle screws (Protasul 100), polyethylene-terephthalate cords (Sulene-PET), and polycarbonate urethane spacers (Sulene-PCU), which fit between the pedicle screw heads (Figure 1). The pedicle screws used in lumbar, thoracolumbar vertebrae, and in the sacrum were 7.2 mm diameter screws. The pedicle entry point was lateral, at the basis of the transverse process. The screws were inserted as deep as possible. So as not to compromise the bone purchase of the screws, given their conical core, we avoided removing and reinserting them in the same hole. Each of the polycarbonate urethane spacers was cut to the desired length and threaded with a polyester cord, which was stretched between and fixed to two adjacent screw heads. Larger spacers were used on the concave side and shorter on the convex side of the scoliosis curve.

Redon drains were applied and maintained for a mean of 3.7 days (range: 3 to 4 days).

## 3. Results

*3.1. Preoperative Data.* One hundred twenty-five consecutive patients were assessed for eligibility: 68 were excluded. Reasons were incomplete radiographic documentation (*n* = 4), previous spinal fusion or instrumentation (*n* = 16), scoliosis Cobb angle >40° (*n* = 20), fixed sagittal imbalance (*n* = 25), and age <60 years (*n* = 3).

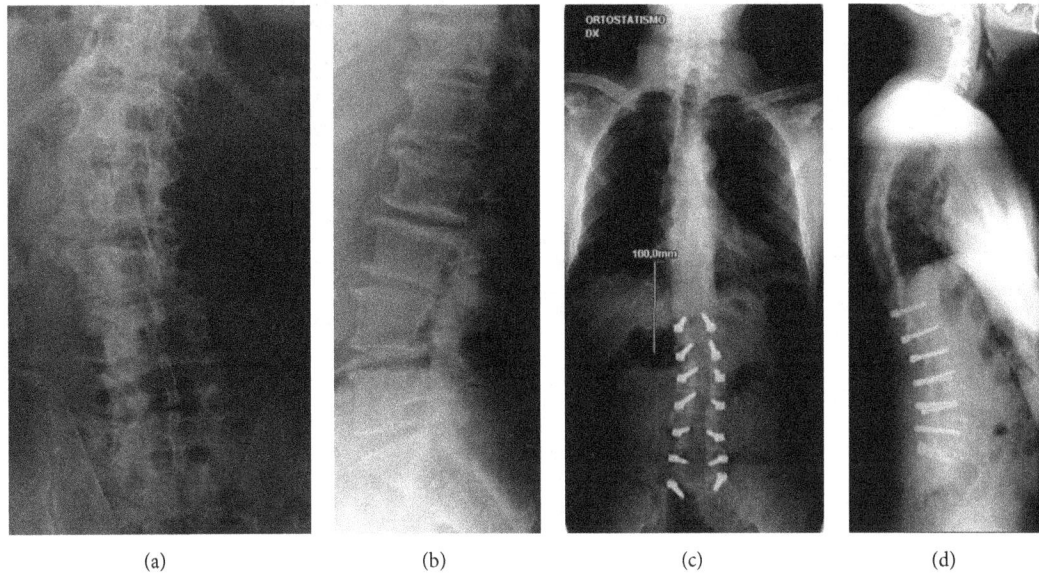

FIGURE 2: A 73-year-old woman. Degenerative lumbar scoliosis with good sagittal balance ((a)-(b)), associated with stenosis of the vertebral canal. Treatment: T12-S1 dynamic stabilization and decompressive laminectomy. Five-year postoperative radiographs showing stable scoliosis correction with maintained sagittal balance ((c)-(d)).

A total of 57 patients were included in the study and reviewed at a mean followup time of 77 months (range: 61 to 91 months) (Table 1). There were 12 men (22%) and 45 women (78%), with a mean age of 68.4 years (range: 66 to 78). At the time of surgery, all 57 patients reported leg pain; 47 (82%) also had neurogenic claudication, and 42 (73%) had back pain. All patients had failed to respond to conservative treatment conducted for at least 12 months.

Average BMI was 26.4 (range: 21 to 36). There were 1.8 ± 0.7 comorbidities per patient, including diabetes mellitus in 25 patients, heart disease in 12, arterial hypertension in 38, liver disease in 13, and pulmonary disease in 16 cases. All patients had degenerative lumbar *de novo* scoliosis (with an average Cobb angle of 17.2°), associated in 52 cases (91%) with vertebral canal stenosis. Twenty-four patients (42%) also presented with degenerative spondylolisthesis, at L2-L3 level in 2 cases, at L3-L4 in 12 cases, at L4-L5 in 7 cases, and at L5-S1 in 3 cases (3 patients had spondylolisthesis at two levels): the mean slippage was 18.9% (range: 12% to 27%). Nineteen patients (33%) had previously undergone lumbar spinal surgery, including decompressions and/or discectomies (seven patients had had 2 previous operation, five had had 2 operations, and 2 patients had had three).

*3.2. Perioperative Data.* All patients had dynamic stabilization without fusion (Figures 2 and 3). Three levels were stabilized in 31 patients (54%: L1-L4 in 6, L2-L5 in 16, and L3-S1 in 9), four levels in 11 patients (19%: L1-L5 in 7, L2-S1 in 4), five levels in 5 cases (8%: T12-L5 in 3, L1-S1 in 2), six levels in 8 patients (15%: T12-S1), and seven levels in 2 patients (4%: T11-S1).

In 52 patients (91%), the stabilization was combined with decompressive laminectomy of 2 levels in 7 cases (14%: L2-L3 in 3, L3-L4 in and 2, L4-L5 in 2), of 3 levels in 14 cases (27%:

TABLE 1: Demographic data.

| Parameters | Value |
| --- | --- |
| Age (yrs) | 68.4 |
| Female gender (%) | 78% |
| Comorbidities | 1.8 ± 0.7 |
| Deg. spondylolisthesis | 42% |
| Stenosis | 91% |
| Prev. spinal surgery | 33% |
| Leg pain | 100% |
| Back pain | 73% |
| Claudicatio | 82% |

L2-L4 in 7, L3-L5 in 7), of 4 levels in 13 cases (25%: L2-L5 in 6, L3-S1 in 7 cases), of 5 levels in 10 cases (19%: L1-L5 in 6, L2-S1 in 4), and of 6 levels in 8 cases (15%: T12-L5 in 6, L1-S1 in 2). If present, the associated spondylolisthesis was always included in the stabilization construct.

Mean operating time was 170 minutes (range: 120 to 210 minutes), mean hospital stay was 6.8 days (range: 6 to 9 days) and mean blood loss was 650 cc (range: 200 to 700 cc). Patients were returned to the upright position at 2.6 days postoperatively (range, 2 to 4 days), with a lumbar orthosis, which was prescribed for 1 month.

*3.3. Clinical Outcome (See Table 2).* The mean preoperative ODI score was 51.6% (range, 28 to 80), mean postoperative score was 27.2 (range, 0 to 66), and the final followup score was 27.7 (range, 0 to 70) ($P < 0.05$), with a mean final improvement of 51.6% (range, 12% to 100%) ($P < 0.05$).

The mean preoperative RMDQ score was 12.4 of 24 (range, 7 to 22), mean postoperative score was 6.0

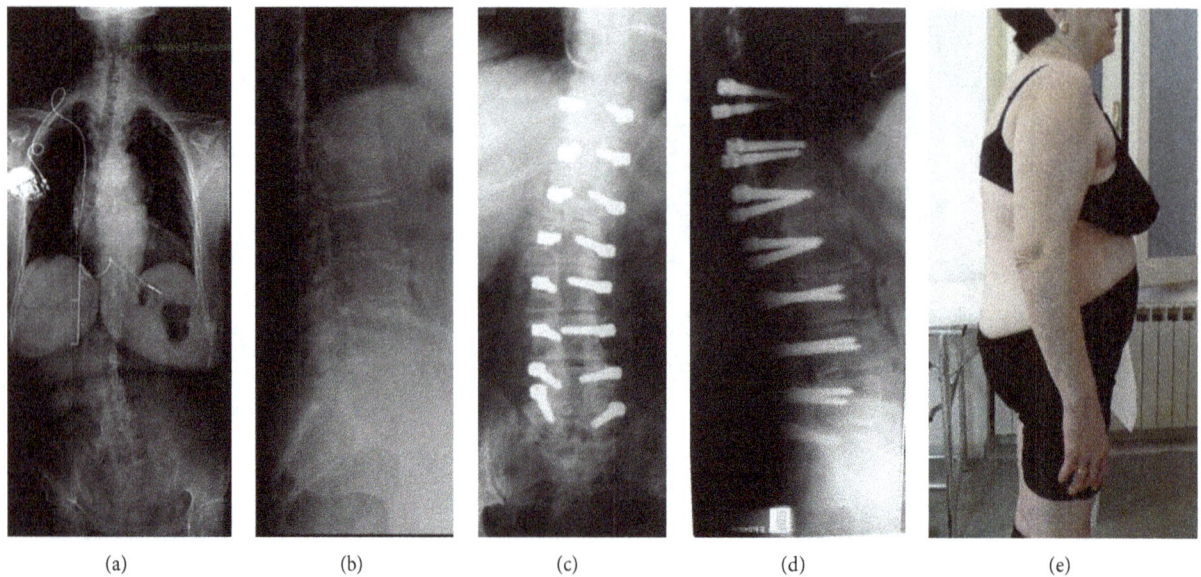

FIGURE 3: A 71-year-old woman. Degenerative lumbar scoliosis associated with stenosis of the vertebral canal: good sagittal balance ((a), (b)). Treatment: T11-S1 dynamic fixation and decompressive laminectomy. Six-year and 9 months postoperative radiographs showing stable scoliosis correction with maintained sagittal balance ((c), (d), and (e)).

TABLE 2: Clinical outcome.

| | Preop | FU | % corr. | $P$ value |
|---|---|---|---|---|
| ODI | 51.6 (28 to 80) | 27.7 (0 to 70) | 51.6 (12 to 100) | <0.05 |
| RMDQ | 12.4 (7 to 22) | 6.3 (0 to 20) | 58.8 (9.1 to 100) | <0.05 |
| VAS "leg score" | 67.5 (30 to 100) | 41.6 (2 to 90) | 51.1 (10 to 96.4) | <0.05 |
| VAS "back score" | 66.7 (30 to 100) | 33.8 (2 to 79) | 57.4 (20 to 97) | <0.05 |

Mean value (range: minimum to maximum).

(range: 0 to 19), and final followup score was 6.3 (range, 0 to 20) ($P < 0.05$), with a mean final improvement of 58.8% (range: 9.1% to 100%) ($P < 0.05$).

The mean leg pain VAS decreased from a preoperative score of 67.5 (range: 30 to 100) to a mean postoperative score of 40.1 (range: 2 to 90) and to a score of 41.6 (range: 2 to 90) at the last followup ($P < 0.05$), with a mean final improvement of 51.1% (range, 10% to 96.4%) ($P < 0.05$). The mean back pain VAS decreased from a preoperative score of 66.7 (range: 30 to 100) to a postoperative score of 33.1 (range: 2 to 75) and to a score of 33.8 (range: 2 to 79) at last followup ($P < 0.05$), with a mean final improvement of 57.4% (range: 20% to 97.0%) ($P < 0.05$).

3.4. Radiologic Outcome (See Table 3). The average scoliosis Cobb angle was 17.2° (range: 12° to 38°) before surgery, 11.0° (range, 4° to 26°) after surgery and remained stable, and 11.3° (range: 4° to 26°), at last followup ($P < 0.05$). Lumbar lordosis was −30.6° (range: 3° to −39°) before surgery, −36.8° (range: −12° to −57°) after surgery, and −35.8° (range: −10° to −55°) at last followup ($P < 0.05$), with a mean final improvement of 6.4% (range: 0% to 17%) ($P < 0.05$).

Thoracolumbar junction alignment (TLJA) (T10-L2) was −2.8° before surgery (range: −25° to 23°), −0.2° (range: −18° to 25°) after surgery, and −0.4° (range: −18° to 25°) at last followup.

Apical vertebra lateral listhesis (AVLL) was 1.2 cm (range: 0.2 to 2.0 cm) before surgery, 0.8 cm (range: 0.2 to 1.1 cm) after surgery, and 0.8 cm (range: 0.3 to 1.2 cm) at last followup ($P < 0.05$), with a mean final correction of 30.7% (range: 0% to 44.4%) ($P < 0.05$).

In the patients with associated spondylolisthesis, anterior vertebral translation was 19.5% (range: 12% to 27%) before surgery, 16.7% (range: 0% to 25%) after surgery, and 17.5% (range: 0% to 27%) at followup ($P < 0.05$), for a 14.9% mean correction (range: 0 to 100%) ($P < 0.05$).

3.5. Complications (See Table 4). No neurological complications were observed in any patient: 8 overall complications (14%) occurred.

Six patients (10%) had minor complications. These included two cases of ileus (4%) and two urinary tract infection (4%), which resolved after medical treatment. Another patient (2%) had transient postoperative delirium, which spontaneously resolved after 3 days. One patient (2%) developed dyspnea after surgery, requiring 5 days of recovery in the Intensive Care Unit for complete resolution.

Two patients (4%) had major complications that required revision surgery. One patient (2%) developed severe postoperative sciatica, resistant to medication without neurological deficit, due to a misplaced screw on L5; revision surgery for replacement of the screw was performed 5 days after

TABLE 3: Radiologic outcome*.

| | Preop | FU | % corr | P value |
|---|---|---|---|---|
| Scoliosis (°) | 17.2° (12 to 38) | 11.3° (4 to 26) | 37.3% (13.3 to 61.5) | <0.05 |
| Lordosis | −30.6° (3 to −39) | −35.8° (−10 to −55) | 6.4% (0 to 17) | <0.05 |
| TLJA | −2.8° (−25 to 23) | −0.4° (−18 to 25) | n.a. | n.a. |
| AVLL (cm) | 1.2 (0.2 to 2) | 0.8 (0.3 to 1.2) | 30.7 (0 to 44.4) | <0.05 |
| AVT (%) | 19.5% (12 to 27) | 17.5% (0 to 27) | 14.9% (0 to 100) | <0.05 |

Mean value (range, minimum to maximum).
TLJA: thoracolumbar junction alignment (T10-L2).
AVLL: apical vertebra lateral listhesis.
AVT: anterior vertebral translation.
n.a.: not available.

TABLE 4: Complications.

| Complications | Percentage |
|---|---|
| Overall | 8 (14%) |
| Minor | 6 (10%) |
| Ileus | 2 (4%) |
| Urinary tract infection | 2 (4%) |
| Transient delirium | 1 (2%) |
| Dyspnea | 1 (2%) |
| Major | 2 (4%) |
| Misplaced screw | 1 (2%) |
| Lower junctional disc degeneration | 1 (2%) |

the first operation, with complete resolution of the sciatica. Another patient (2%) developed persistent leg pain, resistant to medication without neurological deficit, 28 months after surgery, due to disc degeneration at the lower junctional level; revision surgery was performed 32 months after the first operation, with decompression and extension of fixation from L5 to S1.

No screw loosening or breakage was observed at followup. However, asymptomatic radiolucent lines up to 2 mm around the thread of pedicle screws in the sacrum without screw loosening were found in 5 patients (9%) at last followup.

## 4. Discussion

The surgical treatment of degenerative lumbar scoliosis in elderly patients presents demanding aspects. The main goals of surgery are pain relief and improvement in quality of life. Some correction of the deformity is desirable, but this is not the most important issue and it is essential to limit the aggressiveness of the surgical procedure as much as possible [10]. Posterolateral fusion with pedicle screw instrumentation in addition to laminectomy [10, 13–15] is the most commonly used procedure. Unfortunately, a high incidence of complications has been reported in older patients [14, 15, 18–20]. Notably, age has been correlated with an increased incidence of complications, with a 20% rate of major complications over 80 years of age [18]. Furthermore, excessive blood loss and the number of levels fused have been found to be associated with higher complication rates [14].

Less invasive than posterior fusion, pedicle screw-based dynamic stabilization without arthrodesis might be a useful alternative in elderly patients with mild degenerative lumbar scoliosis without sagittal imbalance. Previously, our series of degenerative scoliosis patients often associated with lumbar stenosis has shown that it can prevent progression of scoliosis and postoperative instability, even after laminectomy [23]. In that report, operative duration time was short, blood loss was reduced, and there was no screw loosening or breakage at followup. The present study confirms at midterm followup these results with limited blood loss and short operative time. Moreover, dynamic fixation provided substantial stability by preserving against further scoliosis progression or translation of associated spondylolisthesis, despite use of decompressive laminectomy. By applying asymmetric spacers, larger on the concave side and shorter on the convex side of scoliosis, it was possible to obtain a mild reduction of the scoliosis Cobb angle, albeit less than with fusion constructs, reported in the literature [13–15]. There was no case of screw loosening or breakage during followup. In five of the patients (9%), asymptomatic radiolucent lines up to 2 mm did appear around the thread of pedicle screws in S1 at last X-rays control; however, it was not observed a screw mobilization or a loss of scoliosis correction and the patients were asymptomatic, so we did not classify these cases as "unstable". The overall complication rate was low (14%) with an even markedly lower incidence of major complications (14%).

A frequent complication observed in elderly patients after posterior fusion is adjacent segment disease, which generally occurs proximal to posterior instrumentation and has been reported primarily after short lumbar fusion [15]. Proximal adjacent disease appears to develop more frequently when stopping fusion from T11 to L1 compared with extending it to T10 [14, 24]. In older patients, the advantage for a "short" posterior fusion is obvious, even if the instrumentation should not stop at a junctional zone or adjacent to a rotatory subluxation, spondylolisthesis, or a segment with significant spinal stenosis, because this may lead to spinal instability. In a recent study, Cho et al. [15] compared the results of short posterior fusion, within the deformity, versus long fusion, extended above the upper end vertebra, for degenerative lumbar scoliosis in patients whose mean age was 65.5 years. In this series, there was a trade-off in complications between short fusion and long fusion; whereas all cases of proximal adjacent segment disease developed in the short fusion group, long fusion induced excessive intraoperative blood loss, which was closely related to the development of perioperative complications.

In our series, elderly patients received a short instrumentation, extended up to T11 at most. Only one patient (2%) required subsequent surgery for adjacent segment deasese and a distal junctional disc degeneration 32 months after surgery. At present, there is no consensus on whether or not dynamic instrumentation protects adjacent levels more than fusion. A study concluded that dynamic stabilization can prevent degeneration of the adjacent segment [25]. However, the results of the study of Schnake et al. [26] after Dynesys instrumentation in cases with degenerative spondylolisthesis did not support this theory. The authors found signs of adjacent degeneration in 29% of the patients after 2 years. Although longer followup studies are necessary for definitive conclusions, the theoretical protective effect of dynamic stabilization against adjacent segment degeneration is consistent with our findings, with a 5-year minimum followup.

In different series [13–15], posterior fusion obtained a significative scoliosis correction. In our series there was a scoliosis stabilization at a followup of more than 5 years. However, in *de novo* scoliosis patients the goal of treatment is less for the amount of correction of the curve than its stability over time. The same could be said for final lumbar lordosis; dynamic fixation maintained a stable and satisfying lumbar lordosis at followup. The patient's position on the operating table was always assessed to maintain or to increase the lumbar lordosis. All cases included in this study presented preoperatively a satisfying sagittal balance. In cases of sagittal imbalance, it is very difficult to achieve normal lumbar lordosis by dynamic stabilization or posterior fusion alone. Different surgical techniques such as corrective osteotomy should be considered preoperatively in these patients.

Finally, it's important to underline that, at followup (Table 2) dynamic fixation achieved clinically significant improvement in ODI, RMDQ, and VAS scores.

## 5. Conclusions

The present series must be interpreted in the context of its limitations (the retrospective nature of the review and the fact that patients were not randomized). However, this series of patients is consecutive and they received surgical treatment in the same institution.

In elderly patients with mild degenerative lumbar scoliosis without sagittal imbalance, pedicle screw-based dynamic stabilization permitted to maintain a satisfying balanced spine at follow-up: this procedure resulted less invasive with short operative duration and limited blood loss and low adverse event rates.

Dynamic fixation achieved scoliosis curve stabilization, at an average followup of more than 5 years. Furthermore, functional outcomes resulted were satisfying at last control.

## Acknowledgment

The work should be attributed to the Spine Surgery Department, Istituto Ortopedico Rizzoli, Bologna, Italy.

## References

[1] M. Aebi, "The adult scoliosis," *European Spine Journal*, vol. 14, no. 10, pp. 925–948, 2005.

[2] D. W. Vanderpool, J. I. James, and R. Wynne-Davies, "Scoliosis in the elderly," *Journal of Bone and Joint Surgery. American*, vol. 51, no. 3, pp. 446–455, 1969.

[3] T. Kobayashi, Y. Atsuta, M. Takemitsu, T. Matsuno, and N. Takeda, "A prospective study of de novo scoliosis in a community based cohort," *Spine*, vol. 31, no. 2, pp. 178–182, 2006.

[4] F. Schwab, A. Dubey, L. Gamez et al., "Adult scoliosis: prevalence, SF-36, and nutritional parameters in an elderly volunteer population," *Spine*, vol. 30, no. 9, pp. 1082–1085, 2005.

[5] S. L. Weinstein and I. V. Ponseti, "Curve progression in idiopathic scoliosis," *Journal of Bone and Joint Surgery. American*, vol. 65, no. 4, pp. 447–455, 1983.

[6] J. W. Pritchett and D. T. Bortel, "Degenerative symptomatic lumbar scoliosis," *Spine*, vol. 18, no. 6, pp. 700–703, 1993.

[7] G. C. Robin, E. Y. Span, and R. Steinberg, "Scoliosis in the elderly. A follow-up study," *Spine*, vol. 7, no. 4, pp. 355–359, 1982.

[8] Y. Murata, K. Takahashi, E. Hanaoka, T. Utsumi, M. Yamagata, and H. Moriya, "Changes in scoliotic curvature and lordotic angle during the early phase of degenerative lumbar scoliosis," *Spine*, vol. 27, no. 20, pp. 2268–2273, 2002.

[9] M. Benoist, "Natural history of the aging spine," *European Spine Journal*, vol. 12, no. 2, pp. S86–S89, 2003.

[10] A. Ploumis, E. E. Transfledt, and F. Denis, "Degenerative lumbar scoliosis associated with spinal stenosis," *Spine Journal*, vol. 7, no. 4, pp. 428–436, 2007.

[11] H. Liu, H. Ishihara, M. Kanamori, Y. Kawaguchi, K. Ohmori, and T. Kimura, "Characteristics of nerve root compression caused by degenerative lumbar spinal stenosis with scoliosis," *Spine Journal*, vol. 3, no. 6, pp. 524–529, 2003.

[12] E. D. Simmons, "Surgical treatment of patients with lumbar spinal stenosis with associated scoliosis," *Clinical Orthopaedics and Related Research*, no. 384, pp. 45–53, 2001.

[13] L. Y. Carreon, R. M. Puno, J. R. Dimar, S. D. Glassman, and J. R. Johnson, "Perioperative complications of posterior lumbar decompression and arthrodesis in older adults," *Journal of Bone and Joint Surgery. American*, vol. 85, no. 11, pp. 2089–2092, 2003.

[14] K. J. Cho, S. I. Suk, S. R. Park et al., "Complications in posterior fusion and instrumentation for degenerative lumbar scoliosis," *Spine*, vol. 32, no. 20, pp. 2232–2237, 2007.

[15] K. J. Cho, S. I. Suk, S. R. Park et al., "Short fusion versus long fusion for degenerative lumbar scoliosis," *European Spine Journal*, vol. 17, no. 5, pp. 650–656, 2008.

[16] R. A. Deyo, M. A. Ciol, D. C. Cherkin, J. D. Loeser, and S. J. Bigos, "Lumbar spinal fusion: a cohort study of complications, reoperations, and resource use in the Medicare population," *Spine*, vol. 18, no. 11, pp. 1463–1470, 1993.

[17] G. S. Shapiro, G. Taira, and O. Boachie-Adjei, "Results of surgical treatment of adult idiopathic scoliosis with low back pain and spinal stenosis: a study of long-term clinical radiographic outcomes," *Spine*, vol. 28, no. 4, pp. 358–363, 2003.

[18] C. S. Raffo and W. C. Lauerman, "Predicting morbidity and mortality of lumbar spine arthrodesis in patients in their ninth decade," *Spine*, vol. 31, no. 1, pp. 99–103, 2006.

[19] M. D. Daubs, L. G. Lenke, G. Cheh, G. Stobbs, and K. H. Bridwell, "Adult spinal deformity surgery: complications and outcomes in patients over age 60," *Spine*, vol. 32, no. 20, pp. 2238–2244, 2007.

[20] M. Y. Wang, B. A. Green, S. Shah, S. Vanni, and A. D. Levi, "Complications associated with lumbar stenosis surgery in patients older than 75 years of age," *Neurosurgical Focus*, vol. 14, no. 2, p. e7, 2003.

[21] R. J. Benz, Z. G. Ibrahim, P. Afshar, and S. R. Garfin, "Predicting complications in elderly patients undergoing lumbar decompression," *Clinical Orthopaedics and Related Research*, no. 384, pp. 116–121, 2001.

[22] E. N. Hanley, "The indications for lumbar spinal fusion with and without instrumentation," *Spine*, vol. 20, no. 24, pp. 143S–153S, 1995.

[23] M. Di Silvestre, F. Lolli, G. Bakaloudis, and P. Parisini, "Dynamic stabilization for degenerative lumbar scoliosis in elderly patients," *Spine*, vol. 35, no. 2, pp. 227–234, 2010.

[24] H. Shufflebarger, S. I. Suk, and S. Mardjetko, "Debate: determining the upper instrumented vertebra in the management of adult degenerative scoliosis: stopping at T10 versus L1," *Spine*, vol. 31, no. 19, pp. S185–S194, 2006.

[25] T. M. Stoll, G. Dubois, and O. Schwarzenbach, "The dynamic neutralization system for the spine: a multi-center study of a novel non-fusion system," *European Spine Journal*, vol. 11, no. 2, pp. S170–S178, 2002.

[26] K. J. Schnake, S. Schaeren, and B. Jeanneret, "Dynamic stabilization in addition to decompression for lumbar spinal stenosis with degenerative spondylolisthesis," *Spine*, vol. 31, no. 4, pp. 442–449, 2006.

# 11

# Protocol for Evaluation of Robotic Technology in Orthopedic Surgery

**Milad Masjedi, Zahra Jaffry, Simon Harris, and Justin Cobb**

*MSk Lab, Charing Cross Hospital, Imperial College London, London W6 8RF, UK*

Correspondence should be addressed to Milad Masjedi; m.masjedi@imperial.ac.uk

Academic Editor: Jess H. Lonner

In recent years, robots have become commonplace in surgical procedures due to their high accuracy and repeatability. The Acrobot Sculptor is an example of such a robot that can assist with unicompartmental knee replacement. In this study, we aim to evaluate the accuracy of the robot (software and hardware) in a clinical setting. We looked at (1) segmentation by comparing the segmented data from Sculptor software to other commercial software, (2) registration by checking the inter- and intraobserver repeatability of selecting set points, and finally (3) sculpting ($n = 9$ cases) by evaluating the achieved implant position and orientation relative to that planned. The results from segmentation and registration were found to be accurate. The highest error was observed in flexion extension orientation of femoral implant ($0.4 \pm 3.7°$). Mean compound rotational and translational errors for both components were $2.1 \pm 0.6$ mm and $3 \pm 0.8°$ for tibia and $2.4 \pm 1.2$ mm and $4.3 \pm 1.4°$ for the femur. The results from all processes used in Acrobot were small. Validation of robot in clinical settings is highly vital to ensure a good outcome for patients. It is therefore recommended to follow the protocol used here on other available similar products.

## 1. Introduction

In recent years, robots have become commonplace in industry due to their high accuracy and repeatability especially during procedures that require movement that is beyond the human control [1, 2]. As imaging and robotic technology has advanced, there is real potential to use these capabilities in the field of surgery, from planning to performing the procedure. This is especially useful in operations such as unicompartmental knee arthroplasty (UKA) where previous studies have shown the substantial effect of implant position inaccuracy [3–5].

The robotic procedures can be fully controlled (active) [6], can be shared as control or semiactive, where the robot monitors surgeon performance and provides stability and support through active constraint [7], they can be telesurgical where the surgeon performs the operation from a console distant to operating table [8]. The input to the robot can vary from the actual imaging data of the patient to statistical shape models (SSM) [9] or active shape models (ASM) [10, 11] that are based on a few point estimates of

the patient's morphology. The main problem with the latter is that these models are often created based on a normal anatomy dataset, and using them for pathological subjects can be problematic [12]. Audenaert et al. described the estimated accuracy of imageless surgery as poor because of the significant difference between the actual location of the probe during surgery and what is displayed on the navigation platform screen [13].

The Acrobot Sculptor (Stanmore Implants Worldwide Ltd.) is a semiactive robot, uses the computer tomography (CT) data as input, and could assist with bone resection for UKA surgery in a consistent manner to minimise variability [14]; however, the repeatability and accuracy of this robot in clinical settings are yet to be determined. In this study, we have set up various steps to determine the accuracy and repeatability of the Stanmore Sculptor which we believe will also be applicable to a wide range of other available similar products.

There are a number of processes involved in the use of the Sculptor, as with most robotic systems, with potential for error. Surgeons often use the imaging technology such as computed tomography (CT) to identify the pathology and plan the surgery virtually. During the surgery, a registration process takes place that matches the preoperative plan and imaging data to the patient [15]. This means the transformation between the virtual environment and the patient is known and any points in the plan can be located during the surgery. Results can be affected by both the software and hardware used by the robot [16].

The patient's CT scan is often segmented using available commercial software (e.g., Acrobot Modeller for Acrobot Sculptor). This software can generate the surface structure of the specified bones. It is possible to use these three-dimensional (3D) images to diagnose the pathology even though the surface geometry is not accurate or in scale. However, in robotic procedures, the accuracy of these surfaces has a direct influence on the outcome of surgery. This surface model is then loaded onto Acrobot Planner software to carry out preoperative planning. The Sculptor has a cutting burr attached to its three degrees of freedom (DoF) arm which can sculpt the bone based on a predefined plan. A tracking arm is pinned to the bone so that the system is aware of the 3D position of that bone relative to the robot at all times. Following attachment of the bone to the tracking arm, the intraoperative procedure also requires registration of points on the bone surfaces [15].

Other than the validity of the software, potential sources of error which can influence the outcome of the surgery include (1) the inaccuracy in position of sculpting arm or tracking arm (poor calibration), (2) inaccuracy in the registration algorithms to match the CT data to the bone, and finally (3) the robotic control system that constrains the surgeon to resect only on the safe zone area. Additionally, there may be other errors arising from surgeons in charge such as poor fixture of bones to tracking arm or inaccuracies in the use of tools [16].

The accuracy of registration, specifically, is an aspect that remains to be determined. There are a number of methods through which registration can take place, such as use of X-ray or ultrasound [17]. Some systems use fiducial markers in order to register the bone and some use landmarks on the bone such as discrete identifiable points or the ridge line [17]. Each is subject to a certain type of error including fiducial localization and registration error and target registration error [18]. The Acrobot Sculptor uses a mechanical digitizer (a secondary use of the robotic arm) to register the surface, where the tip of the cutter (ball point) is used as a probe which has a 2 mm diameter. As a result of inaccuracy in calibration or radius of the ball point, the captured data can be displaced from the true surface.

Validation of robot is vital to ensure a good outcome and highlight their value in use with patients [19]. Although there are several technical papers that have talked in detail about the accuracy of registration algorithms and robotic manipulations [20], there is no real simple method to test the accuracy of the robot in a clinical environment, and the main reference point simply remains the manufacturer's information. In this study, we aim to evaluate the above possible cause of errors in a clinical setting.

## 2. Materials and Methods

In order to evaluate the accuracy of the Acrobot Sculptor, the following steps were taken.

The initial step was determining the accuracy of the segmentation procedure. We compared the segmentation result of Modeller (Stanmore Implants, London, UK) from a single femur using various software used to convert CD data to 3D models. These are Mimics (Materialise, Leuven, Belgium) and Robin 3D (Cavendish Medical, London UK) [14]. These surfaces were then matched together using 3-matic (Materialise, Leuven, Belgium) software and the differences in size were analysed.

The second step in determining the reliability and reproducibility of the Sculptor was by placing a set of points (using a marker pen) on the dry bone femur that was CT scanned. A total of 45 points were selected randomly on the distal part of the femur, focussed on for medial UKA procedures and four observers used the Sculptor to register these points. The root mean squared (RMS) error of the registration process was recorded for each observer. In order to check the effect of different tracking and sculpting arm positions, the same procedure was repeated by changing the fixation of the femur. The positions mimicked those found in surgical operations for various patients' size or surgeons' preference.

The last step is to measure the accuracy of constraints set at the planning stage during bone resection. A senior surgeon (JPC) was recruited to plan the operation using the Planner Software. Uniglide implants (Corin, Cirencester, UK) were chosen (a size four tibial component and size three femoral component) to restore the natural joint line, incorporating a seven-degree posterior slope in the tibial component. Nine UKAs were implanted on identical dry bone knee models (Imperial knee, Medical Models Company, Bristol, UK) by three experienced users of the Sculptor (three each). The models used were CT-based replicas of a patient's arthritic knee consisting of a capsule, replica ligaments, and muscle tissues. Following implantation, the knee joint was separated from femur and tibia and each bone was individually scanned using the NextEngine Desktop 3D scanner (NextEngine, Santa Monica, CA, USA). Prior to implantation, the implant was painted in white enamel paint to improve pick-up of the laser spot from the scanner on the metal surface.

These scans were exported as Stereolithography (STL) files to 3-matic software. The positions of the tibial and femoral components were then compared to those of the ideal plan by recording the coordinates of four points on the planned implants versus the achieved implants (Figure 1). Using MATLAB, a local frame of reference was created using these four points for the achieved implant and was compared to that of the planned in all six DoF. These coordinates were created so that they follow the anatomical frame of reference such that the $x$-, $y$- and $z$-axes correspond to mediolateral, anteroposterior, and superoinferior directions accordingly. The magnitude of translational (a combination of the medial-lateral, anterior-posterior, and superior-inferior directions errors) and rotational (a combination of the axial, flexion-extension, and coronal alignment errors) errors were calculated for each case for both tibial and femoral components.

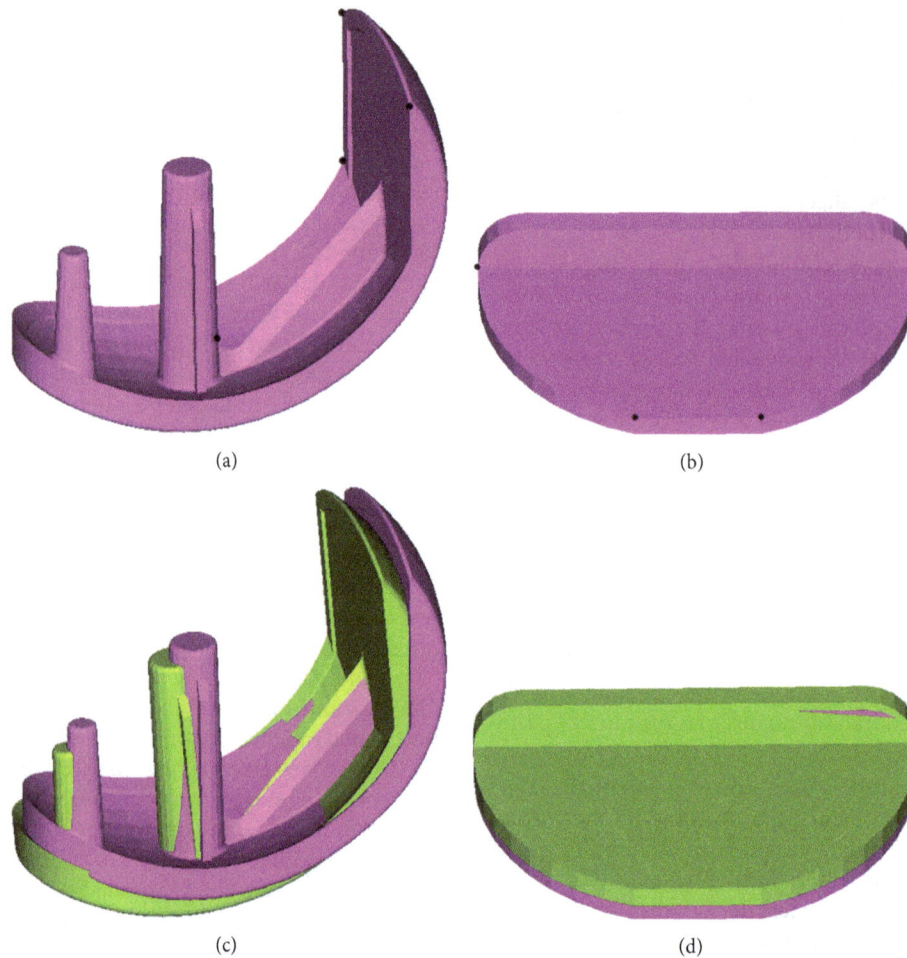

FIGURE 1: Four points selected on the (a) femoral and (b) tibial implants to construct the local frame of reference. Comparison of the planned versus achieved rotational and translational errors based on the local frame of reference for (c) femoral and (d) tibial implants.

TABLE 1: Translational and rotational error values in UKA implant placement ($n = 9$).

|  | Tibia | | | | | | Femoral | | | | | |
|  | Translational error (mm) | | | Rotational error (°) | | | Translational error (mm) | | | Rotational error (°) | | |
|  | Lateral medial | Anterior posterior | Distal proximal | Flexion extention | Varus valgus | Axial rotation | Lateral medial | Anterior posterior | Distal proximal | Flexion extention | Varus valgus | Axial rotation |
|---|---|---|---|---|---|---|---|---|---|---|---|---|
| Mean | 0.0 | −0.9 | 0.8 | 2.1 | −0.8 | 0.4 | 0.6 | −1.5 | −1.1 | 0.4 | −0.5 | 0.9 |
| SD | 1.5 | 0.5 | 1.1 | 0.6 | 1.6 | 1.4 | 0.9 | 1.4 | 1.0 | 3.7 | 0.9 | 2.6 |
| Max | 1.8 | −0.2 | 2.1 | 2.2 | 2.2 | 3.1 | 1.9 | 0.4 | −0.1 | 5.3 | 0.5 | 5.3 |
| Min | −2.8 | −1.6 | −1.7 | −3.3 | −1.3 | −2.4 | −1.2 | −3.2 | −3.5 | −4.7 | −1.9 | −2.1 |

## 3. Results

The results from segmentation using different software were almost identical. The measurements were performed in 3-matic software, and the difference was far less than 0.5 mm at all points.

The results for the registration repeatability (second step) showed a consistent mean RMS error were of 0.5 mm while the maximum error among all subjects was found to be 1.8 mm with mean maximum being $1.53 \pm 0.2$ mm.

The results for implantation are shown in Table 1. Placement of the femoral component in general was more prone to error with a maximum error of 5.3° around the $x$- and $z$-axes. Mean compound rotational and translational errors for tibia component were $2.1 \pm 0.6$ mm and $3 \pm 0.8$° and for femoral component were $2.4 \pm 1.2$ mm and $4.3 \pm 1.4$°

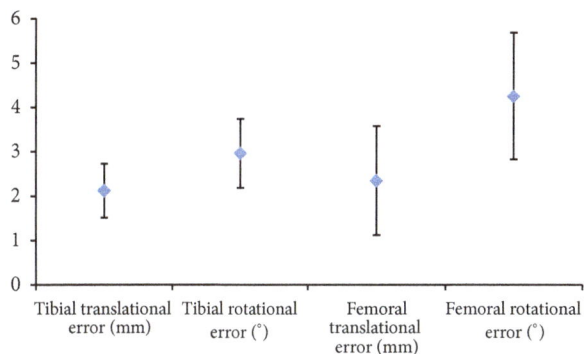

FIGURE 2: Magnitude of resultant rotational and translation error for tibial and femoral components when compared to planned positions.

(Figure 2). The highest error was found in rotational elements for both components.

## 4. Discussion

In this study, we set protocols that make it possible to evaluate robot's accuracy in house, which include testing both software and hardware and are applicable to a variety of similar products on the market. Robotics technology can improve surgical outcomes by providing the surgeon with the greatest amount of accuracy and precision regardless of long surgical training [21]. The robot gives the surgeon more control in terms of the position and alignment of the tools. The accompanied software can also assist in the planning of the surgery and also during the operation by supplying information on direction and amount of cut by enabling the surgeon to visualise these on the screen. These robots are prone to errors both systematic and those due to the operator. Validating the accuracy of image guided surgery is therefore an important issue that needs to be addressed.

The initial step was determining the accuracy of the segmentation procedure. There are numerous techniques available to create the bone surface from CT images. In lack of any available straight forward method, in this study we used comparative validation and found almost identical data using different software. For the second part we evaluated the landmarks that create the frame of reference. In this study, we found that placement of landmarks can be inaccurate. It is therefore important for surgeons to rely on their own experience for planning the procedure as well as the suggested values given by software for the implant position.

In this study, rotational error was found to be the highest source of error in both femoral and tibial components. This we believe is actually not only depends on the cut made by robot but also, when the implant is hammered into the plastic bone. This is on especially important with use of plastic bone, as it is possible to deform this under higher loads which may increase the error seen here. Nevertheless, these errors were accepted, far superior to what has been reported for conventional surgeries [14, 22], and similar to other robots available. For example, Dunbar et al. [22] found that

the MAKO robot's mean RMS errors for the tibia were 1.4 mm and 2.6° and for the femur 1.2 mm and 2.1°. Furthermore, the ranges found are within the safe range reported by Biomet [23].

We recognise the inherent limitations of our study, one of which is the use of dry replica bones rather than patients. To compensate, the dry bones were replicas of a patient's arthritic tibia and femur, with replica ligaments as well as a surrounding capsule attached and hence were as realistic to a real patient as possible. Fixation of the tracking arm to the bone may also cause inaccuracy if fixation pins bend or loosen due to stress on the fixation point. It is therefore important to design fixtures that are robust and rigid and not loosened (i.e., no movement between the tracking device and the anatomy should be allowed). Furthermore, if after screwing the fixtures, the anatomy of the subject deforms due to overloading of the segment, the possible error as a result of this needs to be evaluated for each robot. In the Sculptor, the tracking arm is quite light, and therefore we assumed stress on the fixation point because the weight of the arm would be minimal.

We acknowledge that during the planning phase, landmarks used to define reference frames are located manually by the surgeon. Srivastava et al. [24] describe the effects of landmark placement variability on kinematic descriptions of the knee. The positions of these landmarks may be open to placement inaccuracy and variability between surgeons. In addition to the accuracy measurements described above, a sensitivity analysis should be performed to determine the likely variability in frame of reference orientations and implant position relative to these introduced by the human operator during planning.

Often in the literature, errors are based on the translational or angular location of the implant and cuts; however, Simon et al. [17] argued that there are ambiguities associated with these data due to a dependence upon the selected coordinate system. It is therefore anticipated in the future for the implant manufacturer to provide a standard protocol for evaluation of location of the implant. The use of dry bones meant that soft tissue balancing could not be recreated and the tibio-femoral angle could not be measured. Although this is an important measure of functional outcome following a UKA, it is widely accepted that component alignment is a major influence on the limb's tibiofemoral angle [24]. In this study, we used a laser scanner instead of CT to find the position of the implant postoperatively since a metallic implant will create artefact in the CT scan and inaccuracy in segmentation. There could also be inaccuracies during segmentation and in CT data itself; however, this is not part of the system and would be operator error, not that of the software.

## 5. Conclusions

Overall our results of segmentation, registration, and cuts made by robot were satisfactory for both components using the Acrobot Sculptor. It is possible to apply the full or part of this protocol in this study in a variety of other products available on the market for better understanding and validation of robotic technology.

## Acknowledgments

The authors would like to thank Wellcome trust and EPSRC for funding part of this study.

## References

[1] A. D. Pearle, D. Kendoff, and V. Musahl, "Perspectives on computer-assisted orthopaedic surgery: movement toward quantitative orthopaedic surgery," *The Journal of Bone & Joint Surgery A*, vol. 91, no. supplement 1, pp. 7–12, 2009.

[2] W. L. Bargar, "Robots in orthopaedic surgery: past, present, and future," *Clinical Orthopaedics and Related Research*, no. 463, pp. 31–36, 2007.

[3] P. Hernigou and G. Deschamps, "Alignment influences wear in the knee after medial unicompartmental arthroplasty," *Clinical Orthopaedics and Related Research*, no. 423, pp. 161–165, 2004.

[4] P. Hernigou and G. Deschamps, "Posterior slope of the tibial implant and the outcome of unicompartmental knee arthroplasty," *The Journal of Bone & Joint Surgery A*, vol. 86, no. 3, pp. 506–511, 2004.

[5] E. M. Mariani, M. H. Bourne, R. T. Jackson, S. T. Jackson, and P. Jones, "Early failure of unicompartmental knee arthroplasty," *The Journal of Arthroplasty*, vol. 22, supplement 2, no. 6, pp. 81–84, 2007.

[6] T. Hananouchi, N. Nakamura, A. Kakimoto, H. Yohsikawa, and N. Sugano, "CT-based planning of a single-radius femoral component in total knee arthroplasty using the ROBODOC system," *Computer Aided Surgery*, vol. 13, no. 1, pp. 23–29, 2008.

[7] J. E. Lang, S. Mannava, A. J. Floyd et al., "Robotic systems in orthopaedic surgery," *The Journal of Bone & Joint Surgery B*, vol. 93, no. 10, pp. 1296–1299, 2011.

[8] R. Agganval, J. Hance, and A. Darzi, "Robotics and surgery: a long-term relationship?" *International Journal of Surgery*, vol. 2, no. 2, pp. 106–109, 2004.

[9] S. Schumann, M. Tannast, L.-P. Nolte, and G. Zheng, "Validation of statistical shape model based reconstruction of the proximal femur—a morphology study," *Medical Engineering and Physics*, vol. 32, no. 6, pp. 638–644, 2010.

[10] J. C. Baker-LePain, K. R. Luker, J. A. Lynch, N. Parimi, M. C. Nevitt, and N. E. Lane, "Active shape modeling of the hip in the prediction of incident hip fracture," *Journal of Bone and Mineral Research*, vol. 26, no. 3, pp. 468–474, 2011.

[11] G. Zheng and S. Schumann, "3D reconstruction of a patient-specific surface model of the proximal femur from calibrated x-ray radiographs: a validation study," *Medical Physics*, vol. 36, no. 4, pp. 1155–1166, 2009.

[12] J. Schmid and N. Magnenat-Thalmann, "MRI bone segmentation using deformable models and shape priors," in *Proceedings of the 11th International Conference on Medical Image Computing and Computer-Assisted Intervention (Miccai '08)*, vol. 5241 of *Lecture Notes in Computer Science*, part 1, pp. 119–126, 2008.

[13] E. Audenaert, B. Smet, C. Pattyn et al., "Imageless versus image-based registration in navigated arthroscopy of the hip: a cadaver-based assessment," *The Journal of Bone & Joint Surgery B*, vol. 94, no. 5, pp. 624–629, 2012.

[14] J. Cobb, J. Henckel, P. Gomes et al., "Hands-on robotic unicompartmental knee replacement: a prospective, randomised controlled study of the acrobot system," *The Journal of Bone & Joint Surgery B*, vol. 88, no. 2, pp. 188–197, 2006.

[15] B. L. Davies, F. M. Rodriguez y Baena, A. R. W. Barrett et al., "Robotic control in knee joint replacement surgery," *Journal of Engineering in Medicine H*, vol. 221, no. 1, pp. 71–80, 2007.

[16] M. Masjedi, K. Davda, S. Harris et al., "Evaluate your robot accuracy," in *Proceedings of the Hamlyn Symposium on Medical Robotics*, London, UK, 2011.

[17] D. Simon, R. V. O'Toole, M. Blackwell et al., "Accuracy validation in image-guided orthopaedic surgery," in *Proceedings of the 2nd International Symposium on Medical Robotics and Computer Assisted Surgery*, pp. 185–192, Baltimore, Md, USA, 1995.

[18] J. M. Fitzpatrick, "The role of registration in accurate surgical guidance," *Journal of Engineering in Medicine H*, vol. 224, no. 5, pp. 607–622, 2010.

[19] C. A. Willis-Owen, K. Brust, H. Alsop, M. Miraldo, and J. P. Cobb, "Unicondylar knee arthroplasty in the UK National Health Service: an analysis of candidacy, outcome and cost efficacy," *Knee*, vol. 16, no. 6, pp. 473–478, 2009.

[20] P. L. Yen and B. L. Davies, "Active constraint control for image-guided robotic surgery," *Proceedings of the Institution of Mechanical Engineers H*, vol. 224, no. 5, pp. 623–631, 2010.

[21] M. Karia, M. Masjedi, B. Andrews et al., "Robotic assistance enables inexperienced surgeons to perform unicompartmental knee arthroplasties on dry bone models with accuracy superior to conventional methods," *Advances in Orthopedics*, vol. 2013, Article ID 481039, 7 pages, 2013.

[22] N. J. Dunbar, M. W. Roche, B. H. Park, S. H. Branch, M. A. Conditt, and S. A. Banks, "Accuracy of dynamic tactile-guided unicompartmental knee arthroplasty," *The Journal of Arthroplasty*, vol. 27, no. 5, pp. 803.e1–808.e1, 2012.

[23] Biomet. Oxford partial knee-manual of the surgical technique, 2012.

[24] A. Srivastava, G. Y. Lee, N. Steklov, C. W. Colwell Jr., K. A. Ezzet, and D. D. D'Lima, "Effect of tibial component varus on wear in total knee arthroplasty," *The Knee*, vol. 19, no. 5, pp. 560–563, 2011.

# 12

# Anterior Glenohumeral Instability: Classification of Pathologies of Anteroinferior Labroligamentous Structures Using MR Arthrography

**Serhat Mutlu,**[1] **Mahir Mahıroğullari,**[2] **Olcay Güler,**[3] **Bekir Yavuz Uçar,**[4] **Harun Mutlu,**[5] **Güner Sönmez,**[6] **and Hakan Mutlu**[6]

[1] *Kanuni Sultan Suleyman Education and Research Hospital, Department of Orthopaedic Surgery, Istanbul, Turkey*
[2] *Istanbul Medipol University, Istanbul, Turkey*
[3] *Nisa Hospital, Istanbul, Turkey*
[4] *Dicle University, Diyarbakır, Turkey*
[5] *Taksim Education and Research Hospital, Istanbul, Turkey*
[6] *Gülhane Military Medical Academy Education Hospital, Istanbul, Turkey*

Correspondence should be addressed to Serhat Mutlu; serhatmutlu@hotmail.com

Academic Editor: Panagiotis Korovessis

We examined labroligamentous structures in unstable anteroinferior glenohumeral joints using MR arthrography (MRA) to demonstrate that not all instabilities are Bankart lesions. We aimed to show that other surgical protocols besides classic Bankart repair are appropriate for labroligamentous lesions. The study included 35 patients (33 males and 2 females; mean age: 30.2; range: 18 to 57 years). MRA was performed in all patients. The lesions underlying patients' instability such as Bankart, anterior labral periosteal sleeve avulsion (ALPSA), and Perthes lesions were diagnosed by two radiologists. MRA yielded 16 diagnoses of Bankart lesions, 5 of ALPSA lesions, and 14 of Perthes lesions. Albeit invasive, MRA seems to be a more reliable and accurate diagnostic imaging modality for the classification and treatment of instabilities compared to standard MRI.

## 1. Introduction

Anterior shoulder instability is one of the most common orthopedic problems. Glenohumeral (GH) instability occurs mostly in young, active males and is usually caused by traumatic injury. Recurrent subluxations and dislocations of the GH joint occur as a result of changes in bone, cartilage, and soft tissues and are referred to as habitual dislocation of the shoulder [1, 2]. This problem, which causes severe morbidity that interferes with daily and sporting activities, is associated with many bone and soft tissue changes. The glenohumeral ligament, its inferior part in particular, is one of the most important passive stabilizers of the shoulder. The glenoid labrum contributes to stability of the shoulder by deepening the glenoid fossa with ligamentous attachments [3, 4]. A number of anterior instabilities can be associated with glenohumeral ligament lesions and with lesions of complex ligamentous structures that the glenohumeral ligament forms with neighboring tissues. The main instabilities are Bankart lesion (avulsion of the anterior glenoid labrum from the bone), glenoid edge fracture, Hill-Sachs lesion (osseous defect due to dislocation of the posterosuperior lateral humeral head), and loose body [1]. In addition, the Perthes lesion, a labroligamentous avulsion in which the scapular periosteum remains intact, and the ALPSA lesion, a medial displacement of the anteroinferior labral ligamentous complex with an intact scapular periosteum, should be considered potential causes of shoulder instability [5, 6].

The identification of anterior labral avulsion, capsular laxity, and other pathologies of the GH joint is of great significance in treatment planning. The methods used to identify these pathologic changes include shoulder radiography with different angles of view as well as computerized tomography (CT), CT arthrography (CTA), magnetic resonance (MR), and magnetic resonance arthrography (MRA)

[7–11]. Osseous changes such as lesions of the glenoid and humeral head can be imaged by CT, whereas soft tissue changes such as labral and ligamentous avulsion and capsular laxity can be identified most clearly by MR. Nonetheless, the utility of MRA for precise localization of glenohumeral lesions and identification of the relationships between bone and soft tissue is beyond doubt [12, 13].

The purpose of this study was to show that not all instabilities result from Bankart lesions by in-depth evaluation of bone and soft tissue changes in unstable anterior-inferior glenohumeral joints by MRA and to draw attention to other lesions causing instabilities and to the various treatment approaches.

## 2. Patients and Methods

After standard MRI, MRA was performed in 35 shoulders of 35 patients with recurrent shoulder dislocation (at least three dislocations) who were diagnosed clinically with GH instability between June 2006 and October 2012. Thirty-three patients were males and two were females (mean age: 30.2; range: 18–57 years). These patients were selected from 47 patients with chronic shoulder instabilities. Twelve of forty-seven patients were diagnosed with Bankart lesion based on MR imaging results, whereas pathology involving labroligamentous structures could not be diagnosed with certainty in the 35 patients included in the study. MRA images from the 35 patients were evaluated independently by two radiologists.

This study was planned as a retrospective patient file analysis with the permission of the ethics committee. Before MRA, contrast material was injected via the posterior arthroscopic portal by an orthopedist under the guidance of radiologist-operated ultrasound. Injections were performed following topical anesthesia (prilocaine hydrochloride 2% Citanest) while patients were in a semiprone position with the arm held flexed perpendicular to the body for the duration of imaging. The ultrasound probe was placed parallel to the humerus, along the same axis as the infraspinatus in the posterior direction, and angled to visualize the humeral head and posterior glenoid rim. Under the guidance of ultrasound, a 20-gauge spinal needle was inserted through fatty planes and the infraspinatus muscle and advanced between the humeral head and posterior glenoid rim through the capsule. After the capsule was entered, ~12–16 mL of gadolinium diluted 4/1000 in isotonic solution was administered. Distension of the capsule was evaluated by ultrasound. The process took ~10 min. After the intra-articular injection, the shoulder joint was moved to allow the contrast material to spread inside the capsule.

Ten to fifteen minutes after administration of contrast agent, MRA was performed using a 1.5 Tesla imaging scanner. While patients were in a supine position with the arm externally rotated (for effective evaluation of the rotator cuff and glenohumeral ligaments), selective fat-suppressed axial, coronal, and sagittal T1A-weighted (repetition time: 713 ms, echo time: 12 ms) images were obtained using a shoulder coil.

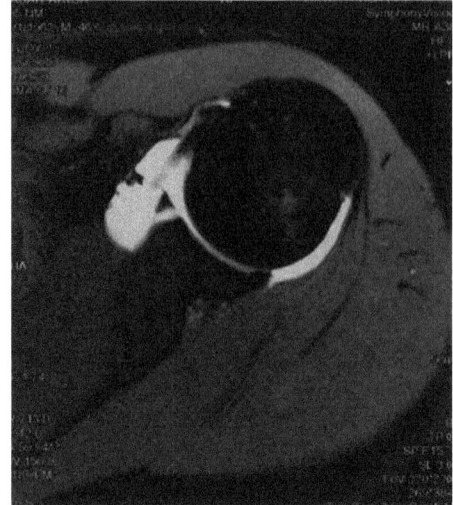

FIGURE 1: Bankart lesion.

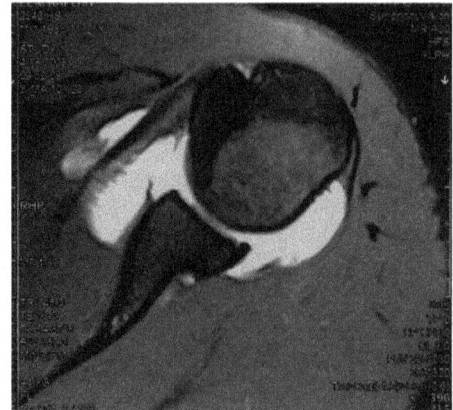

FIGURE 2: ALPSA lesion.

The image matrix was 256 × 256 pixels, section thickness was 4 mm, the gap was 1 mm, and the field of view was 220 mm.

## 3. Results

MRA images revealed capsular distension due to the injection of radioopaque contrast material. Based on the results of MRA, 16 patients were diagnosed with Bankart lesions (Figure 1), 5 with ALPSA lesions (Figure 2), and 14 with Perthes lesions (Figure 3). Twenty-nine patients also had Hill-Sachs lesions due to shoulder dislocation in the posterior surface of the corpus humeri.

MRA images were interpreted and reported separately by two radiologists; their diagnoses agreed completely (100%). The diagnoses were categorized and the results are presented as percentages (Table 1).

## 4. Discussion

The glenohumeral joint has the largest range of motion of all joints in the human body. The joint capsule, ligaments, and

TABLE 1: Distribution of lesions underlying shoulder instability, as diagnosed by MRA.

| | |
|---|---|
| Bankart lesion | 16 (45.72%) |
| Perthes lesion | 14 (40%) |
| ALPSA lesion | 5 (14.28%) |

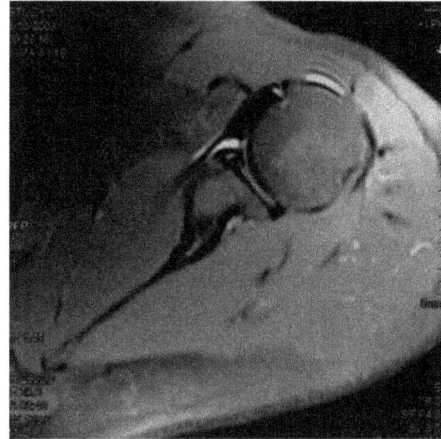

FIGURE 3: Perthes lesion.

muscles help to resolve the incongruity between the humeral head and the glenoid cavity in the glenohumeral joint. Therefore, the shoulder joint is prone to recurrent dislocation [1, 14, 15]. The most common shoulder dislocation is traumatic anterior unidirectional glenohumeral instability, which occurs most often after acute anterior shoulder dislocation [2, 14]. The identification of labroligamentous and capsular pathologies by radiological methods after the acquisition of patient history and a detailed physical examination is of great importance in treatment planning. GH instability after acute dislocation is more common among young adults [2, 7, 14]. Conventional radiographic and CT examinations of the shoulder, though inefficient for the evaluation of soft tissues, are important for the evaluation of bone structures in shoulder dislocations [7, 16].

A prospective analysis of 121 MR arthrograms by Palmer and Caslowitz reported that MRA detects labral abnormalities with a sensitivity of 92% and a specificity of 92%. In another study, Chandnani et al. [17] compared MR and CT arthrography with MRA in the same patient group and reported that MRA was superior.

Because the superiority of MR imaging in the detection of soft tissue lesions of the shoulder is beyond doubt, it is the most widely used diagnostic method before treatment. We propose that MRA is superior to MR imaging because it detects lesions that can be missed by MR imaging, through the expansion of the capsule by the contrast material, which reveals ligament cleavage. MRA can therefore better guide selection of the optimum treatment approach.

Gartsman divided anterior labrum tears into three types: Type A, in which the labrum is separated from the glenoid bone but remains at the level of the glenoid joint, Type B, in which the labrum is separated from the glenoid bone and retracted medially, and Type C, in which the labrum is separated from the glenoid bone, retracted, and has healed medially on the glenoid, equivalent to an ALPSA lesion. Gartsman also reported that surgical dissection should be performed before repair and the labrum should be mobilized to the superolateral region in Type B and Type C lesions [18]. In this study, as also reported by Gartsman, we attempted to underline the fact that not all anterior-inferior labroligamentous lesions are Bankart lesions; that is, some might be other Bankart-like lesions. Even though these lesions can be diagnosed by imaging during surgery, preoperative identification of these lesions helps surgeons plan the intervention, guiding the choice of which lesion to target.

Because MRA is associated with swelling and tightening of the joint, it is highly effective in the identification of labroligamentous structures. Even though, unlike standard MRA, MRA of the shoulder is invasive, it is considerably useful in the classification of lesions. Preoperative identification of labroligamentous structures is of great importance because accurate diagnosis is required to identify the appropriate surgical procedure, which may not be Bankart repair as would be assumed from noninvasive MR imaging. Provencher reported that ALPSA-type lesions are associated with twofold higher bone loss during surgical procedures compared to anterior instability alone [19].

Habermeyer et al. suggested that the evolution of ALPSA lesions depends on time and recurrence and that ALPSA lesions do not usually occur with first-time dislocations [20]. In the study presented here, all patients experienced three or more recurrences of dislocation.

MRI with intra-articular contrast material is more specific and sensitive than other imaging methods in the identification of Bankart and more complex lesions (Perthes and ALPSA). The importance of preoperative identification of lesions in reducing postoperative recurrence risk is evident. The failure rate after surgical repair has been reported to be twice as high in ALPSA lesions compared to that in Bankart repair [21]. Habermeyer et al. reported that the ALPSA lesion is chronic by nature [20], which, along with increased bone loss during surgery, likely underlies increased posttreatment failure [22]. Thus, MRA patients diagnosed with ALPSA and their relatives should be informed of the risk of failure prior to acquiring informed consent for surgical procedures.

ALPSA lesions are more challenging than other lesions to visualize arthroscopically from the standard posterior portal. Since the labroligamentous complex has healed medially, it cannot be visualized from the point where the labral tissue is separated. These lesions are more accurately diagnosed by visualization from the anterosuperior portal. Upon imaging from this view, ALPSA lesions would be repaired by elevating the labroligamentous complex of the scapular neck and bringing it back to the anatomic position on the glenoid face [23].

Perthes lesions, also referred to as partial labral detachments, can be missed on routine MRI and even on arthroscopy because they can heal spontaneously through the synovial membrane, granulation tissues, and periosteal fibers. Thus, there may be no clinical findings despite symptoms of shoulder instability, in which case MRA is superior for diagnosis and guiding treatment because it can visualize partial tears revealed by contrast material-induced tension within the capsule [24].

The number of cases in this study was limited, so the distribution and variety of lesions may not be representative of a larger population. However, even in this small series, there was a wide variety, supporting our initial hypothesis that many types of lesions underlie shoulder joint instability. Another limitation of this study is that MRA diagnoses were not confirmed surgically.

In conclusion, MRA is an efficient technique for the diagnosis and classification of anteroinferior labroligamentous lesions in shoulder joint instability. Although degenerative changes and fibrous tissues make the diagnosis of chronic cases difficult, MRA is beneficial before planning arthroscopic surgical intervention.

## References

[1] S. H. Liu and M. H. Henry, "Anterior shoulder instability: current review," *Clinical Orthopaedics and Related Research*, no. 323, pp. 327–337, 1996.

[2] F. A. Matsen, S. C. Thomas, C. A. Rockwood, and M. A. Wirth, "Glenohumeral instability," in *The Shoulder*, C. A. Rockwood and F. A. Matsen, Eds., vol. 2, pp. 611–689, W.B. Saunders, Philadelphia, Pa, USA, 2nd edition, 1998.

[3] P. W. O'Connell, G. W. Nuber, R. A. Mileski, and E. Lautenschlager, "The contribution of the glenohumeral ligaments to anterior stability of the shoulder joint," *American Journal of Sports Medicine*, vol. 18, no. 6, pp. 579–584, 1990.

[4] J. Ovesen and S. Nielsen, "Stability of the shoulder joint: cadaver study of stabilizing structures," *Acta Orthopaedica Scandinavica*, vol. 56, no. 2, pp. 149–151, 1985.

[5] T. J. Neviaser, "The anterior labroligamentous periosteal sleeve avulsion lesion: a cause of anterior instability of the shoulder," *Arthroscopy*, vol. 9, no. 1, pp. 17–21, 1993.

[6] T. J. Neviaser, "The GLAD lesion: another cause of anterior shoulder pain," *Arthroscopy*, vol. 9, no. 1, pp. 22–23, 1993.

[7] A. Blum, H. Coudane, and D. Molé, "Gleno-humeral instabilities," *European Radiology*, vol. 10, no. 1, pp. 63–82, 2000.

[8] M. Rafii, H. Firooznia, and J. J. Bonamo, "Athlete shoulder injuries: CT arthrographic findings," *Radiology*, vol. 162, no. 2, pp. 559–564, 1987.

[9] M. Rafii and J. Minkoff, "Advanced arthrography of the shoulder with CT and MR imaging," *Radiologic Clinics of North America*, vol. 36, no. 4, pp. 609–633, 1998.

[10] B. Roger, A. Skaf, A. W. Hooper, N. Lektrakul, L. Yeh, and D. Resnick, "Imaging findings in the dominant shoulder of throwing athletes: comparison of radiography, arthrography, CT arthrography, and MR arthrography with arthroscopic correlation," *American Journal of Roentgenology*, vol. 172, no. 5, pp. 1371–1380, 1999.

[11] K. J. Stevens, B. J. Preston, W. A. Wallace, and R. W. Kerslake, "CT imaging and three-dimensional reconstructions of shoulders with anterior glenohumeral instability," *Clinical Anatomy*, vol. 12, pp. 326–336, 1999.

[12] W. E. Palmer and P. L. Caslowitz, "Anterior shoulder instability: diagnostic criteria determined from prospective analysis of 121 MR arthrograms," *Radiology*, vol. 197, no. 3, pp. 819–825, 1995.

[13] S. Waldt, A. Burkart, A. B. Imhoff, M. Bruegel, E. J. Rummeny, and K. Woertler, "Anterior shoulder instability: accuracy of MR arthrography in the classification of anteroinferior labroligamentous injuries," *Radiology*, vol. 237, no. 2, pp. 578–583, 2005.

[14] C. R. Rowe, B. Zarins, and J. V. Ciullo, "Recurrent anterior dislocation of the shoulder after surgical repair: apparent causes of failure and treatment," *Journal of Bone and Joint Surgery A*, vol. 66, no. 2, pp. 159–168, 1984.

[15] S. J. Turkel, M. W. Panio, J. L. Marshall, and F. G. Girgis, "Stabilizing mechanisms preventing anterior dislocation of the glenohumeral joint," *Journal of Bone and Joint Surgery A*, vol. 63, no. 8, pp. 1208–1217, 1981.

[16] L. Pancione, G. Gatti, and B. Mecozzi, "Diagnosis of Hill-Sachs lesion of the shoulder: comparison between ultrasonography and arthro-CT," *Acta Radiologica*, vol. 38, no. 4, part 1, pp. 523–526, 1997.

[17] V. P. Chandnani, T. D. Yeager, T. DeBerardino et al., "Glenoid labral tears: prospective evaluation with MR imaging, MR arthrography, and CT arthrography," *American Journal of Roentgenology*, vol. 161, no. 6, pp. 1229–1235, 1993.

[18] M. Gary and M. D. Gartsman, *Shoulder Arthroscopy*, Chapter Glenohumeral Instability, 2nd edition, 2008.

[19] M. T. Provencher, "Glenoid bone loss in patients with instability: the significance of an ALPSA lesion," in *Proceedings of the American Academy of Orthopaedic Surgeons Annual Meeting*, New Orleans, La, USA, 2010.

[20] P. Habermeyer, P. Gleyze, and M. Rickert, "Evolution of lesions of the labrum-ligament complex in posttraumatic anterior shoulder instability: a prospective study," *Journal of Shoulder and Elbow Surgery*, vol. 8, no. 1, pp. 66–74, 1999.

[21] M. Ozbaydar, B. Elhassan, D. Diller, D. Massimini, L. D. Higgins, and J. J. P. Warner, "Results of arthroscopic capsulolabral repair: bankart lesion versus anterior labroligamentous periosteal sleeve avulsion lesion," *Arthroscopy*, vol. 24, no. 11, pp. 1277–1283, 2008.

[22] A. Bernhardson, "Glenoid bone loss in patients with shoulder instability: the significance of the ALPSA (anterior labroligamentous periosteal sleeve avulsion) lesion," in *Proceedings of the American Academy of Orthopaedic Surgeons Annual Meeting*, New Orleans, La, USA, 2010.

[23] M. T. Provencher and A. A. Romeo, *Shoulder Instability, A Comprehensive Approach*, Chapter 6 Findings and Pathology Associated with Anterior Shoulder Instability, 2010.

[24] M. T. Provencher and A. A. Romeo, *Shoulder Instability, A Comprehensive Approach*, Chapter 8 Radiographic Studies and Findings, 2010.

**13**

# Intervertebral Disc Rehydration after Lumbar Dynamic Stabilization: Magnetic Resonance Image Evaluation with a Mean Followup of Four Years

Li-Yu Fay,[1,2,3] Jau-Ching Wu,[1,2,3] Tzu-Yun Tsai,[4,5] Tsung-Hsi Tu,[1,2] Ching-Lan Wu,[6] Wen-Cheng Huang,[1,2] and Henrich Cheng[1,2,3]

[1] Department of Neurosurgery, Neurological Institute, Taipei Veterans General Hospital,
  Taipei 11217, Taiwan
[2] School of Medicine, National Yang-Ming University, Taipei 11221, Taiwan
[3] Institute of Pharmacology, National Yang-Ming University, Taipei 11221, Taiwan
[4] Department of Ophthalmology, National Taiwan University Hospital, College of Medicine, National Taiwan University,
  Taipei 10002, Taiwan
[5] Department of Ophthalmology, New Taipei City Hospital, New Taipei City 241, Taiwan
[6] Department of Radiology, Taipei Veterans General Hospital, Taipei 11217, Taiwan

Correspondence should be addressed to Jau-Ching Wu; leofay1978@gmail.com

Academic Editor: Mehdi Sasani

*Objective.* To compare the clinical and radiographic outcomes in patients of different ages who underwent the Dynesys stabilization. *Methods.* This retrospective study included 72 patients (mean age 61.4 years) with one- or two-level lumbar spinal stenosis who underwent laminectomy and the Dynesys (Zimmer Spine, Minneapolis) dynamic stabilization system. Thirty-seven patients were younger than 65-year old while the other 35 were older. Mean followup was 46.7 months. Pre- and postoperative radiographic and clinical evaluations were analyzed. *Results.* The mean calibrated disc signal (CDS) at the index level was significantly improved from $60.2 \pm 25.2$ preoperatively to $66.9 \pm 26.0$ postoperatively ($P > 0.001$). Screw loosening occurred in 22.2% of patients and 5.1% of screws. The improvement in CDS at index level was seen to be significant in younger patients but not in older patients. Overall, the mean visual analogue scale (VAS) of back pain, VAS of leg pain, and the Oswestry disability index (ODI) scores improved significantly after operation. There were no significant differences in pre- and postoperative VAS and ODI and screw loosening rates between the younger and older patients. *Conclusions.* There is significant clinical improvement after laminectomy and dynamic stabilization for symptomatic lumbar spinal stenosis. Intervertebral disc rehydration was seen in younger patients.

## 1. Introduction

Instrumented spinal fusion is the treatment of choice for degenerative spondylosis with instability refractory to conservative treatment [1, 2]. Spine surgeons have also used modern biologics such as recombinant human bone morphogenetic protein-2 to increase the rate of spinal fusion in selected patients [3–7]. However, using biologics to enhance spinal fusion has been sometimes reported with complications postoperatively and during followup. Moreover, even autograft has been repeatedly reported with adverse events, such as donor site morbidity. Not to mention that loss of segmental motion and subsequent adjacent segmental degeneration have also been concerned for the spinal fusion surgery [8–10].

In the recent years, there is the emerging option of dynamic stabilization to spare spinal fusion and still yield satisfactory outcomes in the surgical management of lumbar spondylosis and back pain. Fischgrund and colleagues reported application of the Dynesys (Zimmer Spine, Minneapolis, USA), a pedicle-based lumbar dynamic stabilization system, as an effective alternative to treat lumbar spondylosis in 1994 [11–16]. Theoretically Dynesys can unload the intervertebral disc while providing a restricted range of motion and thus alleviates symptoms in the indexed level of spine. Although its long-term effect on the adjacent segment is still uncertain, there are reports demonstrating improved clinical outcomes with acceptably low rate of screw loosening when Dynesys is used in degenerative disc diseases (DDD), lumbar stenosis, and some spondylolisthesis [13, 17]. Despite the common nature of spondylosis in the diseases treated, quite some disparity exists among these patients, who have variable age and bone quality that could affect the screw anchoring in the nonfused constructs. However, there is a paucity of data addressing the differences of age and clinical outcomes in these patients treated by dynamic stabilization with Dynesys.

This study aims to compare the clinical and radiographic outcomes in patients of different ages who underwent surgical decompression and Dynesys stabilization. This is the first study focusing on the discrepancies between the elderly and the younger patients. The pre- and postoperative magnetic resonance imaging (MRI) especially of each patient were compared to evaluate the condition of the discs at the index segments. All clinical data was prospectively collected and outcomes were measured by standardized parameters with more than two years of followup.

## 2. Methods

*2.1. Patient Enrollment.* From September 2007 to August 2009, the study enrolled 88 consecutive patients who underwent surgical decompression and dynamic stabilization with Dynesys (Zimmer Spine, Minneapolis, MN) in the authors' service. The clinical and radiological data were collected prospectively and then analyzed retrospectively. Three experienced spine surgeons performed all operations in a very similar fashion by the same technique.

The inclusion criteria were the patients who had lumbar DDD with persistent symptoms such as intermittent claudication, low back pain, buttock pain, leg pain, or any combination of the above. Each patient underwent preoperative MRI to confirm the diagnosis and had failed medical treatment for longer than 12 weeks. The exclusion criteria were degenerative scoliosis, prior lumbar surgery, disc diseases requiring discectomies, and spondylolisthesis worse than grade II. Patients with psychiatric disorders, cerebral vascular accidents, coexisting cervical or thoracic myelopathy, or neoplasms were also excluded. Among the 88 patients enrolled in this cohort, 72 completed the follow up for more than 24 months and were thus analyzed. These patients were divided into two groups according to the age at operation: young age (<65 years) and old age ($\geqq$65 years).

*2.2. Operative Technique.* Patients were placed in prone position under general anesthesia. Fluoroscopy was used routinely before sterilization to confirm the treated level and keep the lumbar spine in a neutral lordotic curve. Prophylactic antibiotics were infused thirty minutes before incision. After midline incision by subperiosteal dissection, the laminae and spinous process were exposed. The facet joints capsules were preserved intact. Standard total laminectomies and foraminotomies with resection of hypertrophic

spur and ligamentum flavum were performed carefully to preserve the complex structure of the facet joints. The exiting and traversing nerve roots were probed through to confirm the adequate decompression without any bony fragment. Bilateral fascial incisions were made by subdermal dissection through the same wound. Along the Wiltse and Spencer intermuscular plane, the titanium alloy screws were placed transpedicularly without destruction of the facet joints [18]. The modular spacers were cut appropriately and the tension cords were assembled to reach 300 N for dynamic stabilization. Fluoroscope was used to assure the correct position of each screw. Drainage catheters were left and the wound was closed layer by layer.

*2.3. Clinical Assessment.* The Oswestry disability index (ODI) scale was used for functional assessment. The 0–10 visual analogue scale (VAS) was used for back and leg pain evaluation. The patients themselves completed the ODI and VAS questionnaire preoperatively and at 1.5-, 3-, 6-, 12-, and 24-month followup regularly. Preoperative scores were compared to postoperative scores.

*2.4. Radiographic Assessment.* Standard anterior/posterior and lateral radiographs, computed tomography (CT), and magnetic resonance imaging (MRI) studies were routinely performed in preoperative assessment. Radiographs were taken regularly at 1.5-, 3-, 6-, 12-, and 24-month followup.

The presence of "halo zone sign" or "double halo sign" on anteroposterior radiographs was defined as screw loosening during followup (Figure 1). CT was used to determine questionable screw loosening. The halo zone sign was defined as a radiolucent zone alone the screws with 1 mm in width and in any length. The double halo sign was further defined as a radiolucent zone with a radiopaque rim alone the screws.

Pre- and post-operative MRI images were compared focusing on the condition of the discs, including the indexed and adjacent segments. Due to the lack of an absolute unit of measuring the signal intensities on MRI, for example, the Hounsfield unit used in computed tomography to describe radiodensity, these signals of the same patient are difficult to compare. Ideally the pre- and post-operative MRI studies need to be taken by the very same MRI machine to unify the signal intensity references. We tried to allocate the same MRI machine to each patient; however, not every patient achieved the goal. To address this issue, the digital signal in central intervertebral disc of the levels T12-L1 in T2-weighted image (T2WI) was designated as a reference (Figure 2). The signal intensity in the center of the discs in the lumbar spine of each patient was recorded and compared to each patient's own signal intensity recorded at the levels of T12-L1 in T2-weighted MRI (T2WI). The ration differences of signal intensity were calculated and defined as the calibrated disc signal (CDS). The pre- and post-operative CDS of bridged levels were thus all compared and analyzed.

*2.5. Statistical Analysis.* Clinical and radiographic assessments were compared and analyzed using Student's *t*-test, chi-square, and Mann-Whitney *U* test, where appropriate. All

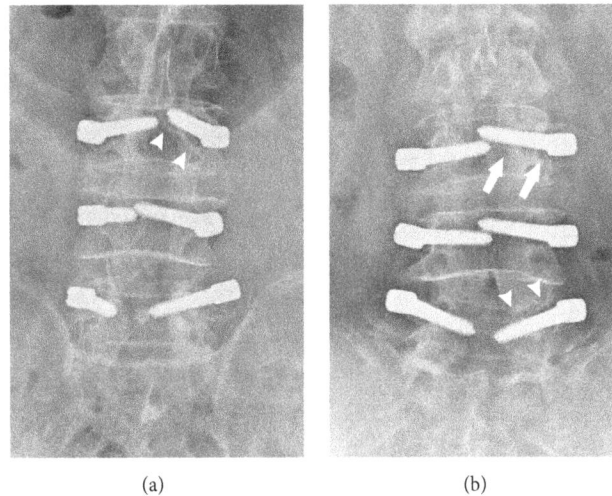

(a)                                                    (b)

FIGURE 1: Anteroposterior radiographs. (a) A 61-year-old female who underwent Dynesys stabilization at 12-month postoperation. The double halo sign indicated loosening of the left L3 pedicle screw. (b) A 75-year-old male who underwent Dynesys stabilization, at 2-year postoperation. The double halo sign indicated screw loosening of the left L5 and the halo sign indicated screw loosening of the left L3 screws. Arrowhead, double halo sign; arrow, halo sign.

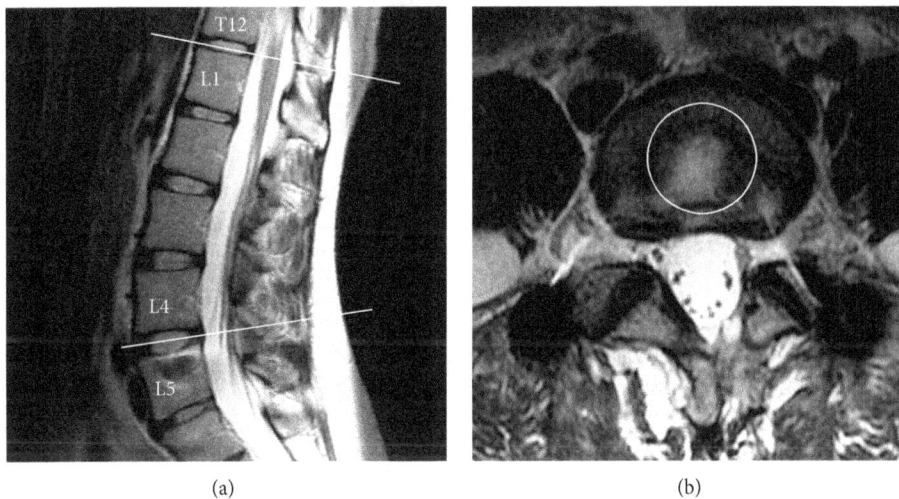

(a)                                                    (b)

FIGURE 2: MRI T2-weighted image of a 34-year-old female. (a) Sagittal view. (b) Axial view. The axial view of each disc was retrieved in correspondence with the center of each disc in sagittal view. A circle of one centimeter in radius, region of interest (ROI), was drawn in the geometrical center of each disc. The mean signal intensity of ROI was then measured and recorded. The mean signal intensity of ROI of each level (e.g., L4-5) divided with reference level (i.e., T12-L1) was called CDS.

data analysis was processed with the statistical software, SPSS version 17.0 (SPSS, Inc., Chicago, IL). Statistical significance was set at $P$ value $< 0.05$.

## 3. Results

Of the 88 consecutive patients with lumbar spondylosis who underwent 1- or 2-level dynamic stabilization with the Dynesys system, 72 patients (81.8%), in whom 370 screws were placed, completed the clinical and radiological evaluations for at least 24 months postoperatively. There were 37 men (51.4%) and 35 women (48.6%) whose mean age was $61.4 \pm 11.3$ (31–82) years at the time of surgery (Table 1).

The mean followup duration was $46.7 \pm 7.8$ (33–58) months. In the 72 patients, 31 (43.1%) underwent a 1-level and 41 (56.9%) underwent a 2-level stabilization. The distributions of index levels were as follows: 3 (4.2%) at L3-4; 23 (31.9%) at L4-5; 5 (6.9%) at L5-S1; 1 (1.4%) at L2-3-4; 33 (45.8%) at L3-4-5; and 7 (9.7%) at L4-5-S1 (Table 2).

Overall there were 15 (20.8%) patients diagnosed of type 2 (diabetes mellitus) DM and 9 (12.5%) patients of hypertension. There were more diabetic patients in older age group (34.3%) than in young age group (8.1%) in current study ($P = 0.006$). The hypertensive patients in both groups had similar prevalence rates (10.8% versus 14.3%, $P = 0.656$) (Table 3).

TABLE 1: Clinical and demographic characteristics ($n = 72$).

| Characteristic | Value |
| --- | --- |
| Gender | |
| Male | 37 (51.4%) |
| Female | 35 (48.6%) |
| Age (years) mean | 61.4 ± 11.3 (31–82) |
| Follow-up (months) mean | 46.7 ± 7.8 (33–58) |
| Number of instrumented levels | |
| 1-level | 31 (43.1%) |
| 2-levels | 41 56.9%) |

TABLE 2: Distribution of treated levels.

| Instrumentation | Level | Number of patients |
| --- | --- | --- |
| | L3-4 | 3 (4.2%) |
| 1-level ($n = 31$) | L4-5 | 23 (31.9%) |
| | L5-S1 | 5 (6.9%) |
| | L2-3-4 | 1 (1.4%) |
| 2-levels ($n = 41$) | L3-4-5 | 33 (45.8%) |
| | L4-5-S1 | 7 (9.7%) |

### 3.1. Clinical Outcomes.
The overall mean VAS for back pain improved with statistical significance, from 6.3 ± 3.3 preoperatively to 2.8 ± 2.9 postoperatively ($P < 0.001$). There was significant improvement in both the young age group (6.1 ± 3.4 preoperatively to 2.9 ± 2.9 postoperatively; $P < 0.001$) and the old age group (6.4 ± 3.1 preoperatively to 2.7 ± 2.9 postoperatively; $P < 0.001$) (Table 3). There were no significant differences in pre- and postoperative VAS between the young and old age groups ($P = 0.811$ and $P = 0.754$, resp.) (Figure 1).

The overall mean VAS for leg pain improved with statistical significance, from 7.0 ± 2.7 preoperatively to 2.6 ± 3.2 postoperatively ($P < 0.001$). There was significant improvement in both the young age group (6.7 ± 3.0 preoperatively to 2.7 ± 3.1 postoperatively; $P < 0.001$) and the old age group (7.4 ± 2.3 preoperatively to 2.4 ± 3.2 postoperatively; $P < 0.001$) (Table 3). There were no significant differences in pre- and postoperative VAS between the young and old age groups ($P = 0.497$ and $P = 0.474$, resp.) (Figure 1).

The overall ODI functional scores significantly improved from 51.1 ± 19.6 preoperatively to 23.4 ± 21.4 postoperatively ($P < 0.001$). The young age group specifically improved from 50.4 ± 21.3 preoperatively to 21.8 ± 22.0 postoperatively ($P < 0.001$) and the old group from 51.7 ± 17.8 preoperatively to 25.2 ± 20.8 postoperatively ($P < 0.001$) (Table 3). There were no significant differences in pre- and postoperative ODI scores between the young and old groups ($P = 0.612$ and $P = 0.291$, resp.) (Figure 1).

### 3.2. Radiographic Outcome of Screw Loosening.
There was screw loosening in 16 out of 72 patients (22.2% per patient) and 19 out of 370 screws (5.1% per screw). Specifically, there were 8 of 37 patients (21.6%) and 9 of 188 screws (4.8%) found loosened in the young age group. In contrast, there were 8 of 35 patients (22.9%) and 10 of 182 screws (5.5%)

TABLE 3: Comparison between young age and old age.

| Variables | Total | Age | | P values |
| --- | --- | --- | --- | --- |
| | | <65-year old | ≥65-year old | |
| Number of patients | 72 | 37 | 35 | |
| Age (years) | 61.4 ± 11.3 | 53.0 ± 9.0 | 70.3 ± 4.8 | <0.001* |
| Gender | | | | |
| Male | 37 | 23 (62.2%) | 14 (40.0%) | 0.060 |
| Female | 35 | 14 (37.8%) | 21 (60.0%) | |
| Number of instrumented levels | | | | |
| One | 31 | 17 (45.9%) | 14 (40.0%) | 0.611 |
| Two | 41 | 20 (54.1%) | 21 (60.0%) | |
| Mean pre-op scores | | | | |
| VAS back pain | 6.3 ± 3.3 | 6.1 ± 3.4 | 6.4 ± 3.1 | 0.811 |
| VAS leg pain | 7.0 ± 2.7 | 6.7 ± 3.0 | 7.4 ± 2.3 | 0.497 |
| ODI (%) | 51.1 ± 19.6 | 50.4 ± 21.3 | 51.7 ± 17.8 | 0.612 |
| Mean 24-month post-op scores | | | | |
| VAS back pain | 2.8 ± 2.9 | 2.9 ± 2.9 | 2.7 ± 2.9 | 0.754 |
| VAS leg pain | 2.6 ± 3.2 | 2.7 ± 3.1 | 2.4 ± 3.2 | 0.474 |
| ODI (%) | 23.4 ± 21.4 | 21.8 ± 22.0 | 25.2 ± 20.8 | 0.291 |
| Serum glucose status | | | | |
| Type 2 DM | 15 | 3 (8.1%) | 12 (34.3%) | 0.006* |
| Euglycemia | 57 | 34 (91.9%) | 23 (65.7%) | |
| Blood pressure | | | | |
| Hypertensive | 9 | 4 (10.8%) | 5 (14.3%) | 0.656 |
| Normotensive | 63 | 33 (89.2%) | 30 (85.7%) | |

Mean values are presented ± SD.
* $P < 0.05$, statistically significant.
DM: diabetes mellitus.
VAS: visual analogue scale.
ODI: Oswestry disability index.

found loosened in the old age group. There was no statistically significant difference found between the two groups in the rates of screw loosening per patient or per screw ($P = 0.900$, $P = 0.739$, resp.) (Table 4).

### 3.3. Radiographic Outcome of Bridged Disc Signal.
The mean overall CDS at bridged level improved (i.e., increased) with statistical significance, from 60.2 ±25.2 preoperatively to 66.9 ± 26.0 postoperatively ($P = 0.014$). There was significant increase in the young age group (58.9 ± 24.7 preoperatively to 67.6 ± 28.7 postoperatively; $P = 0.013$) (Figure 3). However, the change in the old age group was not significant (62.1 ± 26.1 preoperatively to 65.9 ± 22.2 postoperatively; $P = 0.366$). There were no significant differences in pre- and post-operative bridged level CDS between the young and old age groups ($P = 0.732$ and $P = 0.800$, resp.) (Table 4).

TABLE 4: Comparison of disc signal change between young age and old age.

| Variables | Total | Age | | P values |
| --- | --- | --- | --- | --- |
| | | <65-year old | ≥65-year old | |
| Number of patients | 72 | 37 | 35 | |
| Screw loosening per patient | | | | |
| Yes | 16 | 8 (21.6%) | 8 (22.9%) | 0.900 |
| No | 56 | 29 (78.4%) | 27 (77.1%) | |
| Screw loosening per screw | | | | |
| Yes | 19 | 9 (4.8%) | 10 (5.5%) | 0.739 |
| No | 351 | 179 (95.2%) | 172 (94.5%) | |
| CDS of bridged disc | | | | |
| Pre-op | 60.2 ± 25.2 | 58.9 ± 24.7 | 62.1 ± 26.1 | 0.732 |
| Post-op | 66.9 ± 26.0** | 67.6 ± 28.7** | 65.9 ± 22.2 | 0.800 |

Mean values are presented ± SD.
** $P < 0.05$, the post-op value compared with the pre-op value demonstrated significant difference.
CDS: calibrated disc signal.

## 4. Discussion

The current study collected total 72 patients with lumbar spondylosis who underwent decompression and dynamic stabilization. A total 370 screws of Dynesys were placed during the operations. In a mean follow-up period of 46.7 months, the results of both the young age (<65 years old, $n$ = 37) and the old age (≥65 years old, $n$ = 35) groups demonstrated satisfactory improvement in clinical outcomes. The overall screw loosening rate was 22.2% per patient (16 in 72 patients) and 5.1% per screw (19 in 370 screws). The rate of screw loosening was slightly higher in the old age patients. Regarding disc signal, in the overall CDS of bridged discs, the change significantly improved from 60.2±25.2 preoperatively to 66.9 ± 26.0 postoperatively ($P$ = 0.014). However, the change in the young age group (58.9 ± 24.7 to 67.6 ± 28.7, $P$ = 0.013) appeared to be more obvious than in the old age group (62.1 ± 26.1 to 65.9 ± 22.2, $P$ = 0.366).

Using the 10% difference as minimal clinically important difference (MCID) of the ODI defined by Hägg et al., and the 1.2 unit improvement of VAS reported by Copay et al., overall there were 68.1% (49/72) of patients had MCID of VAS back pain, 84.7% (61/72) had MCID of VAS leg pain, and 81.9% (59/72) had MCID of ODI [19, 20]. Therefore, a significant number of patients had clinically significant improvement in the present series at a mean followup of 47 months.

According to the population projections of the United Nations, the number of elderly patients (older than 65 years) in the world will increase from 8 to 14 percent and the percentage will increase far more to 25 percent in more developed nations between 2010 and 2040. Low back pain and lumbar spondylosis is a common problem in the elderly patients which may greatly affect their quality of life. Pain, numbness, claudication, and risk to fall are the frequent symptoms of the patients. The prevalence of lumbar spondylosis will increase as the population ages [21, 22]. Conservative treatment such as medication, physical therapy, or manual therapy may be the first-line treatment for most patients and surgical intervention can still achieve satisfactory improvement in selected patients refractory to conservative treatment [23]. Weinstein et al. conducted a cohort study, spine patient outcome research trial (SPORT), to analyze the pain improvement and functional outcomes. They enrolled a randomized cohort of 304 patients and an observational cohort of 303 patients for analysis. They concluded that patients with degenerative spondylolisthesis and spinal stenosis treated surgically, decompression with or without fusion, would maintain greater pain relief and functional improvement [24].

Regarding the influence of age, Deyo et al. reported that complications associated with procedures were primarily related to patients' age [25]. The mortality and morbidity, length of hospitalization, and hospital charge all increased with the ages of the patients. Wang et al. conducted a retrospective study to analyze the clinical outcomes and complications associated with lumbar stenosis surgery in elderly patients (>75 years) in 2003. Eighty-eight patients older than 75 years of age who underwent lumbar spondylosis surgery were collected and fifty-two (59.1%) patients received spinal fusion. Among them, 76% experienced complete or partial improvement of back pain, 85% experienced complete or partial relief of leg pain, and 61% of 33 patients with preoperative gait disturbance experienced at least one point on the ambulatory scale. They concluded that lumbar spinal surgery could be conducted safely and with satisfactory outcomes as in young age patients [26]. For more complicated spinal degeneration, Daubs et al. surveyed forty-six patients older than 60 years of age in 2007. These elderly patients with mean age of 67 years underwent spinal deformity surgery to perform thoracic or lumbar arthrodesis procedures of 5 levels or more. The overall complication rate is 37%, including dura tear in 4, iliac vein injury in 4, misplaced pedicle screw in 1, and nerve root injury in 1 patient. The overall mean ODI improvement is 24 points which is statistically significant ($P$ < 0.001). They concluded that increasing age was a predicting factor for complication. However, the presence of complications had no association with final clinical outcomes [27].

Dynamic stabilization, Dynesys, is an alternative surgical treatment for lumbar spondylosis. It aims to change the mechanical loading of lumbar spinal segments. Several studies have proved the safety and efficacy of dynamic stabilization but there were only few series involving the Dynesys in the elderly patients [12, 13, 15, 16, 28–30]. Di Silvestre et al. reported that to use this pedicle screw-based system in elderly patients with degenerative scoliosis was able to achieve significant improvement of clinical outcome at last followup. In twenty-nine elderly patients, with mean age of 68.5 years, 51.6% of them had improvement in

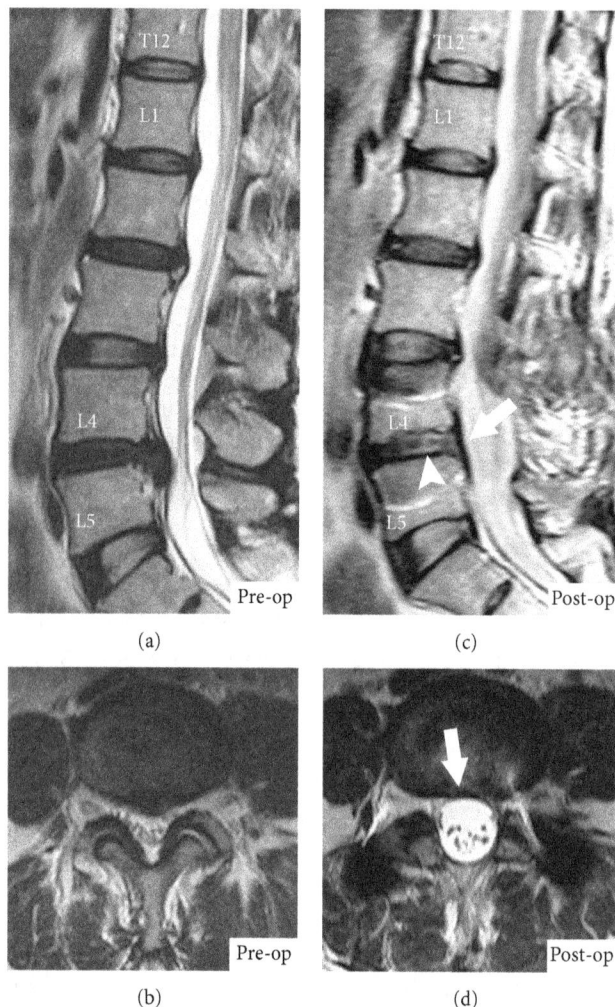

FIGURE 3: MRI T2-weighted image of a 56-year-old female. ((a) and (c)) Sagittal view. ((b) and (d)) Axial view. The significant increase in CDS was seen in L4-5 level (preoperative 0.44 to postoperative 0.92) at 24-month followup. Meanwhile, the signal intensity of T12-L1 demonstrated to be similar brightness. Arrow, reduced bulging disc after stabilization; arrowhead, significant increase in CDS.

ODI and 58.2% had improvement in Roland Morris score. The mean improvement was 51.7% and 57.8% in VAS for back and leg pain, respectively. The scoliosis and associated spondylolisthesis remained stable at the last followup [31]. Wu et al. conducted a study to investigate risk factor and outcomes associated with screw loosening of Dynesys. They collected 126 patients with more than 24-month followup. Besides diabetes mellitus, they concluded that old age was identified as major risk factors for screw loosening. Screw loosening can be asymptomatic to clinical outcomes [17].

However, there was no comparative study to discuss the outcomes between young and elderly patients. To date, there is a paucity of long-term data for the application of Dynesys in the elderly patients. The current retrospective study specifically aimed to compare the cohort of young to old age patients with lumbar spondylosis who underwent dynamic stabilization. Regarding the low back pain, the prevalence may be quite high and it may be often underestimated due to inconsistent study design and definition. Cho et al. reported the lifetime prevalence of low back pain was as high as

53.8% in the Asian population [22]. In our study, between the young and elderly patients, the preoperative VAS for back pain was the same ($6.1 \pm 3.4$ versus $6.4 \pm 3.1$, $P = 0.811$). After decompression and Dynesys implant, they both had significant improvement. Regarding the improvement of VAS back pain, 64.9% (24/37) of patients in young age group had MCID and 71.4% (25/35) of patients in old age group had MCID. The treatment of back pain in elderly seems to be as effective as in young patients. The results of VAS leg pain were similar to back pain. Between the two groups, the preoperative VAS for leg pain was the same ($6.7 \pm 3.0$ versus $7.4 \pm 2.3$, $P = 0.497$). After surgery, 78.4% (29/37) of patients in young age group had MCID and 91.4% (32/35) of patients in old age group had MCID. The elderly group seemed to have much better result than the young age group.

The preoperative ODI scores were similar between the two groups ($50.4 \pm 21.3$ versus $51.7 \pm 17.8$, $P = 0.612$). Thirty in 37 (81.1%) young patients and 29 in 35 (82.9%) old patients had MCID in ODI. Both groups had significant improvement after surgery.

Ko et al. reported the screw loosening rate was 19.7% per patient and 4.6% per screw at last followup in 2010. They collected 71 patients with a mean age of 59.2 years and concluded that screw loosening was not associated with clinical outcomes. Most patients with screw loosening were more than 55-year old [13]. Later Wu et al. conducted a study of 126 patients with 658 screws in 2011 and they reported the screw loosening rate as 19.8% per patient and 4.7% per screw. The patients with screw loosening may be asymptomatic at last followup as 37 months long. They concluded that hyperglycemia and old age may be the risk factors of screw loosening [17]. In current study the overall screw loosening rate was 22.2% per patient and 5.1% per screw which were similar to previous studies. The screw loosening rate in the old age group was higher than the young age group in per patient (22.9% versus 21.6%) and per screw (5.5% versus 4.8%). Even the difference did not reach statistically significant but the result was consistent with previous reports. The smaller patient numbers and uncertain cut value of age both could affect the $P$ value. Further study with larger number of patients will be required for this question.

In concern of the bridged disc degeneration, Kumar et al. collected 32 patients with lumbar spondylosis who underwent Dynesys stabilization and completed 2-year follow-up MRI in 2008. Till now, there were only few in vivo reports to discuss disc change. By using Woodend scores to define the degeneration classification, they found that there was a significant increase in the scores from preoperative 1.95 to postoperative 2.52 ($P < 0.001$) at the treated levels. The data demonstrated progressive disc degeneration at bridged level after dynamic stabilization. The authors concluded that the degeneration may be due to natural disease progression [32]. Regarding this topic, Vaga et al. collected ten patients with low back pain who underwent Dynesys and analyzed the quantification of glycosaminoglycan (GAG) concentration by MRI at followup. The GAG was increased in 61% of bridged level discs and the result suggested that dynamic stabilization was able to stop or partially reverse the degeneration. Interestingly they thought Pfirrmann grading, even achieved excellent intra- and interobserver agreement, is not sensitive enough to detect the disc change in their study [33]. In 2001, Pfirrmann et al. conducted a study for classification of lumbar disc degeneration. They collected 60 patients with 300 intervertebral discs for analysis. They have established a reliable classification on routine T2-weighted MRI [34]. However, the same protocol for MRI evaluation was not practicable in routine clinical followup. Our study evaluated the disc signal on T2WI series in pre- and post-operative imaging study. Regarding the different MRI machines at each study, we used the CDS which referred to compare the target disc signal with the least mobile level. The significant increase in bridged level CDS, which was consistent to Vaga's report, represented the Dynesys to stop and reverse the disc degeneration. In detail, the young patients had much more improvement than the old patients had.

There were limitations to this study. The cohort composition was not strictly uniform. The old age patients had much higher prevalence of type 2 diabetes which may have some influence on the outcomes. Smoking habit, osteoporosis

profile, and body mass index may also have some adverse effect on the outcomes. There were also two iatrogenic dura tear in the old age group (5.7%), but no related symptom was recorded. No other complications (i.e. wound infection) or reoperations have happened to date in the current series.

## 5. Conclusions

There was significant clinical improvement after laminectomy and dynamic stabilization with the Dynesys for symptomatic lumbar spinal stenosis in both the young and old age patients. The screw loosening rate was slightly higher in the old age patients. Disc degeneration may stop or reverse in the young age patients but not for the elderly patients. Further studies are needed to evaluate the regenerative effect of dynamic stabilization on the intervertebral discs.

## Disclosure

No funds were received in support of this work and no benefits in any form have been or will be received from a commercial party related directly or indirectly to the subject of this paper.

## References

[1] S. D. Glassman, L. Y. Carreon, M. Djurasovic et al., "Lumbar fusion outcomes stratified by specific diagnostic indication," Spine Journal, vol. 9, no. 1, pp. 13–21, 2009.

[2] A. R. Vaccaro and S. R. Garfin, "Internal fixation (pedicle screw fixation) for fusions of the lumbar spine," Spine, vol. 20, no. 24, pp. 157S–165S, 1995.

[3] V. Arlet, L. Jiang, T. Steffen, J. Ouellet, R. Reindl, and M. Aebi, "Harvesting local cylinder autograft from adjacent vertebral body for anterior lumbar interbody fusion: surgical technique, operative feasibility and preliminary clinical results," The European Spine Journal, vol. 15, no. 9, pp. 1352–1359, 2006.

[4] K. H. Bridwell, T. A. Sedgewick, M. F. O'Brien, L. G. Lenke, and C. Baldus, "The role of fusion and instrumentation in the treatment of degenerative spondylolisthesis with spinal stenosis," Journal of Spinal Disorders, vol. 6, no. 6, pp. 461–472, 1993.

[5] Z. Ghogawala, E. C. Benzel, S. Amin-Hanjani et al., "Prospective outcomes evaluation after decompression with or without instrumented fusion for lumbar stenosis and degenerative Grade I spondylolisthesis," Journal of Neurosurgery, vol. 1, no. 3, pp. 267–272, 2004.

[6] H. N. Herkowitz and L. T. Kurz, "Degenerative lumbar spondylolisthesis with spinal stenosis: a prospective study comparing decompression with decompression and intertransverse process arthrodesis," Journal of Bone and Joint Surgery A, vol. 73, no. 6, pp. 802–808, 1991.

[7] A. R. Vaccaro, D. G. Anderson, T. Patel et al., "Comparison of OP-1 putty (rhBMP-7) to iliac crest autograft for posterolateral lumbar arthrodesis: a minimum 2-year follow-up pilot study," Spine, vol. 30, no. 24, pp. 2709–2716, 2005.

[8] J. C. Banwart, M. A. Asher, and R. S. Hassanein, "Iliac crest bone graft harvest donor site morbidity: a statistical evaluation," Spine, vol. 20, no. 9, pp. 1055–1060, 1995.

[9] A. Çakmak, A. Gyedu, I. Kepenekçi, C. Özcan, and A. E. Ünal, "Colon perforation caused by migration of a bone graft following a posterior lumbosacral interbody fusion operation: case report," *Spine*, vol. 35, no. 3, pp. E84–E85, 2010.

[10] M. D. Rahm and B. B. Hall, "Adjacent-segment degeneration after lumbar fusion with instrumentation: a retrospective study," *Journal of Spinal Disorders*, vol. 9, no. 5, pp. 392–400, 1996.

[11] J. S. Fischgrund, M. Mackay, H. N. Herkowitz, R. Brower, D. M. Montgomery, and L. T. Kurz, "Degenerative lumbar spondylolisthesis with spinal stenosis: a prospective, randomized study comparing decompressive laminectomy and arthrodesis with and without spinal instrumentation," *Spine*, vol. 22, no. 24, pp. 2807–2812, 1997.

[12] D. Grob, A. Benini, A. Junge, and A. F. Mannion, "Clinical experience with the dynesys semirigid fixation system for the lumbar spine: surgical and patient-oriented outcome in 50 cases after an average of 2 years," *Spine*, vol. 30, no. 3, pp. 324–331, 2005.

[13] C. C. Ko, H. W. Tsai, W. C. Huang et al., "Screw loosening in the Dynesys stabilization system: radiographic evidence and effect on outcomes," *Neurosurgical Focus*, vol. 28, no. 6, article E10, 2010.

[14] S. Schaeren, I. Broger, and B. Jeanneret, "Minimum four-year follow-up of spinal stenosis with degenerative spondylolisthesis treated with decompression and dynamic stabilization," *Spine*, vol. 33, no. 18, pp. E636–E642, 2008.

[15] K. J. Schnake, S. Schaeren, and B. Jeanneret, "Dynamic stabilization in addition to decompression for lumbar spinal stenosis with degenerative spondylolisthesis," *Spine*, vol. 31, no. 4, pp. 442–449, 2006.

[16] T. M. Stoll, G. Dubois, and O. Schwarzenbach, "The dynamic neutralization system for the spine: a multi-center study of a novel non-fusion system," *The European Spine Journal*, vol. 11, no. 2, pp. S170–S178, 2002.

[17] J. C. Wu, W. C. Huang, H. W. Tsai, C. C. Ko, C. L. Wu, T. H. Tu et al., "Pedicle screw loosening in dynamic stabilization: incidence, risk, and outcome in 126 patients," *Neurosurgical Focus*, vol. 31, no. 4, article E9, 2011.

[18] L. L. Wiltse and C. W. Spencer, "New uses and refinements of the paraspinal approach to the lumbar spine," *Spine*, vol. 13, no. 6, pp. 696–706, 1988.

[19] A. G. Copay, S. D. Glassman, B. R. Subach, S. Berven, T. C. Schuler, and L. Y. Carreon, "Minimum clinically important difference in lumbar spine surgery patients: a choice of methods using the Oswestry Disability Index, Medical Outcomes Study questionnaire Short Form 36, and Pain Scales," *Spine Journal*, vol. 8, no. 6, pp. 968–974, 2008.

[20] O. Hägg, P. Fritzell, and A. Nordwall, "The clinical importance of changes in outcome scores after treatment for chronic low back pain," *The European Spine Journal*, vol. 12, no. 1, pp. 12–20, 2003.

[21] H. B. Bressler, W. J. Keyes, P. A. Rochon, and E. Badley, "The prevalence of low back pain in the elderly: a systematic review of the literature," *Spine*, vol. 24, no. 17, pp. 1813–1819, 1999.

[22] N. H. Cho, Y. O. Jung, S. H. Lim, C. K. Chung, and H. A. Kim, "The prevalence and risk factors of low back pain in rural community residents of Korea," *Spine*, vol. 37, no. 24, pp. 2001–2010, 2012.

[23] K. M. Backstrom, J. M. Whitman, and T. W. Flynn, "Lumbar spinal stenosis-diagnosis and management of the aging spine," *Manual Therapy*, vol. 16, no. 4, pp. 308–317, 2011.

[24] J. N. Weinstein, J. D. Lurie, T. D. Tosteson et al., "Surgical compared with nonoperative treatment for lumbar degenerative spondylolisthesis: four-year results in the Spine Patient Outcomes Research Trial (SPORT) randomized and observational cohorts," *Journal of Bone and Joint Surgery A*, vol. 91, no. 6, pp. 1295–1304, 2009.

[25] R. A. Deyo, D. C. Cherkin, J. D. Loeser, S. J. Bigos, and M. A. Ciol, "Morbidity and mortality in association with operations on the lumbar spine. The influence of age, diagnosis, and procedure," *Journal of Bone and Joint Surgery A*, vol. 74, no. 4, pp. 536–543, 1992.

[26] M. Y. Wang, B. A. Green, S. Shah, S. Vanni, and A. D. Levi, "Complications associated with lumbar stenosis surgery in patients older than 75 years of age," *Neurosurgical Focus*, vol. 14, no. 2, article e7, 2003.

[27] M. D. Daubs, L. G. Lenke, G. Cheh, G. Stobbs, and K. H. Bridwell, "Adult spinal deformity surgery: complications and outcomes in patients over age 60," *Spine*, vol. 32, no. 20, pp. 2238–2244, 2007.

[28] M. Putzier, S. V. Schneider, J. F. Funk, S. W. Tohtz, and C. Perka, "The surgical treatment of the lumbar disc prolapse: nucleotomy with additional transpedicular dynamic stabilization versus nucleotomy alone," *Spine*, vol. 30, no. 5, pp. E109–E114, 2005.

[29] W. C. Welch, B. C. Cheng, T. E. Awad et al., "Clinical outcomes of the Dynesys dynamic neutralization system: 1-year preliminary results," *Neurosurgical Focus*, vol. 22, no. 1, article E8, 2007.

[30] C. C. Würgler-Hauri, A. Kalbarczyk, M. Wiesli, H. Landolt, and J. Fandino, "Dynamic neutralization of the lumbar spine after microsurgical decompression in acquired lumbar spinal stenosis and segmental instability," *Spine*, vol. 33, no. 3, pp. E66–E72, 2008.

[31] M. di Silvestre, F. Lolli, G. Bakaloudis, and P. Parisini, "Dynamic stabilization for degenerative lumbar scoliosis in elderly patients," *Spine*, vol. 35, no. 2, pp. 227–234, 2010.

[32] A. Kumar, J. Beastall, J. Hughes et al., "Disc changes in the bridged and adjacent segments after Dynesys dynamic stabilization system after two years," *Spine*, vol. 33, no. 26, pp. 2909–2914, 2008.

[33] S. Vaga, M. Brayda-Bruno, F. Perona et al., "Molecular MR imaging for the evaluation of the effect of dynamic stabilization on lumbar intervertebral discs," *The European Spine Journal*, vol. 18, no. 1, supplement, pp. S40–S48, 2009.

[34] C. W. A. Pfirrmann, A. Metzdorf, M. Zanetti, J. Hodler, and N. Boos, "Magnetic resonance classification of lumbar intervertebral disc degeneration," *Spine*, vol. 26, no. 17, pp. 1873–1878, 2001.

# 14

# Late Prosthetic Shoulder Hemiarthroplasty after Failed Management of Complex Proximal Humeral Fractures

**A. Panagopoulos,**[1] **P. Tsoumpos,**[1] **K. Evangelou,**[1]
**Christos Georgiou,**[1] **and I. Triantafillopoulos**[2]

[1] *Department of Shoulder & Elbow Surgery, Orthopaedic Clinic, University Hospital of Patras, Papanikolaou 1, 26504 Patras, Greece*
[2] *Department of Shoulder & Elbow Surgery, Metropolitan Hospital Athens, Medical School, University of Athens, Ethnarxou Makariou & El. Benizelou 1, N. Faliro, 18547 Piraeus, Greece*

Correspondence should be addressed to A. Panagopoulos; andpan21@gmail.com

Academic Editor: Allen L. Carl

*Background.* The purpose of this study was to report our experience with shoulder hemiarthroplasty in the context of old trauma. *Methods.* 33 patients with failed treatment for a complex proximal humeral fracture underwent prosthetic hemiarthroplasty. There were 15 men and 18 women with a mean age of 58.1 years. The average period from initial treatment was 14.9 months. Sequelae included 11 malunions, 4 nonunions, 15 cases with avascular necrosis (AVN) and 3 neglected posterior locked dislocations. Follow up investigation included radiological assessment and clinical evaluation using the Constant score and a visual analogue pain scale. *Results.* After a mean follow up of 82.5 months the median Constant score was 75.7 points, improved by 60% in comparison to preoperative values. Greater tuberosity displacement, large cuff tears and severe malunion were the factors most affected outcome. No cases of stem loosening or severe migration were noted. 60% of the patients were able to do activities up to shoulder level compared with 24% before reconstruction. *Conclusions.* Late shoulder hemiarthroplasty is technically difficult and the results are inferior to those reported for acute humeral head replacement, nonetheless remains a satisfactory reconstructive option when primary treatment fails.

## 1. Introduction

Shoulder hemiarthroplasty is a technically challenging procedure which can predictably restore shoulder-level function in patients with 4-part fractures, some 3-part fractures, fracture dislocations, head-splitting fractures, and impaction fractures of the humeral head with involvement of more than 50% of the articular surface [1–4]. Early surgical intervention within 2 weeks postinjury, accurate tuberosity reconstruction, and appropriate height and retroversion of the prosthesis are the factors with the greatest impact on functional outcome [5–8].

In contrast, outcomes of internal fixation [9, 10] and non-operative treatment [11, 12] for these complex fractures are quite controversial, with the initial management considered critically important. Krappinger et al. [13] showed in a recent study that multifragmentary fracture patterns in old patients with low local BMD are prone for fixation failure. Revision osteosynthesis or late prosthetic shoulder arthroplasty in these complex fractures is fraught with complications, and functional results are usually disappointing [14, 15]. Bone loss, malunion, ectopic ossification, avascular necrosis, associated rotator cuff tears, and severe contractions of soft tissues are some of the factors that prevent appropriate prosthesis placement and postoperative rehabilitation, thus currently a reverse shoulder arthroplasty is considered as the treatment of choice for these injuries.

The aim of this study is to present the long-term outcome of 33 late prosthetic shoulder replacements carried out on patients who had failed conservative or operative treatment for complex fractures of the proximal humerus.

## 2. Materials and Methods

Between 2004 and 2007, thirty-eight patients underwent shoulder hemiarthroplasty after failed conservative or operative treatment for complex proximal humeral fractures in our department. Three patients were lost from followup, and two died from reasons unrelated to the fracture leaving a cohort of 33 patients, with a minimum followup of 5 years, for the outcome analysis. There were 18 women and 15 men with a mean age of 58.1 years old (range, 34 to 83 years old) at implantation. The dominant arm was involved in 23 (69.7%) cases. Seven patients performed heavy or manual labor, fifteen were sedentary, and eleven were retired.

The type of initial fracture according to Neer classification [5] was a 2-part surgical neck fracture in 2 patients, a 3-part fracture in 5, a 4-part fracture in 12, a 3- or 4-part fracture dislocation in 7, and a neglected "locked" posterior fracture dislocation in 3. Four patients who have been referred to us by other hospitals had no immediate postinjury radiographs, and the type of fracture could not be identified. The initial treatment was conservative in 16 patients and surgical in 17. In the open group, 6 patients had been managed with transosseous suturing fixation [16] (all in our department), 8 patients with plate-screw osteosynthesis, and 2 patients with screw-wiring osteosynthesis (Table 1). Additional operations prior to hemiarthroplasty have been performed in 5 patients: a plate-screws exchanged osteosynthesis after suturing fixation due to nonunion, an open release of the shoulder joint due to adhesive capsulitis after suturing fixation, a hardware removal, and surgical debridement after a persistent deep infection and a McLaughlin procedure for a neglected "locked" posterior dislocation. Another case underwent hardware removal in another center prior to final referral.

With the exception of the "locked" posterior dislocations, the main complication of initial treatment was malunion in eleven cases, nonunion in four, avascular necrosis (AVN) in fourteen, and septic AVN in one but without evidence of active infection (Figure 1). All patients underwent prosthetic hemiarthroplasty in an averaged delay period from the original injury of 12.7 months (range, 2 to 32 months).

Prior to arthroplasty and at the last followup appointment, subjective pain and overall function were evaluated with a visual analog scale (from 0 (maximum pain) to 10 (no pain at all)) and according to the parameters of Constant-Murley score, respectively, Pain, performance of daily activities, range of motion, and strength were scored on a scale of 1 to 100, with 100 being an excellent score. The isometric power of the shoulder was assessed by assigning a maximum of 25 points when a patient could resist a maximal weight of 12 kg at 90° of shoulder abduction or when the resisted weight was lesser but equal to the resisted weight on the contralateral noninjured arm.

An excellent or very good result was considered if the patient expressed none or little pain, reported normal use of his arm and had an objective improvement of shoulder function by at least 75% or 50%, respectively, when these values were compared with the preoperative ones. Unsatisfactory results comprised those cases with moderate or severe pain and objective improvement of shoulder function less than 25% in contrast to the preoperative values. Patients who had values between these limits (25%–50%) were considered as having a moderate outcome. Clinical evaluation was performed by two independent with the project observers (PT and KE). Finally, all patients were asked about their satisfaction with the final result and if they were agreed to undergo the procedure again under similar circumstances.

Radiological evaluation was performed with standardized "trauma series" views of good quality both preoperatively and postoperatively (Figure 1). Additional CT scans with three-dimensional reconstruction were performed in 18/33 patients for further assessment of malunion, articular incongruence, and bone stock quality. A $^{99m}$Tc-bone scan was performed in one patient to exclude the presence of active infection. The most recent radiographs were reviewed by a senior of us (I.T.) not involved in the initial treatment to determine the presence of periprosthetic loosening and heterotopic ossification and to evaluate the stem properties and greater tuberosity position.

## 3. Surgical Technique

Our surgical technique was similar to that original described by Neer [5, 17]. As there were not any preoperative indications or intraoperative findings of severe glenoid degeneration, all patients were managed with shoulder hemiarthroplasty without glenoid replacement. Two types of prosthetic implants were used (Neer II and Biomet). The deltopectoral approach was used in all cases. In 9 cases, diffuse adhesive capsulitis was noted requiring extended capsular release for achieving a functional range of motion. Full-thickness rotator cuff tears were noted in 4 cases (2 of supraspinatus tendon and two of both supraspinatus and infraspinatus tendons), whereas partial-thickness tears was detected in 7 cases; all tears were repaired with non-absorbable Ethibond-2 sutures. The biceps tendon was normal in 20 cases, frayed or degenerative in 11, and complete ruptured in 2 cases. Biceps tenodesis was performed in 8 cases. Greater tuberosity osteotomy was performed in 7 cases and double osteotomy of both tuberosities in 3 cases. Two to three pairs of heavy nonabsorbable sutures (Ethibond no.5) were applied to each tuberosity near the insertion of the adjacent tendon prior to removal of the humeral head. The later was carefully showed off in its anatomical neck, and the humeral canal was prepared without aggressive reaming. Two 2.7 mm drill-holes were created in each side of the diaphysis both laterally and medially, and two pair of sutures were placed for tuberosity fixation. Humeral component was placed after cementing the canal at the appropriate height, with 30°–35° of retroversion. Tuberosity fixation was performed thereafter with the horizontal intertuberosity sutures incorporated to the lateral fins of the prosthesis and the vertical diaphyseal tuberosity sutures in a cruciate tension band fashion that ensures stable fixation of the construct and adequate balance of the adjacent rotator cuff tendons. Additional cancellous bone grafting was placed into the proximal humeral space in 6 cases for filling the spaces between the implant and the tuberosities. Finally, the rotator cuff interval was closed with

Table 1: Overview of clinical data.

| Patient name | Age, gender | Side | Type of fracture | Initial treatment or reoperation | Time from injury to arthroplasty/m | Type of sequelae operative findings | Followup (months) | Constant score | | Pain scale | |
|---|---|---|---|---|---|---|---|---|---|---|---|
| | | | | | | | | Preop | Fup (*) | Preop | Fup |
| (1) KE | 38, m | R | 4-part | SF, capsular release | 36 | AVN, M, RCT | 84 | 55 | 80 (45%) | 4 | 9 |
| (2) TH | 62, m | R | 3-part | SF, PLO | 12 | N, RCT, GTO, LTO | 92 | 47 | 80 (70%) | 5 | 10 |
| (3) SB | 67, f | R | 2-part surg. neck | SF | 7 | AVN | 90 | 45 | 80 (70%) | 3 | 9 |
| (4) LX | 72, f | R | 3-part disloc. | PLO, HDR (elsewhere) | 18 | N, EO, BL | 96 | 48 | 80 (66%) | 2 | 10 |
| (5) KI | 49, m | R | No specified | SWO (elsewhere) | 7 | AVN, M, HMF, GTO | 72 | 56 | 90 (60.7%) | 5 | 10 |
| (6) TP | 47, f | R | No specified | PLO (elsewhere) | 28 | AVN, M, HMF | 65 | 55 | 81 (47%) | 4 | 9 |
| (7) MH | 53, m | R | 4-part fr/dis | C (elsewhere) | 2 | M, EO, GTO | 70 | 45 | 65 (44%) | 5 | 6 |
| (8) XE | 72, f | L | 4-part fr/dis | SF | 13 | M, RCT | 92 | 55 | 75 (36%) | 4 | 8 |
| (9) KM | 77, f | L | 4-part fr/dis | C (elsewhere) | 4 | M, EO, | 90 | 43 | 86 (100%) | 5 | 9 |
| (10) MB | 70, f | R | 4-part | C (elsewhere) | 32 | AVN, EO | 91 | 47 | 85 (80%) | 4 | 10 |
| (11) LB | 67, f | L | No specified | SWO + IMW (elsewhere) | 32 | AVN, M, GTO, LTO | 86 | 45 | 85 (88%) | 2 | 8 |
| (12) DX | 50, f | L | No specified | PLO (elsewhere) | 5 | M, HMF, BL | 92 | 35 | 83 (100%) | 3 | 9 |
| (13) AF | 35, m | R | 4-part | C (elsewhere) | 2 | AVN | 75 | 52 | 87 (67%) | 5 | 10 |
| (14) PE | 61, f | R | 4-part disloc. | C (elsewhere) | 4 | AVN | 65 | 54 | 79 (46%) | 3 | 7 |
| (15) BN | 34, m | R | 4-part | C (elsewhere) | 2 | AVN, M | 61 | 51 | 82 (40%) | 4 | 8 |
| (16) ZS | 83, m | R | 3-part disloc | C (elsewhere) | 2 | M, GTO, LTO | 80 | 43 | 70 (62%) | 3 | 9 |
| (17) DM | 68, f | L | 4-part disloc. | C (elsewhere) | 3 | M, AVN, EO | 89 | 44 | 78 (77%) | 3 | 7 |
| (18) TE | 62, f | R | 2-part surg. neck | C (elsewhere) | 4 | M, EO | 85 | 52 | 76 (46%) | 4 | 8 |
| (19) TB | 65, m | L | 3-part | C (elsewhere) | 12 | M, AVN, GTO | 92 | 54 | 65 (20%) | 5 | 9 |
| (20) KE | 62, f | L | 4-part | PLO, infection, HDR | 40 | AVN, M, RCT | 85 | 47 | 55 (17%) | 4 | 3 |
| (21) AB | 59, m | R | 4-part | C (elsewhere) | 6 | M, AVN, BL, EO | 77 | 53 | 75 (41%) | 5 | 10 |
| (22) KX | 48, m | R | PLFD, neglected | McLaughlin procedure | 24 | D, RCT, block of rotation | 96 | 38 | 70 (84%) | 5 | 8 |

Table 1: Continued.

| Patient name | Age, gender | Side | Type of fracture | Initial treatment or reoperation | Time from injury to arthroplasty/m | Type of sequelae operative findings | Followup (months) | Constant score | | Pain scale | |
|---|---|---|---|---|---|---|---|---|---|---|---|
| | | | | | | | | Preop | Fup (*) | Preop | Fup |
| (23) FT | 34, m | R | PLFD, neglected | C (elsewhere) | 15 | D, block of rotation | 89 | 47 | 85 (80%) | 5 | 8 |
| (24) PE | 67, f | L | 3-part | C (elsewhere) | 12 | M, AVN, GTO | 88 | 30 | 32 (6%) | 4 | 0 |
| (25) KM | 59, m | R | 4-part | SF | 21 | AVN | 64 | 43 | 54 (25%) | 5 | 5 |
| (26) AA | 70, f | R | 4-part | PLO (elsewhere) | 2 | M, EO | 72 | 47 | 82 (75%) | 4 | 8 |
| (27) DB | 61, f | L | 3-part | C (elsewhere) | 7 | N, EO | 91 | 49 | 80 (63%) | 5 | 9 |
| (28) TA | 46, m | R | 4-part | SF | 14 | AVN | 80 | 52 | 82 (57%) | 4 | 9 |
| (29) MX | 44, f | L | 4-part | PLO (elsewhere) | 8 | N, AVN, EO | 80 | 50 | 77 (54%) | 3 | 7 |
| (30) KP | 62, m | R | PLFD, neglected | C (elsewhere) | 13 | D, block of rotation | 67 | 42 | 76 (80%) | 5 | 8 |
| (31) TE | 49, m | L | 4-part | PLO | 11 | AVN | 84 | 53 | 85 (60%) | 5 | 8 |
| (32) DS | 60, f | R | 4-part | C (elsewhere) | 3 | AVN, M | 90 | 52 | 67 (29%) | 3 | 6 |
| (33) KS | 65, f | R | 3-part | PLO | 18 | AVN | 91 | 54 | 74 (37%) | 4 | 8 |

C: conservative treatment, D: dislocation, SF: suturing fixation, PLO: plate-osteosynthesis, M: malunion, N: nonunion, AVN: avascular necrosis, RCT: rotator cuff tear, EO: ectopic ossification, GTO: greater tuberosity osteotomy, LTO: lesser tuberosity osteotomy, HDR: hardware removal, BL: bone loss, SWO: screw-wiring osteosynthesis, HMF: hard material failure, IMW: intramedullary wiring, and PLFD: posterior "locked" fracture dislocation.

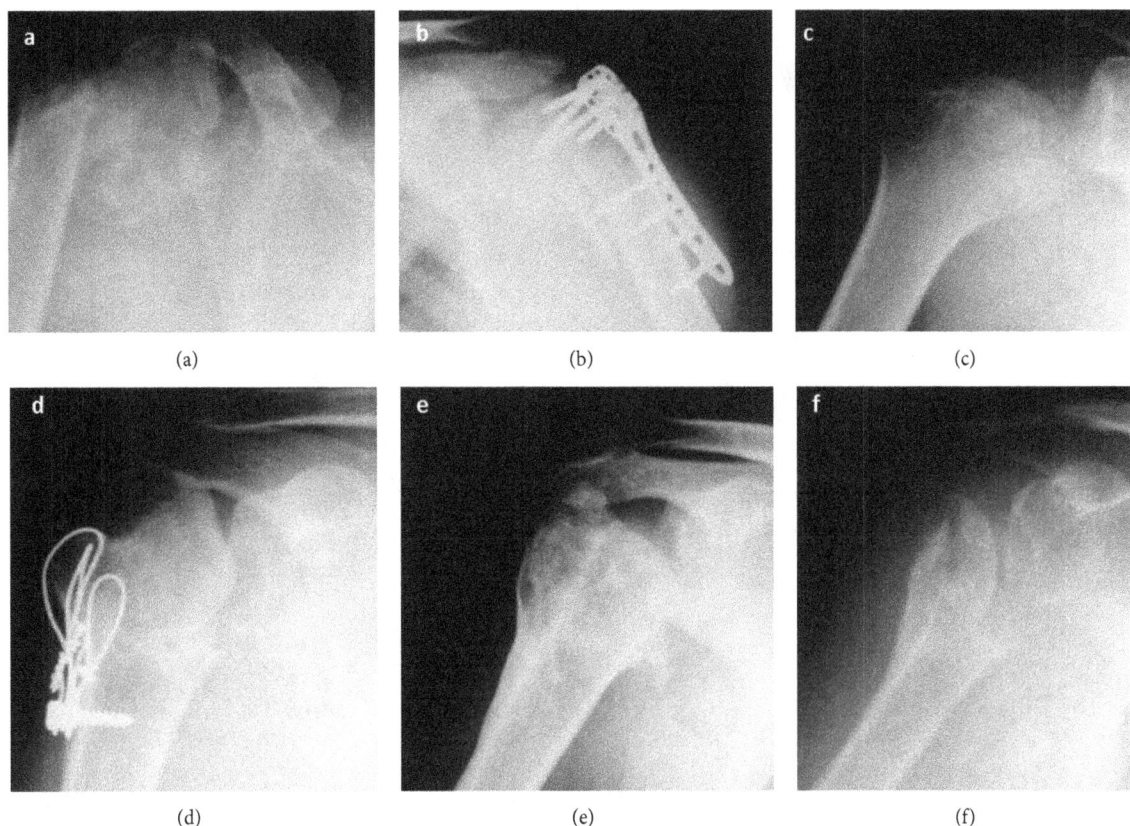

FIGURE 1: Types of sequelae of proximal humeral fractures after initial treatment. (a) Conservative, (b) plate osteosynthesi, (c) neglected locked posterior dislocation, (d) screw-wiring osteosynthesis, and (e) and (f) transosseous suturing [16].

separate sutures and the deltopectoral space with absorbable sutures in a figure of eight manner. The arm was rested in internal rotation in a simple sling with the elbow at the side for 4–6 weeks or was immobilized in abduction in a special brace if a full-thickness rotator cuff or tuberosity osteotomy had been performed.

A closely monitored 3-phase rehabilitation program given to all patients initially consisted of pendulum exercises starting on the 2nd postoperative day until the 3rd to 4th postoperative week. The second phase includes passive assisted exercises in the supine position as the patient is trying to reach the bed, supporting his injured shoulder by the healthy arm or special designed sticks. Until the 6th to the 7th postoperative week, forward elevation and external rotation are performed in the supine position while internal rotation in the standing one with the aid of sticks. As the union of the tuberosities is completed, active exercises using gradually increased weights (starting from 1 kg) are administered until the 10th to the 12th postoperative week. If the patient was capable of forward elevating three kilos in the supine position, active dynamic shoulder motion, and strengthening exercises are administered in the standing position until the 5th to the 6th postoperative month. Preservation of shoulder motion and strength is maintained for another 3 to 4 months. The patient is seen every single week for the first 2 to 3 postoperative months and is instructed and guided by us.

We believe that a simple prescription of physiotherapy does not help the patient as much as this close and monitoring consultation with his surgeon.

## 4. Results

The mean followup period was 82.5 months (range, 61 to 96 months). The median Constant score was 75.7 points, improved by 60% in comparison to preoperative values (mean, 47.9 points). In the pain analogue scale, there was an averaged improvement from 4 to 8 points. According to our criteria, the result was excellent in nine patients, very good in eleven, moderate in ten and unsatisfactory in four. Active forward elevation increased from 56 degrees to 100 degrees, active external rotation increased from 12 degrees to 35 degrees, and finally, active internal rotation increased from the ability of the thumb to reach the sacrum (range, greater trochanter to the first lumbar vertebral body) to the second lumbar vertebral body (range, trochanter to T7). Sixty per cent of the patients were able to do activities up to shoulder level compared with 24% before arthroplasty (Figure 2). Overall, 79% of the patients were satisfied with the final outcome and said that they would repeat the operation in similar circumstances (Figures 2, 3, and 4).

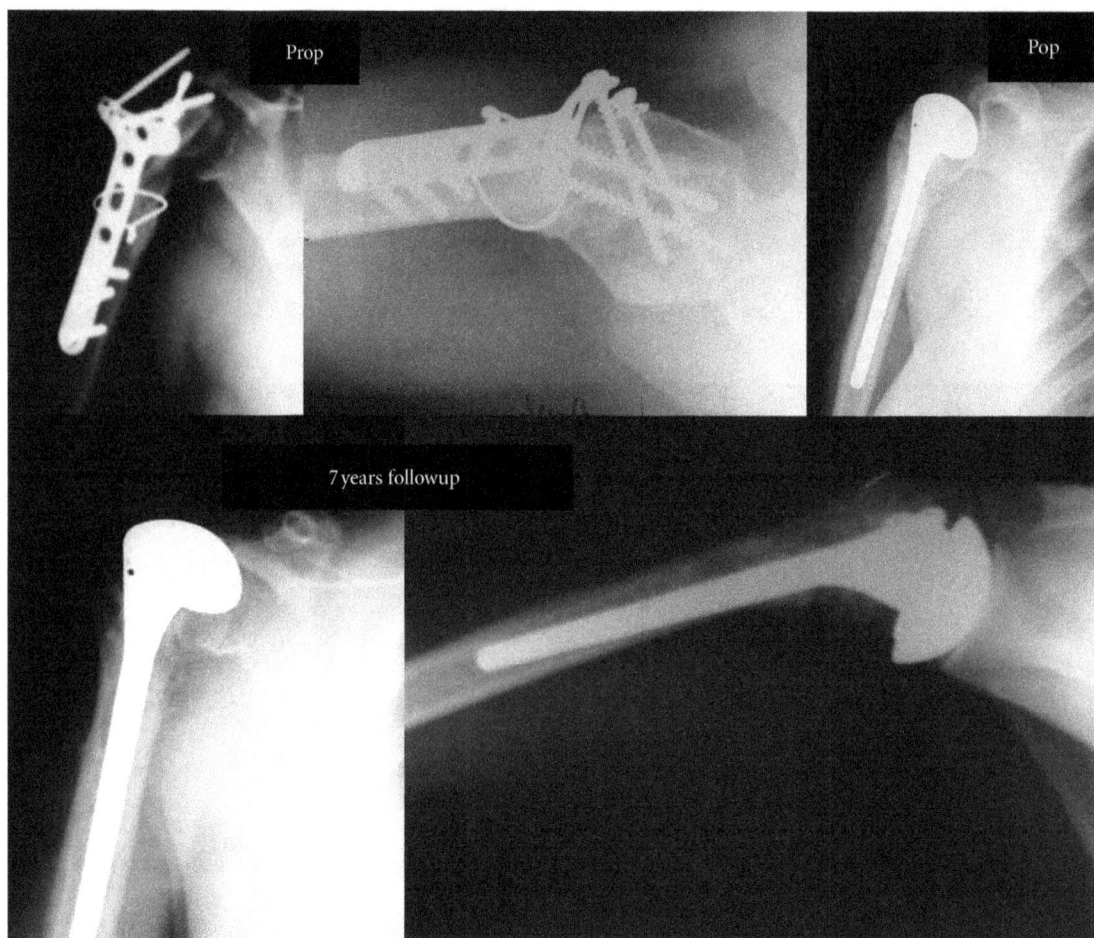

FIGURE 2: Patient no. 31: hemiarthroplasty after failed internal fixation with plate-screws osteosynthesis. Very good radiological and clinical result (Constant score = 85) seven years postoperatively.

Periprosthetic ossification was present in 7 cases. It was minimal in 4 cases, predominant at the humeral side in 2, and near the glenoid in 1. All the humeral implants were normally positioned, except two that were placed in valgus orientation. Slight upward positioning of the implant was noted in three cases and partial anterior subluxation in two. Early loss of greater tuberosity fixation or GT nonunion was not noted, but osteolysis was detected in 3 cases and malunion in two who expressed an unsatisfactory outcome. Four humeral components had radiolucent lines without evidence of loosening.

## 5. Discussion

Complications after proximal humeral fracture fixation are some of the most difficult situations to manage in shoulder reconstruction. An anticipated and reliable functional result is difficult to obtain because of the complexity of bone pathology and the impaired soft tissue envelope, especially if the patient had already undergone surgery. The surgeon has to deal with malunion, nonunion or AVN of the proximal humerus, displacement of the tuberosities, rotator cuff tears, and associated soft-tissue contractures. In the presence of

sever osteoporosis, significant bone loss, articular incongruity, and glenoid erosion, the only indication is prosthetic replacement of the proximal humerus. Generally, a satisfactory result may be expected in 20% to 75% of the cases, with pain relief obtained in more than 85% [6, 18, 19]. Kontakis et al. [3] in a systematic review of 810 early hemiarthroplasties in 808 patients for proximal humeral fractures not only concluded that most patients had no pain or only mild pain but also that the level of function before injury was almost never regained. In the present study of late hemiarthroplasties for proximal humeral fractures, 29/33 patients had a good or acceptable, even moderate outcome, whereas improvement of pain was up to 80%.

The results of shoulder replacement for old trauma are much less favorable than those of primary osteoarthritis or hemiarthroplasty performed for acute fractures [6, 20, 21]. Fevang et al. [22] in a large series of 1.825 shoulder arthroplasties of the Norwegian Registry found that the risk of revision was the highest for patients with sequelae after fracture compared to those with acute fractures. Several other factors have been proposed to alter final outcome such as the age of the patient, initial treatment (conservative or surgical), the type of the sequelae (malunion, nonunion, AVN, and

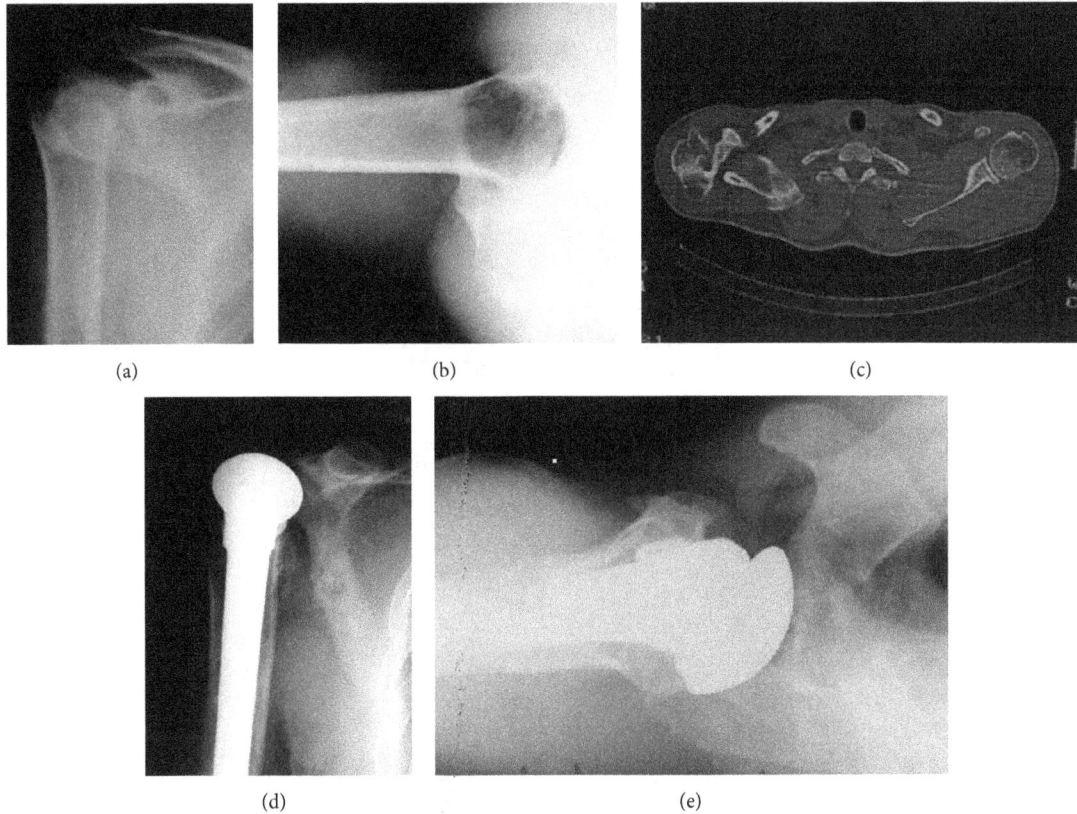

FIGURE 3: Patient no. 30: neglected posterior locked dislocation treated conservatively elsewhere. Very good result 5.5 years postoperatively with a Constant score of 76 points.

glenoid erosion), the need for tuberosity osteotomy, associated rotator cuff tears, and the condition of soft tissues.

In contrast to similar reports [16, 22, 23], the age of the patient did not influence the final outcome in the present study. Bosch et al. [24] stated that what seems to be more important for rehabilitation is the cooperation and mental status of patients, rather than their age. If the patient is closed monitored and instructed by his surgeon the results are more predictable, because the physiotherapy can be focused to the most impaired function.

Norris et al. [14] emphasized the crucial role of the initial fracture treatment for the final results of arthroplasty; the patients who had been managed conservatively had a better result than those who have been operated. We did not notice any difference in our study regarding the initial treatment. From the 17 cases that had been treated operatively, six were managed solely with transosseous sutures, and the consequences of sequelae of the proximal humerus were minimal. Accordingly, these patients were closed monitored as they had received initial treatment in our department, and a good rate of shoulder motion had been achieved prior to arthroplasty; four of them had signs of AVN, and their main complain was pain and not restriction of motion. On the other hand, most of the patients that had been managed in other centers with metallic internal fixation referred to us also for their pain due to AVN or nonunion. Finally, most of the patients that had been treated conservatively elsewhere showed moderate or severe malunion, but as they referred to us early (2-3 months later), the quality of bone, soft tissues, and rotator cuff tendons were less disturbed.

The type of complication after failed initial treatment of a proximal humerus fracture is considered as a crucial factor for the final outcome [6, 20, 25]. Dines et al. [15] reported better results in fractures with AVN in comparison to nonunited or malunited fractures. The present study showed that the results were slightly better in fractures that had complicated mainly with AVN, but the difference was not important. A satisfactory outcome was noted also in all the three cases with neglected posterior "locked" fracture dislocations. The average functional improvement was up to 84%, a result similar to Neer [17] who reported excellent results in 76% of the patients with postdislocation arthropathy.

Glenoid replacement is another predisposing factor of the final outcome [26, 27]. Dines et al. [15] in a recent study of modular prosthesis showed a better result for hemiarthroplasty, in contrast to total shoulder replacement. The survivorship analysis of Fevang et al. [22] showed that for hemiprostheses, the major cause of revision was pain, seen in 15 of 439 cases with rheumatoid arthritis but in none of the 422 cases with acute fractures. None of our patients received total shoulder replacement, although mild erosion of the glenoid was detected in two of them. We do not suggest glenoid replacement even in cases with slight abnormal

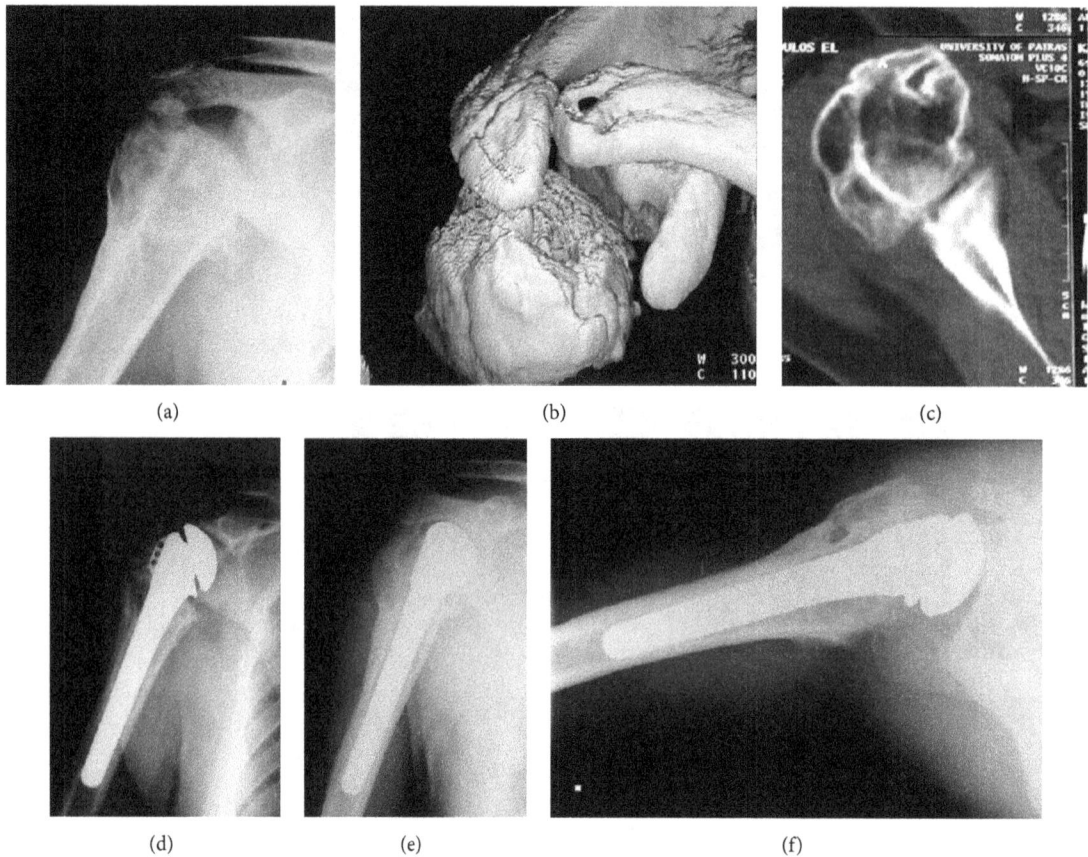

(a)                                                          (b)                                                          (c)

(d)                                                          (e)                                                          (f)

FIGURE 4: Patient no. 1: AVN of the humeral head after trasosseous suturing fixation for a 4-part valgus impacted fracture initially managed to our department. Anteroposterior radiographs in external and internal rotation showed excellent tuberosity healing 7 years postoperatively, although there were slight upward migration of the prosthesis and eccentric position in the axillary view. Despite that, the patient was clinically pain free with a Constant score of 80 points.

cartilage degeneration, especially when the condition of soft tissues and rotator cuff tendons are severely disturbed.

Finally, the negative effect of tuberosity osteotomy and subsequent malunion and/or nonunion in prosthetic replacement of the shoulder has been suggested by many authors [6–8, 21, 24, 28]. Neer [17] has already suggested that in borderline malunions it is better to use prosthesis with a small stem and a small head, in a varus position, to avoid having to perform a greater tuberosity osteotomy. Franta et al. [29] in a multifactorial analysis of 282 unsatisfactory arthroplasties reported that patients with a proximal humerus nonunion were at 20 times greater risk for tuberosity failure than all other diagnoses. In addition, tuberosity failure was found to be significantly associated with humeral component loosening. In the present study, GT osteotomy was performed in 7/33 cases, but only two patients had unsatisfactory results. The amount of GT osteotomy and mainly the type and adequacy of fixation seem to influence the final outcome.

Our study has several limitations: the number of involved patients is quite small, and although have been managed similarly they represent a mixed group of various sequelae of proximal humeral fractures including both conservative and operative treated cases. One can expect better results in

the first group as well as in those patients treated with head preserving surgery, but this was not true in our study and statistical differences could not be established. Furthermore, the data were derived from only one practice with great experience in shoulder reconstruction and, as such, may not be generalizable to all practices.

## 6. Conclusion

Shoulder hemiarthroplasty for management of posttraumatic complications of fracture of the proximal humerus is a technically demanding procedure with unpredictable results. The high rate of complications is often related to technical difficulties, a scarred deltoid, adhesions of rotator cuff tendons, and malunion of the tuberosities. Careful selection of the patients, detail preoperative planning, and meticulous surgical technique are essential elements for a successful outcome. The postoperative rehabilitation program should be modified based on the surgical findings and the technique used. In this manner, certain possible secondary complications could be avoided, and the long-term results will be more favorable.

# References

[1] L. U. Bigliani and G. M. McCluskey III, "Prosthetic replacement in acute fractures of the proximal humerus," *Seminars in Arthroplasty*, vol. 1, no. 2, pp. 129–137, 1990.

[2] P. Dimakopoulos, N. Potamitis, and E. Lambiris, "Hemiarthroplasty in the treatment of comminuted intraarticular fractures of the proximal humerus," *Clinical Orthopaedics and Related Research*, no. 341, pp. 7–11, 1997.

[3] G. Kontakis, C. Koutras, T. Tosounidis, and P. Giannoudis, "Early management of proximal humeral fractures with hemiarthroplasty: a systematic review," *Journal of Bone and Joint Surgery B*, vol. 90, no. 11, pp. 1407–1413, 2008.

[4] B. D. Solberg, C. N. Moon, D. P. Franco, and G. D. Paiement, "Surgical treatment of three and four-part proximal humeral fractures," *Journal of Bone and Joint Surgery A*, vol. 91, no. 7, pp. 1689–1697, 2009.

[5] C. S. Neer II, "Displaced proximal humeral fractures. II. Treatment of three-part and four-part displacement," *Journal of Bone and Joint Surgery A*, vol. 52, no. 6, pp. 1090–1103, 1970.

[6] P. Boileau, C. Trojani, G. Walch, S. G. Krishnan, A. Romeo, and R. Sinnerton, "Shoulder arthroplasty for the treatment of the sequelae of fractures of the proximal humerus," *Journal of Shoulder and Elbow Surgery*, vol. 10, no. 4, pp. 299–308, 2001.

[7] J. Liu, S. H. Li, Z. D. Cai et al., "Outcomes, and factors affecting outcomes, following shoulder hemiarthroplasty for proximal humeral fracture repair," *Journal of Orthopaedic Science*, vol. 16, pp. 565–572, 2011.

[8] E. Farng, D. Zingmond, L. Krenek, and N. F. SooHoo, "Factors predicting complication rates after primary shoulder arthroplasty," *Journal of Shoulder and Elbow Surgery*, vol. 20, no. 4, pp. 557–563, 2011.

[9] B. Schliemann, J. Siemoneit, Ch. Theisen, C. Kösters, A. Weimann, and M. J. Raschke, "Complex fractures of the proximal humerus in the elderly–outcome and complications after locking plate fixation," *Musculoskeletal Surgery*, vol. 96, supplement 1, pp. S3–S11, 2012.

[10] P. Helwig, C. Bahrs, B. Epple, J. Oehm, C. Eingartner, and K. Weise, "Does fixed-angle plate osteosynthesis solve the problems of a fractured proximal humerus? A prospective series of 87 patients," *Acta Orthopaedica*, vol. 80, no. 1, pp. 92–96, 2009.

[11] A. Misra, R. Kapur, and N. Maffulli, "Complex proximal humeral fractures in adults—a systematic review of management," *Injury*, vol. 32, no. 5, pp. 363–372, 2001.

[12] J. E. Bell, B. C. Leung, K. F. Spratt et al., "Trends and variation in incidence, surgical treatment, and repeat surgery of proximal humeral fractures in the elderly," *Journal of Bone and Joint Surgery A*, vol. 93, no. 2, pp. 121–131, 2011.

[13] D. Krappinger, N. Bizzotto, S. Riedmann, C. Kammerlander, C. Hengg, and F. S. Kralinger, "Predicting failure after surgical fixation of proximal humerus fractures," *Injury*, vol. 42, pp. 1283–1288, 2011.

[14] T. R. Norris, A. Green, and F. X. McGuigan, "Late prosthetic shoulder arthroplasty for displaced proximal humerus fractures," *Journal of Shoulder and Elbow Surgery*, vol. 4, no. 4, pp. 271–280, 1995.

[15] D. Dines, R. Warren, D. Altchek, and B. Moeckel, "Posttraumatic changes of the proximal humerus: malunion, nonunion, and osteonecrosis -treatment with modular hemiarthroplasty or total shoulder arthroplasty," *Journal of Shoulder and Elbow Surgery*, vol. 2, pp. 11–21, 1993.

[16] P. Dimakopoulos, A. Panagopoulos, and G. Kasimatis, "Transosseous suture fixation of proximal humeral fractures: surgical technique," *Journal of Bone and Joint Surgery A*, vol. 91, supplement 2, part 1, pp. 8–21, 2009.

[17] C. S. Neer II, "Glenohumeral arthroplasty," in *Shoulder Reconstruction*, C. S. Neer II, Ed., pp. 143–269, Saunders, Philadelphia, Pa, USA, 1990.

[18] S. A. Antuña, J. W. Sperling, J. Sánchez-Sotelo, and R. H. Cofield, "Shoulder arthroplasty for proximal humeral malunions: long-term results," *Journal of Shoulder and Elbow Surgery*, vol. 11, no. 2, pp. 122–129, 2002.

[19] P. K. Beredjiklian, J. P. Iannotti, T. R. Norris, and G. R. Williams, "Operative treatment of malunion of a fracture of the proximal aspect of the humerus," *Journal of Bone and Joint Surgery A*, vol. 80, no. 10, pp. 1484–1497, 1998.

[20] P. Mansat, M. R. Guity, Y. Bellumore, and M. Mansat, "Shoulder arthroplasty for late sequelae of proximal humeral fractures," *Journal of Shoulder and Elbow Surgery*, vol. 13, no. 3, pp. 305–312, 2004.

[21] C. A. Compito, E. B. Self, and L. U. Bigliani, "Arthroplasty and acute shoulder trauma: reasons for success and failure," *Clinical Orthopaedics and Related Research*, no. 307, pp. 27–36, 1994.

[22] B. T. Fevang, S. A. Lie, L. I. Havelin, A. Skredderstuen, and O. Furnes, "Risk factors for revision after shoulder arthroplasty: 1,825 shoulder arthroplasties from the Norwegian Arthroplasty Register," *Acta Orthopaedica*, vol. 80, no. 1, pp. 83–91, 2009.

[23] F. Kralinger, R. Schwaiger, M. Wambacher et al., "Outcome after primary hemiarthroplasty for fracture of the head of the humerus," *Journal of Bone and Joint Surgery B*, vol. 86, no. 2, pp. 217–219, 2004.

[24] U. Bosch, M. Skutek, R. W. Fremerey, and H. Tscherne, "Outcome after primary and secondary hemiarthroplasty in elderly patients with fractures of the proximal humerus," *Journal of Shoulder and Elbow Surgery*, vol. 7, no. 5, pp. 479–484, 1998.

[25] J. P. Ianotti and M. L. Sidor, "Malunions of the proximal humerus," in *Complex and Revision Problems in Shoulder Surgery*, J. P. Warner, J. P. Ianotti, and C. Gerber, Eds., pp. 245–264, Lippincott-Raven, Philadelphia, Pa, USA, 1997.

[26] I. M. Parsons, P. J. Millett, and J. J. P. Warner, "Glenoid wear after shoulder hemiarthroplasty: quantitative radiographic analysis," *Clinical Orthopaedics and Related Research*, no. 421, pp. 120–125, 2004.

[27] R. M. Carroll, R. Izquierdo, M. Vazquez, T. A. Blaine, W. N. Levine, and L. U. Bigliani, "Conversion of painful hemiarthroplasty to total shoulder arthroplasty: long-term results," *Journal of Shoulder and Elbow Surgery*, vol. 13, no. 6, pp. 599–603, 2004.

[28] J. S. Coste, C. Trojani, P. M. Ahrens, and P. Boileau, "Humeral prosthesis for fracture: analysis of tuberosity complications," *Journal of Bone & Joint Surgery, British Volume*, vol. 86, supplement 1, p. 29, 2004.

[29] A. K. Franta, T. R. Lenters, D. Mounce, B. Neradilek, and F. A. Matsen III, "The complex characteristics of 282 unsatisfactory shoulder arthroplasties," *Journal of Shoulder and Elbow Surgery*, vol. 16, no. 5, pp. 555–562, 2007.

# 15

# Pirogow's Amputation: A Modification of the Operation Method

**M. Bueschges,**[1] **T. Muehlberger,**[2] **K. L. Mauss,**[1] **J. C. Bruck,**[3] **and C. Ottomann**[1]

[1] *Sektion für Plastische Chirurgie und Handchirurgie, Intensiveinheit für Schwerbrandverletzte,*
   *Universitätsklinikum Schleswig Holstein Campus Lübeck, Ratzeburger Allee 160, 23560 Lübeck, Germany*
[2] *Abteilung für Plastische Chirurgie, DRK Kliniken Berlin, Berlin, Germany*
[3] *Abteilung für Plastische Chirurgie, Martin Luther Krankenhaus, Caspar-Theyß-Straße 27-31, Grunewald, 14193 Berlin, Germany*

Correspondence should be addressed to M. Bueschges; michaelbueschges@gmx.de

Academic Editor: Patrizio Petrone

*Introduction.* Pirogow's amputation at the ankle presents a valuable alternative to lower leg amputation for patients with the corresponding indications. Although this method offers the ability to stay mobile without the use of a prosthesis, it is rarely performed. This paper proposes a modification regarding the operation method of the Pirogow amputation. The results of the modified operation method on ten patients were objectified 12 months after the operation using a patient questionnaire (Ankle Score). *Material and Methods.* We modified the original method by rotating the calcaneus. To fix the calcaneus to the tibia, Kirschner wire and a 3/0 spongiosa tension screw as well as a Fixateur externe were used. *Results.* 70% of those questioned who were amputated following the modified Pirogow method indicated an excellent or very good result in total points whereas in the control group (original Pirogow's amputation) only 40% reported excellent or very good result. In addition, the level of pain experienced one year after the completed operation showed different results in favour of the group being operated with the modified way. Furthermore, patients in both groups showed differences in radiological results, postoperative leg length difference, and postoperative mobility. *Conclusion.* The modified Pirogow amputation presents a valuable alternative to the original amputation method for patients with the corresponding indications. The benefits are found in the significantly reduced pain, difference in reduced radiological complications, the increase in mobility without a prosthesis, and the reduction of postoperative leg length difference.

## 1. Introduction

In his original article from 1854, Nikolai Iwanowitsch Pirogow reported on hundreds of lower limb amputations he carried out during the Crimean war [1] (Figure 1). The Crimean war was fought between Imperial Russia on one side and an alliance of France, the United Kingdom, the Kingdom of Sardinia, and the Ottoman Empire on the other. The goal of the anti-Russian alliance was to break the Russian position of power around the Black Sea and to put a halt to Russian expansion into the Balkan territory of the Ottoman Empire. The war broke out in 1853 on the Crimean peninsula and ended in 1856 with Russia's loss. The battles fought were not the only cause of the numerous lives lost during the war. Medical care during the war was incredibly substandard, causing the British nurse Florence Nightingale to construct and reorganize numerous military hospitals and care stations.

The Crimean war saw an increased use of mines, and injuries to the foot and leg were becoming a more common occurrence. Due to this fact, Pirogow independently searched for a way to avoid an amputation of the limb below the knee [2]. He developed a method of amputation at the level of the ankle, which offers the patient a variety of benefits compared to the previously used transtibial amputation [3]. This method of amputation at the ankle reduced the mortality rate, which at that time laid between 25% and 50% of patients undergoing lower leg amputation [4]. A further important benefit was the significantly decreased difference in leg length, which allowed the patient to be mobile without the use of a prosthesis [5]. Due to the low level of prosthetic care at the time, this significantly reduced the patient's level of disability. In the scope of a Pirogow amputation, the average difference in leg length in comparison to the healthy extremity amounts to 2.8 cm [6]. Due to the fact that the original literature from

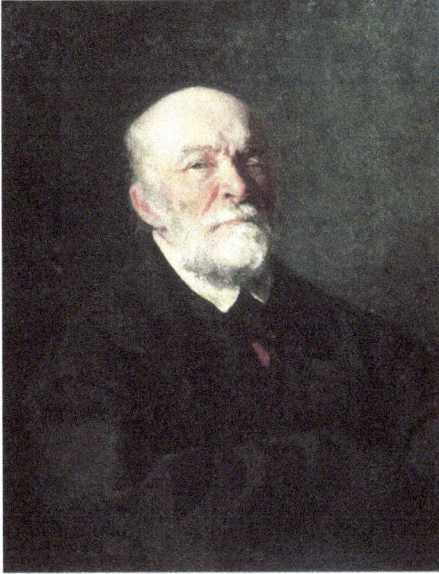

Figure 1: Nikolai Iwanowitsch Pirogow painted by Ilja Jefimowitsch Repin, 1881.

Table 1: Indications and contraindications for an amputation following the Pirogow method [6, 7].

| Indications | Contraindications |
| --- | --- |
| Congenital foot deformity | Severe circulatory problems |
| Forefoot and metatarsal damage due to soft tissue or bone tumors | Open lesions or traumatic damage in the area of the heel and calcaneus |
| Osteomyelitis | Severe immune suppression, cachexy |
| Burns and frostbite | Acute and chronic infections of the ankle and hindfoot |
| Persistent ulcerating soft tissue defects stemming from cardiovascular diseases | Low prospects regarding the expected walking ability |
| Forefoot and metatarsal damage through trauma | Haemodynamically relevant stenosis or closure of the anterior tibialis |

## 2. Indications and Contraindications of the Pirogow Method of Amputation

The indications and contraindications of the Pirogow method of amputation are listed in Table 1.

*2.1. Surgical Technique.* It is recommended to perform an angiography on patients to show the supply of blood to the lower extremities in the heel area when an intact perfusion of the tibialis posterior is doubted. The goal of the amputation technique presented is the complete preservation of the plantar fascia and a large part of the calcaneus in order to preserve the full length of the leg, the mechanically stable skin of the heel with preservation of the original sensation, and the subcutaneous tissue in this area as a contact surface that is well cushioned against shear force and walking processes [9]. Disruptions to wound healing during the postoperative phase are mostly attributable to disrupted circulation in the plantar fascia, and a failure of the calcaneus to fuse with the tibia, which is why a nontraumatic operational technique protecting the tibialis posterior as much as possible, can be seen as a prerequisite [10]. A modified fish-mouth incision is drawn. Two points 1 cm plantar and ventral to the lateral and medial malleolus serve as key points of the incision. These points are joined plantarly and dorsally and result in the edges of the excision, angled to the thigh at 90°. It is recommended to leave at least 6 cm soft tissue of the sole to allow for the wound edges to be reduced as needed during the course of the operation. One begins with the incision at the dorsal marking between the key points along the fascia. The tendons of the foot extensor including the m. tibialis anterior are shortened. The a. dorsalis pedis or the a. tibialis anterior, if necessary, are ligated during the course of the procedure. After the plantar incision is made, the n. suralis and the n. tibialis should be cut through as proximally as possible. Afterward the plantar fascia as well as the foot flexors should be cut while under traction. Afterwards, the midtarsal joint is disarticulated [11]. In order to remove the talus bone, the anterior talocalcaneal ligament deep in the sinus tarsi

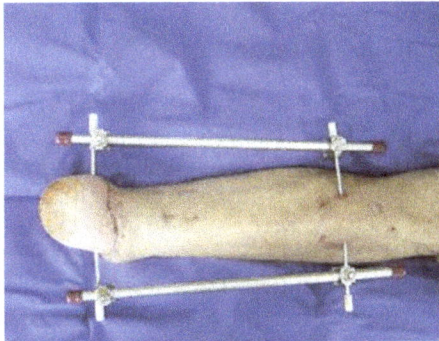

Figure 2: Temporary fixation by fixateur externe.

Pirogow was not written in English, this method spread very slowly [7]. Even today this method is only rarely performed. A publication by AOK Germany from 2003 indicated that out of a total of 44,000 amputations on lower extremities performed, an amputation based on the Pirogow method was only carried out 44 times, which amounts to only 0.1% [8]. In contrast, a lower leg amputation was performed 8321 times in 2003, which amounts to 18% [8]. The authors claim that the original method of Pirogow's amputation can be advanced by rotating and fixing the calcaneus and by obtaining the operation goal by fixing the bones with a Fixateur externe (Figure 2).

Whether these modifications in Pirogow amputation were truly beneficial, ten patients were investigated postoperatively using a questionnaire. These results were compared to a control group of ten patients who were amputated using the original method.

TABLE 2: Modified Ankle and Hindfoot Score (AOFAS) with consideration given to the lack of ankle function and more weight given to functional and radiological criteria based on Taniguchi (Ankle Score) [15].

| Criteria | Assessment (point total) | | | |
|---|---|---|---|---|
| Pain | Pain free (40) | Light (30) | Moderate (20) | Strong (10) |
| Functional criteria | | | | |
|    Walking distance | Unrestricted (20) | 2 km (15) | 500 m–2 km (10) | At home (5) |
|    Limping | | No Limping (4) | Moderate (2) | Unable to walk (0) |
|    Going up stairs | | Unrestricted (4) | Holding the railing (2) | N.m. (0) |
|    Going down stairs | | Unrestricted (4) | Holding the railing (2) | N.m. (0) |
|    Standing on one leg | | Unrestricted (4) | With support (2) | N.m. (0) |
|    Cross-legged | | Unrestricted (4) | With support (2) | N.m. (0) |
| Radiological criteria | | | | |
|    Bone atrophy | | None (5) | Trabecula atrophy (3) | Necrosis (0) |
|    Plantar soft tissue | | >2 cm (5) | 1-2 cm (3) | <1 cm (0) |
| Leg length difference | | None (5) | <2 cm (3) | >2 cm (0) |
| Mobility w/out a prosthesis | | Unrestricted (5) | >10 m (3) | <10 m (0) |
| Total points (100) | Excellent (>80) | Good (60–79) | Satisfactory (40–59) | Unsatisfactory (<40) |

must be cut through. Now, we modify the original method through anchoring the calcaneus by horizontally drilling a Steinmann nail 2 cm cranial and anterior to the calcaneal spur to allow the use of an external fixator. Additionally, a further Steinmann nail is drilled horizontally approx. 20 cm proximal through the front edge of the tibia. The calcaneus together with the plantar heel lobe is then turned at a 60–90 degree angle to correspond with the associated distal tibia surface, whereas Pirogow did not rotate the calcaneus. In order to achieve an adequate degree of rotation, it is advantageous to incise the Achilles tendon or cut it through completely [12]. As a further modification to ensure a stable bone jointment of tibia and calcaneus, a fixateur externe is used (Figure 2) and, after temporarily fixating the calcaneus to the tibia, osteosynthesis is carried out using a Kirschner wire and a 3/0 spongiosa tension screw. After ample haemostasis, the wound can be closed using strong and deep backstitch sutures upon inserting Redon drains.

*2.2. Prosthetic Care after Pirogow Amputation.* An interim prosthesis can be fitted after the fourth postoperative week. This enables the patient to become mobile with slight pressure to the stump before the bone has fully healed [13]. For the permanent prosthesis, we prefer to use an inside tube made from hardened foam, which is made form-fitting using a plaster mould and encompasses the entire lower leg. The prosthesis itself is made from a hard cover and a prosthetic foot is attached to the distal end. This enables the patient to wear normal shoes. From a biomechanical perspective, shear force as little as possible should be applied to the distal area of the amputated stump, especially in the first period of mobility, to prevent a dislocation of the calcaneus. The prosthetic shoe should be placed lightly lateral to the midline at the coronary level to enhance lateral stability. Permanent prosthetic care can be implemented upon removal of the external fixator, usually after the third postoperative month. Our experience shows that the mobilisation of the patient usually occurs

without problems. Even older patients quickly learn to walk with the prosthesis and rate the level of disability in everyday life as low [14].

## 3. Materials and Methods

Between the years 2000 and 2006, 27 patients were operated on in the Department of Plastic Surgery in the Martin Luther Hospital in Berlin. 20 of the 27 total patients amputated using the Pirogow method were included in the study 12 months after the operation and were evaluated using the Ankle Score from Taniguchi et al. [15]. Five of the seven patients included in the study had to undergo lower leg amputations due to postoperative complications (wound healing dysfunctions), and two patients could no longer be reached at the time of the followup 12 months after the amputation. The Ankle Score is based on the Ankle and Hindfoot Score from the American Orthopaedic Foot and Ankle Society (AOFAS) with regard to loss of ankle function and is more heavily weighted for functional and radiological criteria based on Taniguchi (Table 2). Using a point system, the criteria pain, functional and radiological assessment, difference in leg length, and mobility without a prosthesis were rated on a scale from 0 to 100. The functional assessment is divided into the categories walking range, limping, the ability to go up and down stairs, the ability to stand on one leg, and the ability to sit cross-legged. The radiological points are attributed based on the level of bone atrophy and the assessment of the plantar soft tissue layer. With regard to difference in leg length, the points are given based on length in cm, mobility without a prosthesis and based on the walking range. The maximum value possible is 100 points, and a value above 80 points is rated as an "excellent" result, a value between 60 and 79 points as a "good" result, between 40 and 59 points as an "satisfactory" result, and less than 40 points as a "unsatisfactory" result (Table 2). The Ankle Score Questionnaire was given to 10 patients 12 months (plus or minus 2 weeks) after undergoing

TABLE 3: The analysis of the Ankle Scores (AS) from the group of patients using the modified method based on Pirogow.

| Point total | Result | Number of patients | Percent |
|---|---|---|---|
| >80 | Excellent | 2 | 20% |
| 60–79 | Good | 5 | 50% |
| 40–59 | Satisfactory | 3 | 30% |
| <40 | Unsatisfactory | 1 | 10% |

TABLE 4: The analysis of the Ankle Scores (AS) from the group of patients that underwent the original Pirogow's amputation.

| Point total | Result | Number of patients | Percent |
|---|---|---|---|
| >80 | Excellent | 2 | 20% |
| 60–79 | Good | 2 | 20% |
| 40–59 | Satisfactory | 3 | 30% |
| <40 | Unsatisfactory | 3 | 30% |

the modified amputation based on the Pirogow method. The control group, consisting of 10 patients who underwent the original amputation, was given the same questionnaire in the same time frame (12-month follow-up).

# 4. Results

The average age of patients who underwent the modified amputation based on the Pirogow method (modified and original) was 58.6 years, with the youngest patient being 32 years old and the oldest patient 76 years old. 15 patients were males (75%), and 5 were females (25%). In 6 of the cases, the right extremity was operated on (60%), in 4 cases the left extremity (40%). 14 of all patients (70%) were operated on based on the indication of diabetes mellitus with necrosis/gangrene in the front or middle foot area causing an amputation to be necessary. In 2 cases (10%), the indication of an amputation based on the Pirogow method was osteomyelitis. One patient (5%) exhibited osteosarcoma in the forefoot, and one patient (5%) was amputated following the Pirogow method due to a severe case of PAOD (IV°) with an ulcer stemming from a forefoot amputation which had been previously carried out.

The analysis of the Ankle Scores (ASs) from the group of patients that were successfully amputated using the modified Pirogow method resulted in the following point totals (Table 3): 20% report an excellent and 50% a good result (together 70%) compared to 30% claiming an satisfactory and unsatisfactory result. If we examine the individual subcategories of the total AS, we see the following results with regard to the level of pain experienced after being modified amputated: 5 patients (50%) indicated in the 12-month follow-up experiencing no pain (pain free), 4 patients (40%) indicated experiencing light or moderate pain, and one patient (10%) indicated experiencing a high level of pain. If one defines a good result regarding the functional result with a point total >20 with a maximum point total of 40, then 6 patients (60%) indicated a positive functional result 12 months postoperatively. Radiological criteria led to a minimum point total of 0 points; at 12 months after the Pirogow amputation, a trabecula atrophy or bone necrosis persisted. One patient (10%) exhibited this condition. With regard to the difference in leg length, our examination led to the following results: one patient had no difference (10%), 7 patients exhibited a difference <2 cm (70%), and 3 patients exhibited a difference >2 cm (30%). With regard to the level of mobility without a prosthesis, two patients indicated complete mobility (20%), 6 patients (60%) indicated >10

meters, and only 2 patients (20%) indicated being able to move less than 10 meters.

In the control group, consisting of patients having undergone the original amputation method described by Pirogow, the analysis of the Ankle Scores (AS) resulted in the following point totals (Table 4): 20% report an excellent and 20% a good result (together 40%), whereas 60% report a satisfactory or unsatisfactory result. If we examine the individual subcategories of the total AS, we see the following results in regard to the level of pain experienced after being amputated using the original method: 4 patients (40%) indicated in the 12-month follow-up experiencing no pain (pain free), 2 patients (20%) indicated experiencing light pain, one patient (10%) moderate pain, and one patient (10%) indicated experiencing a high level of pain. If one defines a good functional result with a point total >20 with a maximum point total of 40, then 6 patients (60%) indicated a positive functional result 12 months postoperatively, comparable to the modified method. Differences are shown along radiological criteria in the control group: two patients (20%) exhibited an atrophy of bone trabeculae which was radiologically traceable, one patient a bone necrosis (10%). With regard to the difference in leg length, our examination revealed a major drawback to the original amputation method, namely, that all patients exhibited a difference >2 cm resulting in an invariable point total of 0 points. Patients having undergone the original Pirogow's amputation indicated a decreased level of mobility without a prosthesis <10 m of 4 patients (40%).

# 5. Discussion

The problems stemming from lower leg amputations induced N.I. Pirogow to describe a new method of amputation in his original article from 1854. When examining the medical situation from a historical perspective, one can undoubtedly state that the level of prosthetic care towards the end of the 19th century was in no way comparable to the options available today. Simple wooden prostheses or the complete absence of prosthetic care of any kind were the main forms of rehabilitation available at the time of the Crimean War [1, 3]. Using the method of amputation at ankle level, Pirogow successfully enabled patients to stay mobile without a prosthesis. Neither the original article nor further literary research reveals any information regarding the level of mobility as far as distance is concerned. If one examines the information gathered from the patients of the modified Pirogow operation method participating in our study, 20% indicated unrestricted mobility. 40% of the patients indicated a mobility distance of greater than 10 meters. In this case, one could criticise the assessment criteria of the Ankle Score, seeing as how it is unclear if a patient who can walk 3 km without a prosthesis after undergoing an amputation based on the modified Pirogow method assesses this as unrestricted, complete mobility, or merely greater than 10 meters. Adding the option of unrestricted mobility (20%) with the option of mobility greater than 10 meters (40%) shows that 60% of the patients could walk more than 10 meters without a prosthesis, which is an important advantage in particular for mobility in and around the home because although prosthetic care today has been much improved, it is sometimes still necessary to be mobile without a prosthesis, for instance, when going to the bathroom in the middle of the night. In the control group of the original operated patients, 40% indicated a mobility without prothesis <10 m. The patients in both groups were explicitly informed that information given when answering the Ankle Score Questionnaire should only be given regarding mobility without any type of walking assistance (i.e., walkers, crutches, etc.).

A further advantage of the modified Pirogow amputation method is the fixation of the calcaneus carried out using a Kirschner wire and a 3/0 spongiosa tension screw. Additionally, the calcaneus was anchored by drilling Steinmann nails cranial and anterior to the calcaneal spur to allow the use of an external fixator. These leads to a secure fracture healing. According to our results, radiological complications could be seen in 30% of the patients of the control group in comparison to 10% in the modified group. Because of the fact that we rotated the calcaneus as an additional modification, we saw a decreased difference in the postoperative leg length. The longer length of the lower extremity after undergoing the modified amputation based on the Pirogow method must be seen as another advantage of this method. Taniguchi et al. describe a significantly reduced level of physical strain placed on patients amputated with a difference in length <2 cm [7]. If one examines the results of the patient survey conducted with regard to the final results, one sees different results for the modified method of Pirogow's amputation and original method. 70% of the patients undergoing the modified Pirogow's amputation indicated an excellent or good result, whereas 40% of the patients indicated these results after the original amputation procedure. In addition, the assessment of pain felt after the different amputation methods showed different results: 50% of those patients amputated by the modified procedure indicated being completely pain free (40% light or moderate pain), while 40% of those original amputated indicated being completely pain free (30% light or moderate pain). The functional results in both patient groups were similar; however, it must be noted that the functional results with regard to mobility were indicated with the help of a prosthesis. The rate of complications must be examined critically. A direct comparison between the two groups regarding the respective complication rate cannot be made, due to the fact that the group's sample size was adjusted with respect to the common criterion "postoperative complications." The rate of complications following a Pirogow's amputation can be reduced by strictly restricting patients based on indications [16]. For this reason, the authors especially recommend the modified Pirogow method for patients without vascular damage and particularly for patients with traumatic forefoot lesions where preservation of the forefoot through free or vascularised microsurgical flap transplantation is not possible. However, if the modified Pirogow's amputation is carried out successfully, it would present a significant increase in the patient's quality of life due to decreased radiological complications with pain relief, the increased mobility without a prosthesis, and the minimal difference in leg length.

## 6. Summary

The modified method compared to the original method is characterized by rotating the calcaneus. The calcaneus is relocated vertically 60°–90° to the plantar level approx. 3 cm proximal to the calcaneocuboid joint surface. To fix the calcaneus to the tibia, osteosynthesis can be carried out using a Kirschner wire and a 3/0 spongiosa tension screw. For additional modification, the calcaneus is anchored by drilling Steinmann nails cranial and anterior to the calcaneal spur to allow the use of an external fixator. Ten patients who underwent an amputation based on this modified Pirogow method were surveyed 12 months postoperatively using the Ankle Score (AS) patient questionnaire from Taniguchi et al., based on the Ankle and Hindfoot Score from the American Orthopedic Foot and Ankle Society (AOFAS). Using a point system (0–100 points), the criteria pain, functional and radiological assessment, difference in leg length, and mobility without a prosthesis were recorded and evaluated. An identical questionnaire was given to the control group after the same 12-month time period postoperative; this group consisted of ten patients who had undergone the original Pirogow's amputation method. The modified Pirogow's amputation presents a valuable alternative to the original amputation method for patients with the corresponding indications. The benefits are found in the significantly reduced pain, difference in reduced radiological complications, the increase in mobility without a prosthesis, and the reduction of postoperative difference in leg length.

## References

[1] O. Malakhova, "Nikolay Ivanovich Pirogow (1810–1881)," *Clinical Anatomy*, vol. 17, no. 5, pp. 369–372, 2004.

[2] N. I. Pirogow, *Questions of Life: Diary of an Old Physician*, Science History Publications, Sagamore Beach, Mass, USA, 1992.

[3] I. Voloshin and P. M. Bernini, "Nickolay Ivanovich Pirogow. Innovative scientist and clinician," *Spine*, vol. 23, no. 19, pp. 2143–2146, 1998.

[4] N. I. Pirogow, "Resection of bones and joints and amputations and disarticulations of joints. 1864," *Clinical Orthopaedics and Related Research*, no. 266, pp. 3–11, 1991.

[5] R. Baumgartner and P. Botta, *Amputationschirurgie und Prothesenversorgung*, Thieme Stuttgart, 2007.

[6] R. I. Harris, "Syme's amputation; the technical details essential for success," *The Journal of Bone and Joint Surgery. British*, vol. 38, no. 3, pp. 614–632, 1956.

[7]  A. Taniguchi, Y. Tanaka, K. Kadono, Y. Inada, and Y. Takakura, "Pirogow ankle disarticulation as an option for ankle disarticulation," *Clinical Orthopaedics and Related Research*, no. 414, pp. 322–328, 2003.

[8]  Publikation des Wissenschaftlichen Institutes der AOK (WidO), "Häufigkeit der Amputationen der unteren Extremität," Erscheinungsjahr, 2003.

[9]  S. Rammelt, A. Olbrich, and H. Zwipp, "Hindfoot amputations," *Operative Orthopädie und Traumatologie*, vol. 4, pp. 265–279, 2011.

[10] M. Steen, "Flap surgery for stump improvement of the lower extremity," *Fuß & Sprunggelenk*, vol. 5, no. 4, pp. 246–253, 2007.

[11] G. Warren, "Conservative amputation of the neuropathic foot— the Pirogow procedure," *Operative Orthopadie und Traumatologie*, vol. 9, no. 1, pp. 49–58, 1997.

[12] R. van Damme and C. Limet, "Amputation in diabetic patients," *Clinics in Podiatric Medicine and Surgery*, vol. 24, no. 3, pp. 569–582, 2007.

[13] A. R. Edwards, "Study helps build functional bridges for amputee patients," *Biomechanics*, vol. 1, pp. 17–19, 2004.

[14] M. Berlemont, R. Weber, and J. P. Willot, "10 years of experience with immediate application of prosthetic devices to amputees of the low extremities on the operating table," *Prosthetics and Orthotics International*, vol. 3, pp. 8–18, 1969.

[15] A. Taniguchi, Y. Tanaka, K. Kadono et al., "The modified Ankle disarticulation score," *Journal of Foot and Ankle Surgery*, vol. 45, no. 5, pp. 98–103, 2002.

[16] G. T. Aitken, "Surgical amputation in children," *The Journal of Bone and Joint Surgery. American*, vol. 45, pp. 1735–1741, 1963.

# 16

# The Variable Angle Hip Fracture Nail Relative to the Gamma 3: A Finite Element Analysis Illustrating the Same Stiffness and Fatigue Characteristics

**Amir Matityahu,[1] Andrew H. Schmidt,[2] Alan Grantz,[3] Ben Clawson,[3] Meir Marmor,[1] and R. Trigg McClellan[1]**

[1] *Department of Orthopaedic Surgery, UCSF/SFGH Orthopaedic Trauma Institute, 2550 23rd Street, 2nd Floor, San Francisco, CA 94110, USA*

[2] *Department of Orthopaedic Surgery, University of Minnesota, Hennapin County Medical Center, Minneapolis, MN 55454, USA*

[3] *Anthem Orthopaedics VAN, LLC, Santa Cruz, CA 95060, USA*

Correspondence should be addressed to Amir Matityahu; matityahua@orthosurg.ucsf.edu

Academic Editor: Allen L. Carl

Ten percent of the 250,000 proximal femur fractures that occur in the United States each year are malreduced into a varus position after treatment. Currently, there is no cephalomedullary nail available that allows the physician to dynamically change the lag-screw-to-nail angle. The Variable Angle Nail (VAN) was designed to allow movement of the lag screw relative to the shaft of the nail. This study compared the characteristics of the VAN to the Gamma 3 nail via finite element analysis (FEA) in stiffness and fatigue. The results of the FEA model with the same loading parameters showed the Gamma 3 and the VAN with lag-screw-to-nail angle of 120° to have essentially the same stiffness values ranging from 350 to 382 N/mm. The VAN with lag-screw-to-nail angles of 120°, 130°, and 140° should be able to withstand more than 1,000,000 cycles from 1,400 N to 1,500 N loading of the tip of the lag screw. The Gamma 3 should be able to last more than 1,000,000 cycles at 1,400 N. In summary, the VAN is superior or equivalent in stiffness and fatigue when compared to the Gamma 3 using FEA.

## 1. Introduction

More than 250,000 proximal femur fractures occur in the United States each year [1]. Due to aging of the population and the increasing number of elderly persons, the incidence of hip fractures is predicted to double over the next 15 to 20 years [1]. Since their introduction over 15 years ago and subsequent widespread adoption, the so-called cephalomedullary nails that incorporate fixation into the femoral head have become a standard treatment for these proximal femur fractures [2–7]. Despite their popularity, the technology associated with these nails has only been incrementally advanced over the last 10–15 years, with most of the design changes having been done to lessen the likelihood of intraoperative fracture of the femur and cutout of the lag screw [8, 9].

Reports of the results of the stabilization of proximal femoral fractures with cephalomedullary nails indicate that more than 10% of cases demonstrate varus malreduction, with neck-shaft angles that are more than 10° of varus relative to the contralateral side [10, 11]. Varus malreduction contributes to failure of fracture fixation and causes limb shortening and compromised function [12, 13]. Given the number of patients treated by this method, as many as 20,000 individuals per year may have a suboptimal result due to malreduction, and some of these patients may require further surgery [1, 7, 10, 11]. It is recognized that patient outcomes, fracture nonunion, and implant failure are largely dependent on the fracture reduction and less on which specific intramedullary implant is used [14–17]. The etiology of functional impairment following the surgical treatment of intertrochanteric hip fractures is multifactorial. However altered biomechanics are likely to be a contributing factor to poor functional outcomes. Healing with shortening or varus malreduction alters the abductor lever moment arm and femoral head offset. Compromised abductor strength may result in a residual deficit in gait and can have a significant impact on the functional outcome and may require corrective surgery [18]. Satisfactory functional outcomes with near normal gait restoration have been demonstrated in patients with intertrochanteric hip fractures treated with a trochanteric entry nail and accurate anatomic reduction [19–28].

Unfortunately, despite incremental design advances over the last 15 years, surgeons still do not have a means of correcting intraoperative varus malreduction in situ when it occurs. Current implant designs incorporate a static lag-screw-to-nail angle curtailing the ability of the surgeon to change the reduction of the fracture once the implant is placed. The Variable Angle Nail (Anthem Orthopaedics VAN, LLC, Los Altos, CA) has been designed as a solution for the problem of intraoperative proximal femur varus neck-shaft angle malreduction. Because the lag-screw-to-nail angle can be changed intraoperatively to correct malreductions, one can choose the correct angle for the patient's anatomy. However, because the mechanism within the nail is unique, with multiple parts, and is dynamic rather than static, there is need to demonstrate the ability of the implant to withstand expected mechanical loads during clinical use of slightly more than 2 body weights [29–32]. Moreover, because there is a mobile internal apparatus, load transfer may be different between the lag screw, internal apparatus, and nail relative to current static designs. Additionally, the site of internal material stress and potential failure of the novel implant may be different relative to current designs. In current designs of cephalomedullary nails there are compressive forces laterally and medially that cause shear stress at the anterior and posterior aspect of the nail [33]. However, because of the nature of the internal mechanism of the VAN, there may be differences in force transfer from the lag screw to the nail.

The purpose of this finite element analysis study was to describe the areas of high stress and location of failure in the VAN as compared to the Gamma 3 (Stryker, Kalamazoo, MI). Of special interest were areas of high stress concentration at the interface between the lag screw and the nail aperture and internal mechanisms for both the VAN and Gamma 3.

## 2. Methods

Finite element analysis (FEA) of the VAN and Gamma 3 intramedullary nails was performed in several steps. Modeling the implants, testing parameters, material characteristics, static calculations, and fatigue calculations were performed as described in the following.

*2.1. VAN Description.* The Variable Angle Nail (VAN) is comprised of a nail, a lag screw, and an internal mechanism that dynamically moves the lag screw from 120° to 140° of lag-screw-to-nail angles (Figure 1). The surgeon may be able to intraoperatively and in situ move the lag screw to a desired position, thereby accommodating any patient-specific anatomic variations. Unlike the Gamma 3, which has a proximal lateral bend of 4°, the proximal aspect of the VAN

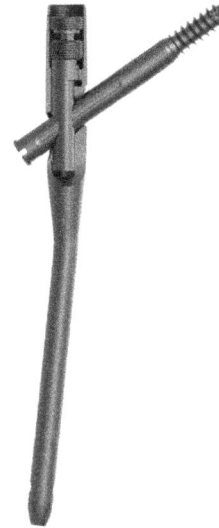

FIGURE 1: The Variable Angle Nail (VAN) with internal mechanism that gives the surgeon the opportunity to move the lag screw relative to the nail.

is bent 6° laterally. Both proximal nails accommodate for lateral entry point and the proximal femoral anatomy.

*2.2. Modeling.* The FEA model for the VAN and Gamma 3 was built from a SolidWorks computer-aided design assembly (SolidWorks Corporation, Concord, Massachusetts). Autodesk Simulation software was used to build and analyze the model (Autodesk, Inc., San Rafael, CA). The model consists of approximately 165,000 elements. A hybrid-meshing scheme was used in which 8-node brick elements comprise the majority of the volume. Fewer 6-node wedge, 5-node pyramid, and 4-node tetrahedral elements were used to close voids where needed. The material model accounted for plasticity in the nail, lag screw, and insert. The nail, lag screw, and insert were the only parts where yield occurred as a result of contact stresses. Surface-to-surface contact elements were employed between lag screw and nail, lag screw and insert, insert and nail, and insert and adjustment screw. The surface-to-surface contact was designed so that the nodes of either surface were prevented from passing through the nodes defining the other surface. A contact tolerance of 0.02 mm was used to define the gap value below which contact is assumed to occur. Frictionless contact was used, as vibration during cyclic testing was assumed to overcome frictional restraint between the parts. An adaptive contact stiffness algorithm was used by the FEA program to calculate contact stiffness. A nonlinear iterative solution method (Newton-Raphson) was used with line search Scheme. The Newton-Raphson method generates a search direction for new possible solutions, while the line search scheme is used to find a solution in the direction that minimizes the out-of-balance force error. The convergence criterion was displacement since the last time step. The convergence tolerance was $\Delta d/D <$ 0.005 with contact and <0.0001 without contact.

TABLE 1

| Material properties of Ti-6Al-4V ELI | Strength in MPa |
| --- | --- |
| Ultimate tensile strength | 860 |
| Tensile yield strength | 790 |
| Compressive yield strength | 860 |
| Ultimate bearing strength | 1,740 |
| Bearing yield strength | 1,430 |

Three versions of this first model set were built with aperture angles of 120°, 130°, and 140° between the lag screw and the nail.

A separate, second model of the interaction between the insert, adjustment screw, and nail was built and analyzed as well to delineate any high stress areas that may be transferred proximally from the lag screw to the insert and then to the adjustment screw and its threads that interact with the nail. This second one, or submodel, was created for the VAN design so that the stress levels in the threads and other features of the adjustment screw and its interface to the nail could be accurately modeled. Accurately modeling the contact elements in the threads of the adjustment screw to nail interface would have resulted in an unacceptably large model. In the full VAN model, contact elements are used between all the parts except the adjustment screw to nail interface and the nail to potting compound (both considered bonded). In the VAN model there were 12 sets of mating surfaces with contact elements.

The adjustment screw was considered bonded to the nail in the first model of the VAN in order to focus on the interactions of the lag screw and the insert laterally and the lag screw and the nail medially. A third model (two versions) was created for the Gamma 3 nail with the aperture angles of 120° and 130° angles between the lag screw and the nail.

*2.3. Set-Up.* A potted base was modeled to simulate the plastic mount for the nail used during in vitro testing. A hose clamp was emulated with multiple springs placed between the end of the truncated lag screw and the medial side of the nail distal to the lag screw aperture in order to constrain the lag screw from sliding laterally. Five springs were used with a stiffness of 1000 N/mm for each spring (Figure 2). The parts and loads were symmetric about the $Y$-$Z$ plane. The load was offset 50 mm from the lower axis of the nail (Figure 3).

*2.4. Material Characteristics.* The VAN and Gamma 3 are both made from a titanium alloy (Ti-6Al-4V ELI). The stress-strain curve used in the FEA model was derived from a curve for annealed Ti-6Al-4V found in the Atlas of Stress-Strain Curves [34]. The curve is modified to account for the yield stress of the ELI alloy of 790–795 MPa and the necking during stressing that occurs during loading. It is also important to note that the following values were taken into account in regard to material properties of Ti-6Al-4V ELI (Table 1).

Since the areas of high contact in the Gamma 3 and VAN nail are bearing type stresses, the local yield stresses may be exceeded without causing component failure.

*2.5. Static Loading and Stiffness Calculations.* The Gamma 3 was tested at the worst-case scenario of 120° lag-screw-to-nail angle with a load of 1400 N directed distally on the lag screw. We chose the 120° because the resultant force vector loading the nail is more horizontal. Therefore, there is an increase in lever arm affecting the nail with an increased lag-screw-to-nail angle. The VAN was tested at 120°, with 1400 N load, and then at 120°, 130°, and 140° lag-screw-to-nail angles at 1500 N. We chose 1500 N because it is slightly more than two times average body weight.

The stiffness plots for the VAN system were calculated using the 50 mm offset from the tip of the lag screw to the shaft of the nail. By necessity, the length of the lag screws is increased in length as the lag-screw-to-nail angle increased from 120° to 140°. The nail proximal bend angle of the Gamma 3 is 4° versus 6° for the VAN system resulting in a shorter lag screw moment arm length for the Gamma 3 (61 mm) versus the VAN (64 mm). The distance from the intersection of the lag screw axis from the center of the nail to the center of the load applicator was 64 mm, 72 mm, and 86 mm, respectively, for 120°, 130°, and 140° lag-screw-to-nail angles. For purposes of comparison, the stiffness values for both the VAN and Gamma 3 with 64 mm moment arms were used. The predicted stiffness for the Gamma 3 with a 64 mm moment arm is 350 N/mm between 0 and 1500 N.

The measured test results for the stiffness of the VAN system from 0 to 1500 N were 340 N/mm for a 120° lag screw angle and an average value of approximately 310 N/mm for 130° and 140° lag screw angles.

*2.6. Fatigue Calculations.* The level of static tensile stress that should not be exceeded if 1,000,000 load cycles were to be achieved before failure was chosen to evaluate the fatigue capability of the VAN and Gamma 3 designs (see Appendix A).

The data for Ti-6AL-4V lists a fatigue strength of 74,000 psi (510 MPa) at 10,000,000 cycles, and the ultimate strength is 131,000 psi (900 MPa) [35, 36]. Because an average person walks 1 million steps in 3 months, 1,000,000 cycles were chosen as the fatigue longevity of the implants for this FEA [37]. Using the stress range formula (Appendix B), the maximum allowable range of stress for 1,000,000 cycles is 566 MPa and for 200,000 cycles it is 605 MPa.

The potential for compressive fatigue was further evaluated by comparing the von Mises stresses with the maximum and minimum principal stresses in the regions of high compressive loading in the nail and insert. The von Mises stress is most commonly used in noncyclic FEA as the best prediction of the material yield point in a multiaxial stress state. The von Mises calculation utilizes distortion energy to find an equivalent value of uniaxial stress, which can be compared to yield point test data. In fatigue analysis, the failure limits in tension and compression can be quite different. Loading in compression can be significantly higher than loading in tension to achieve the same fatigue lifetime. Figure 8 illustrates that the tensile component (maximum principal stress) is much lower than the magnitude of the compressive component (minimum principal stress). The

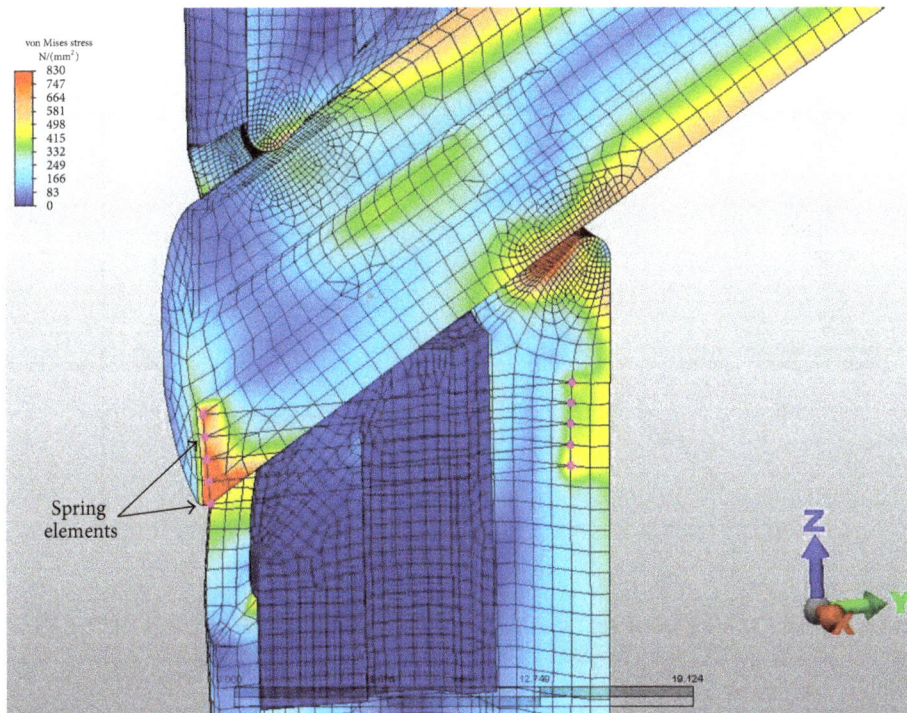

FIGURE 2: FEA model of the interaction between the insert, adjustment screw, and nail showing the spring elements that control collapse of the lag screw within the aperture of the nail.

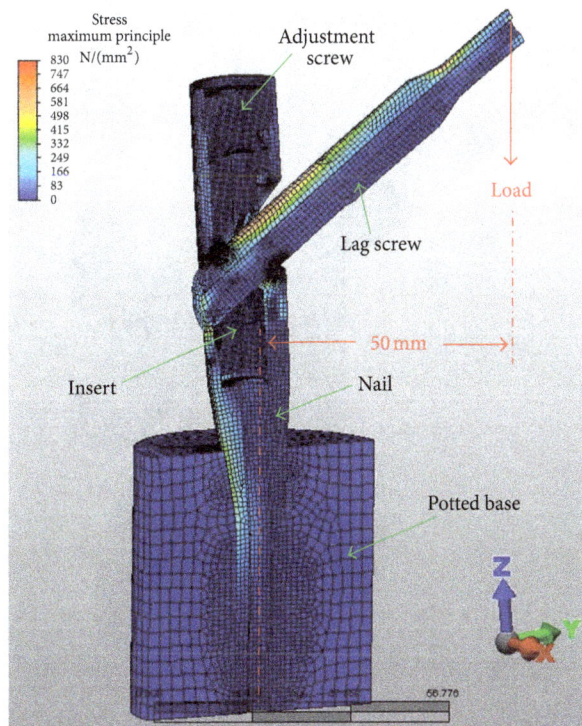

FIGURE 3: FEA model including loading set-up of 50 mm offset from the nail to the point of force application.

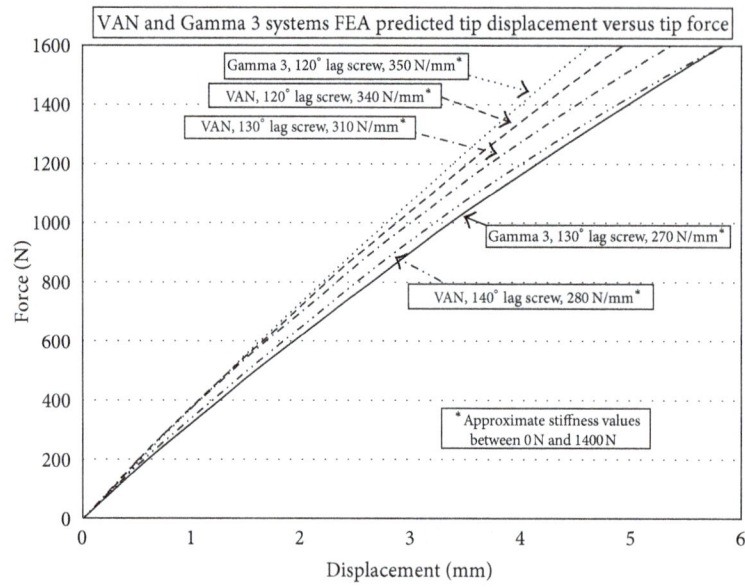

FIGURE 4: Force displacement curve of the VAN at 120°, 130°, and 140° and the Gamma 3 at 120° and 130° lag-screw-to-nail angles. The initial stiffness values were VAN 120°, 340 N/mm; VAN 130°, 310 N/mm; VAN 140°, 280 N/mm; Gamma 3 120°, 350 N/mm; Gamma 3 130°; 270 N/mm.

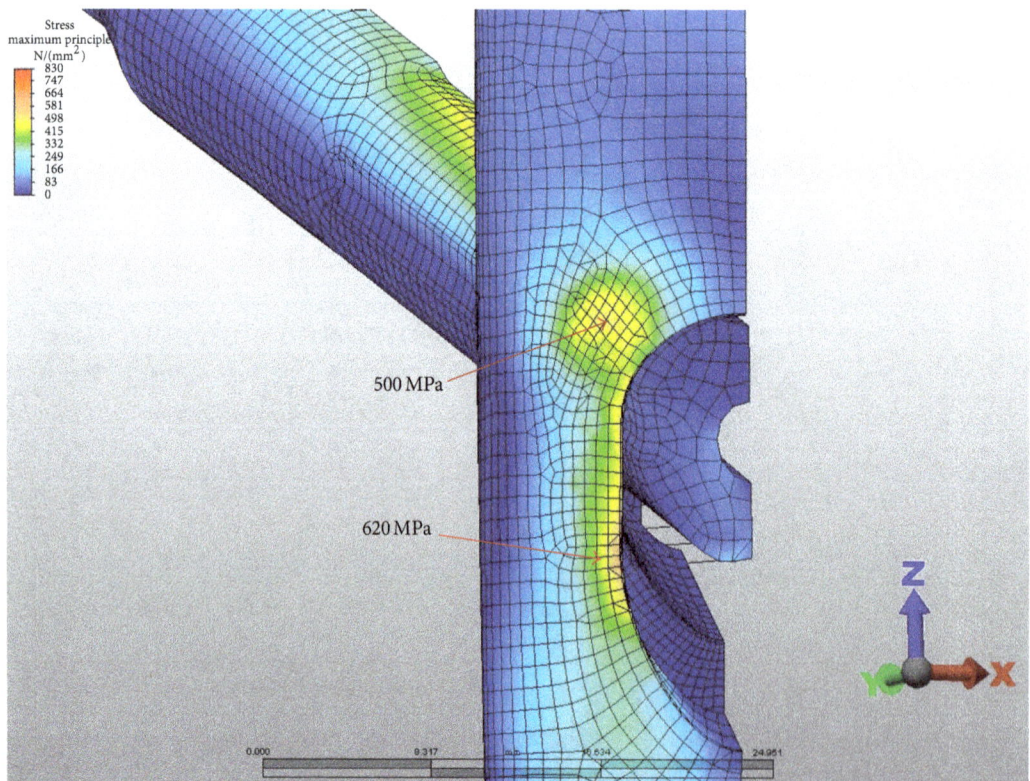

FIGURE 5: 120° lag-screw-to-nail angle VAN stresses. The maximum stress was 500 MPa at the proximal aspects and 620 MPa at the distal aspect of the lateral aperture.

(a)

(b)

(c)

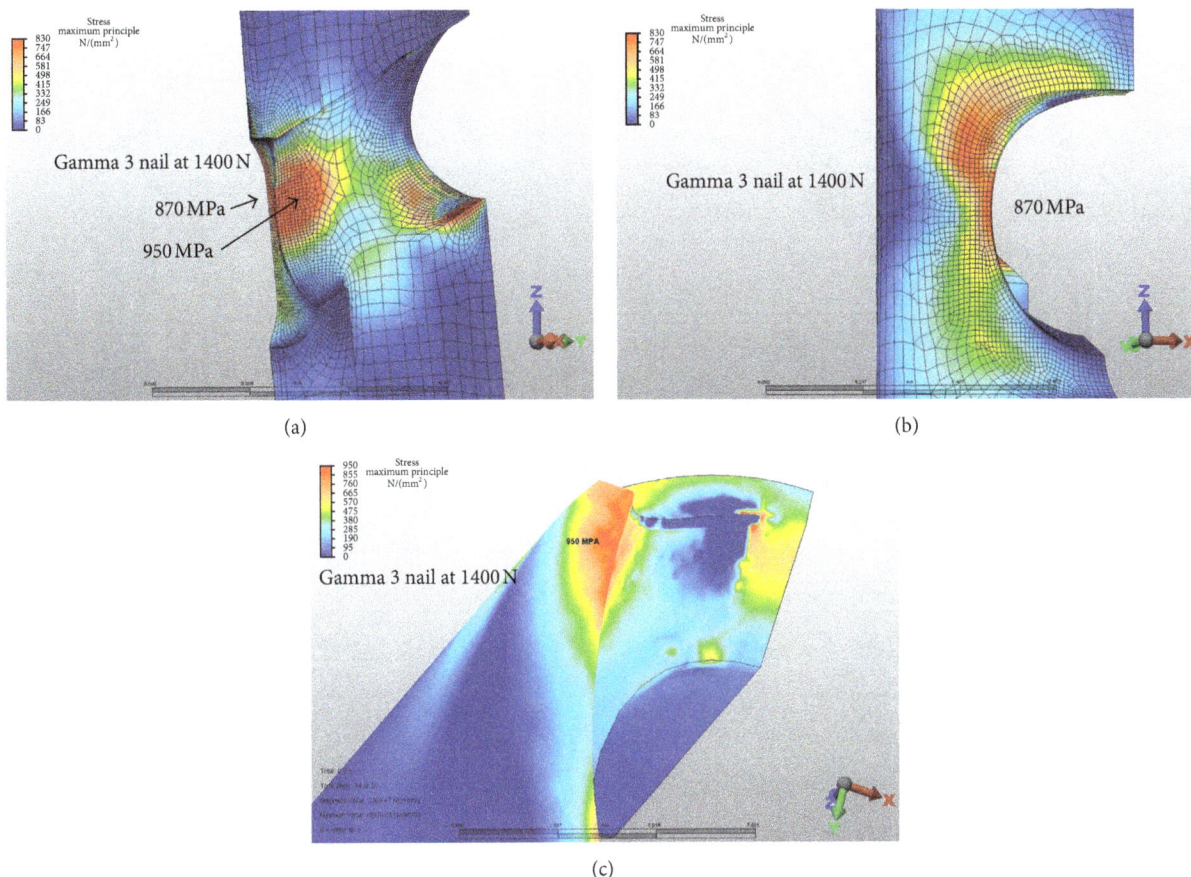

FIGURE 6: 120° lag-screw-to-nail angle Gamma 3 stresses. The maximum stress was 870–950 MPa at the lateral and medial aspect of the nail.

magnitude of the minimum principal stress is approximately equal to the von Mises stress. This shows that the stresses in these regions are predominantly compressive. Using the maximum principal stress component as the basis of the fatigue life calculation explains the test results showing that the VAN system can reach a 1,000,000-cycle fatigue life under high loads. At the actual regions of contact, some plastic deformation occurs, and the loads are redistributed. These contact regions are seen in the bearing stress illustration in Figure 7.

The stress state in the VAN and Gamma 3 analysis are comprised of an average stress and a range stress. In the Soderberg diagram (Appendix C), the average stress is 0.55 Smax, and the range stress is 0.45 Smax.

Therefore, for a fatigue life of 1,000,000 cycles, Se = 566 MPa, and solving for Smax, the maximum tensile stress of the FEA plots should be less than 686 MPa. Moreover, for a fatigue life of 200,000 cycles, the maximum stress on the FEA plots should be less than 711 MPa. In other words, a peak tensile stress of 686 Mpa should not be exceeded at the maximum principal stress areas located on the medial and lateral parts of the nail and nail-insert. This location, the aperture for the lag screw in the Gamma nail, has been found to be the most common location of nail breakage [38, 39]. The highest stresses occur in the contact regions between the lag screw and nail and the lag screw and insert. These regions

are in compression. The compressive yield strength of this Ti alloy is 860 MPa, while the ultimate bearing strength is 1740 MPa. Testing has shown that these regions are not prone to fatigue failure.

## 3. Results

The FEA model illustrated that the 120° Gamma 3 and the 120° VAN had essentially the same stiffness values of 350 N/mm and 340 N/mm, respectively (Figure 4). However; the 130° and 140° VAN was stiffer than the 130° Gamma 3.

Based on the fatigue formula calculations described previously, the peak tensile stress derived by the FEA should not exceed 680 Mpa. At 1400 N of loading, with the VAN set to 120° lag-screw-to-nail angles, the maximum stress was 500 MPa at the proximal aspect and 620 MPa at the distal aspect of the lateral aperture (Figure 5). A Gamma 3 nail with a similar lag-screw-to-nail angle had a maximum stress of 870–950 MPa at the lateral and medial aspect of the nail (Figure 6). At 1500 N of force on the lag screw, subsequent tensile stresses on the VAN at 120°, 130°, and 140° lag-screw-to-nail angles were on average less than 680 Mpa, although local areas of stress approaching the fatigue limit were observed (Figure 7). Figure 8 illustrates that the tensile component (maximum principal stress) is much lower than the magnitude of the compressive component (minimum

(a)

(b)

(c)

(d)

(e)

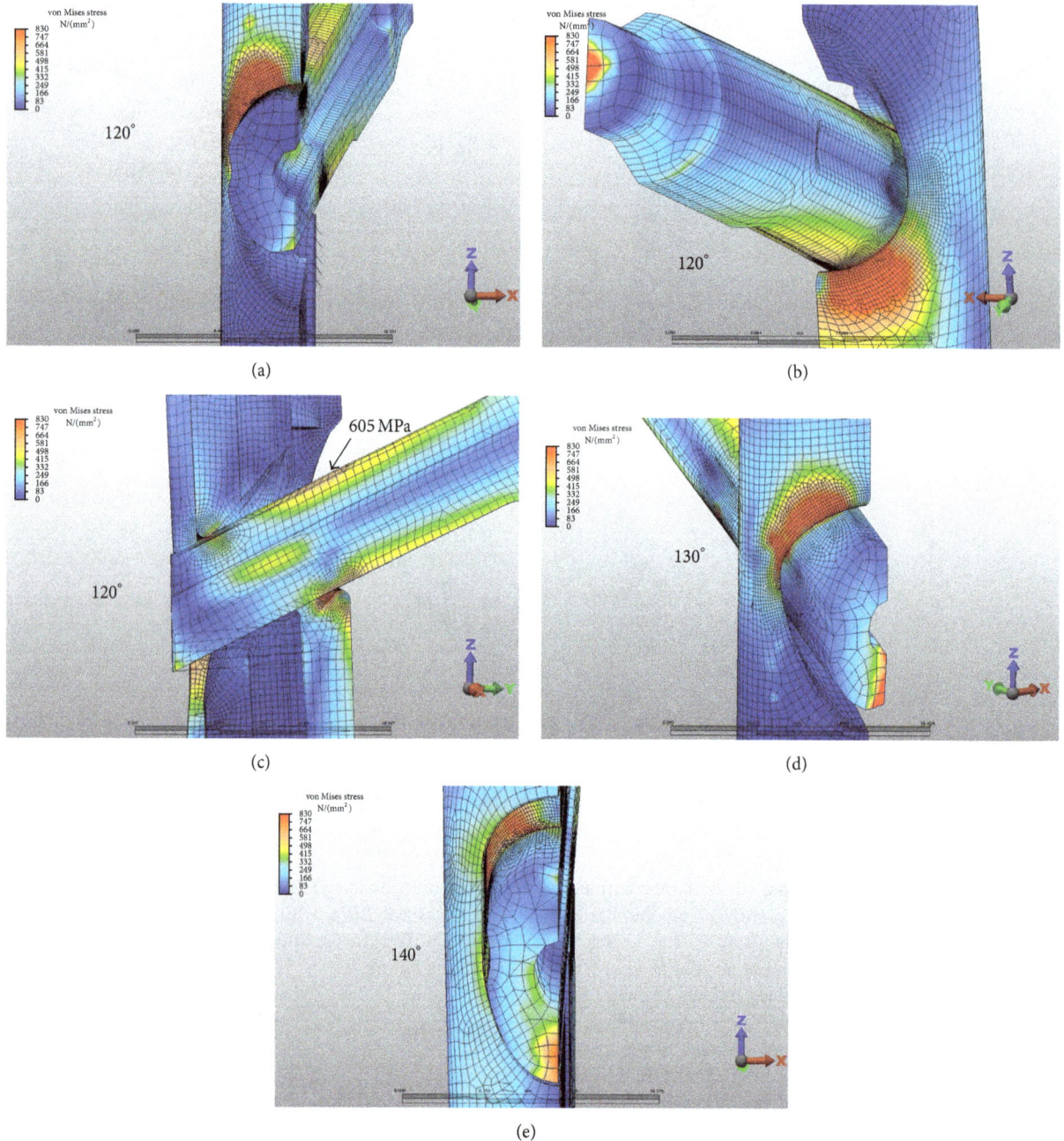

FIGURE 7: 1500 N of force on the lag screw with subsequent stresses on the VAN at 120°, 130°, and 140° lag-screw-to-nail angles.

principal stress). The magnitude of the minimum principal stress is approximately equal to the von Mises stress. This shows that the stresses in these regions are predominantly compressive. Using the maximum principal stress component as the basis of the fatigue life calculation explains the test results showing that the VAN system can reach a 1,000,000-cycle fatigue life under high loads. At the actual regions of contact, some plastic deformation occurs, and the loads are redistributed. These contact regions are seen in the bearing stress illustration in Figure 7. The FEA calculated stresses in the adjustment screw were also below 680 Mpa (Figure 9).

## 4. Discussion

This study was performed to evaluate the mechanical properties of the VAN relative to the Gamma 3. Finite element analysis was performed in order to evaluate the stresses that are transferred from the lag screw onto the VAN during normal loading conditions as compared to the Gamma 3 nail. The analysis suggests that the VAN internal mechanism and nail have a decrease in stresses when compared to the Gamma 3 during nearly similar loading conditions (1400 N and 1500 N).

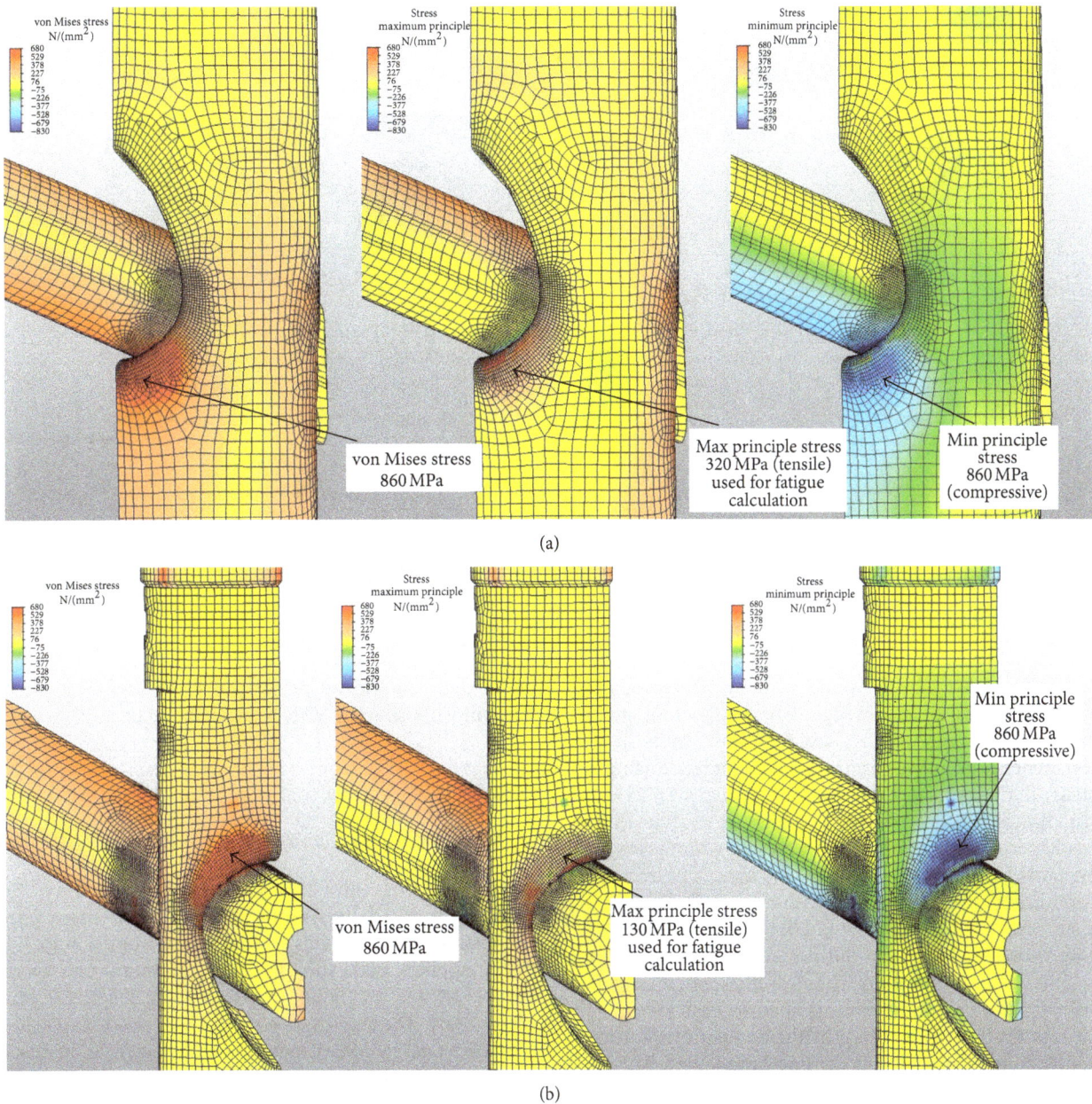

FIGURE 8: 1500 N of force on the lag screw with subsequent von Mises and principal stresses compared at 120° lag screw-to-nail angle.

Typically, Ti alloy nail implants placed in the proximal femur to fix hip fractures fail in tension at the distal aspect of the lateral lag screw aperture (Figure 5). The allowable maximum principal stress for fatigue testing was calculated to be less than 680 MPa. The FEA demonstrated maximal principal tensile stress of up to 620 MPa in the VAN at this location. Calculations of fatigue strength and compression stress indicate that the VAN should be capable of withstanding 1,000,000 cycles at 1400 N at 120°, 130°, and 140°. At 1500 N force on the lag screw, the VAN at 120°, 130°, and 140° neck-shaft angles should pass 1,000,000 cycles, although the lag screw in the 130° setting was approaching the maximum allowable stress. In comparison, the Gamma 3 system is capable of 1,000,000 cycles at 1400 N at 120°.

Given the expected increasing number of proximal femur fractures, variety of anatomic variations in neck-shaft angles and the associated prevalence of varus malreduction following cephalomedullary nailing [1, 10, 11], the VAN may offer a simple intraoperative solution to solve some of these problems.

The limitations of this study may be due to implant modeling, testing set-up assumptions, or computational testing analysis. When designing this study, we sought to minimize any implant modeling error by developing virtual nails from actual implants. The high mesh density of the FEA models resulted in close approximations of the actual nail systems studied. The models consist of approximately 165,000 solid elements, the majority of which are 8-node bricks. In a few

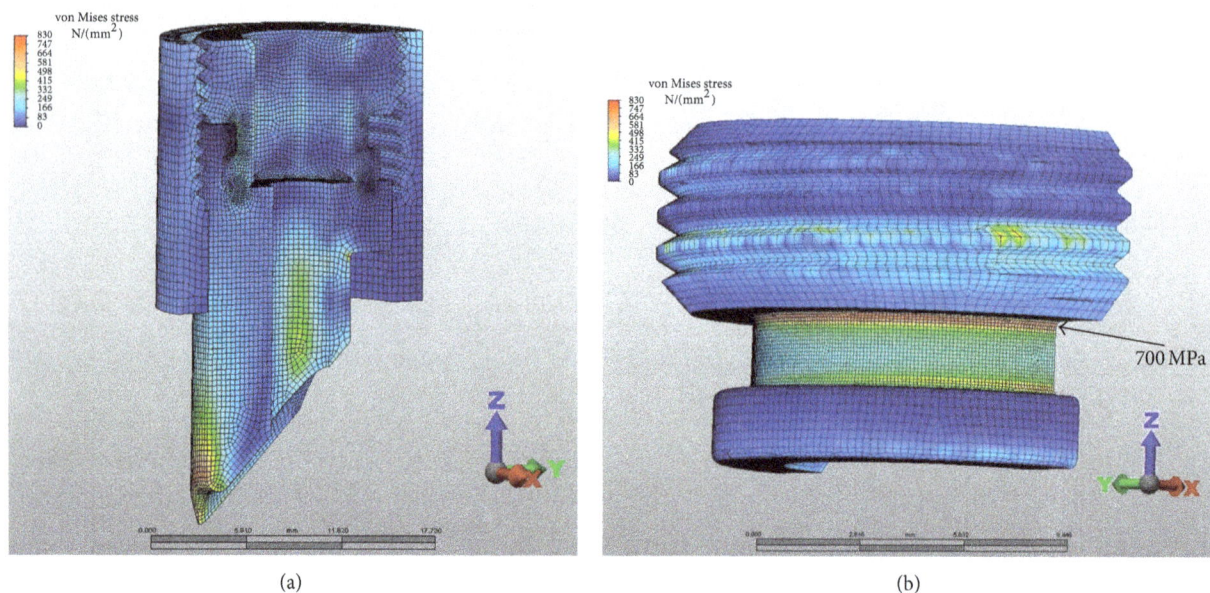

(a)                                                                          (b)

FIGURE 9: Adjustment screw interactions with insert stresses at 1500 N.

regions where 8-node bricks would result in an unacceptably high mesh density, 6-node wedge, 5-node pyramid, and 4-node tetrahedral elements are used to close voids in the model. Material properties were accounted for by allowing for plasticity in the nail, lag screw, and insert.

In clinical practice, the lag screw tends to slide within the nail aperture in patients that are treated with these types of implants. As the lag screw slides, the lever arm decreases and minimizes the stresses seen within the nail. The worst-case situation was emulated by holding the lag screw to the nail by spring elements that did not allow the lag screw to slide. This could change the mechanical environment slightly. However, since the nails were matched to each other, this effect was probably minimized in the comparison between them. By following protocols commensurate with previous studies that evaluated the stiffness and fatigue of implants of this nature, the testing set-up error was minimized. Moreover, established mechanical and FEA testing parameters that exist for proximal femoral fracture nails were employed in order to create uniform testing [33].

One limitation of this study is that there is no previously published mechanical testing of the VAN system. Moreover, there is no in vivo analysis of strain, or even FEA, of the Gamma 3 nail in the unstable hip fracture model that we are aware of. Therefore, although the authors tried to test these two implants relative to each other, the applicability to clinical use is not established as of yet.

In summary, the finite element analysis comparing the Variable Angle Nail (VAN) to the Gamma 3 nail illustrated that there are minimal differences in stiffness or fatigue between the two nails but with the potential advantage changing dynamically the angle between the lag screw and accommodating multiple patient multiple femoral neck-shaft angles with a single nail. Future mechanical testing of strength and fatigue should be performed to further evaluate the feasibility of using the VAN in clinical practice.

## Appendices

### A. Fatigue Range and Total Stress Calculations

Published values of fatigue strength are based on fully reversing induced stresses. In the case of the VAN System, the testing protocol loads the lag screw from 10% to 100% of the applied load. This results in minimum and average stresses of 10% maximum stress and 55% maximum stress respectively. The average stress is (10% of maximum + 100% of maximum)/2 = 55% of maximum. The range, or fluctuating stress is (100% of maximum − 10% of maximum)/2 = + 45% of maximum. The range stress is applied as a sine wave, so the range stress = 45% max stress $*$ sin (wt). The total excursion of the range stress is 90% of the maximum stress. Since the published values of fatigue strength are based on fully reversing stresses, a corresponding maximum allowable stress value must be determined. This maximum allowable stress is then compared to the stress levels predicted by the FEA in order to determine a margin of safety.

Therefore, the total stress = 55% max + 45% max $*$ sin (wt).

### B. Fatigue Strength Calculations

Using a semi-log plot, the fatigue strength, Sr at 1E6 cycles is: Sr = Sult − ((Sult − Se)/7) log 10(N), Sr = 131,000 − ((131,000 − 74,000)/7) log 10($10^6$) = 82,100 psi (566 MPa).

Sr: stress range; Sult: ultimate stress; Se: Se-fatigue endurance stress at 1E7 cycles.

Soderberg diagram

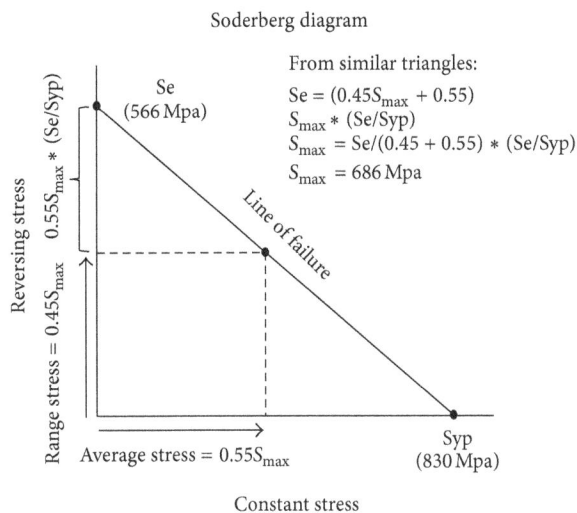

From similar triangles:
$$Se = (0.45S_{max} + 0.55)$$
$$S_{max} * (Se/Syp)$$
$$S_{max} = Se/(0.45 + 0.55) * (Se/Syp)$$
$$S_{max} = 686 \text{ Mpa}$$

FIGURE 10: Soderberg diagram.

Se is the allowable value of fully reversing range stress, Sr.

Since the stress state is not fully reversing, but instead varies from 10% of maximum stress to 100% of maximum stress, we determine the maximum allowable stress, Smax, which results in the same fatigue life (1E6 cycles) as the fully reversing stress, Sr.

## C. Soderberg Diagram

$S_{max}$ is calculated to be 686 MPa (see Figure 10).

## Acknowledgments

Amir Matityahu, MD serves on the speaker's bureau for Synthes, Johnson & Johnson Company, and AO Foundation. They received research funding from OREF, AO Foundation, and Stryker. Amir Matityahu, MD, Andrew Schmidt, MD, and R. Trigg McClellan have stock and/or ownership in Anthem Orthopaedics, LLC, Anthem Orthopaedics VAN, LLC, and 7M Orthopaedics, LLC.

## References

[1] M. R. Baumgaertner, "Intertrochanteric hip fractures," in *Skeletal Trauma: Basic Science, Management and Reconstruction*, P. G. Trafton, Ed., p. 1956, Elsevier, Philadelphia, Pa, USA, 1913.

[2] K. Ozkan, E. Eceviz, K. Unay, L. Tasyikan, B. Akman, and A. Eren, "Treatment of reverse oblique trochanteric femoral fractures with proximal femoral nail," *International Orthopaedics*, vol. 35, no. 4, pp. 595–598, 2011.

[3] S. Şahin, E. Ertürer, I. Ozturk, S. Toker, F. Seçkin, and S. Akman, "Radiographic and functional results of osteosynthesis using the proximal femoral nail antirotation (PFNA) in the treatment of unstable intertrochanteric femoral fractures," *Acta Orthopaedica et Traumatologica Turcica*, vol. 44, no. 2, pp. 127–134, 2010.

[4] M. J. Parker and H. H. Handoll, "Gamma and other cephalocondylic intramedullary nails versus extramedullary implants for extracapsular hip fractures in adults," *Cochrane Database of Systematic Reviews*, no. 9, Article ID CD000093, 2010.

[5] A. H. Ruecker, M. Rupprecht, M. Gruber et al., "The treatment of intertrochanteric fractures: results using an intramedullary nail with integrated cephalocervical screws and linear compression," *Journal of Orthopaedic Trauma*, vol. 23, no. 1, pp. 22–30, 2009.

[6] M. L. Forte, B. A. Virnig, R. L. Kane et al., "Geographic variation in device use for intertrochanteric hip fractures," *Journal of Bone and Joint Surgery A*, vol. 90, no. 4, pp. 691–699, 2008.

[7] J. O. Anglen and J. N. Weinstein, "Nail or plate fixation of intertrochanteric hip fractures: changing pattern of practice—a review of the American Board of Orthopaedic Surgery database," *The Journal of Bone and Joint Surgery—American Volume*, vol. 90, no. 4, pp. 700–707, 2008.

[8] B. Hesse and A. Gächter, "Complications following the treatment of trochanteric fractures with the gamma nail," *Archives of Orthopaedic and Trauma Surgery*, vol. 124, no. 10, pp. 692–698, 2004.

[9] S. Boriani, F. de Lure, L. Campanacci et al., "A technical report reviewing the use of the 11-mm Gamma nail: interoperative femur fracture incidence," *Orthopedics*, vol. 19, no. 7, pp. 597–600, 1996.

[10] J. E. Madsen, L. Næss, A. K. Aune, A. Alho, A. Ekeland, and K. Strømsøe, "Dynamic hip screw with trochanteric stabilizing plate in the treatment of unstable proximal femoral fractures: a comparative study with the gamma nail and compression hip screw," *Journal of Orthopaedic Trauma*, vol. 12, no. 4, pp. 241–248, 1998.

[11] R. K. J. Simmermacher, J. Ljungqvist, H. Bail et al., "The new proximal femoral nail antirotation (PFNA) in daily practice: results of a multicentre clinical study," *Injury*, vol. 39, no. 8, pp. 932–939, 2008.

[12] G. S. Laros and J. F. Moore, "Complications of fixation in intertrochanteric fractures," *Clinical Orthopaedics and Related Research*, vol. 101, pp. 110–119, 1974.

[13] I. B. Schipper, R. K. Marti, and C. van der Werken, "Unstable trochanteric femoral fractures: extramedullary or intramedullary fixation: review of literature," *Injury*, vol. 35, no. 2, pp. 142–151, 2004.

[14] W. J. Jin, L. Y. Dai, Y. M. Cui, Q. Zhou, L. S. Jiang, and H. Lu, "Reliability of classification systems for intertrochanteric fractures of the proximal femur in experienced orthopaedic surgeons," *Injury*, vol. 36, no. 7, pp. 858–861, 2005.

[15] R. Stern, "Are there advances in the treatment of extracapsular hip fractures in the elderly?" *Injury*, vol. 38, supplement 3, pp. S77–S87, 2007.

[16] M. Saudan, A. Lübbeke, C. Sadowski, N. Riand, R. Stern, and P. Hoffmeyer, "Petrochanteric fractures: Is there an advantage to an intramedullary nail? A randomized, prospective study of 206 patients comparing the dynamic hip screw and proximal femoral nail," *Journal of Orthopaedic Trauma*, vol. 16, no. 6, pp. 386–393, 2002.

[17] T. M. Barton, R. Gleeson, C. Topliss, R. Greenwood, W. J. Harries, and T. J. S. Chesser, "A comparison of the long gamma nail with the sliding hip screw for the treatment of AO/OTA 31-A2 fractures of the proximal part of the femur: a prospective randomized trial," *The Journal of Bone and Joint Surgery—American Volume*, vol. 92, no. 4, pp. 792–798, 2010.

[18] J. Bartoníček, J. Skála-Rosenbaum, and P. Doušá, "Valgus intertrochanteric osteotomy for malunion and nonunion of

throchanteric fractures," *Journal of Orthopaedic Trauma*, vol. 17, no. 9, pp. 606–612, 2003.

[19] O. Paul, J. U. Barker, J. M. Lane, D. L. Helfet, and D. G. Lorich, "Functional and radiographic outcomes of intertrochanteric hip fractures treated with calcar reduction, compression, and trochanteric entry nailing," *Journal of Orthopaedic Trauma*, vol. 26, no. 3, pp. 148–154, 2012.

[20] S. Boriani and G. Bettelli, "The Gamma nail. A preliminary note," *La Chirurgia degli Organi di Movimento*, vol. 75, no. 1, pp. 67–70, 1990.

[21] S. Boriani, G. Bettelli, H. Zmerly et al., "Results of the multicentric Italian experience on the Gamma(TM) nail: a report on 648 cases," *Orthopedics*, vol. 14, no. 12, pp. 1307–1314, 1991.

[22] S. H. Bridle, A. D. Patel, M. Bircher, and P. T. Calvert, "Fixation of intertrochanteric fractures of the femur. A randomized prospective comparison of the Gamma nail and the dynamic hip screw," *Journal of Bone and Joint Surgery B*, vol. 73, no. 2, pp. 330–334, 1991.

[23] J. Davis, M. B. Harris, M. Duval, and R. D'Ambrosia, "Pertrochanteric fractures treated with the Gamma(TM) nail: technique and report of early results," *Orthopedics*, vol. 14, no. 9, pp. 939–942, 1991.

[24] R. W. Lindsey, P. Teal, R. A. Probe, D. Rhoads, S. Davenport, and K. Schauder, "Early experience with the gamma interlocking nail for peritrochanteric fractures of the proximal femur," *Journal of Trauma*, vol. 31, no. 12, pp. 1649–1658, 1991.

[25] P. T. Calvert, "The Gamma nail—a significant advance or a passing fashion?" *Journal of Bone and Joint Surgery—British Volume*, vol. 74, no. 3, pp. 329–331, 1992.

[26] S. C. Halder, "The gamma nail for peritrochanteric fractures," *Journal of Bone and Joint Surgery—British Volume*, vol. 74, no. 3, pp. 340–344, 1992.

[27] W. Song, Y. Chen, H. Shen, T. Yuan, C. Zhang, and B. Zeng, "Biochemical markers comparison of dynamic hip screw and Gamma nail implants in the treatment of stable intertrochanteric fracture: a prospective study of 60 patients," *The Journal of International Medical Research*, vol. 39, no. 3, pp. 822–829, 2011.

[28] R. Norris, D. Bhattacharjee, and M. J. Parker, "Occurrence of secondary fracture around intramedullary nails used for trochanteric hip fractures: a systematic review of 13,568 patients," *Injury*, vol. 43, no. 6, pp. 706–711, 2012.

[29] G. Bergmann, G. Deuretzbacher, M. Heller et al., "Hip contact forces and gait patterns from routine activities," *Journal of Biomechanics*, vol. 34, no. 7, pp. 859–871, 2001.

[30] G. Bergmann, F. Graichen, and A. Rohlmann, "Hip joint loading during walking and running, measured in two patients," *Journal of Biomechanics*, vol. 26, no. 8, pp. 969–990, 1993.

[31] G. Bergmann, H. Kniggendorf, F. Graichen, and A. Rohlmann, "Influence of shoes and heel strike on the loading of the hip joint," *Journal of Biomechanics*, vol. 28, no. 7, pp. 817–827, 1995.

[32] N. Helmy, V. T. Jando, T. Lu, H. Chan, and P. J. O'Brien, "Muscle function and functional outcome following standard antegrade reamed intramedullary nailing of isolated femoral shaft fractures," *Journal of Orthopaedic Trauma*, vol. 22, no. 1, pp. 10–15, 2008.

[33] K. Sitthiseripratip, H. van Oosterwyck, J. Vander Sloten et al., "Finite element study of trochanteric gamma nail for trochanteric fracture," *Medical Engineering and Physics*, vol. 25, no. 2, pp. 99–106, 2003.

[34] ASM International, *Atlas of Stress-Strain Curves*, ASM International, Materials Park, Ohio, USA, 2002.

[35] ASM International, *Materials Properties Handbook: Titanium Alloys*, ASM International, Materials Park, Ohio, USA, 1994.

[36] *Structural Alloys Handbook*, CINDAS/Purdue University, West Lafayette, Ind, USA, 1996.

[37] M. M. Sequeira, M. Rickenbach, V. Wietlisbach, B. Tullen, and Y. Schutz, "Physical activity assessment using a pedometer and its comparison with a questionnaire in a large population survey," *American Journal of Epidemiology*, vol. 142, no. 9, pp. 989–999, 1995.

[38] D. B. Álvarez, J. P. Aparicio, E. L. Fernandez, I. G. Mugica, D. N. Batalla, and J. Jiménez, "Implant breakage, a rare complication with the Gamma nail: a review of 843 fractures of the proximal femur treated with a Gamma nail," *Acta Orthopaedica Belgica*, vol. 70, no. 5, pp. 435–443, 2004.

[39] J. L. H. Wee, S. S. Sathappan, M. S. W. Yeo, and Y. P. Low, "Management of gamma nail breakage with bipolar hemiarthroplasty," *Singapore Medical Journal*, vol. 50, no. 1, pp. e44–e47, 2009.

# 17

# Robotic Assistance Enables Inexperienced Surgeons to Perform Unicompartmental Knee Arthroplasties on Dry Bone Models with Accuracy Superior to Conventional Methods

**Monil Karia, Milad Masjedi, Barry Andrews, Zahra Jaffry, and Justin Cobb**

*MSK Lab, Department of Orthopaedics, Charing Cross Hospital, Imperial College London, Fulham Place Road, London W6 8RF, UK*

Correspondence should be addressed to Barry Andrews; b.andrews@imperial.ac.uk

Academic Editor: Michael A. Conditt

Robotic systems have been shown to improve unicompartmental knee arthroplasty (UKA) component placement accuracy compared to conventional methods when used by experienced surgeons. We aimed to determine whether inexperienced UKA surgeons can position components accurately using robotic assistance when compared to conventional methods and to demonstrate the effect repetition has on accuracy. Sixteen surgeons were randomised to an active constraint robot or conventional group performing three UKAs over three weeks. Implanted component positions and orientations were compared to planned component positions in six degrees of freedom for both femoral and tibial components. Mean procedure time decreased for both robot (37.5 mins to 25.7 mins) ($P = 0.002$) and conventional (33.8 mins to 21.0 mins) ($P = 0.002$) groups by attempt three indicating the presence of a learning curve; however, neither group demonstrated changes in accuracy. Mean compound rotational and translational errors were lower in the robot group compared to the conventional group for both components at all attempts for which rotational error differences were significant at every attempt. The conventional group's positioning remained inaccurate even with repeated attempts although procedure time improved. In comparison, by limiting inaccuracies inherent in conventional equipment, robotic assistance enabled surgeons to achieve precision and accuracy when positioning UKA components irrespective of their experience.

## 1. Introduction

Although the benefits of robotic systems in terms of alignment and positioning compared to conventional methods are well established in experienced users [1], the effect of surgical experience and training on the ability to accurately position components with robotic systems is unknown. Conventional unicompartmental knee arthroplasties (UKAs) exhibit a learning curve whereby repetition and experience can lead to improvements in surgical technique, timing, and accuracy [2, 3]. Rees et al. in 2004 demonstrated that a surgeon's UKA performance is significantly worse in their first 10 cases compared to their subsequent 10 cases [3]. Other studies have shown a nonsignificant improvement in accuracy with experience indicating that conventional UKAs have a long learning curve and that even with experience and training obtaining accurate results is difficult [2]. In contrast early

results of a preliminary study by Coon demonstrated that the MAKO robotic system may demonstrate a shorter learning curve and greater accuracy compared to conventional techniques [4]. By comparing their first 36 robot assisted UKA patients to their previous 45 conventional UKA patients, they showed that robotic surgery resulted in a posterior tibial slope accuracy that was 2.5 times better and a varus alignment that was 3.2° better than the conventional group.

Although there are reports of long-term survivorship following UKAs [5] as well as good kinematics [6] and function [7], others have reported a high early failure rate [8]. A variety of factors including patient selection [9] and implant design [10, 11] have been identified as predictors for revision or reoperation of the implant. Incorrect alignments of the tibial and femoral components when performing a UKA have led to poor functional results, high implant wear, and a high revision rate [10–13]. The UKA procedure therefore appears to be more technically demanding, so despite being theoretically both cheaper and better than total knee replacement, its adoption may be limited by surgical skills. Robotic technology has facilitated more accurate and bone preserving methods of UKAs [1, 12, 13] compared to conventional methods which produce inconsistent alignment results [10, 14]. In 2006, Cobb et al. compared the accuracy of Acrobot—a surgical robotic system—to conventional methods of performing a UKA. They showed that all of the 13 robot treated patients had a tibiofemoral coronal alignment within $\pm 2°$ of the plan, whereas only 9 out of 15 patients treated by conventional means had achieved this accuracy ($P = 0.001$) [1]. By providing computer assistance, the spatial locations of the tools and the patient can be tracked and depicted against a preoperatively created plan on a computer screen which is used by the surgeon as guidance. The plan consists of a three-dimensional (3D) computer model of the patient's bone upon which the ideal position of the prosthesis can be determined and placed on the software. It defines regions within which the robot is constrained to avoid cutting critical areas and to facilitate accurate component placement [1]. This mechanism may enable surgeons to perform accurate UKAs in the early stages of their learning curve when inaccurate placement using conventional methods is most likely [3].

The aims of this novel research were twofold:

(1) To assess the accuracy with which surgeons inexperienced in UKAs implant the components using robotic assistance compared to conventional instrumentation.

(2) To assess the effect repetition has on component positioning accuracy in both groups.

We surmised that with robotic assistance surgeons inexperienced in UKA will position components consistently and accurately at every attempt, while with conventional instruments component positioning will be inaccurate and improve with more attempts.

## 2. Methods

*2.1. Subjects.* Sixteen surgeons consented to take part in the study, none of whom had experience in UKAs by neither conventional nor robotic means. Subjects underwent randomisation to one of two groups: conventional UKA or robotic UKA. Each subject performed a UKA once per week for three consecutive weeks by their allocated method on dry bone models. The models used were computer tomography (CT) based replicas of a patient's arthritic knee consisting of a capsule, replica ligaments, and muscle (Medical Models Ltd., London).

Prior to randomization, a CT scan of the dry bone model used in the study was taken and was segmented using the previously validated Stanmore Implants Modeller Software (Stanmore Implants Worldwide (SIW), Elstree, UK) [15]. A plan of the ideal implant positions on the dry bones was created using the Stanmore Implants Planner (SIW, Elstree, UK) which recreated the joint line and was measured to size 3 and size 4 femoral and tibial Corin Uniglide implants,

respectively. The plan was created by a consultant surgeon experienced in UKA and computer-assisted orthopaedic technologies and was designed to be anatomically optimal and achievable using the conventional cutting jig according to the published operative technique.

Subjects in the conventional group were instructed to recreate the plan using the Corin Uniglide UKA standard cutting jigs and instruments. A training video was made to show the group how to perform the procedure correctly prior to their first attempt. Additionally, a conventional UKA operating technique instructional booklet was produced based on the Corin Uniglide operative technique and the preoperative plan, which subjects read prior to the procedure and also referred to during the procedure. The guide detailed the steps the subjects needed to follow in order to achieve component placement that recreated the plan. Subjects in the robotic group were shown a demonstration of the UKA procedure using the Sculptor RGA (Stanmore Implants Worldwide, Elstree, UK) (formerly Acrobot) and were also presented with a robotic UKA guide detailing the methodology.

*2.2. Data Collection and Analysis.* Subjects in both groups were timed during the procedure starting with the initial tibial incision to the insertion of the mobile bearing device. All subjects were provided with feedback in between each repeat detailing the accuracy with which they had implanted the components in their previous attempt.

Once the UKA was complete, the bones were separated into the tibial and femoral parts with the Corin Uniglide implants attached and scanned using a 3D laser scanner which provided a computer generated image of the implanted bone. The completed UKAs were coregistered to their respective plan using the 3-matic software (Materialise, Belgium) [16]. This was initially done visually and then fine-tuned using the 3-matic surface matching function by a researcher blinded as to which group each bone model belonged to. The position of the components on the tibia and femur was then compared to that of the ideal plan by recording the coordinates of four points on the planned implant versus the achieved implant. Using Matlab software, local frames of reference of the planned implants were created and compared to those of the achieved implants in all six degrees of freedom (DoF).

The NextEngine 3D scanner (CA, USA) was used to scan the bones. It is reported to have an accuracy of 0.127 mm and a maximum of 15 samples (points) per millimetre [17]. To validate the accuracy of our methodology, a repeatability study was carried out. Intraobserver reliability involved five repeat measurements of the same bone from which the standard deviation (SD) of the mean translational and rotational errors was reported. Interobserver reliability involved two measurements of the error in six DoF of four randomly chosen bones by two observers from which a Bland-Altman plot was made. The average root mean squared (RMS) differences of three points between the CT-based and laser scanned original bones were also assessed.

The compound rotational errors (calculated as the square root of the sum of the magnitude of the axial, flexion-extension, and coronal alignment errors) and compound translational errors (calculated as the square root of the sum of the magnitude of the medial-lateral, anterior-posterior, and superior-inferior errors) were calculated for each subject for both tibial and femoral components at attempts one, two, and three. A student's $t$-test was used to compare the difference in mean compound rotational and mean compound translational errors between groups at each attempt for each component. A repeated measures ANOVA was used to determine if there was any change in component error within each group between attempts one, two, and three. A post-hoc Bonferroni correction was used for any significant results. Analysis of procedure time was performed by the same statistical methods.

For each subject their RMS error in each of the six DoF was averaged over their three attempts. This was used to calculate the mean RMS error in each DoF for the robot and conventional group using the data from all three attempts combined. We could then compare this mean absolute error from the plan in each of these DoFs between the robot and conventional groups using a student's $t$-test.

All statistics were analysed with Statistical Package for Social Sciences 20 (SPSS 20, Chicago, IL, USA), with statistical significance designated as $P < 0.05$.

## 3. Results

Mean compound rotational error of the tibial component was lower in the robot group compared to the conventional group at all attempts. This difference reached significance at attempts one ($3.0°$ versus $9.7°$) ($P = 0.005$), two ($3.9°$ versus $9.5°$) ($P = 0.001$), and three ($4.0°$ versus $9.0°$) ($P = 0.001$) (Figure 1(a)). The compound translational error was also lower with robotic assistance, reaching significance at attempts one ($2.0$ mm versus $5.2$ mm) ($P = 0.046$) and three ($2.0$ mm versus $4.2$ mm) ($P = 0.005$) (Figure 1(b)). Mean compound rotational error of the femoral component was lower in the robot group, reaching significance at attempts one ($3.3°$ versus $10.8°$) ($P = 0.002$), two ($3.6°$ versus $8.5°$) ($P = 0.002$), and three ($3.6°$ versus $8.9°$) ($P = 0.004$) (Figure 2(a)) as was compound translational error, although this reached significance at attempt three only ($2.0$ mm versus $4.3$ mm) ($P = 0.002$) (Figure 2(b)).

For the tibial component the robotic group had a lower absolute error in each of the three rotational (axial, sagittal, and coronal) and translational (medial-lateral, anterior-posterior, and superior-inferior) DoF compared to the conventional group. This difference failed to reach significance in only the varus-valgus and superoinferior directions. The mean RMS tibial rotational error was $1.8° \pm 1.6°$ for the robot group compared to $4.7° \pm 3.2°$ ($P = 0.0002$) for the conventional group, while the mean RMS tibial translation error was $1.0$ mm $\pm 0.7$ mm for the robot group and $2.1$ mm $\pm 1.5$ mm ($P = 0.021$) for the conventional group.

For the femoral component the robotic group had a lower absolute error in each of the three rotational (axial, sagittal, and coronal) and translational (medial-lateral, anterior-posterior, and superior-inferior) DoF compared to the conventional group. This was significant in all DoF except

for the superoinferior and anteroposterior directions. The mean RMS femoral rotational error was $1.7° \pm 1.7°$ in the robot group compared to $4.7° \pm 3.4°$ ($P < 0.0005$) in the conventional group, while the mean RMS femoral translation error was $1.3$ mm $\pm 1.0$ mm for the robot group and $2.0$ mm $\pm 1.3$ mm ($P = 0.042$) for the conventional group.

Mean procedure time decreased significantly for both robot ($37.5$ mins to $25.7$ mins) ($P = 0.002$) and conventional ($33.8$ mins to $21.0$ mins) ($P = 0.002$) groups with repeated attempts (Figure 3); however, neither group showed a corresponding significant change in rotational (conventional $P = 0.943$, Sculptor RGA $P = 0.724$) or translational (conventional $P = 0.373$, Sculptor RGA $P = 0.184$) component accuracy between attempts.

The results of the intraobserver repeatability study found the mean rotational error of the five repeat bones to be $0.45° \pm 0.40°$ and mean translational error to be $0.23$ mm $\pm 0.15$ mm.

The results of the interobserver repeatability study found the mean difference in observation between the two observers to be $0.07 \pm 1.39$ for each DoF. All measured differences were within $\pm 1.96$ SD of the mean difference and hence were within the acceptable limits of agreement (Figure 4).

RMS errors between the three points on the planned CT bone and laser scanned bone were less than 1 mm for both the femur and tibia.

## 4. Discussion

This randomised study is the first to compare the ability of surgeons to perform accurate UKAs in their initial attempts using both robotic and conventional methods. We have shown that surgeons inexperienced in UKA are able to position components on dry bones when performing a UKA procedure significantly more accurately with the Sculptor RGA than by conventional methods alone and can do so repeatedly and without any prior experience. We have also used a novel method in assessing the accuracy of component positioning in dry bone models which seem robust when judged by our repeatability studies.

The goal of any instrumentation used in arthroplasty should be to allow its user to position the components in a position and orientation which is preoperatively or intraoperatively determined. While there is no precise agreement on the ideal position of implants during a UKA, correct alignment of the femoral and tibial components has been shown to be the most objectively quantifiable factor in determining the wear and longevity of UKAs [12, 18]. This is particularly relevant in the early stages of a surgeon's learning curve when improper component placement is more likely due to the difficulty of the procedure and the relatively little exposure surgeons have to UKAs [3].

In our study, the decrease in time exhibited by both groups between attempts signifies the presence of a learning curve; however, the conventional group did not demonstrate a corresponding increase in accuracy in either rotational or translational alignment between attempts, while robot assistance ensured that accurate placement was consistently

(a)

(b)

(c)

(d)

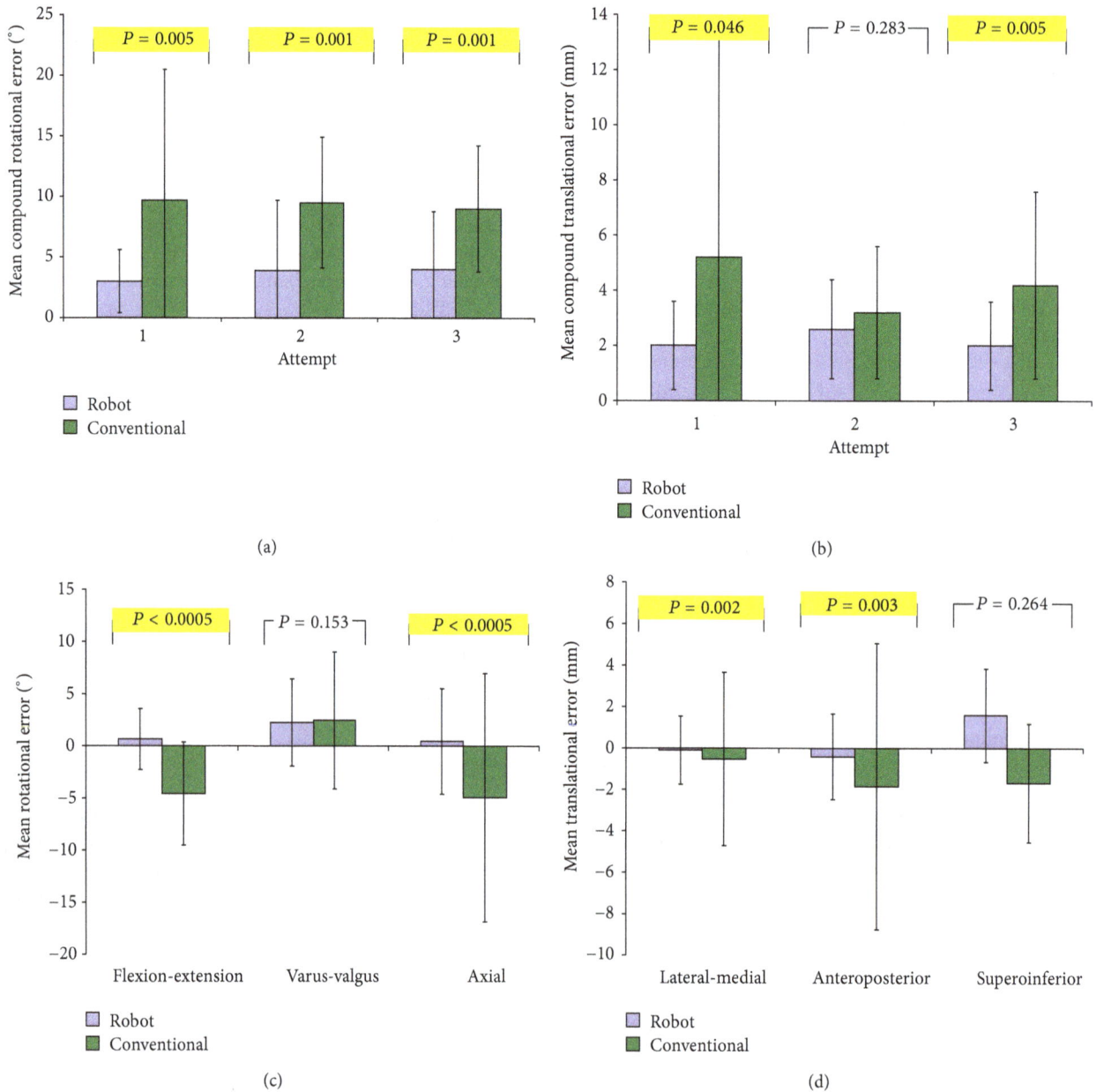

FIGURE 1: Bar graphs comparing tibial component positioning in robot and conventional groups at attempts 1, 2, and 3 by mean (a) compound rotational error, (b) compound translational error, (c) rotational alignment in each DoF, and (d) translational alignment in each DoF. $P$ values compare mean root mean squared errors between groups.

produced at each and every attempt. The lack of improvement in accuracy in the conventional group highlights the need for timely feedback for surgeons in training if they are to produce consistently accurate results. Although we were unable to show any increase in accuracy with repetition in this study, the variability of the component positioning was the highest in the conventional group's first attempt for both tibial (Figure 1) and femoral (Figure 2) components compared to following attempts. This suggests that the precision of component positioning may improve with time, although the study was neither designed nor powered to detect this.

Accuracy of the compound rotational alignment of the tibial component was consistently more accurate than conventional methods over all three attempts. Compound rotational alignment consists of axial rotation, coronal rotation, and the posterior slope, of which the latter is the most reported alignment measure dictating outcomes of a UKA procedure, and as a result posterior slopes greater than 7° should be avoided [12]. The 7° slope built in the conventional jig did not prevent any of the subjects from producing a tibial component placement posterior slope of >7° with errors ranging from +0.5° to +12.6°. Other robotic systems

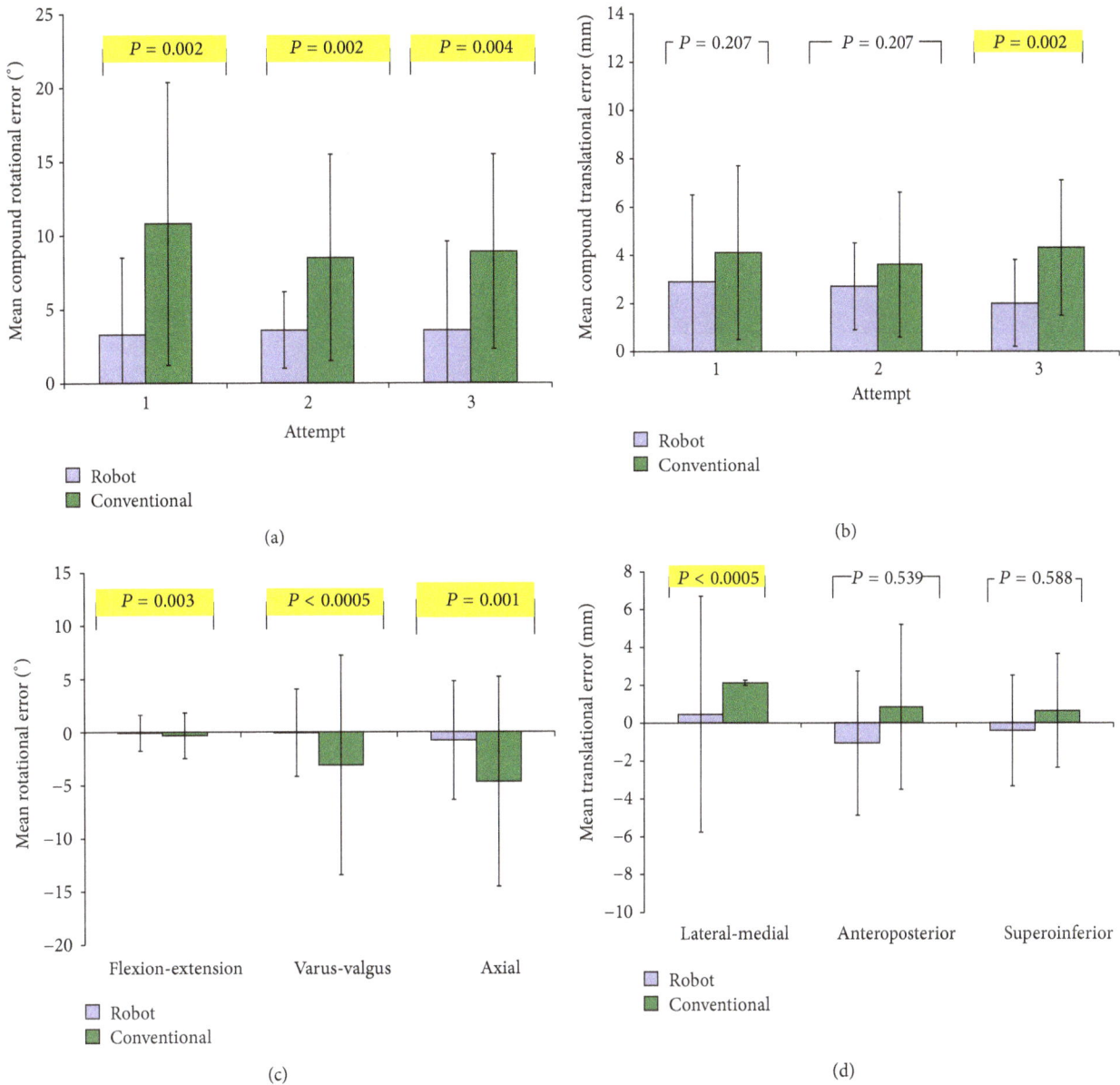

FIGURE 2: Bar graphs comparing femoral component in robot and conventional groups at attempts 1, 2, and 3 by mean (a) compound rotational error, (b) compound translational error, (c) rotational alignment in each DoF, and (d) translational alignment in each DoF. $P$ values compare mean root mean squared errors between groups.

with experienced users have also demonstrated improved sagittal tibial component placement, including the Acrobot [1] and the MAKO robot [4]. This concurs with our results, which showed a significant difference in the magnitude of posterior slope error between the robot group ($1.2° \pm 1.0°$) and conventional groups ($4.6° \pm 2.5°$) ($P < 0.0005$).

Although compound translational errors were higher in the conventional group at every attempt, this was only significant at attempts one and three for the tibial component (Figure 1(b)) and attempt three for the femoral component (Figure 2(b)). Considering the individual femoral translational DoFs only the medial-lateral translation showed a significant difference, while superoinferior and anteroposterior

errors were similar between the two groups (Figure 2(d)). This agrees with previous findings which also found similar results between the robot and conventional groups with experienced users in these DoF [1]. This may be due to the instrumentation used in a conventional UKA. The tibial stylus improves depth control when resecting the tibial plateau which dictates the inferosuperior component error explaining the similar mean robot ($2.0 \text{ mm} \pm 0.9°$) and conventional ($1.7° \pm 0.9°$) errors. During femoral preparation the small reamer can be set to an accuracy of 1 mm, the result of which dictates the superoinferior positioning of the component. Comparatively, the rotational alignment and medial-lateral translational alignment of both components

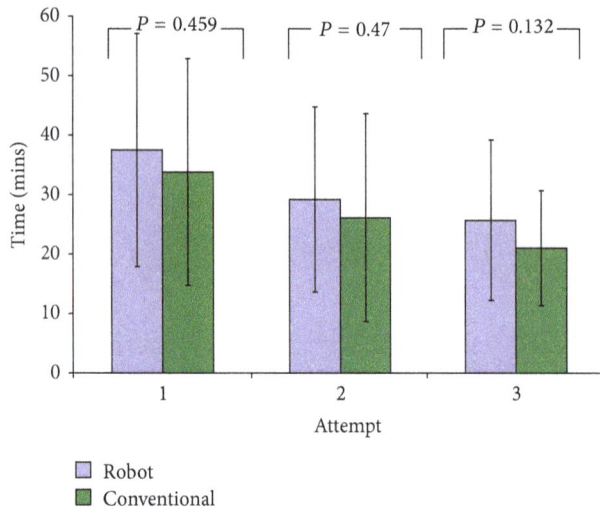

FIGURE 3: Bar graph showing the mean UKA procedure time at each attempt for the robot and conventional groups. P values refer to intergroup analysis. Significant P values are highlighted. Error bars = ± 2SD.

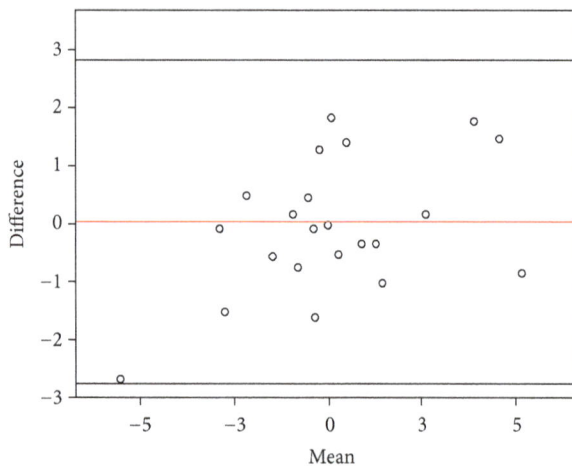

FIGURE 4: Bland-Altman plot of two observer's agreement of component alignment for five different bones. Red line = mean difference, Black lines = ± 1.96 SD.

as well as anteroposterior alignment of the tibial component rely on referencing of bone landmarks, and as a result the instrumentation may lack precision. This can be compared to the TKA procedure whereby the location of transepicondylar axis has been shown to have an interobserver discrepancy of 23° [19], while intraobserver error and interobserver error of 6° and 9°, respectively, in the identification of the epicondylar axis have also been shown [20, 21]. Analogously these discrepancies would exist in a UKA procedure when attempting to align the femoral and tibial jigs using guidelines relying on the patient's anatomy. This reflects our results and others [1] and explains significant differences found in most, but not all, directions of alignment in the conventional group compared to the robot group.

Overall our results of errors in the positioning and orientation of both components using the Sculptor RGA were comparable to results of experienced surgeons operating on real patients: Dunbar et al. [22] found that the MAKO robot's mean RMS errors for the tibia were 1.4 mm and 2.6° and for the femur 1.2 mm and 2.1°, while Cobb et al. [1] reported mean RMS errors using the Acrobot to be 1.1 mm and 2.5° for the tibia and 1.0 mm and 2.6° for the femur. Our robot results using inexperienced UKA surgeons on dry bones are comparable: mean RMS errors of 1.0 mm and 1.8° for the tibial component and 1.3 mm and 1.7° for the femoral component indicate that novice robot users can reproduce experienced surgeons' results. Our slightly lower values may be due to errors introduced during cementing in vivo, which has been reported to give errors of up to 2° in UKAs [23].

We recognise several inherent limitations of our study. It is a small study, using only 3 repetitions to demonstrate learning so may miss an improved performance later in the learning curve, although the largest improvement might be expected to be early in the experience. We did not demonstrate this. It is also a dry bone study. However, the dry bones were replicas of a patient's arthritic tibia and femur with replica ligaments and a capsule attached and hence were as realistic to a real patient as possible. The fact that our accuracy results were comparable to published in vivo data supports the validity of the dry bone model. However, the use of dry bones prevents reproduction of soft tissue balancing and the selection of an appropriate thickness of bearing. Therefore, measurement of the tibiofemoral angle is meaningless. Although this is an important measure of functional outcome following a UKA, component alignment is a major influence of tibiofemoral angle [24, 25], thus justifying the conclusions.

Arthroplasty requires precision and accuracy to be delivered consistently for favourable outcomes. Robotic systems have repeatedly demonstrated superiority over conventional methods when used by experienced users. We have demonstrated that this level of exactitude can be replicated on a dry bone model by surgeons who are unfamiliar with the procedure. Robotic technology, in the form of the Sculptor RGA, enables surgeons to perform this demanding form of arthroplasty accurately without prior experience. It achieves this by removing the inaccuracies inherent in the use of conventional instrumentation.

## Acknowledgments

The authors thank Simon Harris and Adeel Aqil from Imperial College London. They would like to thank Wellcome Trust and EPSRC for funding part of the project.

## References

[1] J. Cobb, J. Henckel, P. Gomes et al., "Hands-on robotic unicompartmental knee replacement: a prospective, randomised controlled study of the acrobot system," Journal of Bone and Joint Surgery B, vol. 88, no. 2, pp. 188–197, 2006.

[2] W. G. Hamilton, D. Ammeen, C. A. Engh Jr., and G. A. Engh, "Learning curve with minimally invasive unicompartmental

knee arthroplasty," *The Journal of Arthroplasty*, vol. 25, no. 5, pp. 735–740, 2010.

[3] J. L. Rees, A. J. Price, D. J. Beard, C. A. F. Dodd, and D. W. Murray, "Minimally invasive Oxford unicompartmental knee arthroplasty: functional results at 1 year and the effect of surgical inexperience," *The Knee*, vol. 11, no. 5, pp. 363–367, 2004.

[4] T. M. Coon, "Integrating robotic technology into the operating room," *American Journal of Orthopedics*, vol. 38, no. 2, pp. 7–9, 2009.

[5] T. J. Heyse, A. Khefacha, G. Peersman, and P. Cartier, "Survivorship of UKA in the middle-aged," *The Knee*, vol. 19, no. 5, pp. 585–591.

[6] D. Hollinghurst, J. Stoney, T. Ward et al., "No deterioration of kinematics and cruciate function 10 years after medial unicompartmental arthroplasty," *The Knee*, vol. 13, no. 6, pp. 440–444, 2006.

[7] M. A. Hassaballa, A. J. Porteous, and I. D. Learmonth, "Functional outcomes after different types of knee arthroplasty: kneeling ability versus descending stairs," *Medical Science Monitor*, vol. 13, no. 2, pp. CR77–CR81, 2007.

[8] B. D. Springer, R. D. Scott, and T. S. Thornhill, "Conversion of failed unicompartmental knee arthroplasty to TKA," *Clinical Orthopaedics and Related Research*, no. 446, pp. 214–220, 2006.

[9] J.-N. A. Argenson, Y. Chevrol-Benkeddache, and J.-M. Aubaniac, "Modern unicompartmental knee arthroplasty with cement: a three to ten-year follow-up study," *Journal of Bone and Joint Surgery A*, vol. 84, no. 12, pp. 2235–2239, 2002.

[10] M. B. Collier, T. H. Eickmann, F. Sukezaki, J. P. McAuley, and G. A. Engh, "Patient, implant, and alignment factors associated with revision of medial compartment unicondylar arthroplasty," *The Journal of Arthroplasty*, vol. 21, no. 6, pp. 108–115, 2006.

[11] P. E. Müller, C. Pellengahr, M. Witt, J. Kircher, H. J. Refior, and V. Jansson, "Influence of minimally invasive surgery on implant positioning and the functional outcome for medial unicompartmental knee arthroplasty," *The Journal of Arthroplasty*, vol. 19, no. 3, pp. 296–301, 2004.

[12] J. H. Lonner, "Indications for unicompartmental knee arthroplasty and rationale for robotic arm-assisted technology," *American Journal of Orthopedics*, vol. 38, no. 2, supplement, pp. 3–6, 2009.

[13] A. D. Pearle, D. Kendoff, V. Stueber, V. Musahl, and J. A. Repicci, "Perioperative management of unicompartmental knee arthroplasty using the MAKO robotic arm system (MAKOplasty)," *American Journal of Orthopedics*, vol. 38, no. 2, supplement, pp. 16–19, 2009.

[14] W. G. Hamilton, M. B. Collier, E. Tarabee, J. P. McAuley, C. A. Engh Jr., and G. A. Engh, "Incidence and reasons for reoperation after minimally invasive unicompartmental knee arthroplasty," *The Journal of Arthroplasty*, vol. 21, no. 6, pp. 98–107, 2006.

[15] M. Masjedi, K. Davda, S. Harris, and J. Cobb, "Evaluate your robot accuracy," in *Proceedings of the Hamlyn Symposium on Medical Robotics*, 2011.

[16] P. Magne, "Virtual prototyping of adhesively restored, endodontically treated molars," *The Journal of Prosthetic Dentistry*, vol. 103, no. 6, pp. 343–351, 2010.

[17] "NextEngine 3D Laser Scanner," http://www.nextengine.com/faq#accuracy.

[18] T. J. Aleto, M. E. Berend, M. A. Ritter, P. M. Faris, and R. M. Meneghini, " Early failure of unicompartmental knee arthroplasty leading to revision," *The Journal of Arthroplasty*, vol. 23, no. 2, pp. 159–163, 2008.

[19] J. Jerosch, E. Peuker, B. Philipps, and T. Filler, "Interindividual reproducibility in perioperative rotational alignment of femoral components in knee prosthetic surgery using the transepicondylar axis," *Knee Surgery, Sports Traumatology, Arthroscopy*, vol. 10, no. 3, pp. 194–197, 2002.

[20] J.-Y. Jenny and C. Boeri, "Low reproducibility of the intraoperative measurement of the transepicondylar axis during total knee replacement," *Acta Orthopaedica Scandinavica*, vol. 75, no. 1, pp. 74–77, 2004.

[21] J. B. Mason, T. K. Fehring, R. Estok, D. Banel, and K. Fahrbach, "Meta-analysis of alignment outcomes in computer-assisted total knee arthroplasty surgery," *The Journal of Arthroplasty*, vol. 22, no. 8, pp. 1097–1106, 2007.

[22] N. J. Dunbar, M. W. Roche, B. H. Park, S. H. Branch, M. A. Conditt, and S. A. Banks, "Accuracy of dynamic tactile-guided unicompartmental knee arthroplasty," *The Journal of Arthroplasty*, vol. 27, no. 5, pp. 803–808, 2012.

[23] R. Sinha and M. Cutler, "Effect of cement technique on component position during robotic-arm assisted unicompartmental arthroplasty (UKA)," in *Proceedings of the International Society for Technology in Arthroplasty (ISTA '10)*, Dubai, UAE, Octobre 2010.

[24] A. Srivastava, G. Y. Lee, N. Steklov, C. W. Colwell Jr., K. A. Ezzet, and D. D. D'Lima, "Effect of tibial component varus on wear in total knee arthroplasty," *The Knee*, vol. 19, no. 5, pp. 560–563, 2011.

[25] P. Hernigou and G. Deschamps, "Posterior slope of the tibial implant and the outcome of unicompartmental knee arthroplasty," *Journal of Bone and Joint Surgery A*, vol. 86, no. 3, pp. 506–511, 2004.

# 18

# The Interspinous Spacer: A New Posterior Dynamic Stabilization Concept for Prevention of Adjacent Segment Disease

**Antoine Nachanakian, Antonios El Helou, and Moussa Alaywan**

*Department of Neurosurgery, Saint George Hospital University Medical Center and Balamand University, Youssef Sursock Street, Rmeil, Beirut 11 00 2807, P.O. Box 166378, Lebanon*

Correspondence should be addressed to Antoine Nachanakian; nachanakian@gmail.com

Academic Editor: Mehdi Sasani

*Introduction*. Posterior Dynamic stabilization using the interspinous spacer device is a known to be used as an alternative to rigid fusion in neurogenic claudication patients in the absence of macro instability. Actually, it plays an important in the management of adjacent segment disease in previously fused lumbar spine. *Materials and Method*. We report our experience with posterior dynamic stabilization using an interspinous spacer. 134 cases performed in our institution between September 2008 and August 2012 with different lumbar spine pathologies. The ages of our patients were between 40 and 72 years, with a mean age of 57 years. After almost 4 years of follow up in our patient and comparing their outcome to our previous serious we found that in some case the interspinous distracter has an important role not only in the treatment of adjacent segment disease but also in its prevention. *Results and Discussion*. Clinical improvement was noted in ISD-treated patients, with high satisfaction rate. At first, radicular pain improves with more than 3/10 reduction of the mean score on visual analog scale (VAS). In addition, disability score as well as disc height and lordotic angle showed major improvement at 3 to 6 months post operatively. And, no adjacent segment disease was reported in the patient operated with interspinous spacer. *Conclusion*. The interspinous spacer is safe and efficient modality to be used not only as a treatment of adjacent segment disease but also as a preventive measure in patients necessitating rigid fusion.

## 1. Introduction

Spinal disorders are among the most common health complaints affecting a large portion of the population in developed and developing countries [1]. Spinal disorders can be treated medically at first and the majority of patients will respond to the latter, whereas others will need surgical treatment for their spinal disease. And though, degenerative disease of the spinal cord became a serious problem with the aging of the population and its management is in continuous evolution.

Spinal stenosis manifested by back or radicular pain and nonresponding to conservative management or evolution to neurogenic claudication necessitates surgical procedure. The management of this pathology changed over time and in case decompressive surgery was not sufficient or the spinal segments degenerated later on, a rigid fusion was used. Rigid fusion was efficient and provided better outcome compared to decompression alone, but it could not resolve the problem of disc degeneration without evident radicular compression [2]. And, overtime, with millions of segmental fusion done, a new pathology known as adjacent segment disease was described. From this evidence for adjacent-segment degeneration emerged the concept of dynamic or nonfusion stabilization of the lumbar spine [3]. The dynamic stabilization hardware functions as shock absorbent at the level above a fused segment and reduces the pressure leading to further degeneration in the spinal cord [4].

Posterior dynamic stabilization was born from the need of normalization of the intersegmental motion [5] and in contrast to the traditional fusion surgery it does not eliminate the mobility of the fused segment [6]. While both procedures treat the microinstability, posterior dynamic stabilization does it in a more physiological manner. By restoring normal motion, mobility is theoretically preserved rather than eliminated, and the forces acting above and below the construct are altered to a lesser extent, reducing the potential undesirable effects of fusion [7].

Interspinous process spacers have been introduced as a possible alternative to spinal decompression and fusion for the treatment of neurogenic intermittent claudication (NIC) and discogenic lower back pain [8]. The interspinous devices work as a shock absorbent device. In addition to intervertebral height restoration, it improves central canal and foraminal stenosis. Interspinous Distracter (ISD) is designed to stabilize the motion segment after neural elements decompression in lumbar stenosis, tolerating flexion and extension in this segment thus preserving the adjacent segment from deterioration [5–8].

## 2. Methods

Our experience is based on 134 cases performed between September 2008 and August 2012 with different lumbar spine pathologies (Table 1). The ages of our patients were between 40 and 72 years, with a mean age of 57 years. All patients were treated with Interspinous Distracter (ISD).

*2.1. Inclusion Criteria.* At the beginning of our usage of ISD, patients were eligible for enrolment if they had the following:

(i) degenerative disk disease and subsequent bilateral foraminal stenosis (Figure 1),

(ii) foraminal-canalar stenosis, due to ligamentum flavum hypertrophy, declared symptoms consisting of neurogenic claudication,

(iii) suspended vertebra shown on X-ray which is due to facet degenerative disease,

(iv) facet joint syndrome.

Then with the development of the techniques and the follow-up results, two indications were added to the above mentioned criteria:

(i) adjacent segment syndrome (Figure 2) which refers to degenerative changes that occur in the mobile segment next to spinal fusion,

(ii) degenerated disc at a level superior to the one necessitating posterior rigid fusion.

After several procedures with successful results in management of adjacent segment syndrome and to avoid later hospitalization and added surgical procedure in previously operated patients with spinal fusion, we started to use ISD as prevention to avoid adjacent segment disease.

*2.2. Exclusion Criteria.* Patients were excluded in cases of more than 2 adjacent levels disease, in the absence of the spinous processes due to previous surgery or fractures, in the presence of spondylolysthesis, and, when severe osteoporosis exists in the lumbar region ($T$ score $< -2.5$ in the lumbar region).

TABLE 1: Number of cases in correlation with disease and sex.

| Number of cases | Pathology | Male/female ratio |
|---|---|---|
| 36 | Biforaminal stenosis | 24/12 |
| 15 | Ligamentum flavum hypertrophy | 8/7 |
| 6 | Suspended vertebrae | 4/2 |
| 3 | Facet syndrome | 0/3 |
| 47 | Adjacent syndrome | 28/19 |
| 27 | Adjacent syndrome prevention | 12/15 |

*2.3. Preoperative Evaluation.* The patients completed the visual analogue scale (VAS) for pain and Oswestry disability index (ODI).

At first, paraclinical evaluation included plain lumbar film, lumbar MRI or CT, and osteodensitometry. Then MRI along with dynamic lumbar X-ray was used and osteodensitometry was done in postmenopause female patients.

The global and segmental lordotic angles (stabilized segments, above and below adjacent segments) were measured using Cobb's method on lateral neutral position lumbosacral spine X-ray.

The segmental lordotic angles (stabilized segments and adjacent segments) were measured from between the upper end plates of the corresponding segments.

### 2.4. Operative Procedure

*2.4.1. Preparation.* The procedure is done under general anesthesia. All patients were operated in a prone position, avoiding hyperlordosis for a better interspinous distraction.

*2.4.2. Product Used.* Different interspinous spacers' types are used in our institution.

*2.4.3. The Instrument Used.* A set of lumbar laminectomy is used. In addition, a set of interspinous spacer measurer is utilized to define the depth and width of the spacer to be used.

*2.4.4. Surgical Note.* The level of the procedure is localized under fluoroscopy after positioning. Surgical exposure is done similar to any lumbar laminectomy procedure. For the insertion of the ISD the interspinous ligament as well as the ligamentum flavum was resected.

After ISD insertion, the depth between it and the dural sac is assessed by 3 mm hook.

In cases where the disc is protruded/herniated, medial discectomy was not done. In cases where degenerative or congenital spondylolysthesis is present, rigid fusion of the spondylotic level was done. The insertion of ISD at the level above was done in patients older than 55 years. In patients younger than 55 years, the decision was made for each case separately. If the level adjacent to the fusion is not degenerated, this level is spared and the ISD is inserted at the level above; whereas if the disc at the adjacent level is degenerated, ISD is used at the latter mentioned level (Figure 3).

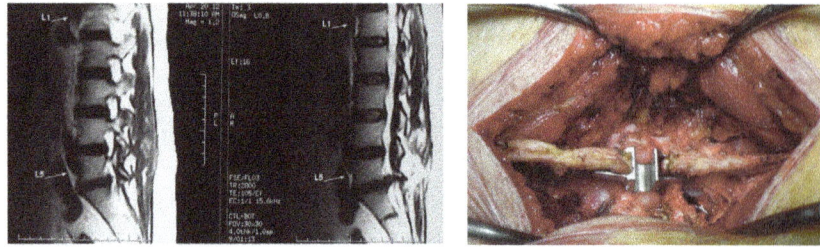

FIGURE 1: On the left, sagittal T2W image MRI of Lumbosacral spine showing extruded L5-S1 disc with degenerated L4-L5 disc. On the right, preoperative view of the same patient showing left L5-S1 laminotomy for disc excision and L4-L5 interspinous distractor.

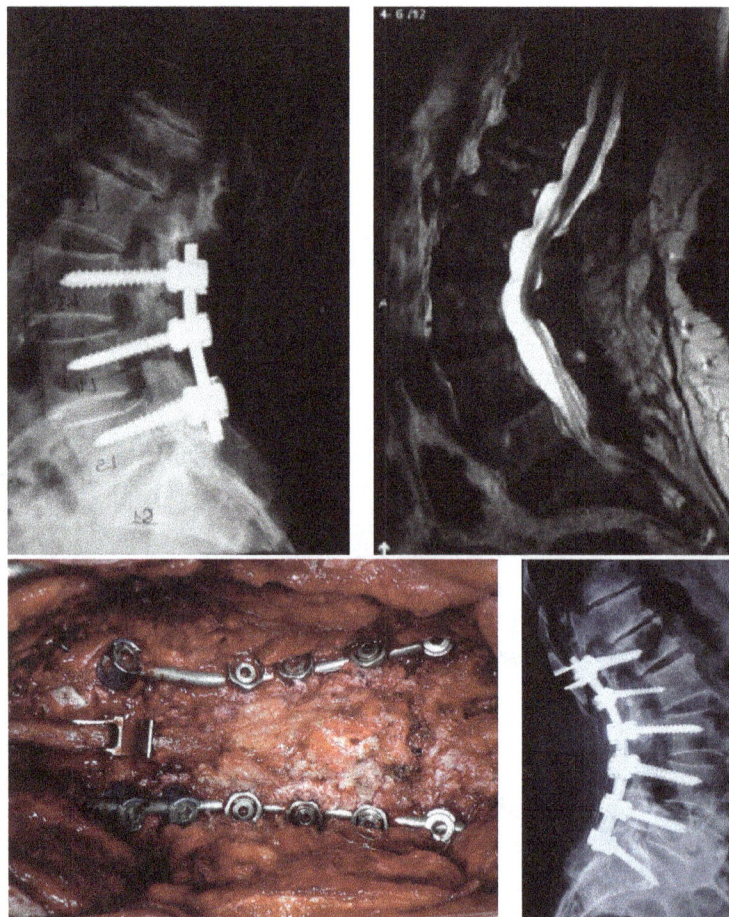

FIGURE 2: Above preoperative spine X-ray with previous instrumented level on the right. On the left, degenerated segments at L1-L2 and L2-L3 levels. Below preoperative view showing the extended fusion from L1 to S1 with Th12-L1 interspinous spacer.

Regular closure of layers and placing of deep hemovac drain ended the surgery.

### 2.5. Follow-Up Evaluation

*2.5.1. Immediate Postoperative Care.* The patient is out of bed the day after surgery and discharged on day 3 after surgery or on day 2 when drain was not inserted. All patients wear a lumbar brace, for a period of one month during their daily activities.

*2.5.2. Late Postoperative Evaluation.* The following data were collected: VAS, ODI, pain medication, complications, and patient satisfaction.

Control lumbosacral X-ray is done in 2 views to evaluate the created distraction.

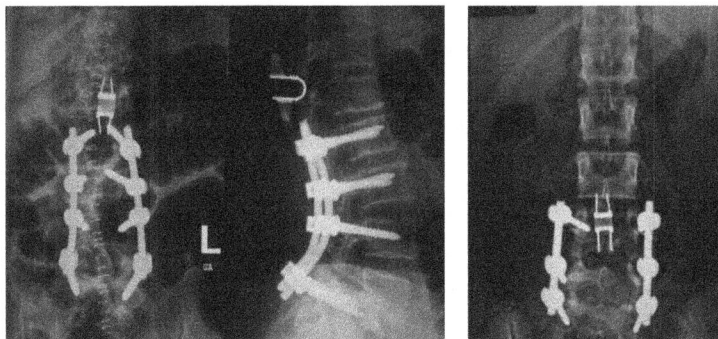

FIGURE 3: Postoperative spine X-ray, on the right, showing multiple level fusions with ISD 1 level skipping the adjacent segment. On the left, ISD used at the level adjacent to the rigid fusion.

The plain radiographs (anteroposterior and lateral standing in neutral position) are obtained at day 1, day 90, and day 180 postoperatively. Disc height and Cobb's angle are measured and compared to the preoperative values.

*2.6. Complications.* In general, materials are well tolerated. The rate of complications is between 1% and 10% in all series. Two sets of complications exist: the early and the delayed.

Early complications include device dislocation/malposition, spinous process fractures, erosion of the spinous process, infection, hematoma, and neurological sequelae.

One case of migration was observed in one series [4]. There were no broken or permanently deformed implants in all series.

In our series, no cases of fracture of the superior spinous process occurred. In our experience, we do osteodensitometry for all patients to assess bone density preoperatively. During operation, we avoid bone erosions of the adjacent spinous processes.

We had one case of recurrent neurological symptoms, and ISD was removed. Microsurgical decompression and posterolateral fusion were done. To avoid this type of complications, a complete posterior decompression through ligamentum flavum excision and discectomy in the presence of herniated disc should be done.

Selection of patients without spondylolysthesis is mandatory to avoid posterolateral fusion later on. And in the presence of spondylotic segment, rigid fusion with insertion of ISD at the superior adjacent level protects from recurrence of neurological symptoms as well as from later adjacent segment disease.

*2.7. Statistical Analysis.* The clinical and radiologic results were analyzed using $t$-test; a $P$ value of less than 0.05 is considered statistically significant. All analyses were carried out using SPSS Ver. 16.00 (IL, Chicago, Inc.).

## 3. Results

*3.1. Pain Assessment.* Overall improvement was noted in ISD-treated patients, with considerable satisfaction in 89% of patients on average.

The patients at first reported an improvement of their radicular pain with a mean reduction of 3.4/10 on visual analog scale (VAS) (scale for 0: absent pain to 10: severe intolerable pain necessitating intravenous treatment).

In the preoperative period, radicular pain had a mean score of 8.6/10 on VAS (5–10). Whereas in the immediate post-op period, the pain mean score was 4.3/10 on VAS (1–7).

Patients achieved maximum improvement after an average period of 6 months, with a mean score of 1.8/10 on VAS (0–5), and up to 83% of patients were pain free (Figure 4).

*3.2. Disability Assessment.* The Oswestry low back disability questionnaire score (ODI) improved from a mean of 68.1% in the pre-op period (23%–91%) to 17.8% at 3 months (0%–52%) and <10% at a 6-month followup ($P < 0.05$) (Figure 5).

*3.3. Disc Height.* The preoperative disc height was measured by MRI, with a mean of 1.2 cm (0.4–1.6 cm) and intervertebral space on lateral X-ray view measured manually had a mean of 1.3 cm (0.7–1.6 cm). Whereas, in post-op evaluation only spine X-ray was done (due to the elevated cost of MRI) and the mean measured intervertebral space was 1.75 cm (1.2–2.4 cm).

Radiologic changes, on lateral views in neutral position in lumbosacral spine X-ray, in the disk height of the stabilized segment, were increased significantly from preoperative to immediate postoperative evaluation ($P < 0.05$). This increase persisted at 3-month followup ($P < 0.05$) (Figure 6).

*3.4. Segmental Lordotic Angles.* The range of motion measured by the segmental lordotic angle in stabilized segment decreased postoperatively ($3.78 \pm 3.1°$) compared to the preoperative measured values ($5.26 \pm 3.68°$). This change was not statistically significant ($P = 0.4$).

Although adjacent segment ROM showed a decrease on post-op X-ray, there was no statistical significance (Figure 6).

*3.5. Operative Characteristics.* The prominent characteristic of this surgery is a low level of postoperative pain. And so, the decompression is done by removal of ligamentum flavum and the reestablishment of the dynamics of the spine plays a

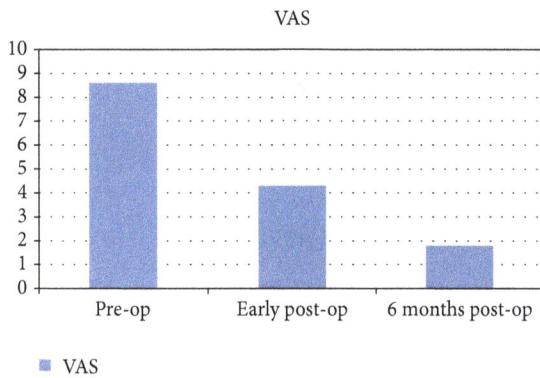

FIGURE 4: Comparative chart of mean VAS from preoperative period, early postoperative, and at 6-month follow up.

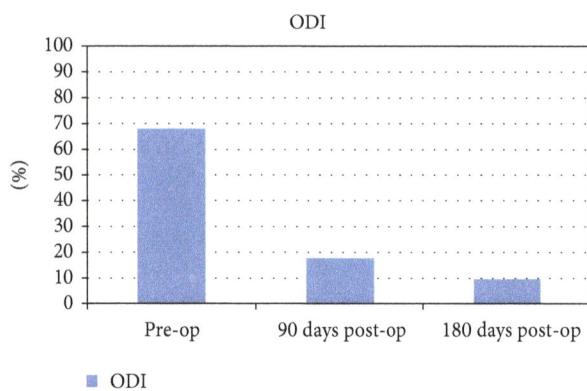

FIGURE 5: Oswestry low back disability score comparing pre-op evaluation to 3 months and 6 months post-op evaluation.

major role in the resolution of back pain. Restoration of the height of the intervertebral disc relieves the pressure on the sinuvertebral nerve which plays a major role in decreasing paraspinal muscles spasm despite the back pain.

In addition, the amount of blood loss with ISD procedure (49.2 cc ± 24.8) compared to rigid stabilization (184.3 cc ± 67.8) was found to be reduced ($P < 0.005$).

## 4. Discussion

Rigid spinal fusion is a mandatory procedure for the management of lumbar instability although it could be associated with different types of complications such as device failure, osteoporosis, and spinal deformity by changing the spinal mechanical activities, leading to adjacent segment disease [9]. The fusion technique shifts the center of rotation of vertebral body over the disc leading to an increase in the stress on the facets and/or disc of the adjacent mobile segment. The increase of stress induces several changes in the mobility of the adjacent segment and elevation of intradiscal pressure [10]. And so, it can lead to disc degeneration which precedes the facet degeneration [11].

Some authors do not agree with the theory of adjacent segment degeneration and in a prospective study conducted

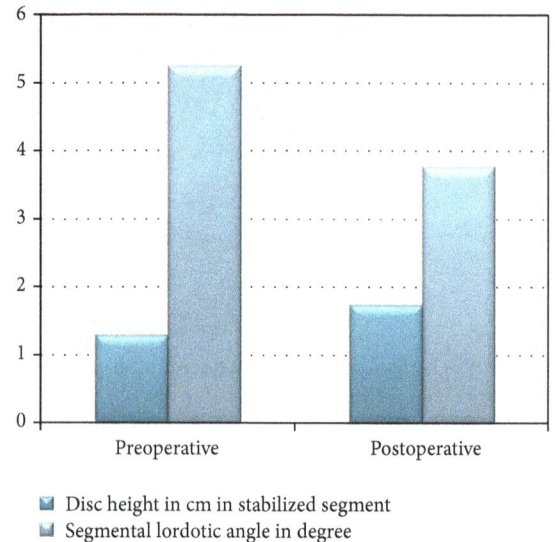

FIGURE 6: Comparative chart between preoperative and postoperative radiological changes.

in Spain, disc degeneration post lumbar fusion appeared homogeneously at several levels cephalad to fusion and seemed to be determined more by individual characteristics than by fusion itself [12].

In our experience, after a long followup period, we have remarked that adjacent segment disease is a serious problem that causes refractory pain to medical treatment, which necessitated long segment fusion which leads to limitation of back motion and spinal deformities [13]. In addition, the refractory pain to medical treatment has high cost both on individual and national levels.

To avoid these adverse effects, the achievement of ideal mobility is important. Thus, dynamic stabilization devices would appear to represent a notable technological advantage.

Posterior dynamic stabilization is done to decrease and/or avoid the harmful effects of rigid fusion, like listhesis, instability, hypertrophic facet joint arthritis, herniated nucleus pulposus, and stenosis.

Several studies comparing interspinal distractor or dynamic pedicular system to posterior lumbar interbody fusion (PLIF) were conducted and showed promising results [14, 15]. We did not try dynamic pedicular system since we had satisfactory results with the interspinous spacer.

The interspinous dynamic stabilization system, with preservation of the disc and facet, creates a favorable environment in the motion segment by reducing the loading on these joints and allowing more normal motion.

The clinical outcomes of patients in our study improved significantly during the follow-up period, not only at 3 and 6 months, but also in the early post-op period.

The system increased the distraction posteriorly and improved the anterior disc space height and articular process pressure which decreased the stenosis, liberated the nerve roots and the foramina [14], and reduced neural pain transmission via the dorsal root ganglia despite decreased overall painful stimuli and transmission [16].

The followup with serial X-rays showed no evidence of osteophytes at articular facets level as noted in rigid fixation. We conclude that ISD not only decreases the load on the facets, but also impairs osteophytes formation. Decreasing the load in addition to the impairment of osteophytes formation is an additional proof that posterior dynamic stabilization is an effective method to treat and to prevent adjacent segment disease. It also shows that this type of fusion not only preserves normal motion, but it prevents further degenerative process by maintaining patient's own lumbar kinematics and reducing instability.

In late postoperative X-ray followup of the patients examined, a mineralization of the spinous process in contact with the implant was found, in particular at its base which appears to absorb high stresses due to lordosis, and this finding was described 10 years ago [17].

Our results concerning disc height and segmental lordotic angles correlate with other studies done in China and Turkey [15, 18]. This means that the ISD is useful regardless of ethnic origin.

Rigid stabilization was found to decrease fiber strain of the intervertebral disc and transfer the load to the rod, changing all the biomechanics of the spinal cord; whereas ISD keeps the natural fiber strain in a physiological manner which was proved by the pre- and postoperative disc height [16].

The ISD system slightly limits the bulging of the disc at the lateral and posterolateral site. This could be due to the decompression effect at the posterior elements by the implant [19]. Compared to rigid stabilization surgery, ISD insertion is associated with less blood loss and shorter surgical time and hospital stay. These criteria have a high impact on postoperative pain, recovery period, and the overall quality of life [20].

## 5. Conclusion

Interspinous spacer insertion after excision of ligamentum flavum showed excellent results in terms of pain control, motion preservation, and prevention of adjacent segment degeneration in previously stabilized lumbar spine segments. It provides restoration of disc height, reduction of vertebral slip and leads to physiological condition concerning disc bulging. We highly recommend its use in treatment as well as in prevention of adjacent segment disease specifically in young patients where spinal fusion for early degenerative disease is needed.

## References

[1] C. S. Chen, C. K. Cheng, C. L. Liu, and W. H. Lo, "Stress analysis of the disc adjacent to interbody fusion in lumbar spine," *Medical Engineering and Physics*, vol. 23, no. 7, pp. 483–491, 2001.

[2] M. Kanayama, T. Hashimoto, K. Shigenobu et al., "Adjacent-segment morbidity after Graf ligamentoplasty compared with posterolateral lumbar fusion," *Journal of Neurosurgery*, vol. 95, no. 1, pp. 5–10, 2001.

[3] S. D. Christie, J. K. Song, and R. G. Fessler, "Dynamic interspinous process technology," *Spine*, vol. 30, no. 16, pp. S73–S78, 2005.

[4] D. Adelt, J. Samani, W.-K. Kim et al., "Coflex Interspinous Stabilisation: clinical and Radiographic results from an international multicenter retrospective study," *Paradigm Spine Journal*, no. 1, pp. 1–4, 2007.

[5] D. L. Kaech, C. Fernandez, and P. Haninec, "Preliminary experience with the interspinous U device," *Rachis*, vol. 13, pp. 303–304, 2001.

[6] D. L. Kaech, C. Fernandez, D. Lombardi-Weber et al., "The interspinous U: a new restabilization device for the lumbar spine," *Spinal Restabilization Procedures*, vol. 30, pp. 355–362, 2000.

[7] D. L. Kaech and J. R. Jinkins, "The interspinous "U": a new restabilization device for the lumbar spine Spinal Restabilization Procedures," *Elsevier Science B.V.*, pp. 355–362, 2002.

[8] C. Bowers, A. Amini, A. T. Dailey, and M. H. Schmidt, "Dynamic interspinous process stabilization: review of complications associated with the X-Stop device," *Neurosurgical Focus*, vol. 28, no. 6, p. E8, 2010.

[9] D. K. Resnick, T. F. Choudhri, A. T. Dailey et al., "Guidelines for the performance of fusion procedures for degenerative disease of the lumbar spine. Part 5: correlation between radiographic and functional outcome," *Journal of Neurosurgery. Spine*, vol. 2, no. 6, pp. 658–661, 2005.

[10] M. N. Kumar, A. Baklanov, and D. Chopin, "Correlation between sagittal plane changes and adjacent segment degeneration following lumbar spine fusion," *European Spine Journal*, vol. 10, no. 4, pp. 314–319, 2001.

[11] J. S. Mehta, S. Kochhar, and I. J. Harding, "A slip above a slip: retrolisthesis of the motion segment above a spondylolytic spondylolysthesis," *European Spine Journal*, vol. 21, no. 11, pp. 2128–2133, 2012.

[12] F. Pellisé, A. Hernández, X. Vidal, J. Minguell, C. Martínez, and C. Villanueva, "Radiologic assessment of all unfused lumbar segments 7.5 years after instrumented posterior spinal fusion," *Spine*, vol. 32, no. 5, pp. 574–579, 2007.

[13] A. Nachanakian, A. El Helou, and M. Alaywan, *Posterior Dynamic Stabilization: The Interspinous spacer, Low Back Pain Pathogenesis and Treatment*, Edited by Y. Sakai, InTech, 2012.

[14] S.-W. Yu, C.-Y. Yen, C.-H. Wu, F.-C. Kao, Y.-H. Kao, and Y.-K. Tu, "Radiographic and clinical results of posterior dynamic stabilization for the treatment of multisegment degenerative disc disease with a minimum follow-up of 3 years," *Archives of Orthopaedic and Trauma Surgery*, vol. 132, pp. 583–589, 2012.

[15] T. Cansever, E. Civelek, S. Kabatas, C. Yılmaz, H. Caner, and M. N. Altinörs, "Dysfunctional segmental motion treated with dynamic stabilization in the lumbar spine," *World Neurosurgery*, vol. 75, no. 5-6, pp. 743–749, 2011.

[16] F. Heuer, H. Schmidt, W. Käfer, N. Graf, and H.-J. Wilke, "Posterior motion preserving implants evaluated by means of intervertebral disc bulging and annular fiber strains," *Clinical Biomechanics*, vol. 27, pp. 218–225, 2012.

[17] K. E. Swanson, D. P. Lindsey, K. Y. Hsu, J. F. Zucherman, and S. A. Yerby, "The effects of an interspinous implant on intervertebral disc pressures," *Spine*, vol. 28, no. 1, pp. 26–32, 2003.

[18] Y. H. Jia and P. F. Sun, "Preliminary evaluation of posterior dynamic lumbar stabilization in lumbar degenerative disease in Chinese patients," *Chinese Medical Journal*, vol. 125, no. 2, pp. 253–256, 2012.

[19] W. Schmoelz, S. Erhart, S. Unger, and C. Alexander, "Disch: biomechanical evaluation of a posterior non-fusion instrumentation of the lumbar spine," *European Spine Journal*, vol. 21, pp. 939–945, 2012.

[20] B. Cakir, B. Ulmar, H. Koepp, K. Huch, W. Puhl, and M. Richter, "Posterior dynamic stabiliziation as on alternative for instrumented fusion in the treatment of degenerative lumbar instability with spinal stenosis," *Zeitschrift fur Orthopadie und Ihre Grenzgebiete*, vol. 141, no. 4, pp. 418–424, 2003.

# 19

# The Costs of Operative Complications for Ankle Fractures: A Case Control Study

**Frank R. Avilucea, Sarah E. Greenberg, W. Jeffrey Grantham, Vasanth Sathiyakumar, Rachel V. Thakore, Samuel K. Nwosu, Kristin R. Archer, William T. Obremskey, Hassan R. Mir, and Manish K. Sethi**

*The Vanderbilt Orthopaedic Institute Center for Health Policy, 1215 21st Avenue S., MCE, South Tower, Suite 4200, Vanderbilt University, Nashville, TN 37232, USA*

Correspondence should be addressed to Manish K. Sethi; manish.sethi@vanderbilt.edu

Academic Editor: Robert F. Ostrum

As our healthcare system moves towards bundling payments, it is vital to understand the potential financial implications associated with treatment of surgical complications. Considering that surgical treatment of ankle fractures is common, there remains minimal data relating costs to postsurgical intervention. We aimed to identify costs associated with ankle fracture complications through case-control analysis. Using retrospective analysis at a level I trauma center, 28 patients with isolated ankle fractures who developed complications (cases) were matched with 28 isolated ankle fracture patients without complications (controls) based on ASA score, age, surgery type, and fracture type. Patient charts were reviewed for demographics and complications leading to readmission/reoperation and costs were obtained from the financial department. Wilcoxon tests measured differences in the costs between the cases and controls. 28 out of 439 patients (6.4%) developed complications. Length of stay and median costs were significantly higher for cases than controls. Specifically, differences in total costs existed for infection and hardware-related pain. This is the first study to highlight the considerable costs associated with the treatment of complications due to isolated ankle fractures. Physicians must therefore emphasize methods to control surgical and nonsurgical factors that may impact postoperative complications, especially under a global payment system.

## 1. Introduction

Healthcare costs in the United States were approximately $2.8 trillion in 2012, representing 17.9% of the national gross domestic product [1]. In an effort to curb the rising costs of care, our healthcare system is moving towards a global payment model in which readmissions for complications may not be reimbursed. Given that ankle fractures, occurring at a rate of 187 per 100,000 people each year, are one of the most common injuries treated by orthopaedic surgeons, it is important to understand the costs of treating the surgical complications that can arise from these injuries and the resultant financial implications that may occur under a bundled or global payment system [2].

Unfortunately, even with the high frequency of these injuries, there is minimal literature regarding the financial costs of ankle fracture complications. For example, in an economic analysis by Belatti and Phisitkul, foot and ankle diseases in the Medicare population were estimated to cost $11 billion in 2011, with treatment secondary to fractures contributing to 31% of these costs [3]. However, these authors did not differentiate ankle fractures from other fractures of the foot and did not analyze the costs secondary to complications. Manoukian et al. investigated ankle fracture costs based on the timing of operation in relation to when patients are admitted to the hospital, but their analysis did not focus on complications or specific areas of costs during the hospitalization [4]. Additionally, Murray and colleagues investigated index hospitalization and readmission costs for ankle fracture patients based on type of surgery; however, the authors did not identify reasons for readmission based on type of complication [5].

Despite studies focusing on various aspects of costs related to ankle fractures, to date, no study has investigated the costs related to the types of complications that these patients with ankle fractures may develop. In a bundled-payment system under which these complications may not be reimbursed, it is vital for the practicing orthopaedic surgeon to understand the financial implications associated with post-surgical complications.

To evaluate the costs associated with ankle fracture complications, we designed a case control analysis where we matched patients who developed complications after ankle fracture surgery ("cases") to those who did not develop complications (controls). The analysis of these cohorts enables us to determine the costs associated with each type of complication. Furthermore, by categorizing the costs associated with different hospital services, we found which factors have the greatest impact on overall expenditures. Therefore, understanding these variations in costs may help drive policymaking to better prepare orthopaedic surgeons for a bundled-payment system.

## 2. Methods

After institutional review board approval, all patients treated at a level I trauma center from January 1, 2000, to January 1, 2010, for ankle fractures were identified through a CPT code search of the university's orthopaedic database. Patient charts were reviewed to include only those who had isolated ankle fractures without any concomitant injuries, including additional fractures, organ injuries, or neurovascular injuries. The charts of these remaining patients were reviewed for basic demographic information including age and gender, as well as type of fracture, fracture location, length of stay for index hospitalization and readmissions, American Society of Anesthesiologist (ASA) score, and complications. Complications included those that resulted in reoperation or readmission and included nonunion, infection, hardware pain, hardware failure, and malunion.

Patients with complications (cases) were matched to those without complications (controls) following principles in orthopaedic literature, which are based on correlating specific factors that may be associated with the outcome of interest. In our study, we matched by ASA score (within one score), age (within 10 years), type of surgery (based on CPT code), and type of fracture (open versus closed) as several studies found correlations between these variables and development of complications [6–8]. Costs for cases and controls were obtained from the university's financial database and included professional and technical charges. Professional charges were subcategorized into costs related to surgery, radiology, and evaluation and management of patients, whereas technical charges included diagnostic, room and board, surgical implant/materials, and pharmacy charges. Wilcoxon ranked-sum tests were performed to compare the differences in costs and length of stay between the case patients and control patients.

TABLE 1: Selected demographics for cases and controls.

| | Cases ($n = 28$) | Controls ($n = 28$) |
|---|---|---|
| Age (years) | | |
| 10–20 | 1 (4%) | 2 (7%) |
| 21–30 | 5 (18%) | 2 (7%) |
| 31–40 | 5 (18%) | 6 (21%) |
| 41–50 | 7 (25%) | 7 (25%) |
| 51–60 | 6 (21%) | 9 (32%) |
| 61–70 | 3 (11%) | 1 (4%) |
| >70 | 1 (4%) | 1 (4%) |
| Gender | | |
| Male | 13 (46%) | 13 (46%) |
| Female | 15 (54%) | 15 (54%) |
| Fracture type | | |
| Closed | 13 (46%) | 13 (46%) |
| Open | 15 (54%) | 15 (54%) |
| ASA score | | |
| 1 | 2 (7%) | 2 (7%) |
| 2 | 18 (64%) | 18 (64%) |
| 3 | 7 (25%) | 8 (29%) |
| 4 | 1 (4%) | 0 (0%) |

## 3. Results

Through a CPT code search, 439 patients presented with isolated ankle fractures, of which 28 developed a post-surgical complication. Basic demographic data, including age, gender, fracture type, and ASA score, for the 28 cases and their corresponding 28 controls is provided in Table 1. The average age of cases was 44 ± 15 years compared to 45 ± 14 years for the control group. Both groups had 15 closed (53.6%) and 13 open (46.4%) fractures, and the average ASA score for cases was 2.14 ± 0.59 compared to 2.21 ± 0.57 for controls. Of the 28 patients with complications, 7 (25.0%) had nonunion, 8 (28.6%) had infection, 10 (35.7%) had hardware pain, 3 (10.7%) had hardware failure, and 1 (3.6%) had malunion.

Table 2 provides the median charges for cases and controls without controlling for type of complication. There were significant differences in median charges between the groups with respect to both professional charges (difference of $8,185) and technical charges (difference of $32,532). Among the professional charges, the median surgical charges specifically differed between the case and control groups ($13,857 and $6,931, resp.). The technical charges associated with implant/materials and pharmacy charges were also significantly higher in the cases when compared to the controls (Table 2). Furthermore, the overall length of stay was greater for the cases (5.5 days) compared to controls (3.0 days) ($P = 0.028$).

Figures 1 and 2 detail the aggregate professional and technical charges, respectively, for the 28 patients within each group. The cases had higher aggregate costs in each category except for radiology charges. In sum, the 28 cases had an aggregate professional and technical charge of $3,090,331 compared to $1,637,589 for the 28 controls.

TABLE 2: Case versus control comparison for *overall* costs.

| | Overall costs (median, IQR) | | P |
| --- | --- | --- | --- |
| | Cases ($n = 28$) | Controls ($n = 28$) | |
| Professional charges | $16,454 ($13,497–$26,648) | $8,269 ($6,554–$11,063) | <0.001 |
| Surgical | $13,857 ($11,269–$22,298) | $6,931 ($4,290–$8,187) | <0.001 |
| Radiology | $688 ($330–$2,080) | $1,789 ($245–$2,197) | 0.940 |
| Evaluation and management | $892 ($573–$1,101) | $669 ($501–$997) | 0.240 |
| Technical charges | $69,162 ($39,849–$112,153) | $36,630 ($31,093–$57,418) | 0.002 |
| Diagnostic | $12,169 ($3,425–$20,920) | $12,446 ($3,339–$18,007) | 0.730 |
| Room and board | $4,845 ($1,354–$14,538) | $2,193 ($1,612–$4,800) | 0.200 |
| Implant/materials | $25,522 ($11,888–$42,816) | $15,244 ($9,551–$25,754) | 0.002 |
| Pharmacy | $12,576 ($5,525–$22,132) | $7,495 ($5,078–$14,527) | 0.006 |
| Total charges | $84,980 ($53,254–$139,950) | $60,538 ($40,606–$98,484) | 0.001 |

TABLE 3: Case versus control comparison for *nonunion* costs.

| | Nonunion costs (median, IQR) | | P |
| --- | --- | --- | --- |
| | Cases ($n = 7$) | Controls ($n = 7$) | |
| Professional charges | $17,863 ($15,683–$30,348) | $8,358 ($6,679–$14,729) | 0.028 |
| Surgical | $16,397 ($14,572–$25,742) | $6,888 ($3,620–$11,481) | 0.003 |
| Radiology | $499 ($347–$1,354) | $2,102 ($1,444–$2,276) | 0.190 |
| Evaluation and management | $765 ($500–$1,556) | $785 ($540–$1,066) | 0.860 |
| Technical charges | $50,508 ($39,405–$141,563) | $46,346 ($38,815–$57,597) | 0.360 |
| Room and board | $3,530 ($2,016–$11,560) | $2,328 ($1,031–3,442) | 0.390 |
| Implant/materials | $25,073 ($13,862–51,470) | $11,210 ($7,260–$20,102) | 0.084 |
| Pharmacy | $5,787 ($5,495–$27,102) | $7,011 ($5,329–$7,495) | 0.500 |
| Total charges | $70,644 ($54,110–$170,775) | $54,453 ($49,196–$68,750) | 0.240 |

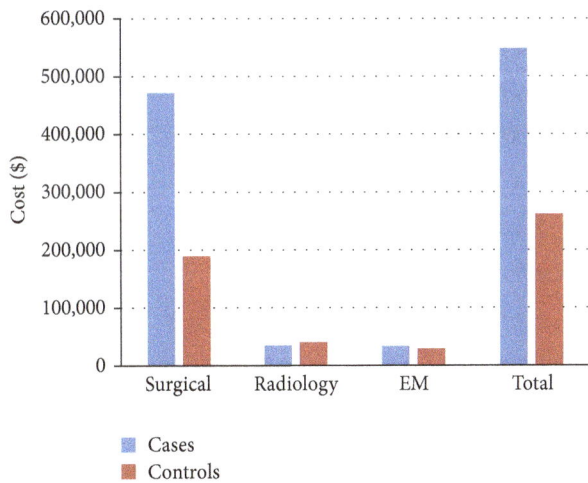

FIGURE 1: Aggregate professional charges for cases and controls are broken down into surgical, radiology, EM (evaluation and management), and total charges. Median values are reported.

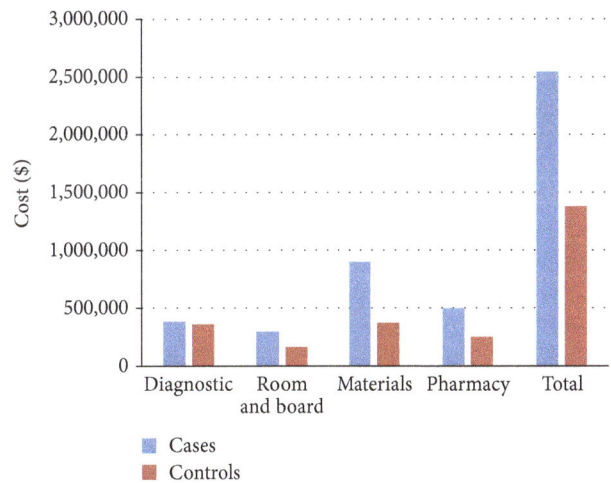

FIGURE 2: Aggregate technical charges for cases and controls are broken down into diagnostic, room at board (R&B), surgical materials and implants (materials), pharmacy, and total charges. Median values are repotted.

Tables 3, 4, 5, and 6 detail costs for matched cases and controls based on type of complication. For nonunions, total professional charges and the subcategory of surgical charges had significantly higher costs associated with the case group compared to the control group ($17,863 versus $8,358, and

$16,397 versus $6,888, resp.). For infections, both professional and technical charges were significantly higher in the patients who presented with this complication, resulting in significantly higher total charges, $128,122 for the cases compared to $49,983 for the controls. These significant differences in

TABLE 4: Case versus control comparison for *infection* costs.

| | Infection costs (median, IQR) | | P |
|---|---|---|---|
| | Cases (*n* = 8) | Controls (*n* = 8) | |
| Professional charges | $25,186 ($14,163–$27,900) | $10,698 ($8,020–$11,208) | 0.004 |
| Surgical | $19,906 ($10,949–$24,480) | $7,947 ($7,069–$9,912) | 0.010 |
| Radiology | $1,566 ($446–$2,080) | $724 ($140–$1,835) | 0.360 |
| Evaluation and management | $898 ($603–$1,494) | $716 ($315–$952) | 0.220 |
| Technical charges | $107,549 ($80,424–$161,665) | $39,068 ($31,924–$51,639) | 0.006 |
| Diagnostic | $18,084 ($11,152–$23,253) | $9,137 ($4,118–$13,194) | 0.072 |
| Room and board | $12,544 ($6,952–$19,894) | $2,058 ($2,031–$3,458) | 0.041 |
| Implant/materials | $31,059 ($21,701–$45,540) | $17,252 ($14,351–$19,285) | 0.093 |
| Pharmacy | $23,554 ($19,325–$31,730) | $8,254 ($5,547–$9,699) | 0.004 |
| Total charges | $128,122 ($106,211–$183,697) | $49,983 ($42,249–$60,529) | 0.006 |

TABLE 5: Case versus control comparison for *hardware pain* costs.

| | Hardware pain costs (median, IQR) | | P |
|---|---|---|---|
| | Cases (*n* = 10) | Controls (*n* = 10) | |
| Professional charges | $13,714 ($12,030–$16,876) | $8,101 ($6,121–$8,960) | 0.006 |
| Surgical | $12,216 ($10,888–$12,644) | $4,478 ($3,939–$7,051) | 0.003 |
| Radiology | $1,424 ($391–$2,404) | $1,832 ($288–$2,177) | 0.510 |
| Evaluation and management | $936 ($677–$1,091) | $614 ($570–$941) | 0.470 |
| Technical charges | $61,165 ($44,829–$76,314) | $32,793 ($27,463–$52,029) | 0.030 |
| Diagnostic | $14,420 ($2,434–$21,170) | $12,100 ($2,766–$17,206) | 0.660 |
| Room and board | $3,502 ($1,379–$14,094) | $2,015 ($1,461–$4,092) | 0.890 |
| Implant/materials | $25,111 ($14,822–$31,141) | $10,560 ($9,360–$13,996) | 0.019 |
| Pharmacy | $11,295 ($9,200–$12,829) | $5,725 ($4,969–$7,236) | 0.030 |
| Total charges | $79,747 ($56,243–93,399) | $40,360 ($35,223–$60,591) | 0.037 |

charges between the groups were driven by greater surgical, room and board, and pharmacy costs for the patients with infections. The length of stay was also 16.0 days for the case group that presented with infection, which was significantly longer than the length of stay calculated for the control group (3.0 days) ($P \leq 0.001$). Similarly for hardware-related pain, the cases presented with both higher professional and technical charges; however, these costs were mainly due surgical and pharmacy charges, respectively. There were no significant differences in all categories of charges between cases and controls for hardware failure, although only 3 patients had this type of complication. Finally, only 1 patient had a nonunion out of our series of 28 patients; therefore a Wilcoxon ranked test was not run. However, this 1 patient did have greater costs in all categories except radiology ($260 versus $2,045) and diagnostics ($13,160 versus $14,478) compared to a similarly matched patient.

Figure 3 provides a comparison of median costs associated with each type of complication. Infection resulted in the greatest expense for patients, whereas hardware failure resulted in the lowest charges.

## 4. Discussion

Our study is the first to report on the specific costs associated with complications related to surgical treatment of patient

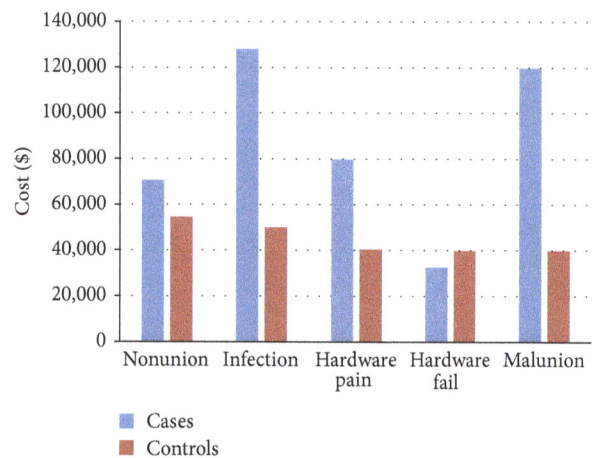

FIGURE 3: The total charges for each complication are compared to controls. *Malunion: only one patient had a malunion.

with an isolated ankle fracture. Based on the results of our study, patients with ankle fractures who develop complications incur significantly greater professional ($16,500 versus $8,300), technical ($69,200 versus $36,300), and total charges ($85,000 versus $60,500) than patients who do not develop complications. Among the specific types of complications,

TABLE 6: Case versus control comparison for *hardware failure* costs.

| | Hardware failure costs (median, IQR) | | P |
| --- | --- | --- | --- |
| | Cases ($n = 3$) | Controls ($n = 3$) | |
| Professional charges | $16,012 ($11,892–$22,453) | $7,231 ($6,120–$13,571) | 0.33 |
| Technical charges | $24,106 ($20,259–$72,818) | $32,539 ($24,799–$131,982) | 0.57 |
| Surgical | $14,871 ($10,919–$19,726) | $4,957 ($4,927–$6,227) | 0.14 |
| Radiology | $272 ($253–302) | $1,614 ($862–$2,861) | 0.57 |
| Evaluation and management | $769 ($633–$1,760) | $660 ($330–$4,450) | 0.85 |
| Diagnostic | $3,618 ($3,232–$8,159) | $12,125 ($6,746–$29,124) | 0.85 |
| Room and board | $651 ($626–$4,758) | $5,250 ($3,602–$24,375) | 0.33 |
| Implant/materials | $7,832 ($4,815–$35,174) | $7,514 ($7,186–$8,916) | 0.85 |
| Pharmacy | $3,565 ($3,487–$12,679) | $4,623 ($3,944–$28,610) | 0.85 |
| Total charges | $32,425 ($31,151–$91,424) | $39,770 ($30,919–$145,553) | 0.85 |

patients who developed infections or had hardware-related pain experienced significantly higher costs compared to their corresponding control patients. Specific subcategories of professional and technical charges, like surgical charges, were higher or lower depending on the type of complication, thereby highlighting areas that may cause the greatest financial risk under a bundled-payment system.

To our knowledge, no other study has compared the costs of all common ankle fracture complications. However, a few studies have investigated costs with certain aspects of ankle fractures and therefore serve as a basis for comparison. In Sanders et al.'s study of 11 open grade IIIB ankle fractures, average inpatient charges were just over $62,000 per patient [9]. This patient cohort consisted of patients with and without complications including soft tissue infection and osteomyelitis. Similarly, in our study we found a median inpatient charge of $61,000 when combining the cases and controls together. Marsh and colleagues investigated 7 patients with supramalleolar nonunions after tibial plafond fractures and found an average patient cost of $66,491 per patient to treat these nonunions [10]. In our analysis, we found a similar result with a slightly higher median value of $70,644 in nonunion patients. Given the similarity of our results to isolated results in the literature, we have some external validation of our data thereby helping the generalizability of our results.

Given that the annual rate of ankle fractures is 187 per 100,000 Americans, then, based on the current US population of approximately 318 million people, nearly 594,650 Americans sustain ankle fractures each year [1, 11]. Based on our study, of those with ankle fractures, about 6.4%, or approximately 38,000 individuals, will develop complications. In fact, this complication rate is conservative compared to other studies that determined complication rates for ankle fractures to be upwards of 30% of patients [11, 12]. Based on the rate of $3 million in aggregate charges per 28 patients with complications in our study, 38,000 complications would cost the US healthcare system $4.1 billion in treatment each year. Complications related to surgical treatment of ankle fractures alone would, therefore, incur a small, yet, significant portion of healthcare costs.

The results of our study identify specific complications that are more likely to increase costs for postsurgical ankle

fracture patients. Orthopaedic surgeons should be aware of the high costs associated with treatment of complications including infection. Such a finding emphasizes the importance of preoperative antibiotics and thorough debridement in open fractures, minimizing soft-tissue stripping intraoperatively, and employing 24 hours of postoperative antibiotics following surgical intervention [13, 14].

Although not specifically assessed in this study, the mode of fixation utilized is known to have variable costs. Murray et al. reported that external fixation of ankle fractures results in greater financial expenditures compared to open reduction internal fixation [5]. Moreover, locking plate technology is more costly than a standard plate. It is the opinion of the authors that every case is unique and the mode of fixation should be geared at effectively attaining and maintaining fracture reduction. In an era of cost-containment, not only is the patient selection important, but also choice of implant should render effective maintenance of fracture reduction while concomitantly limiting potential hardware and soft-tissue complications. The role of optimizing patient's medical comorbidities prior to surgical intervention (e.g., glucose control, selectively discontinuing immunosuppressants, addressing tobacco use, ASA) is essential. Finally, room and board or hospital length costs may be decreased through early operations and identifying patients who are predisposed to longer lengths of stay based on well-established risk factors to facilitate discharge [15–17].

Our study had some limitations. For one, our cost calculations were based only on the type of complication. However, other factors impact ankle surgery costs and may confound the relationship between costs and type of complication. Furthermore, while we matched patients on multiple comorbidities, additional factors such as open fracture grade may have been important to control for given the clear link between open fracture grade and infection risk [18]. It may be difficult to fully generalize our results based on the definitions our institution uses in categorizing costs. As some areas like malunion only had one patient with an isolated injury, it will be important to repeat our analysis with a larger cohort of patients. Additionally, as this study was completed in an academic medical center, the involvement of residents in patient care may bring into question whether this is an independent risk factor for postoperative complication.

Although the evaluation of such trainee involvement has predominantly been addressed in the general surgery literature, a recent report of 13,109 total hip arthroplasty cases shows no increased complication rates within the first 30 days following primary [19–24]. Given the numerous reports as well as the aforementioned large-scale study, resident involvement in these procedures should continue to be encouraged and cultivated. Albeit no surgical intervention is without risk of post-surgical complication, patient and surgeon factors should be mitigated to enable a complication-free outcome.

Our study determined that complications due to isolated ankle fractures greatly increase the cost of treatment. Even though complications cannot be completely prevented in surgery, practicing orthopaedic surgeons should remain vigilant in minimizing factors that potentially lead to complications. Overall, by finding avenues to reduce complications, orthopaedic surgeons can also minimize charges under a bundled-payment system.

## Ethical Approval

This study was performed in accordance with the relevant regulations of the US Health Insurance Portability and Accountability Act (HIPAA) and the ethical standards of the 1964 Declaration of Helsinki. This study has approval from the Vanderbilt IRB.

## Consent

This study used no previously copyrighted materials or signed patient consent forms.

## Conflict of Interests

William T. Obremskey has previously consulted for biometrics, done expert testimony in legal matters, has a grant from the Department of Defense, and has been a Board Member of the OTA and SEFC. For the remaining authors no conflict of interests was declared.

## References

[1] "National health expenditures 2012 highlights," Centers for Medicare and Medicaid Cervices, http://www.cms.gov/Research-Statistics-Data-and-Systems/Statistics-Trends-and-Reports/NationalHealthExpendData/downloads/highlights.pdf.

[2] P. J. Daly, R. H. Fitzgerald Jr., L. J. Melton, and D. M. Ilstrup, "Epidemiology of ankle fractures in Rochester, Minnesota," *Acta Orthopaedica Scandinavica*, vol. 58, no. 5, pp. 539–544, 1987.

[3] D. A. Belatti and P. Phisitkul, "Economic burden of foot and ankle surgery in the US medicare population," *Foot & Ankle International*, vol. 35, no. 4, pp. 334–340, 2014.

[4] D. Manoukian, D. Leivadiotou, and W. Williams, "Is early operative fixation of unstable ankle fractures cost effective? Comparison of the cost of early versus late surgery," *European Journal of Orthopaedic Surgery and Traumatology*, vol. 23, no. 7, pp. 835–837, 2013.

[5] A. M. Murray, S. E. McDonald, P. Archbold, and G. E. Crealey, "Cost description of inpatient treatment for ankle fracture," *Injury*, vol. 42, no. 11, pp. 1226–1229, 2011.

[6] J. W. Busse and W. T. Obremskey, "Principles of designing an orthopaedic case-control study," *Journal of Bone and Joint Surgery A*, vol. 91, no. 3, pp. 15–20, 2009.

[7] K. A. Egol, N. C. Tejwani, M. G. Walsh, E. L. Capla, and K. J. Koval, "Predictors of short-term functional outcome following ankle fracture surgery," *Journal of Bone and Joint Surgery*, vol. 88, no. 5, pp. 974–979, 2006.

[8] S. M. Teeny and D. A. Wiss, "Open reduction and internal fixation of tibial plafond fractures: variables contributing to poor results and complications," *Clinical Orthopaedics and Related Research*, no. 292, pp. 108–117, 1993.

[9] R. Sanders, J. Pappas, J. Mast, and D. Helfet, "The salvage of open grade IIIB ankle and talus fractures," *Journal of Orthopaedic Trauma*, vol. 6, no. 2, pp. 201–208, 1992.

[10] J. L. Marsh, R. E. Rattay, and T. Dulaney, "Results of ankle arthrodesis for treatment of supramalleolar nonunion and ankle arthrosis," *Foot and Ankle International*, vol. 18, no. 3, pp. 138–143, 1997.

[11] N. F. SooHoo, L. Krenek, M. J. Eagan, B. Gurbani, C. Y. Ko, and D. S. Zingmond, "Complication rates following open reduction and internal fixation of ankle fractures," *The Journal of Bone & Joint Surgery*, vol. 91, no. 5, pp. 1042–1049, 2009.

[12] A. Zaghloul, B. Haddad, R. Barksfield, and B. Davis, "Early complications of surgery in operative treatment of ankle fractures in those over 60: a review of 186 cases," *Injury*, vol. 45, no. 4, pp. 780–783, 2014.

[13] P. D. Holtom, L. Borges, and C. G. Zalavras, "Hematogenous septic ankle arthritis," *Clinical Orthopaedics and Related Research*, vol. 466, no. 6, pp. 1388–1391, 2008.

[14] P. Ferrao, M. S. Myerson, J. M. Schuberth, and M. J. McCourt, "Cement spacer as definitive management for postoperative ankle infection," *Foot and Ankle International*, vol. 33, no. 3, pp. 173–178, 2012.

[15] H. Pakzad, G. Thevendran, M. J. Penner, H. Qian, and A. Younger, "Factors associated with longer length of hospital stay after primary elective ankle surgery for end-stage ankle arthritis," *Journal of Bone and Joint Surgery—Series A*, vol. 96, no. 1, pp. 32–39, 2014.

[16] T. Schepers, M. R. De Vries, E. M. M. Van Lieshout, and M. Van der Elst, "The timing of ankle fracture surgery and the effect on infectious complications; a case series and systematic review of the literature," *International Orthopaedics*, vol. 37, no. 3, pp. 489–494, 2013.

[17] P. Pietzik, I. Qureshi, J. Langdon, S. Molloy, and M. Solan, "Cost benefit with early operative fixation of unstable ankle fractures," *Annals of the Royal College of Surgeons of England*, vol. 88, no. 4, pp. 405–407, 2006.

[18] M. J. Patzakis and J. Wilkins, "Factors influencing infection rate in open fracture wounds," *Clinical Orthopaedics and Related Research*, no. 243, pp. 36–40, 1989.

[19] B. D. Haughom, W. W. Schairer, M. D. Hellman, P. H. Yi, and B. R. Levine, "Resident involvement does not influence complication after total hip arthroplasty : an analysis of 13,109 cases," *The Journal of Arthroplasty*, vol. 29, no. 10, pp. 1919–1924, 2014.

[20] S. S. Davis Jr., F. A. Husain, E. Lin, K. C. Nandipati, S. Perez, and J. F. Sweeney, "Resident participation in index laparoscopic general surgical cases: impact of the learning environment on

surgical outcomes," *Journal of the American College of Surgeons*, vol. 216, no. 1, pp. 96–104, 2013.

[21] M. J. Englesbe, Z. Fan, O. Baser, and J. D. Birkmeyer, "Mortality in medicare patients undergoing surgery in july in teaching hospitals," *Annals of Surgery*, vol. 249, no. 6, pp. 871–876, 2009.

[22] M. Bukur, M. B. Singer, R. Chung et al., "Influence of resident involvement on trauma care outcomes," *Archives of Surgery*, vol. 147, no. 9, pp. 856–862, 2012.

[23] R. Fahrner, M. Turina, V. Neuhaus, and O. Schöb, "Laparoscopic cholecystectomy as a teaching operation: comparison of outcome between residents and attending surgeons in 1,747 patients," *Langenbeck's Archives of Surgery*, vol. 397, no. 1, pp. 103–110, 2012.

[24] C. S. Hwang, C. R. Pagano, K. A. Wichterman, G. L. Dunnington, and E. J. Alfrey, "Resident versus no resident: a single institutional study on operative complications, mortality, and cost," *Surgery*, vol. 144, no. 2, pp. 339–344, 2008.

# 20

# Minimally Invasive Sacroiliac Joint Fusion: One-Year Outcomes in 40 Patients

## Donald Sachs[1] and Robyn Capobianco[2]

[1] Center for Spinal Stenosis and Neurologic Care, P.O. Box 8815, Lakeland, FL 33806, USA
[2] SI-BONE Inc., 3055 Olin Ave. Suite 2200, San Jose, CA 95128, USA

Correspondence should be addressed to Robyn Capobianco; spinewriter@gmail.com

Academic Editor: Panagiotis Korovessis

*Background*. SI joint pain is difficult to diagnose due to overlapping symptoms of the lumbar spine, and until recently, treatment options have been limited. The purpose of this retrospective study is to report on the safety and effectiveness of MIS SI joint arthrodesis using a series of triangular, porous plasma coated implants in patients refractory to conservative care. *Methods*. We report on the first 40 consecutive patients with one-year follow-up data that underwent MIS SI joint fusion with the iFuse Implant System (SI-BONE, Inc., San Jose, CA) by a single surgeon. Medical charts were reviewed for demographics, perioperative metrics, complications, pain scores, and satisfaction. *Results*. Mean age was 58 years (range 30–81) and 75% of patients were female. Postoperative complications were minimal and included transient trochanteric bursitis (5%), facet joint pain (20%), and new low back pain (2.5%). There were no reoperations at one year. Mean pain score improved from 8.7 (1.5 SD) at baseline to 0.9 (1.6) at 12 months, a 7.8-point improvement ($P < .001$). Patient satisfaction was very high. *Conclusions*. The results of this case series reveal that MIS SI joint fusion using the iFuse Implant System is a safe and effective treatment option in carefully selected patients.

## 1. Background

Low back pain (LBP) is exceedingly common in modern society, affecting well over 90% of adults at some point in their lives [1]. Apart from the common cold, it is the most common reason for visits to the primary care doctor [1]. Loss of productivity and income combined with medical expenses results in a $60 billion expenditure annually in the US related to low back pain [2]. Successful treatment of low back pain demands identifying the pain generator(s), which can be a significant challenge due to the multifactorial nature of this condition. In the early 1900s, the sacroiliac (SI) joint was suspected as a significant generator of LBP. Over time, as more reliably diagnosed conditions such as herniated discs and facet arthropathy became better understood, less focus was placed on the SI joint [3]. Recently there has been a resurgence in consideration of the SI joint as a low back pain generator. Recent published literature reports that 15–30% of patients presenting with low back pain had SI joint problems [4]. Additionally, up to 75% of postlumbar fusion patients

will develop significant SI joint degeneration after 5 years [5–7]. SI joint pain can mimic discogenic or radicular low back pain, and patients can present with low back, groin, and/or gluteal pain, leading to the potential for inaccurate diagnosis and treatment [1, 8, 9].

Despite the large number of patients with SI joint pain, treatment options have been limited to conservative care involving physical therapy and joint injections or traditional open SI joint arthrodesis surgery until recently. Open arthrodesis procedures reported in the literature require relatively large incisions, significant bone harvesting, and lengthy hospital stays; moreover, they may require nonweight bearing for several months [10–13].

Recent case series reports of a minimally invasive arthrodesis system (iFuse Implant System, SI-BONE Inc., San Jose, CA) have shown excellent outcomes [14–17]. The surgical procedure involves placing a series of triangular, porous plasma spray coated titanium implants placed across the SI joint without the use of second site bone harvesting or graft. We wished to determine if the single center outcomes in the literature were commensurate with our own. The purpose of this retrospective study is to report on the safety and effectiveness of this procedure in a single surgeon's private practice.

## 2. Methods

We report outcomes of the first consecutive 40 patients with one-year follow-up data treated at a single, community-based spine practice between April 2011 and March 2012. Medical charts were reviewed for perioperative metrics, complications, and pain scores using a numerical rating scale (NRS) preoperatively and at 6 weeks, 3-, 6-, and 12-months postoperatively. Patient satisfaction with surgical results (yes or no) was obtained at 12 months post-operatively. IRB approval was obtained before beginning the study.

Mean age was 58 years (range 30–81), and three quarters of the patients were women (75%) (Table 1). Patients were diagnosed with either degenerative sacroiliitis or sacroiliac joint disruption using a combination of history, clinical exam, and positive diagnostic injection. Degenerative sacroiliitis is defined as a degeneration of the joint, either osteoarthritic or as a result of adjacent segment disease after fusion. Sacroiliac joint disruption is a physical separation of the joint, typically as a result of trauma. Patients presented with SI joint pain and all but one complained of low back pain. Additional symptoms were buttock pain (60%) and groin pain (13%). Nearly half (48%) had a history of previous lumbar spine surgery that included: fusion at one or more levels (63%), decompression (16%), discectomy (10.5%), and 10.5% with nonspecific documented procedures.

All patients failed a minimum 6-month course of conservative care consisting of medication optimization, physical therapy, and SI joint injections. A thorough physical and clinical exam was performed on all patients in order to determine the primary pain generator as accurately as possible in this complex back pain population. Positive results on 3 or more provocative physical examination maneuvers (such as FABER, compression, thigh thrust, distraction, and Gaenslen) were used as criteria to guide subsequent diagnostic activities [18]. Diagnostic imaging studies (MRI and/or CT scan) were performed to assess pathology in the lumbopelvic hip complex. When clinical, physical, and imaging examinations were concordant, patients were sent for confirmatory image-guided diagnostic injections of the SI joint using long acting anesthetic. A 75% reduction in pain immediately following injection of local anesthetic was used to confirm the SI joint as a pain generator [7].

Minimally invasive SI joint fusion using the iFuse Implant System (SI-BONE Inc., San Jose, CA) was performed in all cases by a single neurosurgeon in private practice. This system entails the placement of 3 triangular, porous plasma coated titanium implants across the SI joint in order to stabilize and fuse the joint without the need for additional bone graft.

*2.1. Technique Overview.* The procedure is performed with the patient positioned prone on a radiolucent table and under general endotracheal anesthesia. Intermittent fluoroscopy is used to monitor instrument and implant placement. After a 3 cm lateral incision is made into the buttock region, the gluteal fascia is bluntly dissected to reach the outer table of the ilium. A Steinmann pin is passed through the ilium across the SI joint into the center of the sacrum, lateral to the neural foramen. A soft tissue protector is inserted over the pin, and a drill is used to create a pathway and decorticate bone through the ilium to the sacrum. After the drill is removed, a triangular broach is used before the first implant is malleted into place. A total of three implants are placed. (Figure 1). In some cases more than three implants can be used, but in this series all patients had three implants. The most cephalad implant is seated within the sacral ala. A pin-guide system is used to facilitate placement of the subsequent implants. The second implant is generally located above or adjacent to the S1 foramen and the third between the S1 and S2 foramens. The incision is then irrigated, and the tissue layers are closed with Vicryl and Monocryl sutures. Patients are instructed to ambulate with the assistance of a walker for the first 4 weeks after which time toe touch ambulation is recommended for another 4 weeks. After patients have undergone this 8-week program of a gradual return to full weight bearing, they begin 4 weeks of physical therapy.

*2.2. Outcomes.* Pain related to the SI joint was assessed preoperatively and postoperatively at 12 months. Patients were asked to rate their pain using a 0–10 numerical rating scale with 0 representing no pain and 10 representing the worst pain imaginable. Satisfaction was assessed by asking the patient (yes or no) if s/he would have the same surgery again for the same outcome.

## 3. Results

A total of 41 SI joints in 40 patients were treated: 17 right- and 24 left sided. One patient underwent bilateral surgery (Table 2). One patient underwent concomitant L3/4 laminectomy, foraminotomy, and facetectomy. Blood loss was minimal (<50 cc) in all cases, and most patients are kept in the hospital overnight. Surgery time was not available for all patients. We previously reported an operating time of 78 ± 32 minutes in a subset of this cohort [15]. No intraoperative

TABLE 1: Patient demographics.

| Patients | 40 |
|---|---|
| Age | 58 (range 30–81) |
| Gender | 30 F (75%), 10 M (25%) |
| Symptoms | 39 (98%) LBP |
| | 24 (60%) buttock pain |
| | 5 (13%) groin pain |
| Prior lumbar spine surgery | 19 (48%) total |
| | 12 fusion, 3 decompression, 1 unknown, |
| | 2 discectomy, 1 spinal cord stimulator |

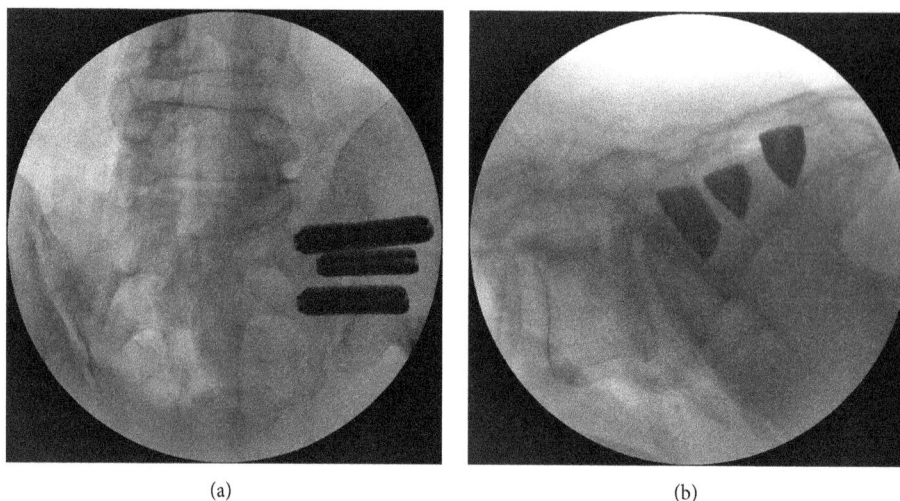

(a)

(b)

FIGURE 1: (a) AP and (b) lateral view of all three implants in place.

complications were observed. At one year, there were no surgical revisions.

### 3.1. Clinical Outcomes.

*3.1. Clinical Outcomes.* Mean (±SD) preoperative pain score as measured using a numerical rating scale (NRS) was 8.7 ± 1.5. Improvement in pain was observed as early as the 6-week follow-up visit (mean 1.2 ± 1.7), and patients continued to have symptom relief at the 3- and 6-month follow-up visits, means 0.6 ± 1.2 and 0.8 ± 1.8, respectively. This improvement was durable through the 12-month followup with a reported mean pain score of 0.9 (±1.6). The mean (±SD) change in pain score was −7.8 (±2.3) points (*t* test, $P < .001$). A subgroup analysis revealed that there was no difference in outcomes between patients with and without prior lumbar spinal fusion. A clinically significant benefit, defined as a >2 point change from baseline, was observed in all but one patient [19]. Patient satisfaction was extremely high with all patients (100%) indicating that they would have the same surgery again for the same result.

*3.2. Complications.* There were no intraoperative complications. Two patients presented with trochanteric bursitis, 1 incident of piriformis syndrome, and 1 episode of new low back pain (Table 3). Eight patients continued to have facet pain, which was present preoperatively. During the postoperative follow-up period, 2 patients with preexisting lower back pain due to degenerative disc disease and severe spinal stenosis underwent lumbar fusion. One patient underwent discectomy at L4/5. All three surgeries were unrelated to the index procedure.

## 4. Discussion

SI joint symptoms can present as pain in the SI joint, low back, hip, groin, or buttock. As a result, a careful and thorough clinical and physical exam must be performed to correctly identify the pain generator(s). Positive provocative physical

TABLE 2: Perioperative characteristics.

| | |
|---|---|
| Joints treated | 41 |
| Right SI joint | 17 |
| Left SI joint | 24 |
| Concomitant spine procedures | 1: L3/4 laminectomy, facetectomy, foraminotomy |

TABLE 3: Postoperative complications and events.

| | |
|---|---|
| Piriformis syndrome | 1 |
| New low back pain | 1 |
| Facet joint pain | 8 |
| Trochanteric bursitis | 2 |
| Discectomy at L4/5 | 1 |
| Lumbar spine fusion | 1 case at L2/3 due to severe spinal stenosis |
| | 1 case at L3/4 for degenerative disc disease |

examination maneuvers (such as FABER, Gaenslen, and Thigh Thrust) combined with marked (e.g., 75% or greater) pain relief after image-guided SI joint injection are a reliable method for diagnosing the SI joint as a pain generator [7, 18, 20].

Recent reports of other MIS approaches to SI joint arthrodesis using screws show relatively good clinical results with room for improvement in outcomes and technique [16]. Al-Khayer et al. reported on 9 patients using a single hollow modular anchorage (HMA) screw packed with bone graft [21]. All patients experienced a clinically significant improvement in VAS pain scores, and all but 1 patient improved in function as measured by ODI. One patient suffered a deep wound infection. Khurana et al. also report on HMA screws with demineralized bone matrix in a cohort of 15 patients with relatively good outcomes [22]. Wise and

Dall reported on 13 patients and 19 joints using $11 \times 25\,\text{mm}$ threaded fusion cages packed with rhBMP-2 with good clinical results [3]. Both of these MIS techniques, which use rhBMP-2 or autologous bone graft, have substantial drawbacks. The use of rhBMP-2 has come under fire for unreported adverse events as well as unapproved uses [23], and autologous iliac crest harvesting can lead to further degeneration of the SI joint [10]. Additionally, the use of cages and screws for SI joint fusion may not be appropriate for patients with a history of instrumented spinal surgery. Mason et al. reported significantly worse outcomes after SI joint fusion using HMA screws in patients with a history of previous lumbar spine surgery [24]. Further studies are needed to assess the incidence of screw loosening, breakage, and need for hardware removal as these events have been reported in association with other spine procedures using orthopedic screws [19].

Several case series reports using the same MIS technique used in this current study report favorable results with minimal complications and no suggestion of implant loosening [14, 15, 17]. In a case series of 50 patients, the author reported clinically and statistically significant improvements in pain and function independent of a prior history of lumbar spine fusion [16]. Similarly, there was no difference in outcomes between patients with and without history of lumbar spinal fusion in our study.

Advantages of MIS SI joint fusion using the iFuse Implant System include a small incision, relatively short operating time, minimal blood loss, a relatively short period of immobilization, and most importantly bone and ligament preservation. The triangular shape combined with an interference fit of the titanium implant used in this cohort was designed to minimize rotation, and micromotion and avoid issues encountered with traditional screws. In our cohort of patients undergoing MIS SI joint fusion, clinical outcomes were favorable with 98% of patients experiencing a clinically significant benefit at 12 months.

Postoperative complications were minimal. Two patients (5%) went on to have fusion surgery for significant degenerative disc disease or spinal stenosis. Both conditions were present prior to SI joint fusion surgery; however the patient's chief complaint was the SI joint necessitating primary attention to this area. There were 2 cases (5%) of transient trochanteric bursitis and 1 episode of piriformis syndrome. These are neither uncommon nor unexpected and can be a result of altered gait pattern due to low back or hip pain, postoperative hip abductor weakness, and other trauma in the region [19]. Facet pain was present in 20% of our patients, but it is unclear whether these patients had symptoms prior to the surgery. These patients were treated with either facet injections or physical therapy, depending on severity and patient preference.

Although our study sample size is small, the results of minimally invasive SI joint surgery appear promising. All patients presented with low back and SI joint pain. Favorable outcomes in these patients underscore the necessity to suspect the SI joint as a pain generator in patients with low back pain. Special attention should be paid to the SI joint after lumbar spine surgery to avoid the potential for inaccurate diagnosis and treatment. Furthermore, this minimally invasive approach may significantly benefit the elderly population, who are not candidates for other conventional techniques due to poor bone quality, delayed healing and reduced mobility. Thirty-eight percent (38%) of our patients were over the age of 65. This segment of the population is not likely to respond well to physical therapy alone in part because of the degenerative nature of SI joint disease. The MIS procedure described herein may afford this segment of the population an opportunity to regain mobility, alleviate SI joint and low back pain caused by SI joint issues, and experience an improved quality of life.

## 5. Conclusion

When conservative measures fail, minimally invasive SI joint fusion using a series of triangular porous plasma coated titanium implants is a safe and effective treatment option in carefully selected patients. Additional prospective controlled trials are underway.

## List of Abbreviations

SI:   Sacroiliac
NRS:  Numerical rating scale
MIS:  Minimally invasive surgery
LBP:  Low back pain.

## Competing Interests

No funds were received for this research. Donald Sachs is a paid consultant for SI-BONE Inc. Robyn Capobianco is an employee of SI-BONE Inc.

## Authors' Contributions

Donald Sachs performed all surgeries, assisted in paper draft, and reviewed final paper. Robyn Capobianco prepared study protocol, IRB documentation, performed data analysis, and drafted paper.

## Authors' Information

Donald Sachs is a board certified neurosurgeon specializing in minimally invasive spine surgery. Robyn Capobianco is a clinical research professional and medical writer.

## Acknowledgments

The authors wish to acknowledge Daniel Cher, MD for data analysis and critical editorial review, Deidre Sachs, and Kristen Ball for data acquisition.

## References

[1] N. Weksler, G. J. Velan, M. Semionov et al., "The role of sacroiliac joint dysfunction in the genesis of low back pain:

the obvious is not always right," *Archives of Orthopaedic and Trauma Surgery*, vol. 127, no. 10, pp. 885–888, 2007.

[2] W. Murray, "Sacroiliac joint dysfunction: a case study," *Orthopaedic Nursing*, vol. 30, no. 2, pp. 126–131, 2011.

[3] C. L. Wise and B. E. Dall, "Minimally invasive sacroiliac arthrodesis: outcomes of a new technique," *Journal of Spinal Disorders and Techniques*, vol. 21, no. 8, pp. 579–584, 2008.

[4] J. N. Sembrano and D. W. Polly, "How often is low back pain not coming from the back?" *Spine*, vol. 34, no. 1, pp. E27–E32, 2009.

[5] K.-Y. Ha, J.-S. Lee, and K.-W. Kim, "Degeneration of sacroiliac joint after instrumented lumbar or lumbosacral fusion: a prospective cohort study over five-year follow-up," *Spine*, vol. 33, no. 11, pp. 1192–1198, 2008.

[6] M. J. Depalma, J. M. Ketchum, and T. R. Saullo, "Etiology of chronic low back pain in patients having undergone lumbar fusion," *Pain Medicine*, vol. 12, no. 5, pp. 732–739, 2011.

[7] J. Y. Maigne, A. Aivaliklis, and F. Pfefer, "Results of sacroiliac joint double block and value of sacroiliac pain provocation tests in 54 patients with low back pain," *Spine*, vol. 21, no. 16, pp. 1889–1892, 1996.

[8] B. S. Foley and R. M. Buschbacher, "Sacroiliac joint pain: anatomy, biomechanics, diagnosis, and treatment," *American Journal of Physical Medicine and Rehabilitation*, vol. 85, no. 12, pp. 997–1006, 2006.

[9] A. C. Schwarzer, C. N. Aprill, and N. Bogduk, "The sacroiliac joint in chronic low back pain," *Spine*, vol. 20, no. 1, pp. 31–37, 1995.

[10] J. M. Buchowski, K. M. Kebaish, V. Sinkov, D. B. Cohen, A. N. Sieber, and J. P. Kostuik, "Functional and radiographic outcome of sacroiliac arthrodesis for the disorders of the sacroiliac joint," *The Spine Journal*, vol. 5, no. 5, pp. 520–528, 2005.

[11] K. A. Giannikas, A. M. Khan, M. T. Karski, and H. A. Maxwell, "Sacroiliac joint fusion for chronic pain: a simple technique avoiding the use of metalwork," *European Spine Journal*, vol. 13, no. 3, pp. 253–256, 2004.

[12] M. N. Smith-Petersen, "Arthrodesis of the sacroiliac joint. A new method of approach," *The Journal of Bone & Joint Surgery*, vol. 3, no. 8, pp. 400–405, 1921.

[13] M. R. Moore, "Surgical treatment of chronic painful sacroiliac joint dysfunction.," in *Movement, Stability, and Low Back Pain: The Essential Role of the Pelvis*, pp. 563–572, Churchill Livingstone, New York, NY, USA, 1997.

[14] L. Rudolf, "Sacroiliac joint srthrodesis-MIS technique with titanium implants: report of the first 50 patients and outcomes," *The Open Orthopaedics Journal*, vol. 6, no. 1, pp. 495–502, 2012.

[15] D. Sachs and R. Capobianco, "One year successful outcomes for novel sacroiliac joint arthrodesis system," *Annals of Surgical Innovation and Research*, vol. 6, no. 1, article 13, 2012.

[16] L. Rudolf, "MIS fusion of the SI Joint: does prior lumbar spinal fusion affect patient outcomes?" *The Open Orthopaedics Journal*, vol. 7, pp. 163–168, 2013.

[17] J. T. Kim, L. M. Rudolf, and J. A. Glaser, "Outcome of percutaneous sacroiliac joint fixation with porous plasma-coated triangular titanium implants: an independent review.," *The Open Orthopaedics Journal*, vol. 7, pp. 51–56, 2013.

[18] K. M. Szadek, P. van der Wurff, M. W. van Tulder, W. W. Zuurmond, and R. S. G. M. Perez, "Diagnostic validity of criteria for sacroiliac joint pain: a systematic review," *Journal of Pain*, vol. 10, no. 4, pp. 354–368, 2009.

[19] A. G. Copay, S. D. Glassman, B. R. Subach, S. Berven, T. C. Schuler, and L. Y. Carreon, "Minimum clinically important difference in lumbar spine surgery patients: a choice of methods using the Oswestry Disability Index, Medical Outcomes Study questionnaire Short Form 36, and Pain Scales," *The Spine Journal*, vol. 8, no. 6, pp. 968–974, 2008.

[20] P.-C. Liliang, K. Lu, C.-L. Liang, Y.-D. Tsai, K.-W. Wang, and H.-J. Chen, "Sacroiliac joint pain after lumbar and lumbosacral fusion: findings using dual sacroiliac joint blocks," *Pain Medicine*, vol. 12, no. 4, pp. 565–570, 2011.

[21] A. Al-Khayer, J. Hegarty, D. Hahn, and M. P. Grevitt, "Percutaneous sacroiliac joint arthrodesis: a novel technique," *Journal of Spinal Disorders and Techniques*, vol. 21, no. 5, pp. 359–363, 2008.

[22] A. Khurana, A. R. Guha, K. Mohanty, and S. Ahuja, "Percutaneous fusion of the sacroiliac joint with hollow modular anchorage screws: clinical and radiological outcome," *Journal of Bone and Joint Surgery B*, vol. 91, no. 5, pp. 627–631, 2009.

[23] E. J. Carragee, A. J. Ghanayem, B. K. Weiner, D. J. Rothman, and C. M. Bono, "A challenge to integrity in spine publications: years of living dangerously with the promotion of bone growth factors," *The Spine Journal*, vol. 11, no. 6, pp. 463–468, 2011.

[24] L. W. Mason, I. Chopra, and K. Mohanty, "The percutaneous stabilisation of the sacroiliac joint with hollow modular anchorage screws: a prospective outcome study," *European Spine Journal*, 2013.

# 21

# Manipulation of Displaced Distal Radial Fractures in the Superelderly: Prediction of Malunion and the Degree of Radiographic Improvement

**N. D. Clement, A. D. Duckworth, C. M. Court-Brown, and M. M. McQueen**

*Department of Orthopaedics and Trauma, The Royal Infirmary of Edinburgh, Little France, Edinburgh EH16 4SA, UK*

Correspondence should be addressed to N. D. Clement; nickclement@doctors.org.uk

Academic Editor: Robert F. Ostrum

Superelderly patients (≥80 years old) account for 20% of all distal radial fractures and are at an increased risk of malunion. The primary aim of this study was to identify predictors of malunion and the degree of improvement in the fracture position offered by closed manipulation of displaced distal radial fractures in the superelderly. We retrospectively identified 228 displaced distal radial fractures in superelderly patients from a prospective database of 4024 distal radial fractures. The inclusion criterion was a patient that underwent closed manipulation as their primary intervention. The majority of patients ($n = 196$, 86%) were defined as having a malunion. A premanipulation dorsal angulation of greater than 25 degrees ($P = 0.047$) and an ulnar variance of 6 mm or more ($P = 0.02$) significantly increased the risk of malunion. The premanipulation dorsal angulation was a significant independent predictor of the degree of improvement in the final dorsal angulation ($P < 0.001$) and ulnar variance ($P = 0.01$). Patients with a high risk of malunion or poor improvement in the fracture position can be identified before manipulation and these patients may benefit from primary surgical intervention.

## 1. Introduction

Fractures of the distal radius account for 16% of all fractures and are the most prevalent fracture that orthopaedic surgeons have to manage [1]. Stable fractures can be managed conservatively with the expectation of a good functional outcome [2, 3]. The management of unstable fractures of the distal radius in the elderly remains controversial [4]. The functional outcome of displaced fractures is generally accepted to correlate with the anatomical reduction of the fracture [2, 3, 5].

It is predicted that there will be an increase in the elderly population over the next decade in the United Kingdom (UK), and currently the fastest growing population is the "oldest old" [6]. It is anticipated that by 2030 the population age of 80 years or more will have doubled [7]. The term "superelderly" has been used in orthopaedics to describe those patients greater than 80 years of age [8, 9]. Superelderly patients account for approximately 20% of all distal radial fractures [10], which will probably increase in the future due to their growing population and will form a greater proportion of the orthopaedic workload.

The primary management of displaced distal radial fractures is close manipulation [11]. However, increasing age, fracture comminution, and dependency are predictors of fracture stability and, if present, are more likely to lead to malunion [12]. These predictors are more likely to be present in the superelderly population and hence are more likely to fail nonoperative management by close manipulation alone. If the risk of malunion and degree of improvement offered by closed manipulation of the fracture could be calculated prior to manipulation, superelderly patients with a high risk of malunion could be identified. These patients may benefit from early operative intervention, avoiding delay and the inconvenience of a failed manipulation.

The primary aim of this study was to identify predictors of malunion and degree of improvement in the fracture position offered by closed manipulation of displaced distal radial fractures in the superelderly. The secondary aim was to describe the epidemiology of superelderly patients with displaced distal radial fractures.

## 2. Patients and Methods

*2.1. Demographic Data.* During a 67-month period 28,376 acute fractures were managed at the study centre, of which distal radial fractures accounted for 4024 (14.2%). A distal radial fracture database was prospectively complied, recording demographics, radiographic data, management, and outcome. The mean age for all patients was 59 (14 to 100) years. There were 574 patients aged 80 years or older identified retrospectively who had sustained a distal radial fracture during the study period, of which 228 were displaced and underwent closed manipulation as their primary intervention. There were 213 (93.4%) females and 15 (6.6%) males with a mean age of 83.7 (80 to 98) years. Two patients sustained bilateral fractures.

*2.2. Database Construction.* Fracture management followed a standard protocol. The emergency-room staff undertook the initial assessment and treatment. Fractures deemed to be in an acceptable position were managed with a dorsal plaster slab. If the fracture position was thought to be unacceptable, the emergency-room staff, prior to application of a dorsal plaster slab, performed closed reduction using intravenous regional anaesthesia. The patients were evaluated clinically and radiographically at one week and six weeks after the injury as per the protocol of the study unit.

At approximately one week following the injury, the patients were reviewed by the senior author (M. M. McQueen) in a dedicated research clinic. The clinical, demographic, and radiographic data were recorded and entered into a database either by the senior author (M. M. McQueen) or a research nurse. The premorbid normal level of function of the patient was categorised as independent if they were able to go shopping without assistance or dependent if assistance was needed. The dorsal slab was completed to a below-the-elbow forearm cast with the wrist in slight flexion and ulnar deviation at one week. Patients with a fracture that was displaced were admitted to the orthopaedic trauma unit for further intervention, unless the patient had low functional demands and operative intervention was deemed inappropriate.

*2.3. Radiographic Measurement Techniques.* All radiographs (presentation, time of reduction, one week, and six weeks) were measured manually with use of a protractor and a ruler to provide values for the dorsal angle and ulnar variance (Figure 1). The fractures were classified using AO/OTA classification [13]. Metaphyseal comminution was recorded, according to the location, as absent or as involving the dorsal metaphysis, volar metaphysis, or both the dorsal and the volar metaphysis. The senior author (M. M. McQueen) alone was responsible for fracture classification and the assessment of comminution. Adequate reduction was defined as dorsal angle of $\leq 0$ degrees and/or $\leq 3$ mm of radial shortening.

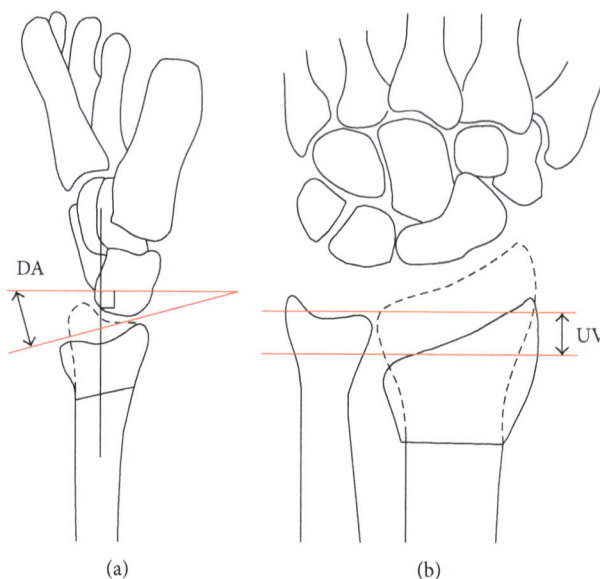

Figure 1: The measurement of dorsal angle (DA) and ulnar variance (UV). These measurements were expressed as a negative for volar angulation and a positive for DA and a positive value for UV if there was radial shortening.

Malunion was defined as a dorsal angle of >10 degrees and/or >3 mm of radial shortening.

*2.4. Statistical Analysis.* SPSS version 16.0 software was used for statistical analysis (SPSS Inc., Chicago, IL, USA). Paired and unpaired $t$-tests were used to compare the improvement in the 6-week dorsal angulation, ulna variance relative to premanipulation dorsal angulation and ulna variance, and the effect of case-mix variables upon the improvement in dorsal angulation and ulna variance, respectively. Pearson's correlation coefficient was used to assess the significance of age and premanipulation dorsal angulation and ulna variance upon the 6-week dorsal angulation and ulna variance. Multiple linear (stepwise methodology) and logistic (forward conditional methodology) regression analyses were used to identify significant independent predictors of improvement in dorsal angulation and ulnar variance and risk of malunion. A $P$ value of $\leq 0.05$ determined statistical significance.

## 3. Results

The majority of patients were female and were independent (Table 1). The mean age of males was 83.2 (range 80 to 88) years and that of females was 83.7 (range 80 to 98) years (unpaired $t$-test $P = 0.58$). Thirty-seven (16%) of patients sustained an associated fracture during the same injury, of which the commonest mode was a simple fall from standing height (Table 1). Dorsal comminution was observed in most patients, and only one patient sustained a partial articular fracture (Table 1). The mean premanipulation dorsal angulation was 25.2 degrees (10 to 56 degrees, SD 14.9) and radial shortening was 2.9 mm (−4 to 16 degrees, SD 3.1).

TABLE 1: Case-mix variables for the study cohort.

| Case-mix variables | $n = $ (%) |
| --- | --- |
| Gender | |
| Male | 15 (6.6) |
| Female | 213 (93.4) |
| Dominant limb | |
| Yes | 93 (40.8) |
| No | 135 (59.2) |
| Independent | |
| Yes | 126 (55.3) |
| No | 102 (44.7) |
| Injury mechanism | |
| Simple fall | 224 (98.2) |
| Fall from height | 1 (0.4) |
| RTA | 2 (0.9) |
| Assault | 1 (0.9) |
| Associated fracture | |
| Yes | 37 (16.2) |
| No | 191 (83.8) |
| AO Classification | |
| A | 123 (53.9) |
| B | 1 (0.4) |
| C | 104 (45.6) |
| Dorsal comminution | |
| Yes | 212 (93.0) |
| No | 16 (7.0) |

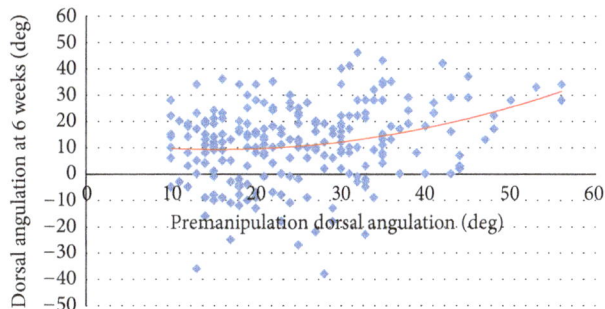

FIGURE 2: Correlation between premanipulation dorsal angulation and dorsal angulation at 6 weeks.

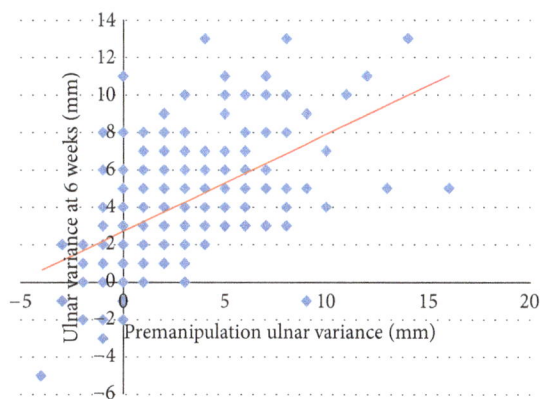

FIGURE 3: Correlation between premanipulation ulnar variance and ulnar variance at 6 weeks.

An adequate reduction of the distal radial fracture was achieved in 87 patients (38%). Overall there was a significant improvement in the position of the fracture, in both the degree of dorsal angulation and the degree of ulnar variance (Table 2). The position of the fracture 6 weeks after injury had deteriorated, resulting in 196 (86%) patients being defined as having a malunion (Table 2).

There was a significant correlation between premanipulation dorsal angulation ($r = 0.24$ and Pearson correlation $P < 0.001$) and ulnar variance ($r = 0.54$, Pearson correlation $P < 0.001$) with that measured at 6 weeks after injury (Figures 2 and 3). Using these correlations on average a mean dorsal angulation of greater than 25 degrees, or an ulnar variance of 6 mm or more, would result in a malunion at 6 weeks (Figures 2 and 3). Using these values as predictors, a dorsal angulation of greater than 25 degrees (odds ratio (OR) 2.3 and chi-square $P = 0.047$) and an ulnar variance of 6 mm or more (OR 1.2 and chi-square $P = 0.02$) both significantly increased the risk of malunion. These two risk factors were additive (OR 2.7 and chi-square $P = 0.014$), and combining these two predictors alone would result in a test that is 52% sensitive and 72% specific for predicting malunion. This test was a significant independent predictor of malunion when adjusting for other confounding variables ($R^2 = 0.05$, OR 2.72, using bivariate regression analysis $P = 0.017$). No other variables were significant and they were not included within the model.

Dorsal comminution, the premanipulation dorsal angulation, and ulnar variance were significant predictors of the degree of improvement in the 6-week dorsal angulation and ulnar variance (Table 3). Premanipulation dorsal angulation was the only significant isolated predictor, after adjusting for other confounding variables, of improvement in the degree of dorsal angulation at 6 weeks (Table 4). Premanipulation dorsal angulation and ulnar variance and dorsal comminution were all significant isolated predictors, after adjusting for other confounding variables, of improvement in the ulnar variance at 6 weeks (Table 4).

## 4. Discussion

We have demonstrated that the majority of displaced distal radial fractures in superelderly patients occur in females, after a simple fall, of which approximately half are functionally independent. Closed manipulation of the distal radial fracture achieved an adequate reduction in one-third of patients, and the majority of patients had an improvement of their fracture position. The degrees of dorsal angulation, ulna variance, and dorsal comminution were independent predictors of improvement in the position of the fracture; however, most patients (86%) went onto a malunion. Those patients with a dorsal angulation of greater than 25 degrees

TABLE 2: Dorsal angulation and ulnar variance pre- and postmanipulation and the statistical significance of improvement relative premanipulation measurement.

| Time point | | Dorsal angulation in degrees (SD) | P value* | Ulnar variance in mm (SD) | P value* |
|---|---|---|---|---|---|
| Premanipulation | | 25.2 (10.1) | — | 2.9 (3.1) | — |
| One week | Absolute | 1.2 (9.4) | <0.001 | 0.9 (2.6) | <0.001 |
| | Improvement | 24.0 | | 2.0 | |
| 6 weeks | Absolute | 11.9 (14.5) | <0.001 | 4.3 (3.0) | <0.001 |
| | Improvement | 13.3 | | −1.4 | |

*Paired $t$-test.

TABLE 3: Predictors of improvement in the dorsal angulation and ulna variance at 6 weeks.

| Case-mix variables | | Improvement in dorsal angulation (degrees) | $r =$ | P value | Improvement in ulnar variance (mm) | $r =$ | P value |
|---|---|---|---|---|---|---|---|
| Gender | Male | 13.7 | — | 0.92* | 1.7 | — | 0.51* |
| | Female | 13.3 | — | | 2.1 | — | |
| Age | | — | 0.05 | 0.46† | — | 0.05 | 0.47† |
| Independent | Yes | 14.2 | — | 0.35* | 1.9 | — | 0.24* |
| | No | 12.3 | — | | 2.3 | — | |
| Dorsal comminution | Yes | 13.4 | — | 0.7* | 2.2 | — | 0.001* |
| | No | 11.9 | — | | 0.1 | — | |
| AO classification | A | 14.0 | — | | 2.0 | — | |
| | B | 16.0 | — | 0.15** | 4.0 | — | 0.7** |
| | C | 12.8 | — | | 2.2 | — | |
| Premanipulation | Dorsal angulation | — | 0.43 | <0.001† | — | 0.34 | <0.001† |
| | Ulnar variance | — | 0.15 | 0.021† | — | 0.70 | <0.001† |

*Unpaired $t$-test.
**ANOVA.
†Pearson correlation.

TABLE 4: Significant predictors of improvement in dorsal angulation and ulna variance at 6 weeks.

| Outcome variable | Risk factor | B | 95% confidence interval | P value* |
|---|---|---|---|---|
| Improvement in dorsal angulation ($R^2 = 0.20$) | Premanipulation dorsal angulation | 0.66 | 0.47 to 0.84 | <0.001 |
| | (constant) | −3.17 | −8.14 to −1.79 | <0.001 |
| Improvement in ulnar variance ($R^2 = 0.31$) | Premanipulation dorsal angulation | 0.03 | 0.01 to 0.06 | 0.01 |
| | Premanipulation ulnar variance | 0.53 | 0.46 to 0.61 | <0.001 |
| | Dorsal comminution | 1.43 | 0.52 to 2.34 | 0.002 |
| | (constant) | −1.62 | −1.88 to −1.35 | 0.002 |

*Linearregression analysis.

and an ulna variance of more than 6 mm at the time of their injury were at the greatest risk of malunion.

Approximately 30% of distal radial fractures occur in men, and 70% are due to falls from standing height [10]. The prevalence of superelderly male patients sustaining displaced distal radial fractures is less, accounting for only 6%, and 98% are due to falls from standing. This probably relates to the increased fragility of the superelderly population, with a greater prevalence of osteoporosis in female patients [14], resulting in more low energy fractures in women. The incidence of distal radial fractures increases with age, with a peak of 1107/10^5/year in superelderly women [15]. If the predicted rise in the population is correct this will result in 44 thousand (population estimate of 6 million [7] with an approximate incidence of 730/10^5/year [10]) distal radial fractures in superelderly patients presenting to orthopaedic trauma services per year in the UK by the year 2030. Assuming 40% will have displaced fractures, as we have demonstrated, this would mean 18 thousand superelderly patients may undergo manipulation. This will have major repercussions upon the orthopaedic trauma workload, and hence efficient and appropriate management of these fragility fractures will be of paramount importance in optimising the care of these patients.

A unique aspect of this study was to define specific cutoff values for dorsal angulation and ulnar variants as independent predictors of malunion of distal radius fractures in the superelderly. Previous studies identifying risk factors for malunion found dorsal comminution to be an independent predictor of malunion [12, 16]. We have also demonstrated that the combination of dorsal angulation of greater than 25 degrees and/or ulnar variance of greater than 6 mm resulted in the greatest risk of malunion in the superelderly patients. The clinical relevance of this is not clear in this low demand group [4]. There is a body of evidence which demonstrates that the functional outcome of distal radial fractures correlates with the end anatomic result [2, 3, 5]. These studies are, however, heterogeneous including patients with a wide age range and include both extra- and intra-articular fracture patterns. Studies focusing on elderly patients and those with low functional demand have shown that malunion does not correlate with an inferior outcome [4]. More recently Grewal and MacDermid [17] demonstrated that for independent elderly patients with displaced extra-articular distal radius fractures, malunion did not result in a diminished functional outcome.

If a malunion does not affect functional outcome then the question could be asked whether it is worth manipulating displaced distal radius fractures in superelderly patients. Beumer and McQueen [18] suggested that for functionally active elderly patients it would be reasonable to assume that functional outcome does correlate with reduction of the fracture, as demonstrated for younger patients. It would also seem reasonable to assume that the degree of malunion may correlate with functional outcome in the elderly. Hence, manipulation of the fracture with improvement in the position, despite being defined as a malunion, may result in an improved outcome. Kelly et al. [19] demonstrated that elderly patients with more than 30 degrees of dorsal angulation and 5 mm of ulnar variance resulted in a poorer outcome. Using our prediction models for improvement in dorsal angulation and ulnar variance for superelderly patients it would be mathematically possible to calculate the improvement potentially offered by manipulation of displaced fractures, for example:

Improvement in dorsal angulation (DA)

$$= (\text{premanipulation DA} \times 0.655) - 3.174 \ (\text{constant})$$

Improvement in ulna variance (UV)

$$= (\text{pre-manipulation UV} \times 0.534)$$
$$+ (\text{pre-manipulation DA} \times 0.032)$$
$$+ 1.433 \text{ if dorsal comminution} - 1.617 \ (\text{constant}).$$

(1)

This would enable a patient's final position to be calculated, identifying those patients who would achieve or fail to achieve the radiographic criteria defined by Kelly et al. [19]. Independent superelderly patients who are predicted to fail to achieve these radiographic criteria may benefit from primary surgical intervention, to avoid a wasted intervention and delay in definitive management.

Superelderly patients with a displaced distal radial fracture managed with closed manipulation alone will result in a malunion for the majority of patients. The position of the fracture will, however, be improved by closed manipulation, but whether this improvement results in an enhanced functional outcome is not known. It would seem reasonable to assume that the improvement in the radiographic position of the fracture correlates with a superior functional outcome. This assumption needs to be confirmed to ensure primary manipulation is of functional benefit to superelderly patients and not a waste of healthcare resources and an inconvenience to our patients.

## Conflict of Interests

The authors declare that there is no conflict of interests regarding the publication of this paper.

## References

[1] C. M. Court-Brown and B. Caesar, "Epidemiology of adult fractures: a review," *Injury*, vol. 37, no. 8, pp. 691–697, 2006.

[2] M. McQueen and J. Caspers, "Colles fracture: does the anatomical result affect the final function?" *Journal of Bone and Joint Surgery Series B*, vol. 70, no. 4, pp. 649–651, 1988.

[3] W. P. Cooney, "Management of Colles' fractures," *Journal of Hand Surgery*, vol. 14, no. 2, pp. 137–139, 1989.

[4] R. J. Diaz-Garcia, T. Oda, M. J. Shauver, and K. C. Chung, "A systematic review of outcomes and complications of treating unstable distal radius fractures in the elderly," *Journal of Hand Surgery*, vol. 36, no. 5, pp. 824–835, 2011.

[5] M. M. McQueen, "Redisplaced unstable fractures of the distal radius. A randomised, prospective study of bridging versus non-bridging external fixation," *The Journal of Bone and Joint Surgery. British Volume*, vol. 80, pp. 665–669, 1998.

[6] C. Tomassini, "The oldest old in Great Britain: change over the last 20 years," *Population Trends*, no. 123, pp. 32–39, 2006.

[7] Parliament UK, http://www.parliament.uk/business/publications/research/key-issues-for-the-new-parliament/value-for-money-in-public-services/the-ageing-population/.

[8] N. D. Clement, S. A. Aitken, A. D. Duckworth, M. M. McQueen, and C. M. Court-Brown, "The outcome of fractures in very elderly patients," *Journal of Bone and Joint Surgery B*, vol. 93, no. 6, pp. 806–810, 2011.

[9] N. D. Clement and C. M. Court-Brown, "Four-score years and ten: the fracture epidemiology of the super-elderly," *Injury Extra*, vol. 40, no. 10, p. 235, 2009.

[10] C. M. Court-Brown, S. A. Aitken, D. Forward, and R. V. O'Toole, "The epidemiology of fractures," in *Rockwood and Greens Fractures in Adults*, R. W. Bucholz, J. D. Heckman, C. M. Court-Brown, and P. Tornetta, Eds., pp. 53–77, Lippincott, Wlliams & Wilkins,, Philadelphia, Pa, USA, 7th edition, 2010.

[11] N. C. Chen and J. B. Jupiter, "Management of distal radial fractures," *The Journal of Bone & Joint Surgery*, vol. 89, no. 9, pp. 2051–2062, 2007.

[12] P. J. Mackenney, M. M. McQueen, and R. Elton, "Prediction of instability in distal radial fractures," *Journal of Bone and Joint Surgery A*, vol. 88, no. 9, pp. 1944–1951, 2006.

[13] J. L. Marsh, T. F. Slongo, J. Agel et al., "Fracture and dislocation classification compendium—2007: Orthopaedic Trauma

Association classification, database and outcomes committee," *Journal of Orthopaedic Trauma*, vol. 21, no. 10, S133 pages, 2007.

[14] R. A. E. Clayton, M. S. Gaston, S. H. Ralston, C. M. Court-Brown, and M. M. McQueen, "Association between decreased bone mineral density and severity of distal radial fractures," *The Journal of Bone & Joint Surgery*, vol. 91, no. 3, pp. 613–619, 2009.

[15] T. Flinkkilä, K. Sirniö, M. Hippi et al., "Epidemiology and seasonal variation of distal radius fractures in Oulu, Finland," *Osteoporosis International*, vol. 22, no. 8, pp. 2307–2312, 2011.

[16] N. H. Jenkins, "The unstable Colles' fracture," *Journal of Hand Surgery*, vol. 14, no. 2, pp. 149–154, 1989.

[17] R. Grewal and J. C. MacDermid, "The risk of adverse outcomes in extra-articular distal radius fractures is increased with malalignment in patients of all ages but mitigated in older patients," *Journal of Hand Surgery*, vol. 32, no. 7, pp. 962–970, 2007.

[18] A. Beumer and M. M. McQueen, "Fractures of the distal radius in low-demand elderly patients: closed reduction of no value in 53 of 60 wrists," *Acta Orthopaedica Scandinavica*, vol. 74, no. 1, pp. 98–100, 2003.

[19] A. J. Kelly, D. Warwick, T. P. K. Crichlow, and G. C. Bannister, "Is manipulation of moderately displaced Colles' fracture worthwhile? A prospective randomized trial," *Injury*, vol. 28, no. 4, pp. 283–287, 1997.

# 22

# The Comprehensive Biomechanics and Load-Sharing of Semirigid PEEK and Semirigid Posterior Dynamic Stabilization Systems

D. K. Sengupta,[1] Brandon Bucklen,[2] Paul C. McAfee,[3] Jeff Nichols,[2] Raghavendra Angara,[2] and Saif Khalil[2]

[1] Dartmouth-Hitchcock Medical Center, One Medical Center Drive, Lebanon, NH 03756, USA
[2] Globus Medical, Inc., Valley Forge Business Center, 2560 General Armistead Avenue, Audubon, PA 19403, USA
[3] Towson Orthopaedic Associates, P.A.—Scoliosis and Spine Center, O'Dea Medical Arts Building, Suite 104, 7505 Osler Drive, Towson, MD 21204, USA

Correspondence should be addressed to Brandon Bucklen; bbucklen@globusmedical.com

Academic Editor: Ali Fahir Ozer

Alternatives to conventional rigid fusion have been proposed for several conditions related to degenerative disc disease when nonoperative treatment has failed. Semirigid fixation, in the form of dynamic stabilization or PEEK rods, is expected to provide compression under loading as well as an intermediate level of stabilization. This study systematically examines both the load-sharing characteristics and kinematics of these two devices compared to the standard of internal rigid fixators. Load-sharing was studied by using digital pressure films inserted between an artificially machined disc and two loading fixtures. Rigid rods, PEEK rods, and the dynamic stabilization system were inserted posteriorly for stabilization. The kinematics were quantified on ten, human, cadaver lumbosacral spines (L3-S1) which were tested under a pure bending moment, in flexion-extension, lateral bending, and axial rotation. The magnitude of load transmission through the anterior column was significantly greater with the dynamic device compared to PEEK rods and rigid rods. The contact pressures were distributed more uniformly, throughout the disc with the dynamic stabilization devices, and had smaller maximum point-loading (pressures) on any particular point within the disc. Kinematically, the motion was reduced by both semirigid devices similarly in all directions, with slight rigidity imparted by a lateral interbody device.

## 1. Introduction

Conventional instrumentation to achieve fusion in the lumbar spine utilizes rigid rods and pedicle screws [1–3]. Rigid rod fixation is criticized to reduce load-sharing and inhibit fusion mass formation because of the stress-shielding effect [4]. Not only does load-sharing influence fusion, but it may also affect a patient's pain level, adjacent segment kinematics, and the potential for device failure following spine surgery [2]. Semirigid instrumentations, such as polyetheretherketone (PEEK) rods and titanium rods with helical grooves, are designed to increase load-sharing in attempt to induce compression on the bone graft and promote bone remodeling as first credited by Wolff [4]. There is certainly evidence of

osteoblastic response to mechanical activation, in various forms, as well as increases in bone formation rate following bouts of loading [5, 6]. Semirigid PEEK instrumentation attempts to allow loading through the anterior column, but most studies show the stiffness of these constructs to be relatively high [7].

One hypothesized benefit of a dynamic device is to restore the loading of the damaged disc to similar thresholds as a normal disc would tolerate. For example, with damage comes reduced proteoglycan content, overload of the annulus, change in homogeneity of material properties, depressurization of the nucleus, and inability of the disc to hydrophilically retain water [3, 8]. Normal physiological loads on a damaged disc will produce stress concentrations higher and more disparate than a corresponding healthy disc. Therefore, one goal of semirigid stabilization should be to reduce and redistribute these loads off the disc to some degree, while trying to maintain a similar loading as what a healthy disc would experience, all in the presence of fusion.

Dynamic stabilization systems may be used as a load-sharing device, to mechanically stimulate bone cells toward fusion. The purpose of the device is to act as semirigid instrumentation, with the ability to dampen the loads as the spine moves. Design of posterior dynamic stabilization devices (PDSs) is very difficult for the reason that every diseased disc is not diseased in the same way and to the same extent as one another. How much offloading is ideal remains a matter of debate. Sengupta et al. suggest that pain alleviation is determined by the uniformity of loading on the disc space, as a fully healthy disc is expected to act as a uniform load bearing structure [3, 8].

In this study, the authors are interested in evaluating the load-sharing and kinematic properties of the spectrum of surgical options, from rigid, using titanium rods, to semirigid, using PEEK rods, to PDS, using polymer-based posterior dampeners. The goal was to quantify load-sharing as well as to determine the distribution of these loads within the interbody space.

## 2. Materials and Methods

There are two arms to this study. The first arm is determining the load-sharing through the anterior column as determined by the type of posterior instrumentation. The second arm is determining the kinematic range-of-motion as determined by the type of posterior instrumentation. Due to difficulty in measuring regional loading through an intervertebral disc *in vivo* or *in vitro*, mechanical testing was conducted on a spine model with a flat disc surface, as to accommodate a pressure sensor on the disc. The range-of-motion characterization was carried out on human cadaveric spines.

### 2.1. Load-Sharing

*2.1.1. Testing Fixtures and Protocol.* Tests were performed on lumbar spine models, prepared according to the ASTM F1717 standard corpectomy model (modified with a construct height of 28 mm from top screw to bottom screw) using ultrahigh molecular weight polyethylene (UHMWPE) blocks. The load-sharing of the vertebral disc was simulated through controlled mechanical testing using a MTS Bionix Servohydraulic Test System (Eden Prairie, MN) with an MTS 661.18 Force Transducer, 2.5 kN maximum. Prior to testing, each construct was soaked in a saline (0.9%) bath at body temperature (37°C) for 1 hour. An axial compressive bending load was applied to the construct at a rate of 10 mm/min in ambient air until 320 N was reached. The moment arm was chosen so that the bending moment, with respect to the posterior instrumentation, in maximum flexion was 12.8 Nm resulting in a 0.04 m moment arm. The constructs were subjected to cyclical loading for three cycles, and the data were captured from the third cycle.

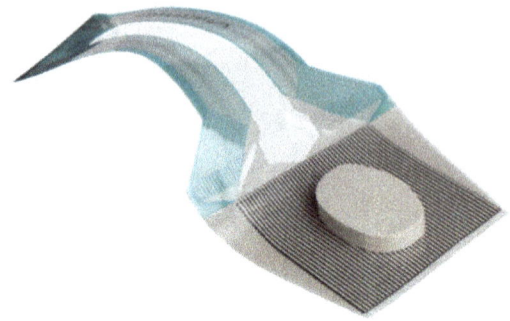

FIGURE 1: Tekscan pressure film used to measure contact pressures on the spacer. Note that during testing the film was placed above the spacer.

The anterior column load was measured using Tekscan pressure mapping software (I-Scan Pressure Measurement System, Boston, MA) and a digital pressure film (Model 5051) placed between the endplate of the polyethylene vertebral body and the modified interbody spacer device (CONTINENTAL, Globus Medical, Audubon, PA) to detect contact pressures. The pressure film consists of a square grid of 44 × 44 sensor cells with a row and column width of 0.03 inches. Each cell registers the force passing through it. Based on the known area of each cell, the software postprocesses pressure as well as other parameters involving regional data averaging.

The spacer was machined from PEEK, and two windows (in the shape of bone graft windows) were milled to a depth of 3 mm on the bottom surface (to ensure consistent location), while the top surface of the spacer remained flat (test surface) (Figure 1). The top surface of the spacer was tested via a profilometer to ensure no preexisting roughness which could cause pressure artifacts. Solid rigid polyurethane foam (Sawbones, density 20 pcf, Vashon, WA) which contained a boss of the same window shape as the spacer was inserted into the bottom test block (UHMWPE). The windows were used to secure a press fit of the spacer onto the bottom polyurethane foam insert, so that the spacer would not move throughout the testing. A flat polyurethane foam insert was used in the upper test block (UHMWPE). The sequence of load transfer was therefore through the MTS machine, upper test block, upper polyurethane foam insert, pressure film, spacer, lower polyurethane foam insert, and lower test block. The pressure film was placed between the spacer and upper polyurethane foam block, according to Figure 2. A fixed clearance was introduced to ensure consistency in the location of first contact. The clearance between the interbody spacer and upper test fixture was chosen at 400 $\mu$m and was measured on all four sides, prior to testing.

*2.1.2. Posterior Stabilization.* Three different posterior instrumentation systems representing rigid (titanium rods, REVERE, Globus Medical, Audubon, PA), semirigid (PEEK rods, LEGACY, Medtronic, Memphis, TN), and semirigid

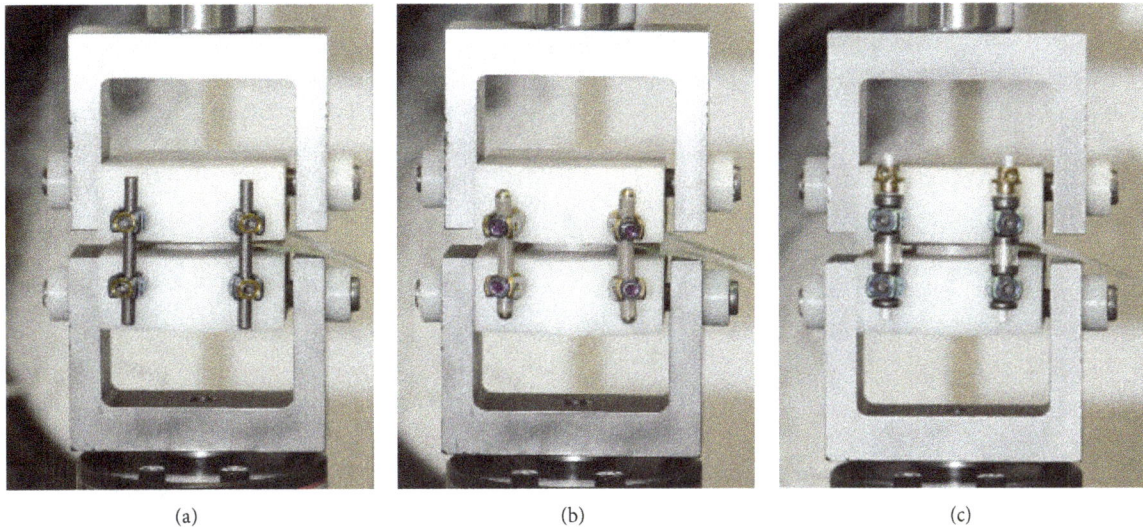

FIGURE 2: Testing constructs loaded in fixtures. Left to right: rigid rods, PEEK rods, and posterior dynamic stabilization. The pressure film can be seen above the spacer.

(dynamic stabilization, TRANSITION, Globus Medical, Audubon, PA) stabilization methods were tested. The pedicle screws were placed with the tulip heads nearly flush with respect to the UHMWPE test blocks with just enough space for polyaxial head toggle. The PDS device, TRANSITION Stabilization System, was evaluated (Figure 3), and it requires some explanation. The device consists of titanium spools over a polyethylene terephthalate (PET) cord which are dropped in between pedicle screws of adjacent levels. A polycarbonate urethane (PCU) polymer spacer surrounds the cord and fits between the spools which is used to buffer compressive forces. The PCU spacer between the pedicle screws is compressible, to allow normal extension with a soft end point, and the PCU bumper is compressible, allowing a dampened flexion motion. A PET cord which is not attached directly to the pedicle screw head but imbedded within titanium spools allows small interpedicular distance (IPD) changes.

Prior to testing, the pressure mapping system was calibrated using loads of 50% and 100% of the maximum load (320 N) without posterior instrumentation in place, in order to correlate the raw sensor readings to standardized pressure units (pounds per square inch). Five samples were tested. Each sample was prepared by assembling the posterior instrumentation on the test fixtures with appropriate test clearance. Following testing, the assembly was deconstructed, soaked in saline, and subsequently reconstructed with the next sample. Data was recorded from the pressure film in real time during the three loading and unloading cycles and saved as a sequence of image files. Data analysis and postprocessing was completed on the pressure profile of the image slice corresponding to the maximum load of 320 N for the last cycle.

*2.1.3. Data Analysis.* The total force passing through the spacer (i.e., pressure film) was used to estimate load-sharing

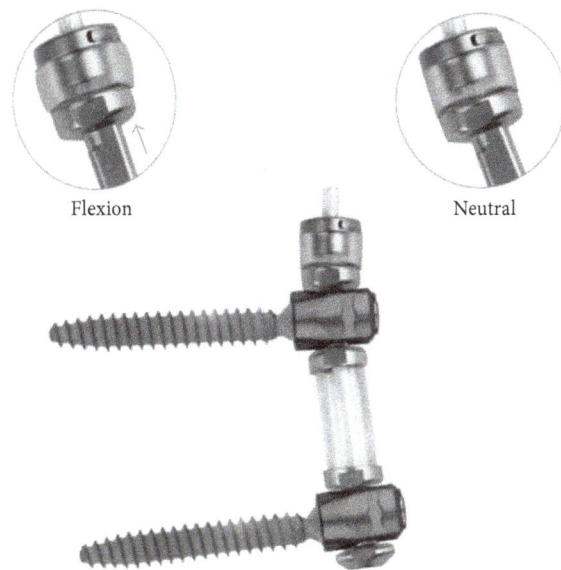

FIGURE 3: The TRANSITION Stabilization System. The cephalad bumper shown in neutral and flexed positions.

between the anterior and posterior column. The load passing through the spacer represented anterior column load-sharing, while the remaining load was assumed to pass through the posterior instrumentation and represented posterior column loading. Subsequent analysis involved splitting the anterior column spacer area into four distinct regions, hereafter referred to as bounding boxes: anterior, posterior, left, and right, according to the symmetrical midlines of the spacer itself (see Figure 4). For each bounding box, the following quantities were tabulated: total force, box pressure, and peak (maximum) box pressure. The total force is the sum of the forces in the rectangular bounding box. Box pressure is the sum of the forces in the rectangular bounding box

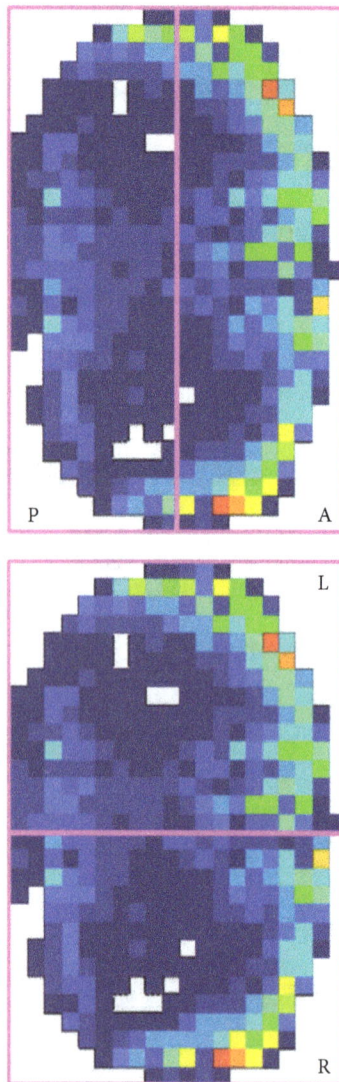

FIGURE 4: Pressure area division by bounding box: anterior (A), posterior (P), left (L), and right (R).

divided by the area of the bounding box. Peak box pressure is the maximum localized pressure in that bounding box. Statistical comparisons were made using two-tailed student's $t$-tests assuming equal variance, with a probability of type I error, $\alpha = 0.05$ ($n = 5$).

### 2.2. Kinematics

*2.2.1. Specimen Preparation and Test Constructs.* Ten human cadaver lumbosacral spines (L3-S1) were tested under a pure moment of 7 N-m, using a 6-degree-of-freedom spine tester in flexion-extension (FE), lateral bending (LB), and axial rotation (AR). The spines were fixed proximally at L3 and distally at S1 in a three-to-one mixture of Bond Auto Body Filler and fiberglass resin (Bondo Mar-Hyde Corp., Atlanta, GA). The specimens were divided into two groups of five, according to the type of semirigid fixation applied. Each type of transpedicular semirigid instrumentation utilized pedicle

screws of a different design and could not be reused on the same specimen without sacrificing screw purchase. Posterior fixation was tested with and without a lateral interbody spacer (TransContinental, Globus Medical) and in the injured state following a lateral discectomy (Figures 5 and 6). Results are presented as a percentage of intact range-of-motion (ROM).

*2.2.2. Test Setup and Data Analysis.* The spine was affixed to a six-degree-of-freedom (6DOF) testing apparatus via magnetization, and pure unconstrained bending moments will be applied in the physiologic planes of the spine at room temperature using a multidirectional hybrid flexibility protocol [9]. The 6DOF machine applies unconstrained loading through three cephalad stepper motors placed in each of the three physiological rotation axes. Moreover, the supports are mounted on air bearings to provide near frictionless resistance to the natural kinematics of the spine. Plexiglass markers, each having three infrared light-emitting diodes, were secured rigidly to each vertebral body via bone screws to track its motion with the Optotrak Certus (NDI, Inc., Waterloo, Canada) motion analysis system. The location of the markers (denoting a rigid body) were aligned approximately sagitally along the curvature of the spine. The Optotrak Certus software superimposes the coordinate systems of two adjacent vertebral bodies in order to inferentially determine the relative Eularian rotations in each of the three planes.

Data analysis was conducted using independent single factor ANOVA, with both groups combined. The data was first normalized to intact motion and underwent a log transformation to remove unequal variances. The Student-Newman-Keuls post hoc test was applied to all eight comparison groups at a level-1 alpha value of 0.05.

## 3. Results

*3.1. Load-Sharing.* A representative example of the recorded data is shown in Figure 7 (during maximum applied loading) for each type of posterior fixation. TekScan software postprocesses the output of each sensor cell into color-coded regions from low to high for easy visualization. A three-dimensional view is useful to assess the distribution and locations of maximum pressure.

The force through the entire spacer was used to determine the percentage of anterior and posterior columns loading as a fraction of the applied load (Figure 8). All load not passing through the pressure film (located in the anterior column) was considered to pass through the posterior instrumentation (located in the posterior column). No energy dissipation due to friction or any form was considered. Anterior column load-sharing was 55%, 59%, and 75%, for rigid rods, PEEK rods, and posterior dynamic stabilization, respectively. The posterior dynamic stabilization system transferred statistically more load than rigid or PEEK rods. Rigid and PEEK rods did not statistically differ from each other in their ability to transfer load through the anterior column. Moreover, of the three instrumentation types tested, the dynamic stabilization most closely approximated the load-sharing of the intact

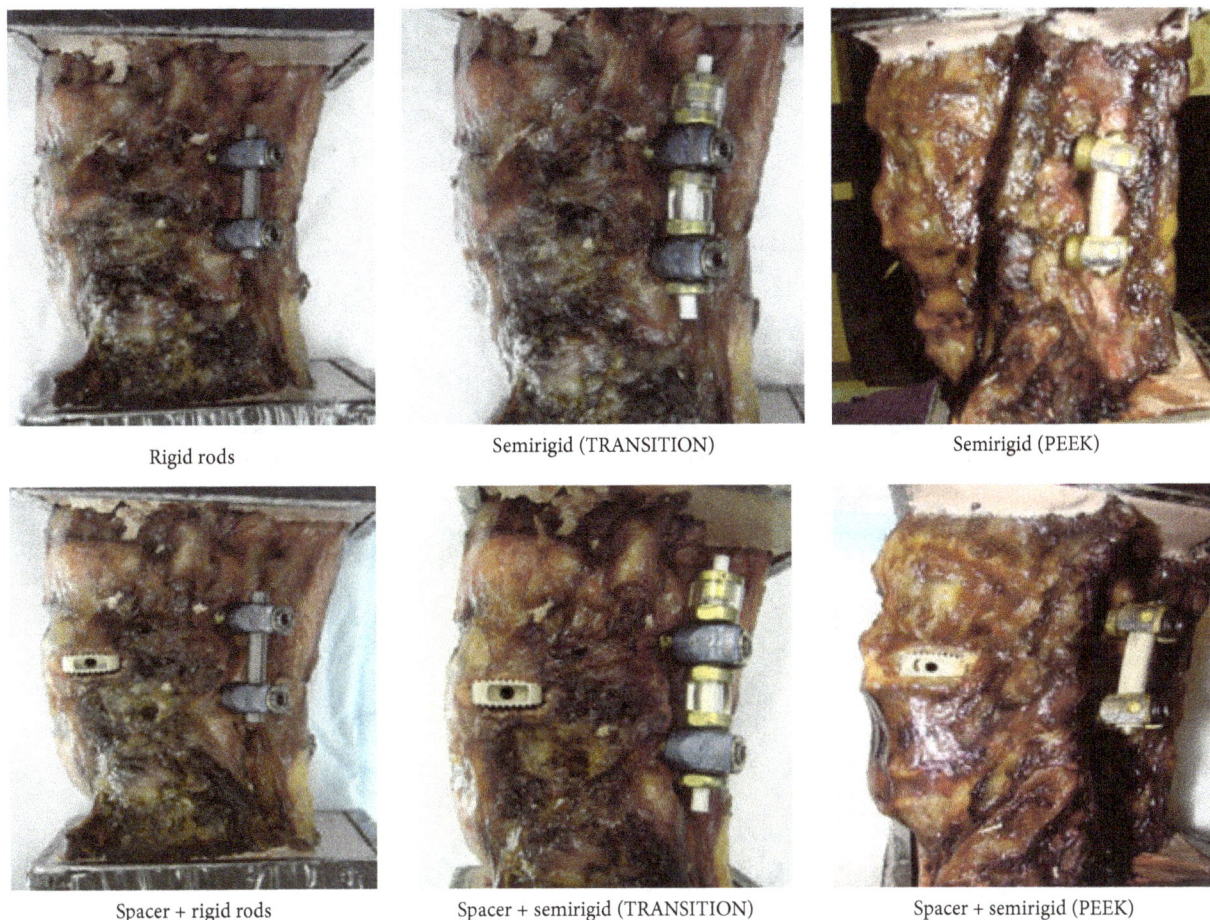

| Rigid rods | Semirigid (TRANSITION) | Semirigid (PEEK) |

| Spacer + rigid rods | Spacer + semirigid (TRANSITION) | Spacer + semirigid (PEEK) |

FIGURE 5: Select test images from flexibility testing, showing rigid and semirigid devices.

lumbar spine as an 80%–20% distribution in the anterior-posterior column as described by White and Panjabi, 1990 [10]. It should be noted that posterior elements and their contribution toward the load-sharing could not be included in the mechanical model.

*3.1.1. Regional Loading.* The spacer area was divided into bounding boxes describing anterior, posterior, left, and right regions. The average (Figure 9) and peak (Figure 10) pressures in each bounding box are reported. The reader should note the distinction between anterior and posterior bounding boxes (Figure 4) and the anterior and posterior columns loading as described previously.

In all types of fixation, the average anterior box pressure was larger than the posterior box pressure, and left and right pressures were similar (Figure 9). The disparity between anterior and posterior pressures was largest for PEEK rod instrumentation (63 PSI) and smallest for posterior dynamic instrumentation (29 PSI). The regional pressure profile created by PEEK rods was similar to that of rigid rods, except that PEEK had a higher anterior pressure. In all cases, posterior dynamic stabilization resulted in statistically higher average pressure readings, in the posterior, left, and right sides of the spacer, than the other posterior fixation groups.

The PEEK rods were the only constructs to result in a statistical difference in left versus right box pressures.

In all types of fixation, the peak anterior box pressure was larger than the peak posterior box pressure, and there were no statistical differences between left and right pressures (Figure 10). The disparity between anterior and posterior peak pressures was largest for PEEK rod instrumentation (312 PSI) and smallest for posterior dynamic instrumentation (65 PSI). The maximum pressure across the entire spacer (denoted by "max" in Figure 10) was the largest for PEEK rods (316 PSI), followed by rigid rods (233 PSI), and smallest for posterior dynamic instrumentation (193 PSI). All three instrumentation types were statistically different.

*3.2. Kinematics.* As per Figure 11, in the without-interbody group, rigid rods achieved the highest level of fixation (FE: 25%, LB: 33%, AR: 52%), with both semirigid systems demonstrating equivalence (TRANSITION; FE: 34%, LB: 54%, AR: 82%; PEEK Rods; FE: 35%, LB: 51%, AR: 65%). The addition of a lateral interbody spacer provided much stability, similar to that of semirigid instrumentation without interbody, in all three loading modes. In the interbody group, rigid rods achieved the highest level of fixation (FE: 16%, LB: 23%, AR: 40%) compared to the semirigid systems

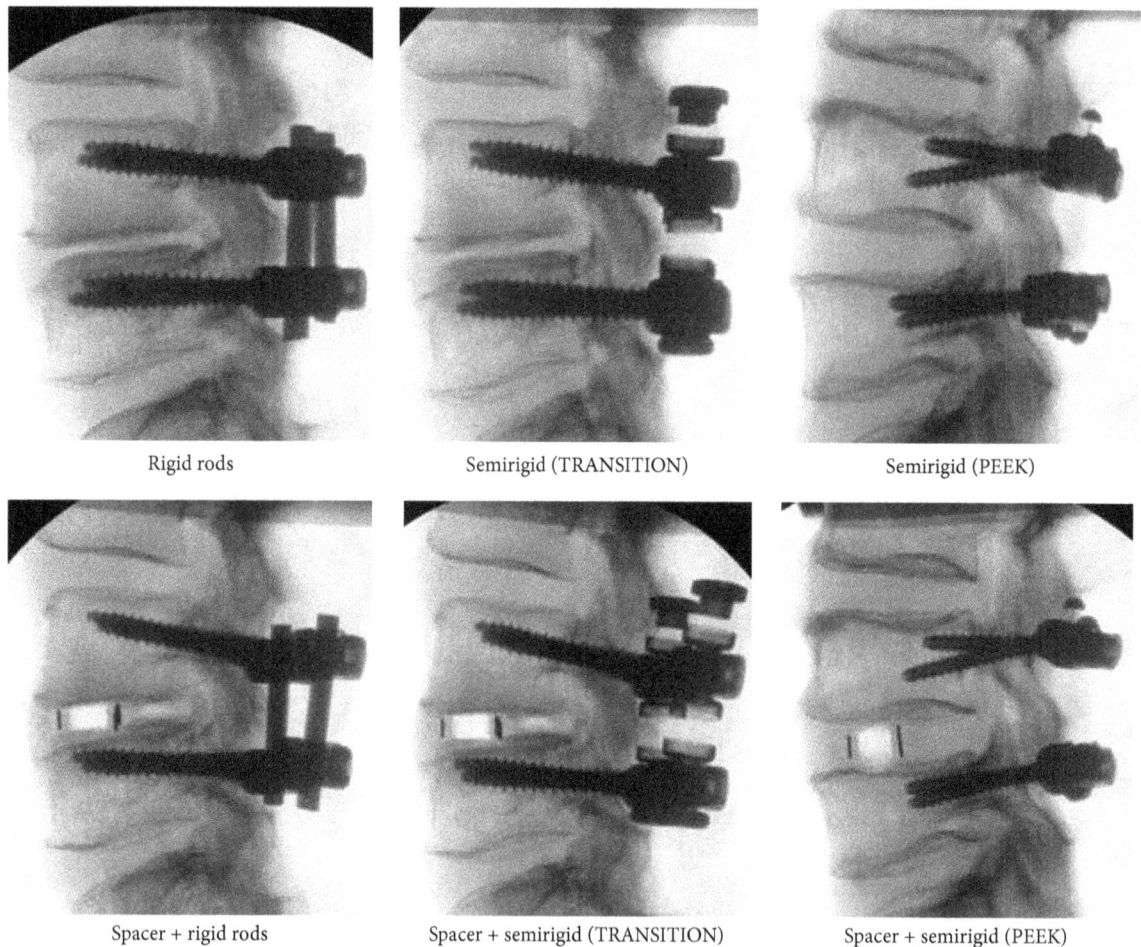

FIGURE 6: Select radiographs from flexibility testing, showing rigid and semirigid devices.

(TRANSITION FE: 20%, LB: 30%, AR: 48%; PEEK Rods FE: 18%, LB: 30%, AR: 47%). Semirigid systems led to gradual decrease of stiffness of 10%, 20%, and 20% in FE, LB, and AR, respectively, when compared to rigid systems without interbody. With the addition of a lateral interbody device, range-of-motion of semirigid systems was reduced by 16%, 22%, and 26%. There were no detectable differences between the semirigid devices tested.

## 4. Discussion

The stiffness of the spine after surgery is a combination of the applied instrumentation and fusion mass. With difficulty in predicting the contribution of the fusion mass, this study investigated the rigidity of posterior instrumentation imparted on the spine and the allowable anterior load-sharing. The benefits of semirigid systems may further contribute to the stiffness of the fusion mass, but could not be evaluated.

The hypothesis was that anterior column load-sharing would be higher for posterior dynamic stabilization (PDS) and PEEK rods than rigid systems. According to Sengupta et al., load-sharing and uniformity of loading are two important factors responsible for mechanical back pain, when occurring abnormally [3, 8]. Load-sharing at the index level is useful to promote fusion by stimulating bone cells to form new bone in the graft space. Most patients complain of acute or short bouts of pain, which could be triggered with peak contact pressures (abnormal load-sharing) or nonuniform pressures on a compromised disc. Load-sharing influences adjacent level motion, which has been considered as contributing to adjacent level disease. While previous biomechanical studies have described the relationship between adjacent level problems and kinematic behavior of PDS devices, there is no reported study that investigated load-sharing, which may prove to be clinically as important as global range-of-motion—though consistent clinical evidence is even lacking for motion [11, 12]. In this study, anterior column load-sharing was improved by the use of a semirigid posterior dynamic stabilization device when compared to semirigid PEEK or rigid fixation. The anterior-posterior column distribution was 55%–45%, 59%–41%, and 75%–25%, for rigid rods, PEEK rods, and posterior dynamic stabilization, respectively. The PDS device approximated the 80%–20% distribution of the normal spine as outlined by White and Panjabi, 1990 [10]. No statistical difference in anterior column loading existed between PEEK or rigid rods,

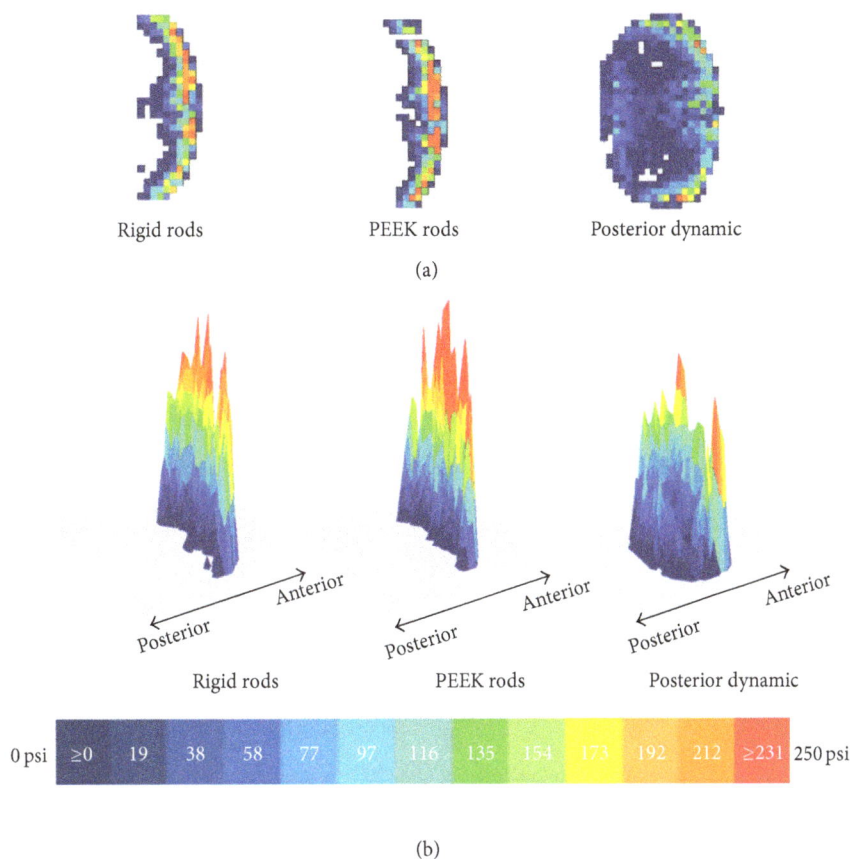

FIGURE 7: Example of pressure film data showing pressure contact area of spacer with blue colors representing low pressures and red colors representing high pressures, in two dimensions (a) and three dimensions (b) for each posterior instrumentation type.

but the PDS device provided statistically more load through the anterior column than both systems.

The load distribution across the interbody spacer area proved to be more uniform with posterior dynamic stabilization when compared to semirigid PEEK or rigid fixation as evidenced by Figures 5, 7, and 8. With rigid and PEEK rods, only nominal load was transferred to the posterior aspects of the spacer. PEEK rods consistently demonstrated larger average and maximum pressures on the anterior region of the spacer, when compared to PDS or rigid fixation. Dynamic stabilization and rigid rods have similar pressures on the anterior region of the spacer but differ dramatically in the posterior, left, and right portions of the spacer, which are much more uniform and statistically higher for PDS when compared to rigid rods. It should be noted, due to the predefined clearance of $400\,\mu m$, that load was first transmitted to the anterior portion of the spacer, to ensure consistency of testing.

Another difference between the PDS design and conventional designs is that the PDS device in this study utilized a PET cord which was not attached directly to the pedicle screw head but imbedded within titanium spools which allow some travel or sliding to compress and engage the soft bumper. This effect may have helped to redistribute the loads. This redistribution seems very evident in Figure 5, where the PDS device shows more coverage and symmetry in loading.

Additionally, the repeatability of the testing was high across all five samples.

Peak or maximum pressures are of great concern and may be mechanically induced pain generators even during normal loading. Ideally, a PDS device would reduce abnormally high pressures as well as reduce disparities between different portions of the interbody space. While total load-sharing with the PEEK device is marginally improved compared to rigid rods, the disparity between anterior and posterior regions of PEEK is the least favorable, with a 312 psi difference. The PDS device has a more favorable profile of maximum pressures which are lower in magnitude and more equally distributed across different regions (largest regional difference 65 psi). Statistically speaking, PEEK rods produced the highest maximum pressures, while the PDS device produced the least.

There are very few literature studies which looked at load-sharing in posterior dynamic stabilization devices, of which the data from the current study could be compared. Analytical finite element studies on L3-L4 spinal segment showed that axial forces across the anterior column would be 29%, 67%, and 59% of the applied loading for rigid rods, PEEK rods, and PDS, respectively[4]. However, the PDS device examined was a nitinol rod, which could not be compared to the current device or conventional devices. The data from this study shows higher overall load transfer, with minimal differences in rigid and PEEK rods. Their data show a stark

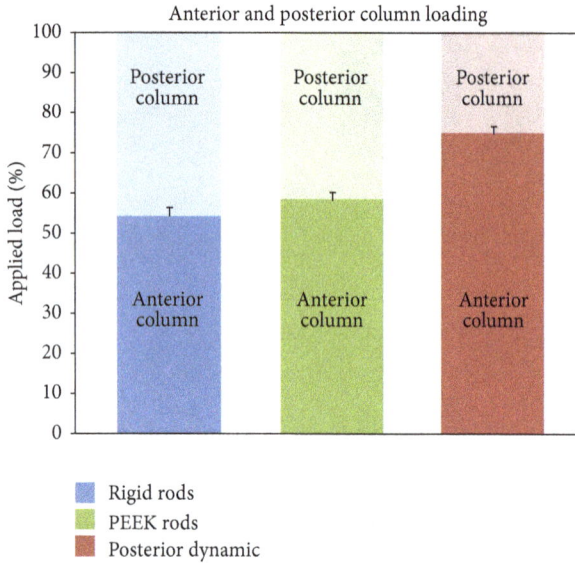

FIGURE 8: Anterior and posterior columns load-sharing. The bars represent standard deviations in measured anterior column load.

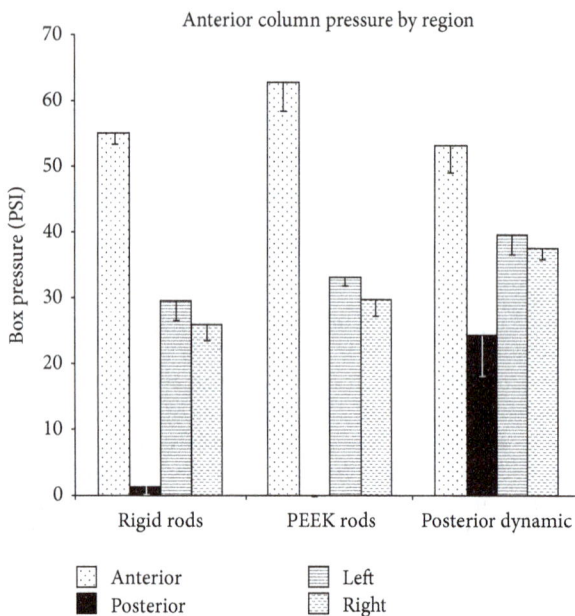

FIGURE 9: Average box pressure of the anterior, posterior, left, and right portions of the spacer as measured through the pressure film (according to Figure 4).

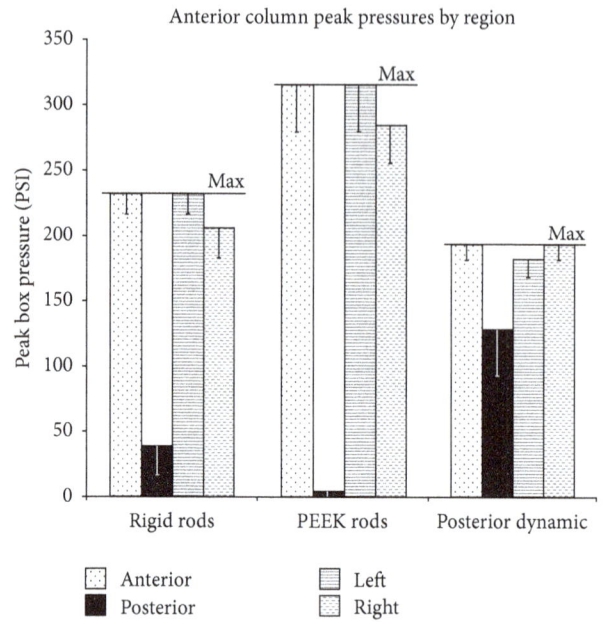

FIGURE 10: Peak (or maximum) box pressure of the anterior, posterior, left, and right portions of the spacer as measured through the pressure film (according to Figure 4).

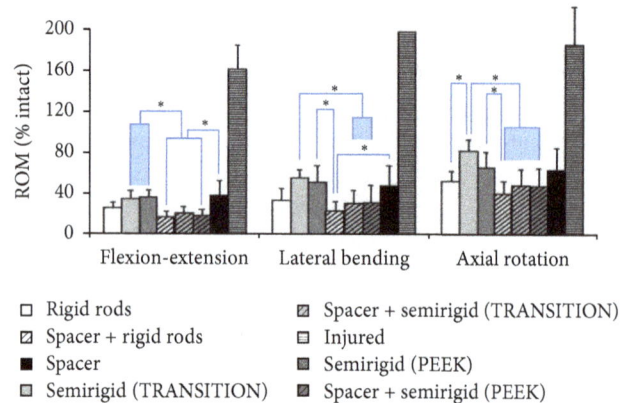

** Note that all constructs are significant w.r.t. injured

FIGURE 11: The biomechanical flexibility results normalized to intact motion (100%) by mode. Statistical indicators are shown with asterisks.

improvement in anterior column load-sharing for PEEK rods which was not observed in the present study.

The kinematics of the two semirigid systems investigated was very similar. There was not much difference in the response of the spine to either device, with or without interbody fusion—in terms of motion output. Nevertheless, as mentioned, there were clear differences in load-sharing. Rigid and semirigid PEEK instrumentation formed concentrated pressures on the area of first contact, while the semirigid dynamic stabilization system redistributed load away from

the initial contact point. Ultimately with the PDS device, the total force through the spacer was larger, but the maximum pressures were reduced. PEEK rods appear to provide some benefit in terms of total force transmission through the interbody space, albeit statistically insignificant, but like rigid rods suffer from very nonuniform regions of loading across the spacer area.

## 5. Conclusion

Load-sharing of the spinal column is an important biomechanical factor which may directly affect a patient's pain level, fusion success, and future disease progression, following spine surgery. In this study, load-sharing and regional load distribution of the interbody area were compared between rigid rods, semirigid PEEK rods, and semirigid dynamic posterior instrumentation with flexion-extension dampening materials. Despite similarities in motion characteristics between PEEK rods and PDS systems, the overall load-sharing was highest for the PDS device, with marginal differences between rigid and semirigid PEEK instrumentation. The PDS system reduced regional pressure gradients and was more uniform in the anterior, posterior, left, and right interbody spaces when compared to the other instrumentation types. The semirigid PEEK rods had the least uniform distribution in contact pressure. The outcomes reported here are encouraging for the use of PDS devices, but more clinical evaluation is needed to understand how load-sharing properties relate to clinical outcomes.

# References

[1] N. Boos and J. K. Webb, "Pedicle screw fixation in spinal disorders: a European view," *European Spine Journal*, vol. 6, no. 1, pp. 2–18, 1997.

[2] P. A. Cripton, G. M. Jain, R. H. Wittenberg, and L. P. Nolte, "Load-sharing characteristics of stabilized lumbar spine segments," *Spine*, vol. 25, no. 2, pp. 170–179, 2000.

[3] R. C. Mulholland and D. K. Sengupta, "Rationale, principles and experimental evaluation of the concept of soft stabilization," *European Spine Journal*, vol. 11, supplement 2, pp. S198–S205, 2002.

[4] Y. H. Ahn, W. M. Chen, K. Y. Lee, K. W. Park, and S. J. Lee, "Comparison of the load-sharing characteristics between pedicle-based dynamic and rigid rod devices," *Biomedical Materials*, vol. 3, no. 4, Article ID 044101, 2008.

[5] P. A. Kokkinos, I. K. Zarkadis, D. Kletsas, and D. D. Deligianni, "Effects of physiological mechanical strains on the release of growth factors and the expression of differentiation marker genes in human osteoblasts growing on Ti-6Al-4V," *Journal of Biomedical Materials Research A*, vol. 90, no. 2, pp. 387–395, 2009.

[6] M. J. Patel, H. C. Kyungh, M. C. Sykes, R. Talish, C. Rubin, and H. Jo, "Low magnitude and high frequency mechanical loading prevents decreased bone formation responses of 2T3 preosteoblasts," *Journal of Cellular Biochemistry*, vol. 106, no. 2, pp. 306–316, 2009.

[7] A. Rohlmann, N. K. Burra, T. Zander, and G. Bergmann, "Comparison of the effects of bilateral posterior dynamic and rigid fixation devices on the loads in the lumbar spine: a finite element analysis," *European Spine Journal*, vol. 16, no. 8, pp. 1223–1231, 2007.

[8] D. K. Sengupta, "Dynamic stabilization devices in the treatment of low back pain," *Neurology India*, vol. 53, no. 4, pp. 466–474, 2005.

[9] M. M. Panjabi, "Hybrid multidirectional test method to evaluate spinal adjacent-level effects," *Clinical Biomechanics*, vol. 22, no. 3, pp. 257–265, 2007.

[10] A. White and M. Panjabi, "Physical properties and functional biomechanics of the spine," in *Clinical Biomechanics of the Spine*, chapter 1, Lippincott Williams & Wilkins, Philadelphia, Pa, USA, 1990.

[11] W. Schmoelz, J. F. Huber, T. Nydegger, L. Claes, and H. J. Wilke, "Influence of a dynamic stabilisation system on load bearing of a bridged disc: an in vitro study of intradiscal pressure," *European Spine Journal*, vol. 15, no. 8, pp. 1276–1285, 2006.

[12] W. Schmoelz, J. F. Huber, T. Nydegger, Dipl-Ing, L. Claes, and H. J. Wilke, "Dynamic stabilization of the lumbar spine and its effects on adjacent segments: an in vitro experiment," *Journal of Spinal Disorders and Techniques*, vol. 16, no. 4, pp. 418–423, 2003.

# 23

# Does Semi-Rigid Instrumentation Using Both Flexion and Extension Dampening Spacers Truly Provide an Intermediate Level of Stabilization?

Dilip Sengupta,[1] Brandon Bucklen,[2] Aditya Ingalhalikar,[2]
Aditya Muzumdar,[2] and Saif Khalil[2]

[1] Dartmouth-Hitchcock Medical Center, Orthopedics, One Medical Center Drive, Lebanon, NH 03756-0001, USA
[2] Globus Medical Inc., Valley Forge Business Center, 2560 General Armistead Avenue, Audubon, PA 19403, USA

Correspondence should be addressed to Brandon Bucklen; bbucklen@globusmedical.com

Academic Editor: Vijay K. Goel

Conventional posterior dynamic stabilization devices demonstrated a tendency towards highly rigid stabilization approximating that of titanium rods in flexion. In extension, they excessively offload the index segment, making the device as the sole load-bearing structure, with concerns of device failure. The goal of this study was to compare the kinematics and intradiscal pressure of monosegmental stabilization utilizing a new device that incorporates both a flexion and extension dampening spacer to that of rigid internal fixation and a conventional posterior dynamic stabilization device. The hypothesis was the new device would minimize the overloading of adjacent levels compared to rigid and conventional devices which can only bend but not stretch. The biomechanics were compared following injury in a human cadaveric lumbosacral spine under simulated physiological loading conditions. The stabilization with the new posterior dynamic stabilization device significantly reduced motion uniformly in all loading directions, but less so than rigid fixation. The evaluation of adjacent level motion and pressure showed some benefit of the new device when compared to rigid fixation. Posterior dynamic stabilization designs which both bend and stretch showed improved kinematic and load-sharing properties when compared to rigid fixation and when indirectly compared to existing conventional devices without a bumper.

## 1. Introduction

Fusion using rigid pedicle screw-rod instrumentation is a conventional surgical treatment for mechanical back pain due to disc degeneration when nonoperative treatment has failed. In spite of this standard, it is associated with implant-related failures such as screw breakage or loosening. Screw breakage or loosening have been reported in the literature to range from 1% to 11.2% of the screws inserted [1–7]. It has been shown to be affected by a number of factors such as screw design, the number of levels fused, anterior column load-sharing, bone density, the presence of pseudoarthrosis, and its use in burst fractures [3, 4, 8–10]. While in multilevel fusion, bone density and burst fracture applications are more related to patient pathology and indications; all other factors are more dependent on implant design and biomechanics. Anterior column load-sharing is negatively affected by the absence of interbody support and higher stiffness of posterior fixation devices [3, 11]. Adjacent segment degeneration (ASD) has also been recognized as a potential long-term complication of rigidly instrumented fusion [12–17]. While there is some debate surrounding the causality of the disease (whether it is mechanical factors or a natural degenerative progression), a review of 271 articles found a higher rate of symptomatic ASD in 12%–18% of patients fused with rigid transpedicular instrumentation. In spite of these disadvantages, it is proven that implant rigidity is required to achieve successful fusion.

The challenge for surgeons, biomechanists, and engineers has been to determine and develop an optimally stiff device that will provide enough rigidity across a destabilized spinal segment while simultaneously sharing load with the fusion mass. Posterior fixation devices have evolved from larger diameters and stiffer materials (6.5 mm cobalt chromium/stainless steel) to smaller diameters and less stiff or semi-rigid materials (5.5 mm poly ether ether ketone (PEEK)), respectively. Semi-rigid fixation or dynamic stabilization devices such as PEEK rods, titanium rods with helical grooves, and polymeric spacers with an interwoven cord tethered between pedicle screws have been designed to increase load-sharing in an attempt to induce compression on the bone graft and accentuate the concept of bone remodeling as first credited by Wolff [18]. Examples of such devices are Isobar TTL (Scient'x, Maitland, FL), a metal rod with disc springs, the CD Horizon Legacy PEEK rod (Medtronic Sofamor Danek, Memphis, TN), and Dynesys Dynamic Stabilization System (Zimmer, Warsaw, IN) consisting of a polymeric dampener and posterior tensioning cord. Semi-rigid fixation devices attempt to offload adjacent levels, but most studies show the stiffness of these constructs to be too high to have much of an effect on adjacent level loading [18–21]. These devices have also been clinically recommended for stabilization and modulation of the load distribution across mildly degenerated discs in an attempt to alleviate discogenic back pain and potentially enable regeneration of disc cells [22, 23].

In this particular study, the TRANSITION Stabilization System (Globus Medical, Inc., Audubon, PA) was utilized as the method of semi-rigid stabilization. The device was designed to bend and stretch by incorporating two polymeric spacers: one strategically placed above the cranial pedicle screw and the other between the pedicle screws, to allow a resistance to flexion, and a natural compression across the joint, respectively. We hypothesize that the compressibility across the surgical level may have implications on both the index and adjacent levels, but to what degree remains unknown.

The aim of this study was to evaluate the implanted and adjacent level kinematics and load-sharing effects of the human lumbosacral spine implanted with a semi-rigid fixation device, TRANSITION, compared to rigid fixation, and the historical performance of conventional semi-rigid devices. In this study, the injury model of the motion segment was created by a decompression involving facetectomy.

## 2. Materials and Methods

*2.1. Specimen Preparation.* All spines were radiographed to ensure the absence of fractures, deformities, and any metastatic disease. The spines were stripped of paravertebral musculature while preserving the spinal ligaments, joints, and disk spaces. Subsequently, they were mounted at L1 rostrally and S1 caudally in a three-to-one mixture of Bond Auto Body Filler and fiberglass resin (Bondo MarHyde Corp., Atlanta, GA). The spine was then affixed to a six degree-of-freedom (6-DOF) testing apparatus, and pure unconstrained bending moments were applied in the physiological planes of the spine at room temperature using a multidirectional hybrid flexibility protocol [24]. The 6-DOF machine applied

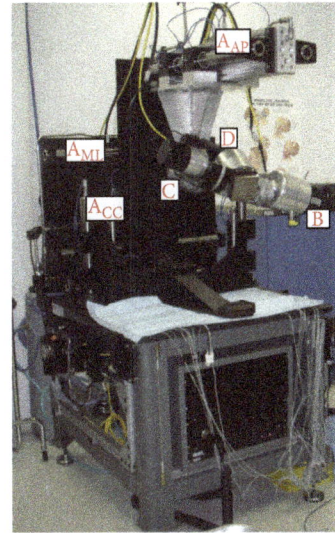

Figure 1: Six degree-of-freedom testing apparatus, allowing unconstrained motion and rotations. Three motors, each placed in a physiological rotation direction providing pure rotations, while translational guide rails allow the forces to redistribute according to the kinematic properties of the spine. $A_{AP}$: guide rail with air bearings (anterior-posterior), $A_{ML}$: guide rail with air bearings (medial-lateral), $A_{CC}$: guide rail with air bearings (cephalad-caudal), B: flexion-extension motor, C: lateral bending motor, and D: axial rotation motor.

unconstrained loading through the application of three cephalad stepper motors placed in each of the three physiological rotation axes (Figure 1). Moreover, the supports were mounted on air bearings to provide near frictionless resistance to the natural kinematics of the spine. Plexiglas markers, each having three infrared light-emitting diodes, were secured rigidly to each vertebral body via bone screws to track its motion with Optotrak Certus (NDI, Inc. Waterloo, Canada) motion analysis system. The location of the markers (denoting a rigid body) was approximately aligned sagitally along the curvature of the spine. The Optotrak Certus software was able to superimpose the coordinate systems of two adjacent vertebral bodies in order to inferentially determine the relative eulerian rotations in each of the three planes.

*2.2. Device Descriptions.* The semi-rigid device which can both bend and stretch (TRANSITION) is composed of titanium, polycarbonate urethane (PCU), and polyethylene terephthalate (PET) (Figure 2). Essentially, instead of a rod, a PCU spacer is placed between the pedicle screws, while a central PET cord, which runs from top to bottom, provides resistance to stretching (namely flexion). The cord is not tethered to the screws, like conventional devices, but is passed through spools which are the attachment point of the pedicle screws. The spools are 5.5 mm thick at the portion which fits into the pedicle screw. Above the cranial pedicle screw is another PCU spacer which is compressed when the cord is in tension (flexion). The rigid rods tested were standard

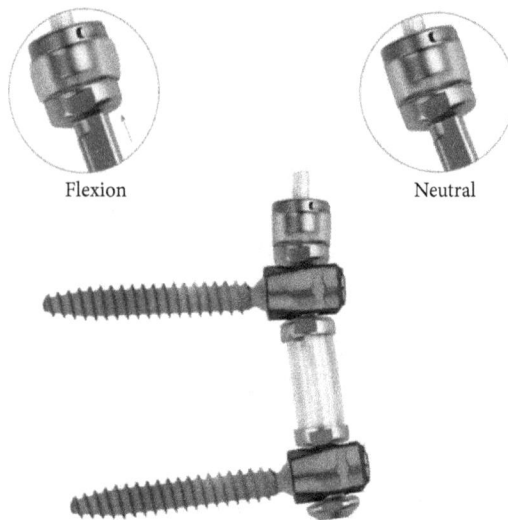

FIGURE 2: The TRANSITION Stabilization System. The cephalad bumper shown in neutral and flexed position.

5.5 mm diameter titanium rods (REVERE Stabilization System, Globus Medical). Both devices were locked in place through the same screws, having the same tulip, and same locking caps. Comparisons to historical controls or so-called conventional dynamic stabilization devices are primarily focused on Dynesys Dynamic Stabilization System (Zimmer, Warsaw, IN) but could also include Isobar TTL (Scient'x, Maitland, FL), CD Horizon Legacy PEEK rod (Medtronic Sofamor Danek, Memphis, TN), or others. Dynesys has been by far the most extensively studied, biomechanically and clinically.

*2.3. Test Groups.* Nine intact fresh human cadaver lumbosacral spines (L1-S1) were tested by applying a pure moment of ±8 Nm, according to the test standards for lumbar spine [25]. The specimens consisted of 6 males and 3 females, with an average age of 53 ± 10 years. The hybrid protocol for testing adjacent level effects was applied, as described by Panjabi [24]. Initially, the total L1-S1 range of motion (ROM) was determined in an individual intact specimen. In all subsequent tests for the respective specimen, the displacement of the spine was ranged to the intact total ROM values in flexion (F), extension (E), lateral bending (LB), and axial rotation (AR). A series of three load/unload cycles were performed for each motion with data analysis based on the final cycle. The first five specimens were tested for unilateral facetectomy and unilateral stabilization of L4-L5 segment in the following sequence (Figure 3): (1) intact; (2) unilateral facetectomy (UF); (3) UF and unilateral TRANSITION PDS device (UF + UT); and (4) UF and bilateral TRANSITION PDS device (UF + BT). All the nine specimens (including the previous five unilateral models) were tested for bilateral facetectomy and bilateral stabilization at the L4-L5 segment in the following sequence: (1) intact; (5) bilateral facetectomy (BF); (6) BF and bilateral TRANSITION PDS device (BF + BT); and (7) BF and bilateral rigid fixation (pedicle screws and titanium rod, REVERE Stabilization System, Globus

Medical) with interbody spacer (Sustain-O, Globus Medical) (BF + S + R). The numbers in parenthesis indicate the construct number identifying the test condition, in the rest of this paper. Disc pressure was measured using miniature pressure transducers (width = 1.5 mm; height = 0.3 mm, Precision Measurement Co., Ann Arbor, MI) inserted at the adjacent levels, in the posterior half of the disc space, confirmed by sagittal radiographs [26]. The transducers were configured using C-DAQ (National Instruments, Austin, TX) data acquisition module.

*2.4. Data Interpretation.* Several comparisons were made to evaluate any statistical differences between constructs 1 and 7. The unilateral model (constructs 1, 2, 3, and 4) was evaluated separately from the bilateral model (constructs 1, 5, 6, and 7). Statistical comparisons were completed using a single factor, repeated measures analysis of variance (ANOVA). In all cases to alleviate inhomogeneity of variance, log transforms in the form of $\log_{10}$ (rawdata + 1) were applied to the raw data. Comparisons were made with a probability of type I error, $\alpha =$ 0.05, using Tukey's *post hoc* comparison for equal sample size ($n$ = 5 unilateral and $n$ = 9 bilateral). Intradiscal pressure (IDP) profiles were normalized according to the neutral zone "base pressure" such that the only changes between the base pressure and the pressure at maximum displacement were recorded according to Schmoelz et al. [13]. When the percentage change is discussed, unless otherwise stated, the percentages are calculated through differences in normalized ROM of surgical groups, when normalized to the intact spine motion (100%).

## 3. Results

*3.1. Unilateral Model.* The range of motion (ROM) was determined for each surgical construct of the unilateral injury model (Figure 4), and *post hoc* comparisons were tabulated. Unilateral facetectomy (UF) did not cause any significant destabilization in flexion, extension, or lateral bending but increased rotation significantly (124% of intact; $Q > Q_{.05}$, 7.9 > 4.2). The stabilization of the unilateral injury with a unilateral TRANSITION (UF + UT) resulted in the reduction of motion which was significant in flexion and axial rotation ($F$: 58% of injury, $Q > Q_{.05}$, 4.4 > 4.2; AR: 87% of injury, $Q > Q_{.05}$, 5.7 > 4.2) but insignificant in extension ($E$: 62% of injury) and lateral bending (LB: 65% of injury). The stabilization of the unilateral injury with a bilateral TRANSITION (UF + BF) resulted in the reduction of motion which was significant in flexion, lateral bending, and axial rotation ($F$: 52% of injury, $Q > Q_{.05}$, 5.4 > 4.2; LB: 57% of injury, $Q > Q_{.05}$, 5.1 > 4.2; AR: 85% of injury, $Q > Q_{.05}$, 6.0 > 4.2) but insignificant in extension ($E$: 65% of injury). With respect to intact, the stabilization with a unilateral TRANSITION (UF + UT) resulted in the reduction of motion which was significant in flexion ($F$: 56% of intact, $Q > Q_{.05}$, 4.6 > 4.2) but insignificant in extension ($E$: 72% of intact), lateral bending (LB: 67% of intact), and axial rotation (AR: 108% of intact). With respect to intact, stabilization with a bilateral TRANSITION (UF + BF) resulted in reduction of

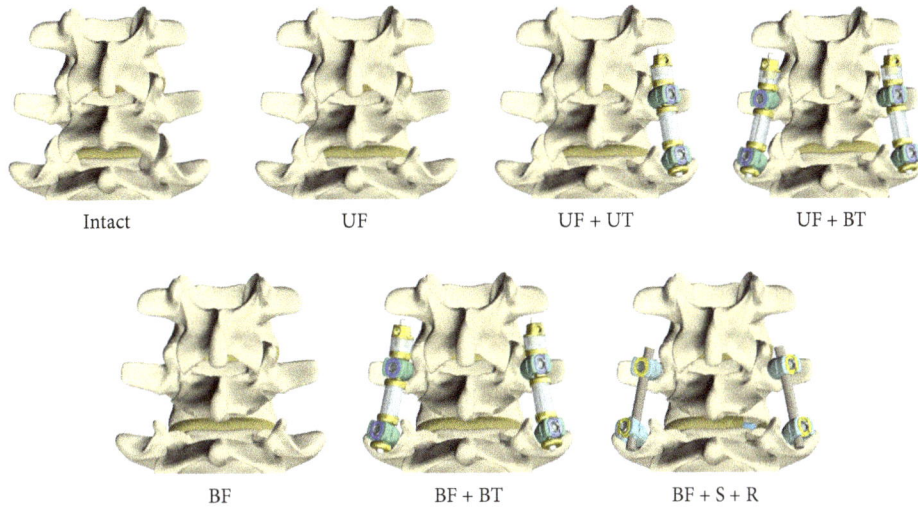

FIGURE 3: Surgical testing sequence. (1) Intact; (2) unilateral facetectomy (UF); (3) UF and unilateral TRANSITION device (UF + UT); (4) UF and bilateral TRANSITION device (UF + BT); (5) bilateral facetectomy (BF); (6) BF and bilateral TRANSITION device (BF + BT); (7) BF and bilateral rigid fixation with interbody spacer (BF + S + R).

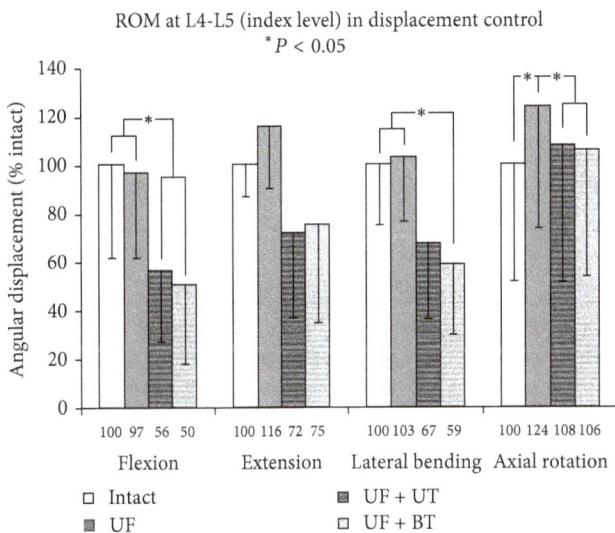

FIGURE 4: Index surgical level results of multidirectional flexibility testing for constructs 1, 2, 3, and 4 (unilateral model).

motion which was significant in flexion and lateral bending ($F$: 50% of intact, $Q > Q_{.05}$, 5.6 > 4.2; LB: 59% of intact, $Q > Q_{.05}$), but insignificant in extension ($E$: 75% of intact) and axial rotation (AR: 106% of intact).

Increased motion due to the UF injury was expected to lead to reduced motions at the immediate adjacent levels in a displacement control protocol (Table 1). This was generally true (especially for L3-L4), but the reduced motions were small and insignificant, except in axial rotation. The stabilization with the PDS system reduced ROM at L4-L5, and, as expected, produced larger ROM at the adjacent levels, which reached significance (with respect to injury) only in lateral bending (L3-L4: UF + UT, 107% of injured, $Q > Q_{.05}$, 4.7 > 4.2; L3-L4: UF + BT, 108% of injured,

$Q > Q_{.05}$, 5.3 > 4.2; L5-S1: UF + UT, 110% of injured $Q > Q_{.05}$, 4.5 > 4.2; L5-S1: UF + BT, 112% of injured, $Q > Q_{.05}$, 5.2 > 4.2) and axial rotation (L3-L4: UF + UT, 104% of injured, $Q > Q_{.05}$, 4.6 > 4.2; L3-L4: UF + BT, 106% of injured, $Q > Q_{.05}$, 5.6 > 4.2). There were few differences between unilateral stabilization (UF + UT) and bilateral stabilization (UF + BT) on adjacent level motion.

With respect to intact, adjacent level motion was significantly increased in lateral bending at L5-S1 by both PDS constructs (UF + UT: 114% of intact, $Q > Q_{.05}$, 6.4 > 4.2; UF + BT: 116% of intact, $Q > Q_{.05}$, 7.1 > 4.2).

Intradiscal pressure measurements of adjacent levels (Table 1) showed greater differences between intact and injury groups than what was seen kinematically. Therefore, even small changes in kinematics may translate to large changes in load-sharing properties. Statistically, in lateral bending, unilateral injury stabilized with a bilateral TRANSITION (UF + BT) was the only construct to produce significantly more adjacent level pressure than the corresponding level of the unilaterally injured spine (L3-L4: 131% of injured, $Q > Q_{.05}$, 7.5 > 4.2) and the intact spine (L3-L4: 127% of intact, $Q > Q_{.05}$, 5.7 > 4.2). With respect to the intact spine, both unilateral TRANSITION (UF + UT) and bilateral TRANSITION (UF + BT) produce significantly more adjacent level pressure in flexion (L5-S1: UF + UT, 161% of intact, $Q > Q_{.05}$, 4.7 > 4.2; L3-L4: UF + BT, 220% of intact, $Q > Q_{.05}$, 5.7 > 4.2; L5-S1: UF + BT, 207% of intact, $Q > Q_{.05}$, 6.7 > 4.2).

*3.2. Bilateral Model.* The range of motion (ROM) was determined for each surgical construct of the bilateral injury model (Figure 5), and *post hoc* comparisons were tabulated. Destabilization after BF increased the ROM in all directions, but this reached statistical significance only in axial rotation (AR: 168% of intact, $Q > Q_{.05}$, 8.0 > 3.9). Again, in flexion and lateral bending, similar statistical trends were seen, revealing that BF + BT provided significant stabilization with respect

TABLE 1: Unilateral model (construct 1, 2, 3, and 4) adjacent level ROM and pressure. Brackets show which construct groups are significant.

| | Intact [1] | UF [2] | UF + UT [3] | UF + BT [4] |
|---|---|---|---|---|
| ROM (% of intact) | | | | |
| Flexion | | | | |
| L3-L4 | Mean 100 (SD 23) [4] | Mean 101 (SD 20) | Mean 109 (SD 24) | Mean 111 (SD 27) [1] |
| L5-S1 | Mean 100 (SD 32) | Mean 98 (SD 26) | Mean 107 (SD 41) | Mean 108 (SD 35) |
| Extension | | | | |
| L3-L4 | Mean 100 (SD 11) | Mean 91 (SD 12) | Mean 101 (SD 16) | Mean 98 (SD 9) |
| L5-S1 | Mean 100 (SD 26) | Mean 118 (SD 28) | Mean 133 (SD 43) | Mean 126 (SD 35) |
| Lateral bending | | | | |
| L3-L4 | Mean 101 (SD 16) | Mean 98 (SD16) [3, 4] | Mean 105 (SD 17) [2] | Mean 106 (SD 20) [2] |
| L5-S1 | Mean 100 (SD 28) [3, 4] | Mean 104 (SD 29) [3, 4] | Mean 114 (SD 31) [1, 2] | Mean 116 (SD 31) [1, 2] |
| Axial rotation | | | | |
| L3-L4 | Mean 100 (SD 31) [2, 3, 4] | Mean 89 (SD 29) [1, 3, 4] | Mean 93 (SD 28) [1, 2] | Mean 94 (SD 28) [1, 2] |
| L5-S1 | Mean 100 (SD 22) | Mean 99 (SD 25) | Mean 110 (SD 27) | Mean 109 (SD 26) |
| Pressure (% of intact) | | | | |
| Flexion | | | | |
| L3-L4 | Mean 100 (SD 42) [4] | Mean 144 (SD 33) | Mean 166 (SD 38) | Mean 220 (SD 76) [1] |
| L5-S1 | Mean 100 (SD 58) [3, 4] | Mean 141 (SD 62) | Mean 161 (SD 53) [1] | Mean 207 (SD 82) [1] |
| Extension | | | | |
| L3-L4 | Mean 100 (SD 21) | Mean 74 (SD 26) | Mean 78 (SD 31) | Mean 99 (SD 24) |
| L5-S1 | Mean 100 (SD 84) | Mean 103 (SD 78) | Mean 120 (SD 89) | Mean 113 (SD 96) |
| Lateral bending | | | | |
| L3-L4 | Mean 100 (SD 54) [4] | Mean 97 (SD 59) [4] | Mean 109 (SD 66) [4] | Mean 127 (SD 76) [1, 2, 3] |
| L5-S1 | Mean 100 (SD 78) | Mean 90 (SD 70) | Mean 90 (SD 65) | Mean 94 (SD 70) |
| Axial rotation | | | | |
| L3-L4 | Mean 100 (SD 44) | Mean 92 (SD 33) | Mean 110 (SD 36) | Mean 81 (SD 21) |
| L5-S1 | Mean 100 (SD 33) | Mean 85 (SD 35) | Mean 100 (SD 45) | Mean 87 (SD 33) |

to intact (F: 44% of intact, $Q > Q_{.05}$, 15.1 > 3.9; LB: 58% of intact, $Q > Q_{.05}$, 7.8 > 3.9) and BF (F: 42% of injury, $Q > Q_{.05}$, 16.2 > 3.9; LB: 56% of injury, $Q > Q_{.05}$, 8.3 > 3.9). In extension, the bilateral injury produced larger motions (119%) when compared to intact.

The trend of index level motion follows the model BF + S + R < BF + BT < BF, where all constructs were statistically different than one another. The stabilization with TRANSITION PDS device reduced the ROM values, which were, in terms of intact, 44% ($Q > Q_{.05}$, 15.1 > 3.9), 62% ($Q > Q_{.05}$, 4.2 > 3.9), 58% ($Q > Q_{.05}$, 7.8 > 3.9), and 125% ($Q < Q_{.05}$, 3.3 < 3.9), while rigid fixation resulted in ROM values of 31% ($Q > Q_{.05}$, 19.5 > 3.9), 29% ($Q > Q_{.05}$, 8.7 > 3.9), 34% ($Q > Q_{.05}$, 13.6 > 3.9), and 77% ($Q < Q_{.05}$, 3.8 < 3.9) in $F$, $E$, LB, AR, respectively. Compared to the BF, and stabilization with TRANSITION PDS device reduced the ROM values, which were, in terms of injury, 42% ($Q > Q_{.05}$, 16.2 > 3.9), 52% ($Q > Q_{.05}$, 5.5 > 3.9), 56% ($Q > Q_{.05}$, 8.3 > 3.9), and 74% ($Q > Q_{.05}$, 4.7 > 3.9), while rigid fixation resulted in ROM values of 30% ($Q > Q_{.05}$, 20.6 > 3.9), 24% ($Q > Q_{.05}$, 10.0 > 3.9), 33% ($Q > Q_{.05}$, 14.1 > 3.9), and 46% ($Q > Q_{.05}$, 11.9 > 3.9) in $F$, $E$, LB, and AR, respectively.

Increased motion due to the BF injury at the index level is expected to lead to reduced motions at the immediate

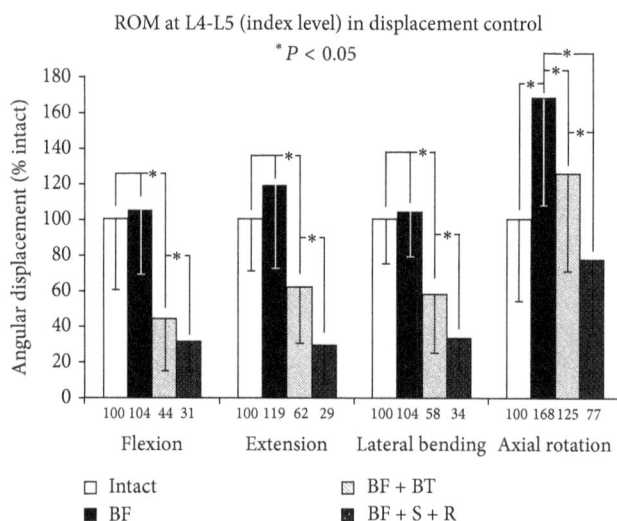

FIGURE 5: Index surgical level results of multidirectional flexibility testing for constructs 1, 4, 5, and 6 (bilateral model).

adjacent levels in a displacement control protocol (Figures 6 and 7). This was generally correct, but the reduced motions

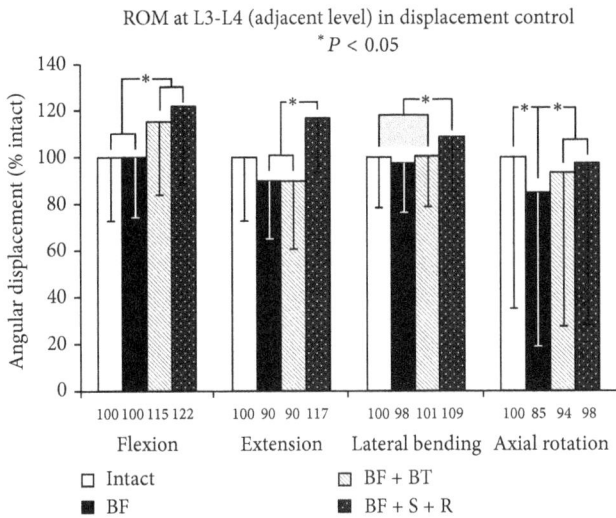

FIGURE 6: Cranial adjacent level results of multidirectional flexibility testing for constructs 1, 5, 6, and 7.

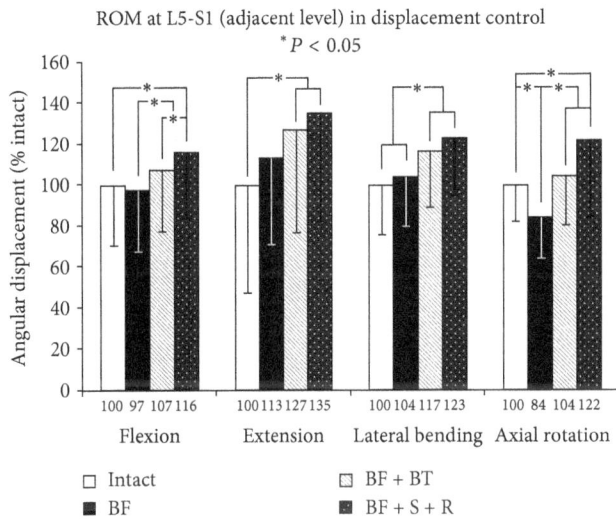

FIGURE 8: Cranial adjacent level intradiscal pressures of multidirectional flexibility testing for constructs 1, 5, 6, and 7.

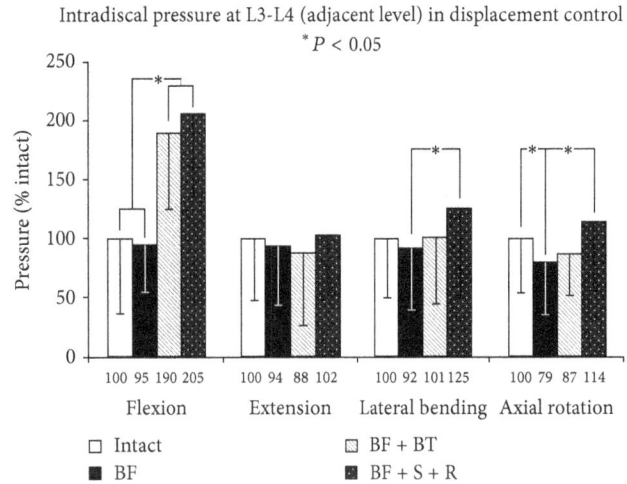

FIGURE 7: Caudal adjacent level results of multidirectional flexibility testing for constructs 1, 5, 6, and 7.

were small and insignificant, except for axial rotation where BF was significantly less than intact ($P < 0.05$) (except for L5-S1). The stabilization at L4-L5 increased the ROM at both the adjacent levels and the trend followed the model BF + S + R ≥ BF + BT ≥ BF for all loading modes at both L3-L4 and L5-S1, indicating the utility of semi-rigid stabilization to offset adjacent level effects caused by rigid instrumentation. Nevertheless, this trend was not always large enough to warrant significance.

The load-bearing effect at the adjacent levels, as measured by intradiscal pressure, (Figures 8 and 9) demonstrated very similar trends to ROM, that is, the IDP was decreased or unchanged after facetectomy at the L4-L5 level and increased with PDS stabilization, with an even greater increase with rigid stabilization. The increase in adjacent segment pressure after rigid stabilization was more pronounced at the cranial

(L3-L4) level than the caudal (L5-S1) level, reaching a significant level, with respect to injury in flexion (209% of injured, $Q > Q_{.05}$, 7.6 > 3.9), lateral bending (136% of injured, $Q > Q_{.05}$, 5.5 > 3.9), and axial rotation (144% of injured, $Q > Q_{.05}$, 5.4 > 3.9) at L3-L4, but only in flexion (192% of injured, $Q > Q_{.05}$, 7.2 > 3.9) at L5-S1. While adjacent segment ROM changes were more pronounced in rotation, the increase in adjacent segment pressure was most noticeable in flexion. At the cranial adjacent level (L3-L4), while the ROM in flexion was increased to 122% after rigid fixation, the corresponding disc pressure was increased to 205% of the intact value. The stabilization with PDS also significantly increased the adjacent segment pressures in flexion, but the increase was smaller (190%) than with rigid fixation ($P < 0.05$). Therefore, though a strong relationship exists between ROM and IDP changes at the adjacent segments, it shows a nonlinear phenomenon in flexion. Additionally, though the use of the particular PDS device reduced the adjacent level pressure, it did not restore it near the intact value in flexion. Whether this would translate into potential alleviation of adjacent level stresses needs to be corroborated with clinical evidence. The remaining ROM and IDP trends are very similar, though higher variation (standard deviations) in the measurement of pressure resulted in very little significance and no significance between BF + BT and BF + S + R in any loading mode.

## 4. Discussion

Conventional rigid fusion in the surgical treatment for chronic low back pain has some negative side effects such as the potential for adjacent segment degeneration and screw loosening. The concept of semi-rigid or dynamic stabilization has evolved to possibly prevent such degeneration, if it is not a function of natural disease progression, mainly through the reduction of stress at the adjacent segments. Soft-stabilization devices were developed to permit load-sharing with the anterior column to accomplish solid fusion and, at the same time, provide a softer posterior implant stiffness.

Intradiscal pressure at L5-S1 (adjacent level) in displacement control
$^*P < 0.05$

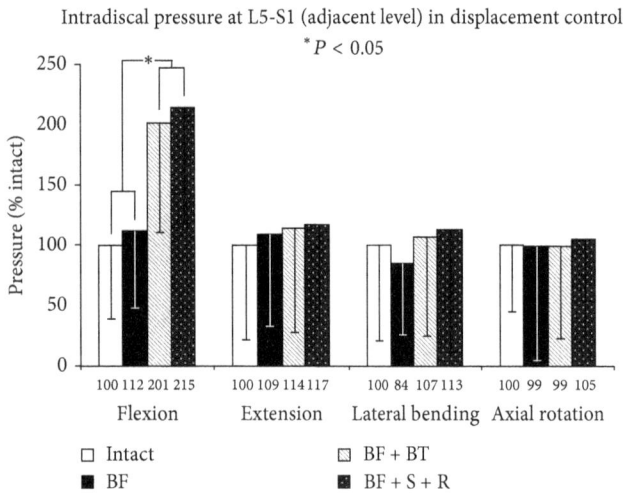

FIGURE 9: Caudal adjacent level intradiscal pressures of multidirectional flexibility testing for constructs 1, 5, 6, and 7.

Consequently, semi-rigid instrumentation is expected to lower screw breakage associated with transmission of forces through posterior instrumentation as opposed to through the anterior column. While there is some disparity between the potential uses of PDS systems (whether they are for reducing adjacent level degeneration or for promoting fusion through load-sharing), the ubiquitousness of such systems cannot be ignored. Their prevalence currently has more to do with dissatisfaction with conventional fusion than a proven efficacy. This study attempts to characterize the biomechanical efficacy of a select system. The clinical efficacy has yet to be determined. It remains to be seen if "soft fusion" can be achieved and if, in the presence of boney ingrowth with weaker mechanical properties, adjacent level effects can be ameliorated.

The purpose of this study was to evaluate the stability of using a posterior dynamic stabilization (PDS) device which differs from conventional PDS devices in two ways: (1) by the addition of both flexion and extension dampening materials; and (2) by the addition of titanium spools (attached to the screw heads) which slide along the PET cord. The primary aim was to compare this device to rigid fixation with pedicle screws and rods. The hypothesis is that the new PDS design will load-share with the surgical level more effectively, therefore minimizing the over-load effect of the adjacent levels compared to the conventional rigid and PDS devices.

Both the PDS and rigid devices produced significant stabilization, but a consistent and significant trend of increased flexibility was observed in all loading modes for BF + BT (TRANSITION) when compared to BF + S + R (rigid). TRANSITION led to ROM values which were, in terms of intact, 44%, 62%, 58%, and 125% in $F$, $E$, LB, and AR, respectively, while rigid fixation resulted in ROM values of 31%, 29%, 34%, and 77%. Gédet et al. reported (load control protocol using a follower load and partial injury including a 25% nucleotomy) that Dynesys system provided stabilization when compared to intact values of ~20%, 40%, 40%, and

100% for $F$, $E$, LB, and AR, respectively [27]. The data from the current study showed a higher ROM baseline because of the facetectomy as opposed to nucleotomy as the injury model but the stabilization effect followed a similar pattern. A separate study, investigating Dynesys in a more severe injury model without axial preload, revealed that PDS restored motion to ~20%, 100%, 27%, and 130% of the intact values [14]. While it is difficult to directly compare the magnitudes reported in the literature sources to the current data, due to differences in test protocols, injury models, and the use of follower loads, the pattern in data is still comparable.

The PDS device used in this study resulted in kinematic and load-sharing trends which appear different when compared to trends observed in conventional PDS designs within the literature [13, 14]. The majority of data in the literature show Dynesys behaves more rigid in flexion, almost comparable to rigid fixation, and less rigid in extension. On the contrary, the data from the present study show a more uniform rigidity in ROM across flexion, extension, and lateral bending. This inference is only based on indirect comparisons. In terms of load-sharing effect, the literature showed Dynesys responds to extension by total load-bearing of the implant, resulting in negative pressure in the disc at the index level [13]. This study cannot comment on load-sharing at the index level because the rigid rod construct was tested with an interbody spacer, precluding the simultaneous use of a pressure transducer. Comparisons of this construct with the PDS construct would not have been possible; therefore, both were excluded. Nevertheless, the adjacent level effects consistently reveal that the hypermobility of rigid fixation was reduced via TRANSITION. Moreover, the amount of reduction was uniform across the loading modes, not favoring extension over flexion. In rotation, more motion was allowed and not limited through the bumper mechanism. Yet, rotation itself is much less of a problem in a degenerated lumbar spine and is infrequently diagnosed as a cause of pain.

In a finite element study by Schmidt et al., the authors predicted the performance of PDS devices in different loading modes, as a function of polymer properties [28]. The material properties of posterior instrumentation were input in the analysis in terms of the bending stiffness and axial stiffness, axial stiffness referring to purely compressing the polymer spacer and bending stiffness similar to folding the spacer. The difference in bending stiffness between a PCU spacer and rigid rod is expected to be larger than their difference in axial stiffness. In that study, the authors concluded that, in each loading mode, the resulting ROM of an L4-L5 segment with posterior instrumentation involved a combination of both bending and axial stiffness. However, in flexion-extension, the relationship was mostly determined through axial stiffness, while in lateral bending and axial rotation, both stiffness parameters played a role. Extrapolating these results to PDS findings helps explain the relative rigidity of PDS devices in flexion-extension, which, despite a polymer spacer, are significantly stabilized with respect to intact values. Moreover, their findings predict that materials with high bending flexibility, such as PCU, would respond with increased motion in lateral bending and axial rotation. These conclusions are consistent with the results reported here as well as other studies. In this study, the extra polymeric material added through the spacer and bumper can be expected to add to the overall flexibility of conventional PDS devices, especially in lateral bending and axial rotation.

The PDS test device reduced adjacent level hypermobility caused by rigid fixation. The trend of adjacent level motions followed the model $BF + S + R \geq BF + BT \geq BF$ for all loading modes at both L3-L4 and L5-S1, indicating the utility of semi-rigid stabilization to offset adjacent level effects. While this trend is encouraging to alleviate adjacent level stresses, its clinical relevance needs to be proven. The question "How much is off-loading ideal?" remains to be answered. Nevertheless, the new PDS device produced significantly smaller motions than rigid fixation at the adjacent levels, in flexion (only at L5-S1), extension (only at L3-L4), and lateral bending (only at L3-L4).

Intradiscal pressure measurements at the adjacent level reflected the same trends as the ROM, but, in flexion, the relationship between ROM and IDP was nonlinear. For example, a 22% increase in L3-L4 level motion caused by L4-L5 rigid fixation, resulted in 105% increase in the IDP value. Moreover, the stabilization with PDS device (BF + BT) was not able to restore these large pressure that increases to near the intact value. If adjacent level disease is indeed related to a physiological imbalance in load-sharing and kinematics of segments juxtaposed to the fusion site, then the role of motion versus pressure on the rate of disease progression needs to be determined. Since these factors are nonlinearly related, restricting the motion may not be sufficient at buffering the load-sharing effects on the adjacent level.

There were certain limitations in this study. One objective was to relate the biomechanical differences observed between this study and those found on the widely studied conventional device, Dynesys. The ideal way to evaluate the difference was to compare TRANSITION versus Dynesys directly. In the current study, this comparison was indirect from the literature data. The reason behind this was that testing TRANSITION and Dynesys on the same specimen was not possible because the pedicle screws are different in the two systems, and the reinsertion of the pedicle screws in the same specimens introduces unacceptable errors because of loosening at the screw-bone interface. Removing the bumper alone from the TRANSITION does not make it comparable to Dynesys. The second limitation of this study was the bilateral facetectomy injury model, which may not be the most common scenario of a decompression clinically. However, facetectomy produced considerable instability, possibly more than what can be achieved by nucleotomy alone. The injury model was chosen because of the benefit of having a greater degree of instability (or worst-case scenario). Thirdly, testing pedicle screws and rods without an interbody device would have provided some information in the comparison of rigid rods and TRANSITION. Nevertheless, the authors were predominately interested in seeing the maximum change in the rigidity between interbody fusion with internal fixation and semi-rigid posterolateral fusion. Lastly, there is a certain amount of error introduced via suboptimal device placement which can occur via difficulty in the anatomy, irregular curvatures, or even screw placement. The PDS device considered made use of individually sized PCU spacers which were trialed to appropriate length. The implants are also pre-assembled with a constant tension of 220 N, so there should never be a case where one side of the disc space is artificially tensioned more than the other. Therefore, device placement was not separately considered in the analysis of variance.

## 5. Conclusion

The semi-rigid fixation/dynamic stabilization device investigated in this study, which utilized posteriorly placed flexion and extension dampening materials, was able to reduce the motion ($P < 0.05$) at the surgical level in all modes, and the reduction in motion was significantly less in comparison to rigid internal fixation. The adjacent levels were off-loaded by the dynamic stabilization device, in terms of both motion and intradiscal pressure, though the effect was often insignificant. The new dynamic device provides more uniform reduction of motion at the surgical level in all directions, especially in flexion, as well as permits more uniform load-sharing when compared to conventional systems like Dynesys. The disc, which is a uniform load-bearing structure of homogeneous material properties, may, likewise, benefit from a device with uniform rigidity.

## Acknowledgments

The authors would like to thank Kurt Faulhaber for his contribution to the artwork in Figure 3. The authors acknowledge the funding and materials provided by Globus Medical, Inc., specifically for their Research Department.

## References

[1] S. H. Davne and D. L. Myers, "Complications of lumbar spinal fusion with transpedicular instrumentation," *Spine*, vol. 17, supplement 6, pp. S184–S189, 1992.

[2] S. I. Esses and D. A. Bednar, "The spinal pedicle screw: techniques and systems," *Orthopaedic Review*, vol. 18, no. 6, pp. 676–682, 1989.

[3] P. C. Jutte and R. M. Castelein, "Complications of pedicle screws in lumbar and lumbosacral fusions in 105 consecutive primary operations," *European Spine Journal*, vol. 11, no. 6, pp. 594–598, 2002.

[4] J. E. Lonstein, F. Denis, J. H. Perra, M. R. Pinto, M. D. Smith, and R. B. Winter, "Complications associated with pedicle screws," *Journal of Bone and Joint Surgery A*, vol. 81, no. 11, pp. 1519–1528, 1999.

[5] H. Pihlajamäki, P. Myllynen, and O. Böstman, "Complications of transpedicular lumbosacral fixation for non-traumatic disorders," *Journal of Bone and Joint Surgery B*, vol. 79, no. 2, pp. 183–189, 1997.

[6] A. D. Steffee and J. W. Brantigan, "The variable screw placement spinal fixation system: report of a prospective study of 250 patients enrolled in Food and Drug Administration clinical trials," *Spine*, vol. 18, no. 9, pp. 1160–1172, 1993.

[7] J. L. West III, J. W. Ogilvie, and D. S. Bradford, "Complications of the variable screw plate pedicle screw fixation," *Spine*, vol. 16, no. 5, pp. 576–579, 1991.

[8] H. Daniaux, P. Seykora, A. Genelin, T. Lang, and A. Kathrein, "Application of posterior plating and modifications in thoracolumbar spine injuries: indication, techniques, and results," *Spine*, vol. 16, supplement 3, pp. S125–S133, 1991.

[9] K. R. Gurr and P. C. McAfee, "Cotrel-Dubousset Instrumentation in adults. A preliminary report," *Spine*, vol. 13, no. 5, pp. 510–520, 1988.

[10] H. J. Hehne, K. Zielke, and H. Bohm, "Polysegmental lumbar osteotomies and transpedicled fixation for correction of long-curved kyphotic deformities in ankylosing spondylitis: report on 177 cases," *Clinical Orthopaedics and Related Research*, vol. 258, pp. 49–55, 1990.

[11] P. Enker and A. D. Steffee, "Interbody fusion and instrumentation," *Clinical Orthopaedics and Related Research*, no. 300, pp. 90–101, 1994.

[12] B. Cakir, C. Carazzo, R. Schmidt, T. Mattes, H. Reichel, and W. Käfer, "Adjacent segment mobility after rigid and semirigid instrumentation of the lumbar spine," *Spine*, vol. 34, no. 12, pp. 1287–1291, 2009.

[13] W. Schmoelz, J. F. Huber, T. Nydegger, L. Claes, and H. J. Wilke, "Influence of a dynamic stabilisation system on load bearing of a bridged disc: an in vitro study of intradiscal pressure," *European Spine Journal*, vol. 15, no. 8, pp. 1276–1285, 2006.

[14] W. Schmoelz, J. F. Huber, T. Nydegger, Dipl-Ing, L. Claes, and H. J. Wilke, "Dynamic stabilization of the lumbar spine and its effects on adjacent segments: an in vitro experiment," *Journal of Spinal Disorders and Techniques*, vol. 16, no. 4, pp. 418–423, 2003.

[15] B. C. Cheng, J. Gordon, J. Cheng, and W. C. Welch, "Immediate biomechanical effects of lumbar posterior dynamic stabilization above a circumferential fusion," *Spine*, vol. 32, no. 23, pp. 2551–2557, 2007.

[16] J. Beastall, E. Karadimas, M. Siddiqui et al., "The dynesys lumbar spinal stabilization system: a preliminary report on positional magnetic resonance imaging findings," *Spine*, vol. 32, no. 6, pp. 685–690, 2007.

[17] K. S. Delank, E. Gercek, S. Kuhn et al., "How does spinal canal decompression and dorsal stabilization affect segmental mobility? A biomechanical study," *Archives of Orthopaedic and Trauma Surgery*, vol. 130, no. 2, pp. 285–292, 2010.

[18] R. C. Huang, T. M. Wright, M. M. Panjabi, and J. D. Lipman, "Biomechanics of nonfusion implants," *Orthopedic Clinics of North America*, vol. 36, no. 3, pp. 271–280, 2005.

[19] S. Schaeren, I. Broger, and B. Jeanneret, "Minimum four-year follow-up of spinal stenosis with degenerative spondylolisthesis treated with decompression and dynamic stabilization," *Spine*, vol. 33, no. 18, pp. E636–E642, 2008.

[20] K. J. Schnake, S. Schaeren, and B. Jeanneret, "Dynamic stabilization in addition to decompression for lumbar spinal stenosis with degenerative spondylolisthesis," *Spine*, vol. 31, no. 4, pp. 442–449, 2006.

[21] A. Rohlmann, N. K. Burra, T. Zander, and G. Bergmann, "Comparison of the effects of bilateral posterior dynamic and rigid fixation devices on the loads in the lumbar spine: a finite element analysis," *European Spine Journal*, vol. 16, no. 8, pp. 1223–1231, 2007.

[22] D. K. Sengupta and H. N. Herkowitz, "Degenerative spondylolisthesis: review of current trends and controversies," *Spine*, vol. 30, supplement 6, pp. S71–S81, 2005.

[23] D. K. Sengupta and R. C. Mulholland, "Fulcrum assisted soft stabilization system: a new concept in the surgical treatment of degenerative low back pain," *Spine*, vol. 30, no. 9, pp. 1019–1030, 2005.

[24] M. M. Panjabi, "Hybrid multidirectional test method to evaluate spinal adjacent-level effects," *Clinical Biomechanics*, vol. 22, no. 3, pp. 257–265, 2007.

[25] V. K. Goel, M. M. Panjabi, A. G. Patwardhan, A. P. Dooris, and H. Serhan, "Test protocols for evaluation of spinal implants," *Journal of Bone and Joint Surgery A*, vol. 88, supplement 2, pp. 103–109, 2006.

[26] P. A. Cripton, G. A. Dumas, and L. P. Nolte, "A minimally disruptive technique for measuring intervertebral disc pressure in vitro: application to the cervical spine," *Journal of Biomechanics*, vol. 34, no. 4, pp. 545–549, 2001.

[27] P. Gédet, D. Haschtmann, P. A. Thistlethwaite, and S. J. Ferguson, "Comparative biomechanical investigation of a modular dynamic lumbar stabilization system and the dynesys system," *European Spine Journal*, vol. 18, no. 10, pp. 1504–1511, 2009.

[28] H. Schmidt, F. Heuer, and H. J. Wilke, "Which axial and bending stiffnesses of posterior implants are required to design a flexible lumbar stabilization system?" *Journal of Biomechanics*, vol. 42, no. 1, pp. 48–54, 2009.

# 24

# Comparison of Conventional Polyethylene Wear and Signs of Cup Failure in Two Similar Total Hip Designs

**Thomas B. Pace,**[1,2] **Kevin C. Keith,**[3] **Estefania Alvarez,**[3]
**Rebecca G. Snider,**[1] **Stephanie L. Tanner,**[1] **and John D. DesJardins**[3]

[1] *Department of Orthopaedics, Greenville Health System, Greenville, SC 29605, USA*
[2] *University of South Carolina SOM, Greenville Health System, P.O. Box 27114, Greenville, SC 29616, USA*
[3] *Department of Bioengineering, Clemson University, Clemson, SC 29634, USA*

Correspondence should be addressed to Thomas B. Pace; tpacemd@aol.com

Academic Editor: Christian Bach

Multiple factors have been identified as contributing to polyethylene wear and debris generation of the acetabular lining. Polyethylene wear is the primary limiting factor in the functional behavior and consequent longevity of a total hip arthroplasty (THA). This retrospective study reviewed the clinical and radiographic data of 77 consecutive THAs comparing in vivo polyethylene wear of two similar acetabular cup liners. Minimum follow-up was 7 years (range 7–15). The incidence of measurable wear in a group of machined liners sterilized with ethylene oxide and composed of GUR 1050 stock resin was significantly higher (61%) than the compression-molded, GUR 1020, $O_2$-free gamma irradiation sterilized group (24%) ($P = 0.0004$). Clinically, at a 9-year average followup, both groups had comparable HHS scores and incidence of thigh or groin pain, though the machined group had an increased incidence of osteolysis and annual linear wear rate.

## 1. Introduction

Ultra high molecular weight polyethylene (UHMWPE) is currently the most widely used polymer for joint replacement prosthesis. Polyethylene mm head were used in all cases. The ceramicwear is the primary limiting factor in the functional behavior and consequent longevity of a total hip arthroplasty (THA). Polyethylene debris has been often linked to the development of osteolysis with subsequent loss of bone stock and implant fixation [1]. Linear wear rate of polyethylene is closely associated with osteolysis following THA, more so than patient weight, femoral head material, or implant design and offset. Acetabular cup loosening due to polyethylene wear is the most frequent reason for long-term revision in THAs, especially in young and active patients [2, 3].

Multiple factors have been identified as contributing to polyethylene wear and debris generation of acetabular lining. These variables include conformity of the articulating surface, polyethylene thickness, femoral head diameter, polyethylene locking mechanism, polyethylene additives [4], sterilization technique [5, 6], manufacturing method [4, 7], and surgical implantation technique [8]. Linear penetration of the femoral head into the polyethylene occurs through creep and wear. Creep occurs at a rate of approximately 0.18–0.2 mm/year and subsides after approximately the first 24 months. The remaining penetration is considered wear from multifactorial sources and typically occurs at reported rates of 0.05–0.18 mm/year for conventional polyethylene in THA, with compression molding having comparatively less wear [9–11]. This study compares linear wear rate of two similar total hip systems that are able to reduce the variables of interest to polyethylene resin, sterilization technique, and manufacturing methods.

The acetabular polyethylene liners of one of the total hip systems were machine fabricated using a bar extrusion technique from GUR 1050 stock resin, before being sterilized with ethylene oxide (EtO). This group will henceforth be referred to as Group 1. The other hip design uses compression molded polyethylene, from GUR 1020, resin and was sterilized using $O_2$-free gamma irradiation. This grouping of polyethylene liners will henceforth be referred to as Group 2. The two hip systems had similar polyethylene locking mechanisms, articulating head surfaces, and articulating head geometry.

In the past decade, there has been significant progress in the development of a more wear and oxidation resistant UHMWPE alternative such as the highly cross-linked UHMWPE. Initial lab and clinical studies have shown that cross-linked polyethylene may be more wear resistant than non cross-linked alternatives [12]. The focus of this study, however, compares two conventional (non highly cross-linked GUR 1050 and 1020) polyethylene liners commonly used at the time the arthroplasties were performed. The goal of this study was to clinically and radiographically compare these two similar acetabular cup liners which differ primarily in machine versus molded with respect to their linear polyethylene wear. There is no associated conflict of interests for any author listed for this study.

## 2. Materials and Methods

Institutional Review Board approval was granted for this study. Criteria for this study included THA cases with at least 7-year followup, with standard polyethylene (with a minimum of 7 mm thickness), with the same diameter femoral heads 28 mm Alumina Ceramic (Al2O3) or Cobalt Chrome (CoCr), and one of two press fit titanium acetabular cups. The CoCr femoral heads of both groups were from the same manufacturer. Seventy-seven THAs, performed by the same surgeon that occurred between February 1996 and August 2003, with these criteria were retrospectively reviewed. Clinical and radiographic data-collected including presurgery diagnosis, patient demographics, pre- and post-surgery Harris Hip Scores (HHS), incidence and severity of polywear, osteolysis, and patient reporting thigh and/or groin pain. Refer to Table 1 for demographical information.

This study compares clinical and radiographic assessment of polyethylene wear of two different acetabular cup liners, Group 1 (Smith and Nephew, Memphis, TN, USA) and Group 2 (Zimmer, formerly Sulzermedica, Warsaw, IN, USA). Each liner studied articulates with either a cobalt chrome femoral head (Zimmer, formerly Sulzermedica, Warsaw, IN, USA) or a ceramic femoral head (Alumina) (CeramTec, Germany) and has effective and similar locking mechanisms within the acetabular cup to minimize backside wear.

All surgeries were performed using a posterolateral approach. Thirty-one press fit Smith and Nephew Reflection acetabular cups (Group 1) and 46 press fit Zimmer Intraop acetabular cups (Group 2) were implanted. Cup screws were used based on surgical indication for cup fixation and stability. The natural hip press fit stem and a corresponding CoCr or Al2O3 28 mm head were used in all cases. The ceramic heads were used primarily in younger male patients with physically demanding jobs. Postoperative rehabilitation included patients being weight-bearing as tolerated with walker support for 3–6 weeks as needed. Venous thrombosis event (VTE) prophylaxis was based on an individual patient VTE risk assessment. For the standard at risk patient included oral warfarin 5 mg the night of surgery and continued daily

TABLE 1: Patient demographical information for the different manufactured polyethylene groups with different material pairings.

| | Group 1 | Group 2 | |
| | CoCr | CoCr | $Al_2O_3$ |
|---|---|---|---|
| Total cases | **31** | **15** | **31** |
| Males | 13 | 4 | 17 |
| Females | 18 | 11 | 14 |
| Median age* (range) | 66 (46–86) | 65 (38–81) | 57 (42–77) |
| Diagnosis | | | |
| Osteoarthritis | 31 | 15 | 27 |
| AVN** | 0 | 0 | 2 |
| Other*** | 0 | 0 | 2 |

* Age at time of surgery.
** AVN: avascular necrosis.
*** Dysplasia and rheumatoid arthritis.

until the ProTime (prothrombin time) reached 15 seconds or the INR (international normalized ratio) reached 1.2–2. Oral warfarin 2 mg was then given daily for a 4-week protocol of 2 mg per day mini-fixed dose oral warfarin regimen. For the patient without higher VTE or bleeding risk assessment, once the hospital ProTime reached 15 seconds or INR (International Normalized Ratio) levels reached 1.2–2.0, post discharge monitoring was not done unless signs or symptoms of bleeding occurred. For higher risk VTE patients, higher dose monitored oral warfarin was used (ProTime of 18–20 seconds or INR range 2.0–2.5). All patients were counseled to avoid dislocation-prone lower extremity positioning of surgical leg internal rotation and adduction and maintain less than 90 hip flexion for 12 weeks following surgery.

Radiographic assessment of osteolysis was performed in each case at the most recent annual clinical follow up-period and classified based on Gruen et al.'s and DeLee and Charnley's classification for the femoral stem and acetabulum respectively [13, 14].

Linear polywear rate and cup abduction/inclination angle were measured on digital radiographs using femoral head size to standardize magnification. Linear wear was assessed with a resolution of 0.1 mm using techniques described and validated by Griffith et al. and Livermore et al. [15, 16]. Linear polyethylene wear was calculated from the most recent AP pelvis X-ray by subtracting the shortest distance from the femoral head to the (superior) inner cup from the original polyethylene thickness. In each case, this calculated difference was adjusted for X-ray magnification using the 28 mm femoral head as a reference. The magnification range varied from 14% 26%. Limitations of this technique do not allow for assessment of volumetric wear. Patients with ≤1 mm of head penetration on AP X-rays were categorized as having progressing creep only and not listed as measurable polyethylene wear. As all patients had a minimum of 7-year follow-up, the polyethylene deformation secondary to creep was felt to be non-contributory after the first two-year wear in period and equal in both study groups. The data was analyzed using Fishers exact probability test ($\alpha = 0.05$).

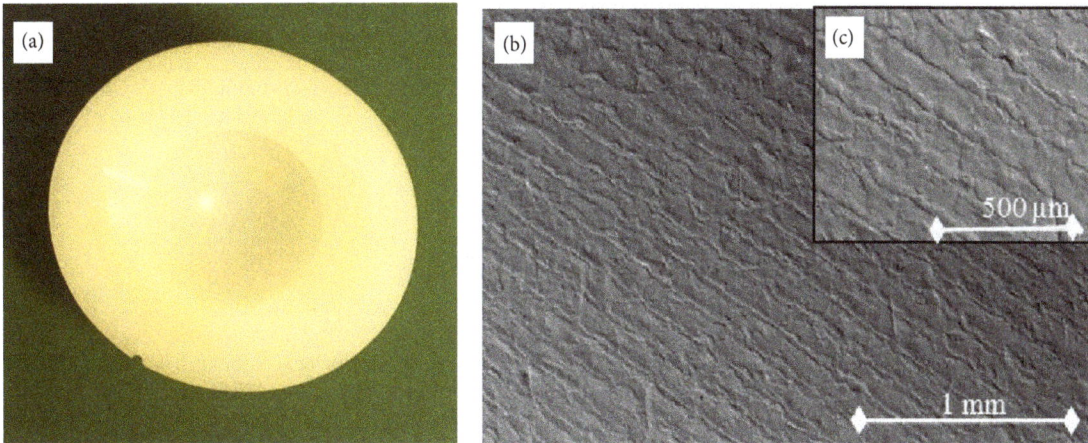

FIGURE 1: (a) The machined polyethylene acetabular cup retrieved at 5.5 years in this study paired with a cobalt chrome head. A photomicrograph of the nonarticulating surface of the retrieved conventional UHMWPE machined liner (b) 40x and (c) 95x (backscattered Topographical mode).

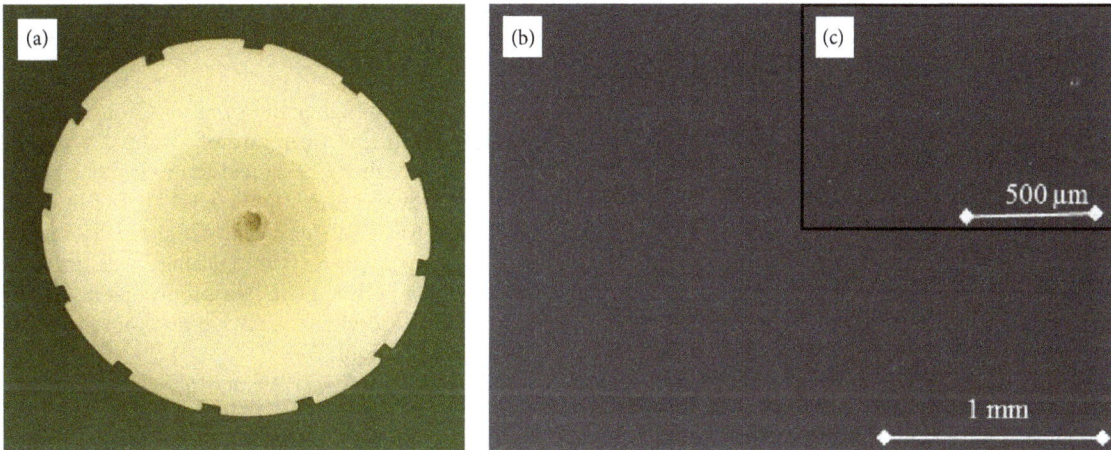

FIGURE 2: (a) The retrieved compression-molded polyethylene acetabular cup retrieved at 7.2 years (in) this study paired with a cobalt chrome femoral head. A photomicrograph of the non-articulating surface of the retrieved UHMWPE compression molded (b) 40x and (c) 95x (backscattered topographical mode).

TABLE 2: Comparison of the characteristics of the acetabular polyethylene.

| | Group 1 | Group 2 |
|---|---|---|
| Stock resin | GUR 1050 | GUR 1020 |
| Manufacturing process | Ram extrusion, final geometry machined | Compression molding |
| Sterilization | Ethylene oxide | Gamma irradiation, oxygen-free environment |
| Polyethylene thickness | Range: 7.0–15.5 mm | Range: 7.0–14.5 mm |

Both titanium cup designs incorporated secure polyethylene inserts with locking mechanisms that significantly restrict both rotational and pistoning motions to minimize backside wear potential. Both cups incorporate hemispherical geometry with roughened outer surfaces for acetabular bone ingrowth. All polyethylene liners were a minimum of 7 mm actual thickness with ranges from 7 to 15.5 mm depending on the size of the individual patient's acetabulum and subsequent cup diameter. The acetabular cups liners differ primarily with respect to stock resin, manufacturing methods, and sterilization techniques (Table 2). Figure 1 shows a photograph of an explanted machined polyethylene and corresponding scanning electron microscope (SEM) image. Figure 2 shows a photograph of an explanted compression molded polyethylene and corresponding SEM.

SEM images were taken using a variable pressure Hitachi 3400 SEM at 20 keV accelerating potential capability at magnification of 40x and 95x. It is equipped with Phillips Secondary Electron Detector 6765/50 complimented by a Hitachis Backscattered Electron.

TABLE 3: Incidence and polyethylene wear rates for both groups of material pairings used in this study.

| | Group 1 (CoCr heads) | Group 2 (CoCr heads) | Group 2 ($Al_2O_3$ heads) |
|---|---|---|---|
| Incidence of >1 mm polywear | 19/31 | 1/15 | 10/31 |
| Average wear rate (range) | 0.24 mm/year (0.11–0.88) | 0.09 mm/year (0.09) | 0.13 mm/year (0.08–0.25) |

TABLE 4: Clinical results for hip scores and pain for both groups material pairings used in this study.

| | Group 1 (CoCr heads) | Group 2 (CoCr heads) | Group 2 ($Al_2O_3$ heads) |
|---|---|---|---|
| Total | 31 | 15 | 31 |
| Preoperation HHS Average (range) | 67 (58–87) | 68 (58–87) | 67 (58–81) |
| Last clinical HHS Average (range) | 99.1 (95–100) | 98.9 (93–100) | 99.5 (95–100) |
| Thigh pain | 2 | 1 | 0 |
| Groin pain | 1 | 0 | 2 |

TABLE 5: Radiographic findings for each acetabular liner articulating against Same CoCr bearing counterface.

| | Group 1 (CoCr heads) | Group 2 (CoCr heads) | P values |
|---|---|---|---|
| Total | 31 | 15 | |
| Calcar erosion | 5 | 1 | 0.65 |
| Osteolysis | 4 | 0 | 0.29 |
| Cup | 1 | 0 | 1 |
| Stem | 3 | 0 | 0.54 |

TABLE 6: Radiographic results for each acetabular liner articulating against different femoral head material.

| | Group 1 (CoCr heads) | Group 2 ($Al_2O_3$ heads) | P values |
|---|---|---|---|
| Total | 31 | 31 | |
| Calcar erosion | 5 | 0 | 0.05 |
| Osteolysis | 4 | 0 | 0.11 |
| Cup | 1 | 0 | 1 |
| Stem | 3 | 0 | 0.24 |

The effect of the manufacturing procedure on the surface of the UHMWPE liners (machined and compression molded) was evaluated using noncontact profilometry using a WYKO NT2000 profilometer (Veeco Corp., Tucson, AZ, USA). Surface characterization was performed after retrieval at a nominal magnification of 25x (field of view 736 × 480 nm, ± 0.1 nm). To best capture the manufactured original surface, Nonarticulating surfaces were characterized for roughness measures arithmetic surface roughness (Ra), average maximum profile peak height (Rpm), and average maximum profile valley height (Rvm). Five measurements were taken on the nonarticulating surface of each polyethylene liner in a linear fashion in order to fully quantify and characterize the component and ensure reliable and repeatable estimate of nonarticulating surface roughness. Statistical analysis (Student's $t$-test with $\alpha = 0.05$) was performed to evaluate whether there was a significant difference between machined and compression molded nonarticulating liner surface roughness.

In order to characterize the surface morphology of the UHMWPE liners, both optical microscopy and SEM analysis were performed on the nonarticulating surface of the UHMWPE liners. The images were taken choosing positions along the Nonarticulating surface using a stereomicroscope (model K400P, Motic Inc., Xiamen, China) with lenses providing 6x to 50x magnification with controlled fluorescent ring illumination and a color digital camera (model infinity 2-1C, Lumenera Corp., Ottawa, ON, Canada).

## 3. Results

With the numbers in this study, no significant difference was found in patient demographics between the two groups. The incidence of measurable wear in the Group 1 (61.3%) was significantly higher than that of Group 2 (23.9%) ($P = 0.0004$). The linear wear rate of Group 1 was additionally significantly higher (2.7 times) than Group 2 polyethylene's with CoCr head group ($P = 0.0014$). The linear wear rate of Group 1 was also significantly higher (1.8 times) than the $Al_2O_3$ Group 2 ($P = 0.0028$). There was no difference in the wear rate between the two subgroups in Group 2 when comparing those with CoCr heads and those with $Al_2O_3$ ($P = 0.071$) (refer to Table 3).

Clinically, at a 9-year average follow-up, both groups were doing equally well with HHS scores and reported thigh or groin pain incidences of 9.7% for the machined polyethylene group and 6.5% in the compression molded group ($P$ values > 0.05) (refer to Table 4). The revision rate for both groups was the same, with one case in each group for recurrent dislocation. While there were no revisions for osteolysis, the incidence of osteolysis was higher in Group 1 (12.9% machined versus 0% compression molded). When assessing focal calcar erosion of ±1 cm, the incidence was higher in Group 1 (16%) than in Group 2 (2%). (refer to Table 5). Typical representative radiographs from each group are presented in Figure 3. Tables 5 and 6 present the radiographic differences in the machined polyethylene and compression molded polyethylene groups.

Nakahara et al. have shown that acetabular cups implanted with >45° abduction have higher polyethylene wear rates than cups implanted with 45° or less [8]. When assessing the cup abduction/inclination (≥45°) as a variable affecting linear wear in each group, there was not a significant difference ($P = 0.777$).

The complications in each group were comparable and no statistical difference was found in the complications in either group (refer to Table 7).

Figure 4 shows surface profiles of the retrieved Group 1 GUR 1050 UHMWPE liner 5.5 years post implantation and

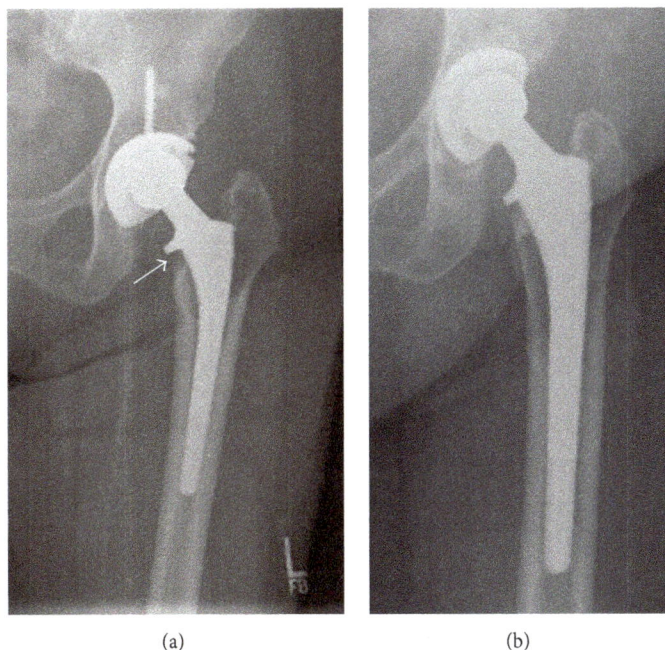

FIGURE 3: (a) AP radiograph of THA with machined polyethylene after 8 years of implantation. The measured polywear was of 4 mm. There is focal stem osteolysis and calcar erosion (arrow). (b) AP radiograph of THA with compression-molded polyethylene after 11 years of implantation. The measured polywear was of 2 mm. There were no significant signs of osteolysis.

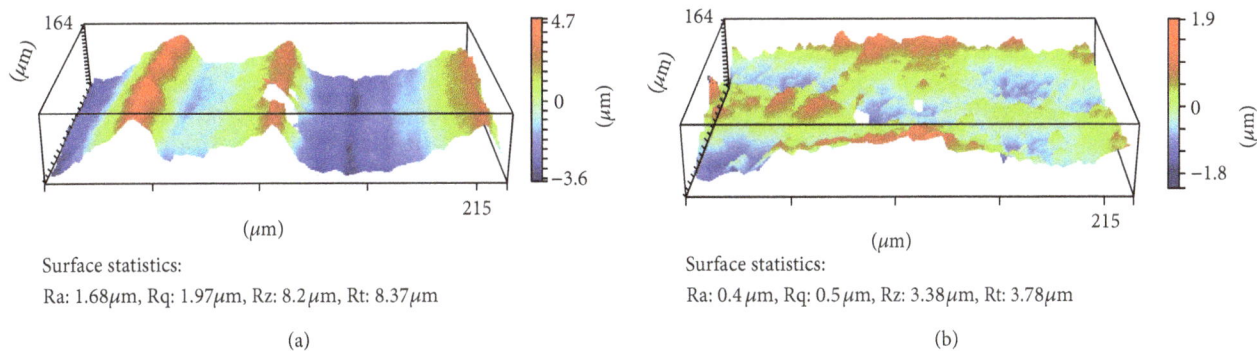

Surface statistics:
Ra: 1.68 $\mu$m, Rq: 1.97 $\mu$m, Rz: 8.2 $\mu$m, Rt: 8.37 $\mu$m

(a)

Surface statistics:
Ra: 0.4 $\mu$m, Rq: 0.5 $\mu$m, Rz: 3.38 $\mu$m, Rt: 3.78 $\mu$m

(b)

FIGURE 4: (a) Nonarticulating surface profile for machined polyethylene. The machining marks are represented by the peaks and valleys illustrated by the color scale. (25x) (b) Nonarticulating surface profile of retrieved compression-molded polyethylene, which has no significant changes in its topography.

Group 2 GUR 1020 UHMWPE liner 7.2 years post implantation. The 3D representative profile shows the machining and compression molded marks as a result of the manufacturing process.

## 4. Discussion

This study examines the clinical polyethylene wear characteristics of two independent total hip systems. Upon comparison, significant statistical differences are found between the polyethylene wear seen within the two systems.

The polyethylene of Group 1, made of GUR 1050 resin, sterilized through the use of ethylene oxide, was manufactured by ram extrusion and machining. Group 2 polyethylene is compression-molded from GUR 1020 resin and is sterilized by means of gamma irradiation in an oxygen free-environment. In vitro studies on tibial inserts for knee arthroplasties have shown that compression molded and oxygen free sterilization reports less wear than machined tibial inserts for total knee arthroplasties [11, 17, 18]. Yet little knowledge is available on the performance of THAs with regard to these same variables.

The polyethylene of Group 2 was sterilized via oxygen-free gamma irradiation. Gamma irradiation in the presence of $O_2$ has shown to increase polyethylene oxidation due to free radical generation and subsequent oxidation, consequently lowering mechanical properties, leading to rapid polyethylene wear. However, gamma irradiation performed in an oxygen free environment has been shown to negate the

TABLE 7: Reported clinical complications for the seventy-seven THR considered in this study.

|  | Group 1 | Group 2 | |
|  | (CoCr heads) | (CoCr heads) | (Al₂O₃ heads) |
| --- | --- | --- | --- |
| Total | 31 | 15 | 31 |
| Total complications | 2 | 3 | 3 |
| Dislocation | 1 | 2 | 2 |
| Infection | 0 | 1 | 0 |
| Symptomatic DVT & PE | 0 | 0 | 0 |
| Major/minor bleeding | 0 | 0 | 0 |
| Heterotopic ossification | 1 (grade 2) | 0 | 1 |
| Revisions | 1 (recurrent dislocation) | 1 (recurrent dislocation) | 0 |

oxidative effects of irradiation [5]. Faris et al. demonstrated that annual linear wear rate significantly increased in a population of gamma irradiated liners in air when compared with a population of similar gamma irradiated hips in an oxygen free vacuum [5].

Each liner was also formed from two different polyethylene resins, GUR 1050 for Group 1 and GUR 1020 for Group 2. The lone difference between the two resins is the average molecular weight, which is around $3.5 \times 10^6$ g/mol for GUR 1020 and $5.5 \times 10^6$ for GUR 1050. Past studies have shown that the higher molecular weight provides better abrasive wear resistance, but only slightly. Kurtz [4] argued that both the impact strength and the wear resistance of each resin increased nonlinearly with increasing intrinsic viscosity of the resin, which is a function of average molecular weight. However, Tipper et al. performed an in vitro cyclic wear test between GUR 1020 and 1050 and demonstrated that while GUR 1050 did have greater wear resistance, it was not considered statistically important [19].

Previous authors have compared the bearing material effect on CoCr versus Al₂O₃ with respect to polyethylene clinical wear rate in THAs [19]. Clinically, the linear wear rate for polyethylene paired with CoCr heads ranges between 0.1 and 0.3 mm/year whereas when compared with Al₂O₃ the range is 0.03–0.15 mm/year [20, 21]. While not statistically significant, there was a trend towards more wear in Group 2 with Al₂O₃ head versus CoCr heads, though the linear wear rates reported in this study fall within the expected range. This may be explained by the practice of using Al₂O₃ heads in younger more active patients. While there was not a difference in average age or range, there was a tendency for more males in the compression molded Al₂O₃ head group. There was a trend towards younger males in the Al₂O₃ head group compared to either group (machined or compression molded) with CoCr. This was not statistically different (Table 1).

The final variable of interest that could significantly affect polyethylene wear is the manufacturing technique. There are various types of fabrication methods that can be employed in the fabrication of polyethylene orthopedic implants. Most

of the acetabular liners used today are machined from extruded bar stock or compression-molded directly from the polyethylene powder resin [4]. Machined polyethylene liners are made by first producing a polyethylene bar stock from the resin, followed by the machining process, which cuts the bar stock to a very precise size and geometry through the use of a lathe. The polyethylene bar stocks themselves are produced through a process known as ram extrusion where the polyethylene resin is simultaneously heated and pressurized within an evacuated chamber. As the solid polyethylene forms, it is extruded through an open extrusion port within the chamber [22]. Because the extrusion process is noncontinuous, inconsistencies can be found within the solid polyethylene bar stock. These zones of polyethylene inconsistencies, or what Bankston et al. referred to as "dead zones," can produce areas of greatly altered molecular weight resulting in altered wear resistance [22]. The alternate process of compression molding is a single-step process where the polyethylene resin is molded directly into the predetermined size and geometry of the acetabular insert.

In addition to the maldistribution of solid-phase polyethylene within the ram extruded bar stock, surface characteristics and topography may have a significant role in polyethylene oxidation. In the machined polyethylene insert, machine marks from the lathe creates numerous micron size grooves and shreds on the bearing surface, which are not found on the surface of the compression molded polyethylene insert. This was confirmed in the current study as shown in Figure 4. Bankston et al. mentioned that not only could this be a source of third body wear, but also the microindentations and scratches on the surface created added surface area to which oxidation could more easily occur [22]. The characteristic surfaces seen in the three-dimensional topographic images of Figure 4 are a result of the manufacturing methods of each polyethylene design. The repeating peak and valley topography in Figure 4 is indicative of the machining marks, which occur during the machining portion of liner formation. The compression molded topographic image in comparison lacks the large surface wave ranges and is flatter owing to the forming process. The micron-level surface differences between each polyethylene cause a higher surface roughness average (Ra) in the machined polyethylene. The representative images show an Ra of 1.68 μm for machined and 0.40 μm for molded surfaces, which are characteristic of these surfaces in UHMWPE implants [12]. Despite the SEM and surface profile findings noted, the gross inspection of each retrieval specimen showed no visible signs of delamination, pitting, scratches, or cracking.

## 5. Conclusion

In summary, the implant design using GUR1050 bar stock, sterilized in ETO, with final articular surface geometry machined had significantly more linear wear and radiographic osteolysis. The implant using GUR 1020 stock powder, compression-molded into final surface geometry without machining, and sterilized in inert gamma irradiation showed significantly less radiographic measured wear and osteolysis. It is beyond the scope of this paper to conjecture which of the differing elements is responsible for the greater linear wear rate in one implant versus the other. PE wear rates have been shown to predict osteolysis, implant longevity, and revision surgery, and it is routine practice to monitor all implants for wear and signs of failure. Most current THA implants are using highly cross-linked PE because of more favorable reported wear rates. However, there are a large number of hip arthroplasty implants using conventional PE that were implanted before highly cross-linked PE was available. Cross-linked PE has also been slow to move into wide-scale implementation on a global scale due to its high cost and low availability outside of the United States. Thus, understanding the fundamental core materials and the manufacturing process for conventional PE implants and having comparative clinical reviews as described here suggest that it may be prudent to monitor some implants more closely than others for polyethylene wear-related signs of problems.

# References

[1] W. H. Harris, "Wear and periprosthetic osteolysis the problem," *Clinical Orthopaedics and Related Research*, no. 393, pp. 66–70, 2001.

[2] E. Garcia-Cimbrelo and L. Munuera, "Early and late loosening of the acetabular cup after low-friction arthroplasty," *Journal of Bone and Joint Surgery A*, vol. 74, no. 8, pp. 1119–1129, 1992.

[3] A. Eskelinen, V. Remes, I. Helenius, P. Pulkkinen, J. Nevalainen, and P. Paavolainen, "Total hip arthroplasty for primary osteoarthrosis in younger patients in the Finnish arthroplasty register: 4 661 primary replacements followed for 0-22 years," *Acta Orthopaedica Scandinavica*, vol. 76, no. 1, pp. 28–41, 2005.

[4] S. M. Kurtz, *UHMWPE Biomaterials Handbook: Ultra-High Molecular Weight Polyethylene in Total Joint Replacement*, Elsevier/Academic, Amsterdam, The Netherlands, 2009.

[5] P. M. Faris, M. A. Ritter, A. L. Pierce, K. E. Davis, and G. W. Faris, "Polyethylene sterilization and production affects wear in total hip arthroplasties," *Clinical Orthopaedics and Related Research*, vol. 453, pp. 305–308, 2006.

[6] E. García-Rey and E. García-Cimbrelo, "Polyethylene in total hip arthroplasty: half a century in the limelight," *Journal of Orthopaedics and Traumatology*, vol. 11, no. 2, pp. 67–72, 2010.

[7] J. B. Meding, M. Keaton, and K. E. Davis, "Acetabular UHMWPE survival and wear changes with different manufacturing techniques," *Clinical Orthopaedics and Related Research*, vol. 469, no. 2, pp. 405–411, 2011.

[8] I. Nakahara, N. Nakamura, T. Nishii, H. Miki, T. Sakai, and N. Sugano, "Minimum five-year follow-up wear measurement of longevity highly cross-linked polyethylene cup against cobalt-chromium or zirconia heads," *Journal of Arthroplasty*, vol. 25, no. 8, pp. 1182–1187, 2010.

[9] H. McKellop, F. W. Shen, B. Lu, P. Campbell, and R. Salovey, "Effect of sterilization method and other modifications on the wear resistance of acetabular cups made of ultra-high molecular weight polyethylene. A hip-simulator study," *Journal of Bone and Joint Surgery A*, vol. 82, no. 12, pp. 1708–1725, 2000.

[10] L. C. Sutula, J. P. Collier, K. A. Saum et al., "Impact of gamma sterilization on clinical performance of polyethylene in the hip," *Clinical Orthopaedics and Related Research*, vol. 319, pp. 28–40, 1995.

[11] B. H. Currier, J. H. Currier, J. P. Collier et al., "Effect of fabrication method and resin type on performance of tibial bearings," *Journal of Biomedical Materials Research A*, vol. 53, no. 2, pp. 143–151, 2000.

[12] G. R. Plank, D. M. Estok, O. K. Muratoglu, D. O. O'Connor, B. R. Burroughs, and W. H. Harris, "Contact stress assessment of conventional and highly crosslinked ultra high molecular weight polyethylene acetabular liners with finite element analysis and pressure sensitive film," *Journal of Biomedical Materials Research B*, vol. 80, no. 1, pp. 1–10, 2007.

[13] T. A. Gruen, G. M. McNeice, and H. C. Amstutz, "Modes of failure of cemented stem-type femoral components. A radiographic analysis of loosening," *Clinical Orthopaedics and Related Research*, vol. 141, pp. 17–27, 1979.

[14] J. G. DeLee and J. Charnley, "Radiological demarcation of cemented sockets in total hip replacement," *Clinical Orthopaedics and Related Research*, vol. 121, pp. 20–32, 1976.

[15] M. J. Griffith, M. K. Seidenstein, D. Williams, and J. Charnley, "Socket wear in Charnley low friction arthroplasty of the hip," *Clinical Orthopaedics and Related Research*, vol. 137, pp. 37–47, 1978.

[16] J. Livermore, D. Ilstrup, and B. Morrey, "Effect of femoral head size on wear of the polyethylene acetabular component," *Journal of Bone and Joint Surgery A*, vol. 72, no. 4, pp. 518–528, 1990.

[17] L. C. Benson, J. D. Desjardins, and M. Laberge, "Effects of in vitro wear of machined and molded UHMWPE tibial inserts on TKR kinematics," *Journal of Biomedical Materials Research*, vol. 58, no. 5, pp. 496–504, 2001.

[18] A. V. Lombardi, B. S. Ellison, and K. R. Berend, "Polyethylene wear is influenced by manufacturing technique in modular TKA," *Clinical Orthopaedics and Related Research*, vol. 466, no. 11, pp. 2798–2805, 2008.

[19] J. L. Tipper, A. L. Galvin, E. Ingham et al., "Comparison of the wear, wear debris and functional biological activity of non-crosslinked and crosslinked GUR 1020 and GUR 1050 polyethylenes used in total hip prostheses," in *Proceedings of the 2nd UHMWPE International Meeting*, Torino, Italy, March 2005, http://www.uhmwpe.unito.it/2005/atti/10%20Tipper.pdf.

[20] M. Semlitsch and H. G. Willert, "Clinical wear behaviour of ultra-high molecular weight polyethylene cups paired with metal and ceramic ball heads in comparison to metal-on-metal pairings of hip joint replacements," *Proceedings of the Institution of Mechanical Engineers H*, vol. 211, no. 1, pp. 73–88, 1997.

[21] J. A. Urban, K. L. Garvin, C. K. Boese et al., "Ceramic-on-polyethylene bearing surfaces in total hip arthroplasty," *Journal of Bone and Joint Surgery A*, vol. 83, no. 11, pp. 1688–1694, 2001.

[22] A. B. Bankston, E. M. Keating, C. Ranawat, P. M. Faris, and M. A. Ritter, "Comparison of polyethylene wear in machined versus molded polyethylene," *Clinical Orthopaedics and Related Research*, vol. 317, pp. 37–43, 1995.

# 25

# Changes in Joint Gap Balances between Intra- and Postoperation in Total Knee Arthroplasty

**Arata Nakajima,**[1,2] **Yasuchika Aoki,**[1] **Masazumi Murakami,**[2] **and Koichi Nakagawa**[1]

[1] *Department of Orthopaedic Surgery, Toho University Sakura Medical Center, 564-1 Shimoshizu, Sakura, Chiba 285-8741, Japan*
[2] *Department of Orthopaedic Surgery, Chiba Aoba Municipal Hospital, 1273-2 Aoba-cho, Chuo-ku, Chiba 260-0852, Japan*

Correspondence should be addressed to Arata Nakajima; a-nakaji@sf7.so-net.ne.jp

Academic Editor: Elizaveta Kon

Achieving correct soft tissue balance and preparing equal and rectangular extension and flexion joint gaps are crucial goals of TKA. Intraoperative gap balances would change postoperatively; however, changes in joint gap balances between pre- and postoperation remain unclear. To explore these changes associated with TKA, we prospectively investigated 21 posterior cruciate ligament retaining TKAs for varus knees. Intraoperative extension gap balance (iEGB) was 2.6 ± 2.0° varus versus postoperative extension gap balance (pEGB) of 0.77 ± 1.8° valgus ($P < 0.01$), while no significant difference between intraoperative flexion gap balance (iFGB) and postoperative flexion gap balance (pFGB) was observed. We also explored correlations between intraoperative and postoperative gap balances but found no significant correlations. These observations indicate that (i) surgeons should avoid excessive release of the medial soft tissue during TKA for varus knees and (ii) intraoperative gap balance may not be necessarily reflected on postoperative gap balance.

## 1. Introduction

Achieving correct soft tissue balance of the knee is fundamental to the success of TKA [1], and an equal joint gap during extension and flexion is a prerequisite for satisfactory soft tissue balance [2–4]. In addition, equalizing the distance from the femoral component to the tibial surface (i.e., the joint gap) throughout the full range of knee motion prevents lift-off of the tibial component and theoretically assists in achieving proper contact pressure and kinematics. Thus, preparing equal and rectangular extension and flexion joint gaps is the most important goal of TKA.

Meanwhile, most surgeons agree that accurate ligament balancing of the knee with varus deformity is difficult especially during posterior cruciate ligament retaining (CR)-TKA. The standard procedure for ligament balancing of the medial side of the knees uses subperiosteal release of the medial collateral ligament (MCL) [5–7]. Despite performing such release of MCL, varus balance is likely to remain in most CR-TKAs because posterior cruciate ligament (PCL) is an important component of the medial supporting mechanism of the knee [8].

Recently, Sekiya et al. reported that residual lateral ligamentous laxity immediately after surgery subsequently corrected itself spontaneously in some instances [9]. This finding suggests that some degree of residual lateral laxity, namely, varus balance, may be tolerable for varus knees so long as proper valgus alignment is maintained. However, it has not been explored whether remaining varus balance is also tolerable for CR-TKAs where intraoperative varus balance is likely to remain.

Sasanuma et al. compared soft tissue balance during TKA with soft tissue balance after TKA and concluded that immediate postoperative coronal laxity correlated positively with intraoperative coronal laxity at 0° (extension) but exhibited no correlation with intraoperative coronal laxity at 90° (flexion) [10]. So far, however, relationship between intraoperative and postoperative gap balance in TKA has not been elucidated fully.

In this study, we hypothesized that intraoperative varus balance would improve postoperatively in CR-TKAs and that intraoperative gap balance would correlate with postoperative gap balance. To verify these hypotheses, we prospectively investigated the posterior cruciate ligament retaining

Extension

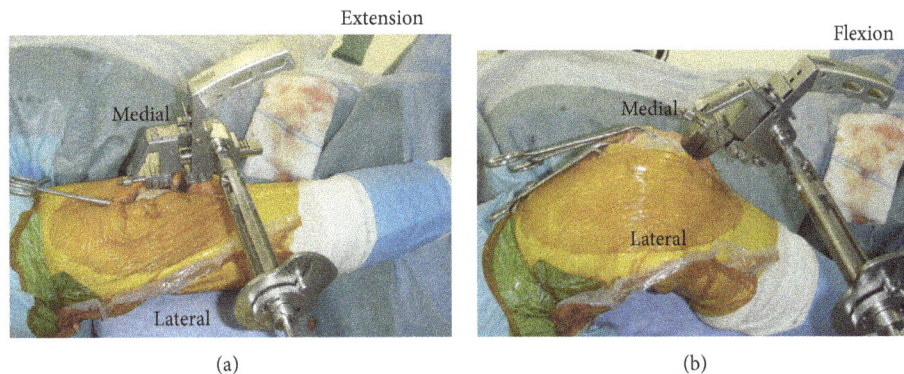

(a)

Flexion

(b)

FIGURE 1: Measurements of intraoperative gap balance for the right knee at 0° (extension) and 90° (flexion) with the patella in a reduced position and a constant 40-pound distracting force being applied between the cut surfaces of the distal femur and the proximal tibia.

(CR)-TKAs for varus-deformed knees. We measured intraoperative tibiofemoral gap balance in knee extension and flexion before implanting femoral and tibial components and consecutively measured tibiofemoral gap balance four to six weeks postoperatively. We then used these measurements to analyze the relationship between intraoperative and postoperative gap balances.

## 2. Patients and Methods

We analyzed 21 selected knees in 20 patients with osteoarthritis (4 men and 16 women with a mean age of 75.0 years, ranging from 61 to 82 years) who had undergone TKA in Chiba Aoba Municipal Hospital between June 2009 and February 2010. Knees with ankylosis or severely limited range of motion (fixed flexion deformity >20 or flexion <90) were excluded from this study. All patients received a CR-type Scorpio NRG (Stryker Orthopedics, Mahwah, NJ).

We performed all operations in accordance with previously published descriptions of the gap technique [11–13] with our modifications. After bone cuts, we measured the joint gap and medial and lateral soft tissue balance at 0° and 90° flexion with the patella reduced (intraoperative gap balance), using a tensor device (Stryker Orthopedics) (Figure 1). We applied a constant 40-pound distracting force between upper and lower plates via a ratchet-type hex wrench which limited the applied force to 40 pounds [14, 15]. Finally, we added medial soft tissue release for all cases according to the staged release reported by Clayton et al. [16] until both extension and flexion gap balances would be within 5° and then recorded the measurements as intraoperative gap balances. We implanted appropriately sized femoral and tibial components along with a polyethylene insert of the appropriate thickness.

Four to six weeks after surgery, we evaluated medial and lateral soft tissue balance at knee extension and flexion positions (postoperative gap balance) in a knee-neutral position. In extension, we took anteroposterior radiographs with patients in a supine position and measured the angle between the cut lines of the distal femur and the proximal tibia. In flexion, we took axial radiographs of the distal femur employing a technique recently described in the literatures [17, 18]. In practice, we measured the angle between the cut

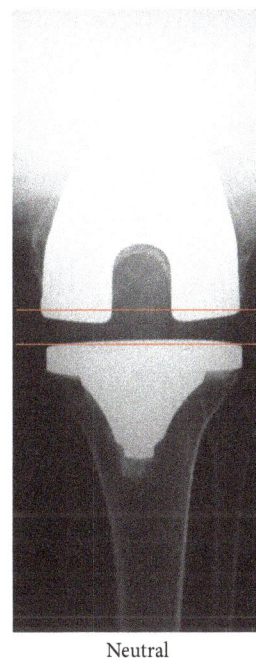

Neutral

FIGURE 2: Postoperative axial radiographs of the left distal femur. Patients sit on a table with their lower legs dependent and a 1.5 kg weight attached to the ankle on the treated side. The angle between the cut lines of the posterior femoral condyles and the proximal tibia represents the flexion gap balance (FGB).

lines of the posterior femoral condyles and the proximal tibia while patients sat on a table with their lower legs dependent and a 1.5 kg weight attached to the ankle on the treated side, an arrangement which facilitated clear visualization of the shape and width of the flexion gap (Figure 2).

Data are expressed as mean ± standard deviation. We used the ANOVA to identify differences between intraoperative and postoperative gap balances both in extension and flexion. Where differences existed in ANOVA, the Fisher-protected least significant difference test was used to determine significance. We also calculated correlation coefficients between intraoperative and postoperative gap balances both

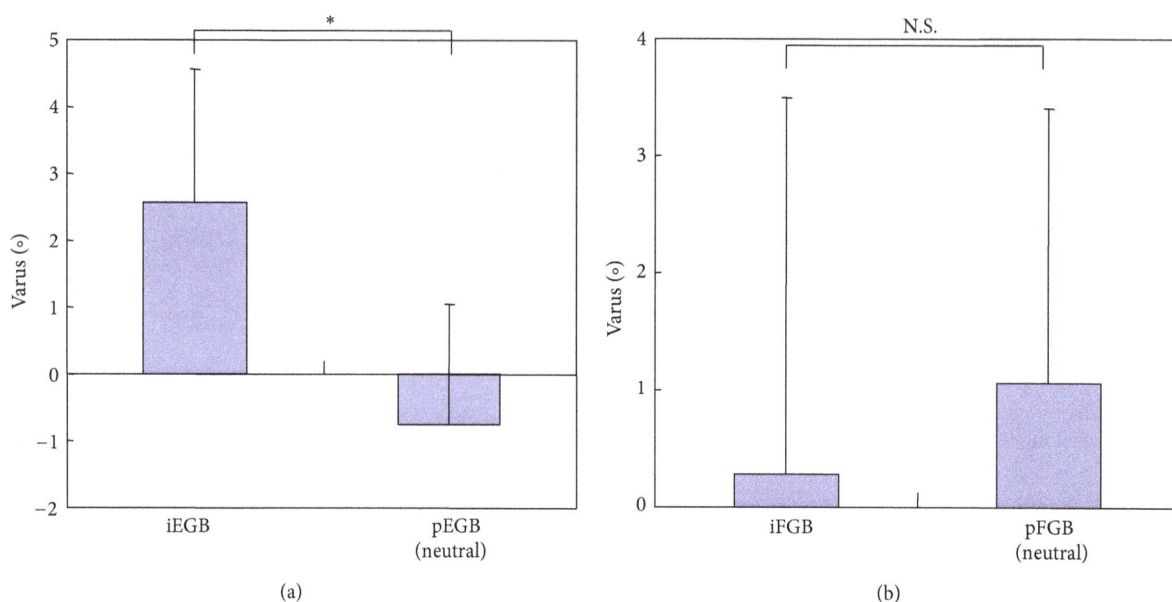

(a)

(b)

FIGURE 3: Changes in joint gap balance between intraoperative and postoperative measurements. (a) Intraoperative extension gap balance (iEGB) of 2.6° varus significantly differs from postoperative extension gap balance (pEGB) of 0.77° valgus in neutral position ($^*P < 0.01$). (b) No significant difference is observed between intraoperative flexion gap balance (iFGB) and postoperative flexion gap balance (pFGB) in neutral position.

in extension and flexion. The level of significance was set at $P < 0.05$ for all analyses.

This study was approved by the Ethical Committee of Chiba Aoba Municipal Hospital and all patients gave their informed consent before their inclusion in this study.

## 3. Results

*3.1. Changes in Joint Gap Balances between Intraoperative and Postoperative Measurements.* Intraoperative extension gap balance (iEGB) was 2.6 ± 2.0° varus versus a postoperative extension gap balance (pEGB) in neutral position of 0.77 ± 1.8° valgus, a statistically significant difference ($P < 0.01$) (Figure 3(a)). On the other hand, intraoperative flexion gap balance (iFGB) was 0.29 ± 3.2° varus versus a postoperative flexion gap balance (pFGB) in neutral position of 1.1 ± 2.3° varus, a difference that was not statistically significant (Figure 3(b)).

*3.2. Correlation between Intraoperative and Postoperative Gap Balance.* To evaluate how well intraoperative gap balances correlate with postoperative gap balances, we performed a correlation analysis between iEGB and pEGB and between iFGB and pFGB. However, we observed no significant correlations between both of them (data not shown).

## 4. Discussion

Achieving proper soft tissue balance is one of the most important requirements for successful TKA; however, controversy persists as to whether the intraoperative joint gap in extension should be equal in all aspects to the intraoperative joint gap in flexion.

Sekiya et al. measured coronal, lateral, or medial ligamentous laxity immediately after TKA and at 3, 6, and 12 months postoperatively in 71 knees with preoperative varus deformity and showed that residual lateral ligamentous laxity immediately after surgery subsequently corrected itself spontaneously in some instances [9]. In our study, mean intraoperative gap balance in extension (mean iEGB = 2.6° varus) improved postoperatively to a mean value of 0.77° valgus. We do not know exact reason for this change in alignment but speculate that the improvement of varus balance was caused by the spontaneous correction of lateral ligament laxity as Sekiya et al. reported [9] and/or by the temporally improved medial ligament tightness because we used the CR-type implants in all cases.

The question then arises as to why the flexion gap balance remained stable after TKA. One plausible explanation is that PCL reduces medial ligamentous laxity in flexion both during and after TKA. During TKA for varus knees, the medial collateral ligament is released frequently and osteophytes at the medial femoral chondyle and tibial plateau were removed to enable proper coronal ligament balance, resulting in an increase in medial ligamentous laxity. Thus, as well as the extension gap balance, the flexion gap balance would change to valgus alignment if we used the PS implants. However, we used the CR implants where PCL functioned as a medial supporting stabilizer, which contributed to the stable valance in flexion.

Prior to starting this study, we had hypothesized that intraoperative gap balances would correlate with postoperative gap balances; however, contrary to our expectation, we observed no significant correlation between intraoperative gap balance and postoperative gap balance both in extension and in flexion (data not shown). Possible explanations for this outcome include the following. First, we employed different methods for our intraoperative and postoperative measurements of joint gap balance. Intraoperatively, we distracted the joint gap by 40 lbs and measured the gap balance, whereas we measured the postoperative gap balance with the patient supine on the table without a distraction force. Moreover, we chose 40 lbs as the distraction force based upon a previous study [15], but we do not know how well 40 lbs distraction force reflects physiological conditions of the knee. Second, the operating conditions of the extensor mechanism substantially differ between intraoperative and postoperative environments. Even with the patella in a reduced position during measurements of the intraoperative gap balance, some degree of impairment of the extensor mechanism, especially in flexion, would still persist, which could result in no significant correlation between intraoperative gap balance and postoperative gap balance. Third, we measured the intraoperative tibiofemoral gap balance before implanting femoral components. Because implanting femoral components strongly affects the joint gap balances especially in extension [19], measurements under presence or absence of the femoral components might affect accurate relation between intraoperative gap balance and postoperative gap balance. Due to the relatively small number of TKA cases comprising our study, further studies are needed to more definitively determine how much correlation, if any, there is between intraoperative and postoperative gap balance both in extension and in flexion.

In conclusion, our results showed that intraoperative gap balance was significantly reduced postoperatively in extension but not significantly altered in flexion. Furthermore, we observed no significant correlation between intraoperative gap balance and postoperative gap balance both in extension and flexion. Despite its limitations, our results presented here indicate the importance of avoiding excessive release of the medial soft tissue during TKA for varus knees. Development of surgical procedures to allow accurate predictions of postoperative joint gap balances based upon intraoperative joint gap balances measurements remains a pressing need.

## Conflict of Interests

The authors declare that they have no conflict of interests.

## References

[1] M. J. Winemaker, "Perfect balance in total knee arthroplasty: the elusive compromise," *The Journal of Arthroplasty*, vol. 17, no. 1, pp. 2–10, 2002.

[2] J. N. Insall, C. S. Ranawat, W. N. Scott, and P. Walker, "Total condylar knee replacement: preliminary report," *Clinical Orthopaedics and Related Research*, no. 120, pp. 149–154, 1976.

[3] J. N. Insall, R. Binazzi, M. Soudry, and L. A. Mestriner, "Total knee arthroplasty," *Clinical Orthopaedics and Related Research*, no. 192, pp. 13–22, 1985.

[4] M. Tanzer, K. Smith, and S. Burnett, "Posterior-stabilized versus cruciate-retaining total knee arthroplasty: balancing the gap," *The Journal of Arthroplasty*, vol. 17, no. 7, pp. 813–819, 2002.

[5] L. A. Whiteside, K. Saeki, and W. M. Mihalko, "Functional medical ligament balancing in total knee arthroplasty," *Clinical Orthopaedics and Related Research*, no. 380, pp. 45–57, 2000.

[6] W. M. Mihalko, K. J. Saleh, K. A. Krackow, and L. A. Whiteside, "Soft-tissue balancing during total knee arthroplasty in the varus knee," *Journal of the American Academy of Orthopaedic Surgeons*, vol. 17, no. 12, pp. 766–774, 2009.

[7] W. M. Mihalko, L. A. Whiteside, and K. A. Krackow, "Comparison of ligament-balancing techniques during total knee arthroplasty," *The Journal of Bone & Joint Surgery A*, vol. 85, supplement 4, pp. 132–135, 2003.

[8] C. Luring, T. Hüfner, L. Perlick, H. Bäthis, C. Krettek, and J. Grifka, "The effectiveness of sequential medial soft tissue release on coronal alignment in total knee arthroplasty: using a computer navigation model," *The Journal of Arthroplasty*, vol. 21, no. 3, pp. 428–434, 2006.

[9] H. Sekiya, K. Takatoku, H. Takada, H. Sasanuma, and N. Sugimoto, "Postoperative lateral ligamentous laxity diminishes with time after TKA in the varus knee," *Clinical Orthopaedics and Related Research*, vol. 467, no. 6, pp. 1582–1586, 2009.

[10] H. Sasanuma, H. Sekiya, K. Takatoku, H. Takada, and N. Sugimoto, "Evaluation of soft-tissue balance during total knee arthroplasty," *Journal of Orthopaedic Surgery*, vol. 18, no. 1, pp. 26–30, 2010.

[11] T. K. Fehring, "Rotational malalignment of the femoral component in total knee arthroplasty," *Clinical Orthopaedics and Related Research*, no. 380, pp. 72–79, 2000.

[12] M. A. Katz, T. D. Beck, J. S. Silber, R. M. Seldes, and P. A. Lotke, "Determining femoral rotational alignment in total knee arthroplasty: reliability of techniques," *The Journal of Arthroplasty*, vol. 16, no. 3, pp. 301–305, 2001.

[13] D. A. Dennis, "Measured resection: an outdated technique in total knee arthroplasty," *Orthopedics*, vol. 31, no. 9, pp. 940, 943–944, 2008.

[14] Y. Kadoya, A. Kobayashi, T. Komatsu, S. Nakagawa, and Y. Yamano, "Effects of posterior cruciate ligament resection on the tibiofemoral joint gap," *Clinical Orthopaedics and Related Research*, no. 391, pp. 210–217, 2001.

[15] R. Gejo, Y. Morita, I. Matsushita, K. Sugimori, and T. Kimura, "Joint gap changes with patellar tendon strain and patellar position during TKA," *Clinical Orthopaedics and Related Research*, vol. 466, no. 4, pp. 946–951, 2008.

[16] M. L. Clayton, T. R. Thompson, and R. P. Mack, "Correction of alignment deformities during total knee arthroplasties: staged soft-tissue releases," *Clinical Orthopaedics and Related Research*, no. 202, pp. 117–124, 1986.

[17] K. Kanekasu, M. Kondo, and Y. Kadoya, "Axial radiography of the distal femur to assess rotational alignment in total knee arthroplasty," *Clinical Orthopaedics and Related Research*, no. 434, pp. 193–197, 2005.

[18] Y. Tokuhara, Y. Kadoya, K. Kanekasu, M. Kondo, A. Kobayashi, and K. Takaoka, "Evaluation of the flexion gap by axial radiography of the distal femur," *The Journal of Bone & Joint Surgery B*, vol. 88, no. 10, pp. 1327–1330, 2006.

[19] H. Muratsu, T. Matsumoto, S. Kubo et al., "Femoral component placement changes soft tissue balance in posterior-stabilized total knee arthroplasty," *Clinical Biomechanics*, vol. 25, no. 9, pp. 926–930, 2010.

# 26

# Union Rate on Hinge Side after Open-Door Laminoplasty Using Maxillofacial Titanium Miniplate

**Koopong Siribumrungwong, Theerasan Kiriratnikom, and Boonsin Tangtrakulwanich**

*Department of Orthopedic Surgery and Physical Medicine, Faculty of Medicine, Prince of Songkla University, Hat Yai, Songkla 90110, Thailand*

Correspondence should be addressed to Koopong Siribumrungwong; koopongs@hotmail.com

Academic Editor: Hiroshi Hashizume

*Background*. One of the important complications of open-door laminoplasty is a premature laminoplasty closure. In order to prevent premature laminoplasty closure many techniques have been described and a titanium miniplate is one of the instruments to maintain cervical canal expansion. This study was performed to evaluate the effectiveness of titanium miniplates on the union rate for open-door laminoplasty. *Materials and Methods*. We performed open-door laminoplasty in 68 levels of fourteen patients using maxillofacial titanium miniplates. Axial computed tomography scans were obtained at 6 months postoperatively to evaluate the union rates of the hinge side. The Japanese Orthopedic Association (JOA) score was used to compare the clinical outcomes before and after surgery. *Results*. Computed tomography scan data was available on 68 levels in 14 patients. There were no premature closures of the hinge or miniplate dislodgements. The union rate on the hinge side was 70.5% (48/68). The mean JOA score increased significantly from 7.0 before surgery to 10.2, 12.2, and 13.0 after surgery at 1, 3, and 6 months, respectively. *Conclusion*. Open-door laminoplasty using maxillofacial titanium miniplates can provide union rates comparable to other techniques. It can maintain canal expansion without failures, dislodgements, and premature closures.

## 1. Introduction

Open-door laminoplasty is a standard procedure for the treatment of multiple levels of cervical spondylotic myelopathy and ossification of posterior longitudinal ligaments (OPLL). There are several techniques to maintain cervical canal expansion such as the Hirabayashi technique [1] which is the classic open-door laminoplasty that maintains cervical canal expansion by suturing to the contralateral soft tissue. The Itoh and Tsuji technique [2] maintains an elevated lamina by a spinous process spacer with suturing to the lateral mass. However, sutures do not provide a rigid fixation [3] and so premature laminoplasty closure is one of the important complications in open-door laminoplasty which results in subsequent restenosis. In one series using suturing techniques, patients developed some degree of reclosure at one or more levels up to 34% [4]. In order to prevent premature laminoplasty closure with a rigid fixation many techniques such as ceramic spacers, bone strut grafts, and plating systems

have been introduced. However, bone struts and ceramic spacers are associated with the potential of graft dislodgement which can lead to reclosure of laminoplasty or neurological deficit if the spacers dislodge into the canal [5, 6]. Plating can provide immediate rigid fixation [7] and there are many types of plates used to maintain cervical canal expansion. In 1996 O'Brien et al. [8] used a maxillofacial miniplate and screws to maintain the canal expansion in an open-door laminoplasty. But this procedure is technically difficult as the assistant and primary surgeon must work together to hold the lamina and plate in place while drilling, tapping, and inserting the requisite screws [7]. A new plating design was developed [7] in an attempt to provide easier fixation. The results showed good effectiveness of the new plate design [9]. There were no plate failures or premature laminoplasty closures. The union rates after using the new plate design were 55%, 77%, and 93% at 3, 6, and 12 months, respectively. But the cost of the new laminoplasty plate is still high. The first advantage of the maxillofacial titanium miniplate over the commercial laminoplasty plate is the lower cost. The second advantage is when the patient has a bony anatomical variation or the open-door laminoplasty site does not match with the commercial laminoplasty plate the maxillofacial titanium miniplate can be adjusted to different lengths. This plate can also bend in all three dimensions to follow the contour of an abnormal anatomy on the open-door side. In our institution, the authors use a maxillofacial titanium miniplate to maintain cervical canal expansion in open-door laminoplasty. However, there are only a few studies evaluating its effectiveness on the union rate of the hinge side. The purpose of this study was to evaluate the effectiveness of the maxillofacial titanium miniplate to maintain cervical canal expansion in open-door laminoplasty.

## 2. Materials and Methods

This was a cohort study of 14 consecutive patients including 8 male and 6 female patients from April 2011 to February 2012 with 68 levels of open-door laminoplasty using maxillofacial titanium miniplates. This study was approved by the Institutional Review Board, Faculty of Medicine, Prince of Songkla University. All patients signed a written consent form before surgery and all patients had a radiographic proven multilevel myelopathy or OPLL on MRI and were indicated for open-door laminoplasty. Inclusion criteria were patients who were diagnosed as multilevel cervical spondylotic myelopathy or OPLL. Eligible patients were aged 40–80 years. All patients underwent open-door laminoplasty using a maxillofacial titanium miniplate to maintain cervical canal expansion at Songklanagarind Hospital. We excluded patients with a history of titanium allergy or spinal cord myelopathy from trauma.

The patients underwent general anesthesia and the surgery was performed by an experienced spine surgeon. The patients were placed in a prone position with Mayfield traction to control the position of the cervical spine. We used a standard midline posterior approach. The number of levels that required decompression depended on the pattern of cord compression. In all cases, a 3 mm high speed burr was used to create the hinge at the junction between the lateral mass and laminar. The hinge side was not grafted. The open side was stabilized with the maxillofacial miniplate and miniscrews (Medtronic Sofamor Danek, Memphis, TN, USA) (Figure 1). The miniplates were cut into appropriate lengths and bent before application at the open-door side to maintain the decompressed spinal canal (Figure 2). We applied the miniplates at all decompressed levels (Figure 3). We did not add strut grafts at the open-door side. One screw was fixed on each side. One redivac drain was placed and removed 48 hours postoperatively.

*2.1. Postoperative Rehabilitation.* Immediately following the surgery, the patients were placed into a soft cervical collar. Although the soft collar did not provide adequate immobilization of the cervical spine, [12] we used the soft collar for resting the cervical spine muscle postoperatively. After discharge from the hospital, the patients were encouraged to

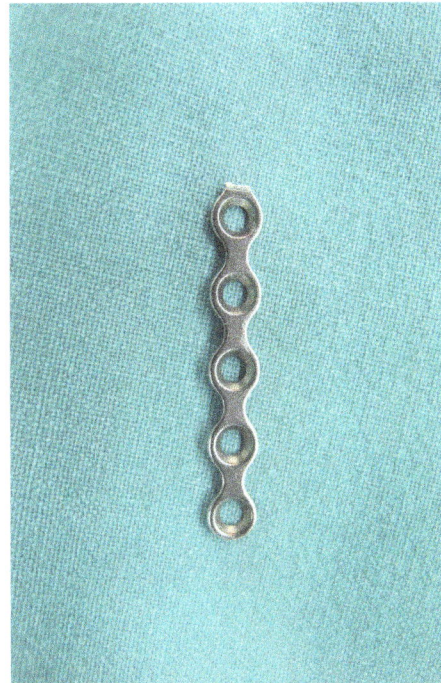

FIGURE 1: Maxillofacial titanium miniplate.

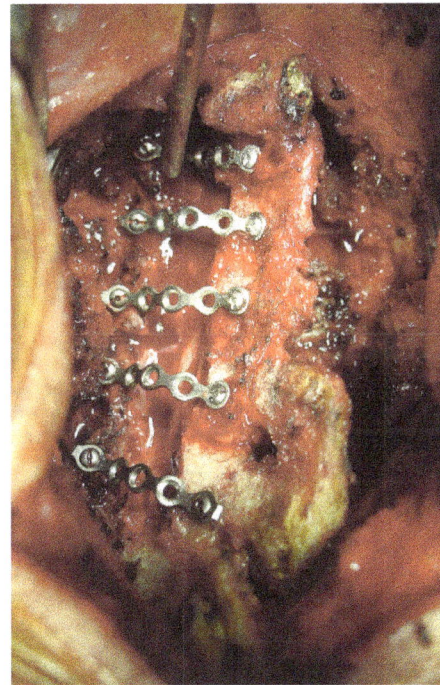

FIGURE 2: Five maxillofacial titanium miniplates were applied at decompressed levels.

engage in range-of-motion exercises of the cervical spine as permitted by wound pain. A soft collar was usually applied to all patients for 4–6 weeks and then removed once the wound pain subsided. Low-strength active resistive exercises were started after the wound pain subsided. A previous study by

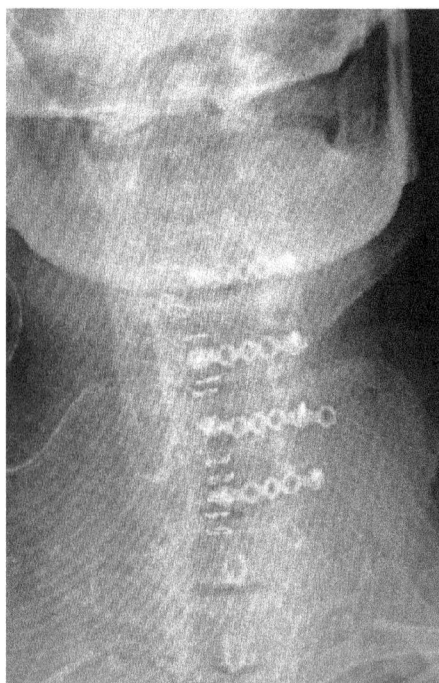

(a)

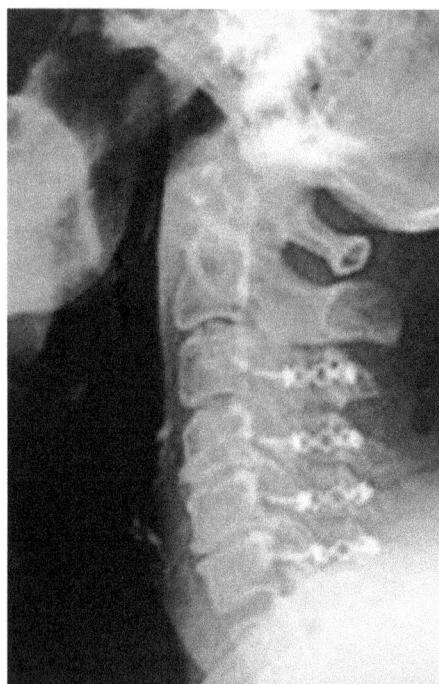

(b)

FIGURE 3: Postoperative AP and lateral film.

Assano et al. [13] showed a decrease in the incidence of axial neck symptoms using this active rehabilitation protocol.

The clinical preoperative and postoperative outcomes were assessed by Japanese Orthopedic Association Scores [14] (JOA scores) at 1, 3, and 6 months. The recovery rate at 1, 3, and 6 months, operative time, and blood loss were also recorded. Reclosure of the lamina or the "spring-back" phenomenon usually occurs postoperatively before 6 months [15]. The union rate at 6 months postoperatively was documented by computed tomography scan (CT). The dorsal and ventral cortices of each hinge were assessed separately for the presence of either cancellous or cortical bone bridging. We defined the union of the hinge side by the presence of bridging bone of both the dorsal and ventral cortices (Figure 4). If only one cortical bridging was noted, the hinge was not defined as a union as we could see whether or not the hinge was perfectly formed as a continuous ventral cortex that immediately appears after surgery (Figure 5) [9]. We used specific criteria to avoid any false positive from an interpretation of the union on the hinge side. Complications such as plate dislodgement, postoperative C5 palsy, and reclosure of laminoplasty were also recorded.

*2.2. Statistical Analysis.* Analysis of variance (ANOVA) test was used to evaluate the statistically significant difference of union rates between levels. The $P$ value was set at 0.05. The statistical analysis was calculated by SPSS program version 14.0.

## 3. Results

There were 14 consecutive patients included in this study with 8 males and 6 females. Sixty-eight levels of open-door laminoplasty were involved using maxillofacial titanium miniplates. The mean age was 58 years ± 5.6. Twelve patients underwent surgery for five levels (C3–C7) and two patients for four levels (C3–C6). All patients received followups at 1, 3, and 6 months. CT scan data was available on 68 levels at 6 months. Mean operative time was 181 ± 36 minutes. Mean blood loss was 330 ± 82 cc. The mean JOA score increased significantly from 7.0 ± 1.0 before surgery to 10.21 ± 1.8, 12.21 ± 1.8, and 13.0 ± 1.3 after surgery at 1, 3, and 6 months, respectively. Mean recovery rates at 1, 3, and 6 months were 32.6%, 52.4%, and 60.15%, respectively. At 6 months the healing rate at C3, C4, C5, C6, and C7 were 71.4%, 64.2%, 64.2%, 71.4%, and 83.3%, respectively. There was no statistically significant difference in the union rates between each level. The mean percentage of all levels of hinges that formed a union at 6 months postoperatively from CT scans was 70.5%; however, there were no cases at any time which showed premature closure of the lamina, plate dislodgement, or broken plates even in the cases with a nonunion hinge (Figure 6). Two of 68 levels (2.9%) had evidence of loosening or reversing of screws on final postoperative follow-up radiographs, but no reclosure of the lamina occurred (Figure 6). Screw back-out was not associated with any neurological consequences. No one developed a cervical kyphotic deformity after surgery.

## 4. Discussion

Open-door laminoplasty is one of the most common decompressive procedures for addressing congenital canal stenosis, multiple levels of cervical spondylotic myelopathy, and OPLL.

TABLE 1: Comparison of the union rates on the hinge side of different types of fixation.

| Authors and year | Fixation technique | Graft | Union rate (6 months) |
|---|---|---|---|
| Tanaka et al. [10], 2008 | Interconnected porous calcium hydroxyapatite spacer | No | 84% |
| | Autogenous graft spacer | Yes | 79% |
| Rhee et al. [9], 2011* | New titanium miniplate | No | 77% |
| Jiang et al. [11], 2012 | New titanium miniplate | Yes | 100% |
| Koopong Siribumrungwong, 2013* | Maxillofacial titanium miniplate | No | 70.5% |

*Measurement of the union rate with the same specific criteria (Union means bridging of both dorsal and ventral cortices).

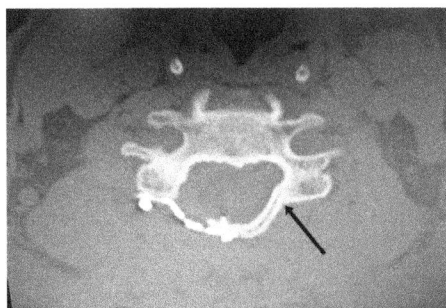

FIGURE 4: Union of hinge side as defined by the union of both dorsal and ventral cortices (arrow).

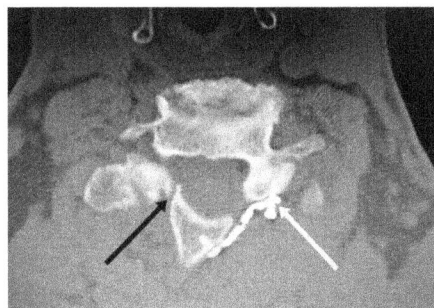

FIGURE 6: Axial CT scan at 6 months demonstrates screw back out (white arrow) and nonunion on the hinge side (black arrow) (no bone bridge at both dorsal and ventral cortices). There was no reclosure of laminoplasty.

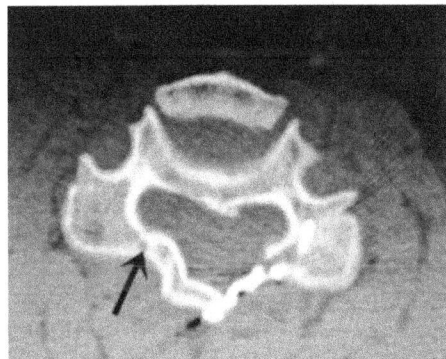

FIGURE 5: The hinge was perfectly formed continuously only at the ventral cortex that immediately appeared after surgery (arrow) that may cause a false positive on interpretation.

It can provide sufficient decompression of the cervical spine by providing sufficient space for the spinal cord to drift in a posterior direction and preserve motion of the cervical spine. There are a number of techniques used to maintain cervical canal expansion. However, currently there is no "best" technique that is recommended. Plating is one type of the fixation techniques that can provide immediate rigid fixation [7] and can allow early mobilization. In this study, we evaluated the results of the maxillofacial titanium miniplate in maintaining cervical canal expansion in open-door laminoplasty with specific criteria. We used the criteria of union based on both dorsal and ventral cortices as described by Rhee et al. [9].

These criteria can avoid a false positive from a perfectly hinged creation (bridging only the ventral cortex).

A new titanium plating design was developed [7] in an attempt to provide easier fixation [16]. But in our hospital the cost of the new titanium plate design is about 800 US dollars/level which is much more expensive than the maxillofacial titanium miniplate (70 US dollars/level). The cost of the new plating design is almost ten times more expensive than the maxillofacial titanium miniplate in levels. Our study of the maxillofacial titanium miniplate showed a union rate of 70.5% on the hinged side at 6 months. That is comparable to a study by Rhee et al. [9] using the new titanium plate design without graft which showed a union rate of 77% at 6 months. Our union rate can also be compared to a study by Tanaka et al. [10] which evaluated bone healing in 88 patients who underwent open-door laminoplasty with hydroxyapatite spacers and autogenous graft spacers with union rates on the hinged side of 84% and 79%, respectively, at six months (Table 1).

Although we reported the lowest union rate of 70.5% compared to other studies (Table 1), there was only one study by Rhee et al. that used specific criteria for a reported union rate of 77% which can be compared with our study.

We compared the mean operative time and estimated blood loss of this study with another open-door laminoplasty technique (Itoh and Tsuji) that was performed in the same hospital and with the same surgeon [17]. The mean operative time was significantly less using the maxillofacial plate (181 ±

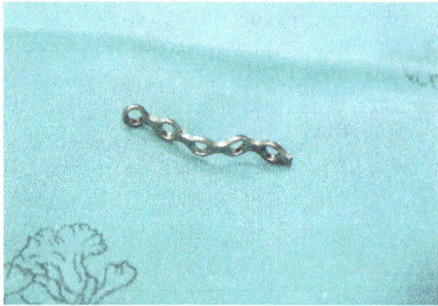

FIGURE 7: The maxillofacial titanium miniplate can be adjusted in length and bent in all three dimensions to fit the contour of the open-door side of the laminoplasty.

36 minutes) compared to Itoh and Tsuji's technique (305 ± 46 minutes). However the mean intraoperative blood loss was significantly less in the Itoh and Tsuji group (240 ± 45 mL) compared with the maxillofacial plate (330 ± 82 mL).

Although there was no statistically significant difference in the union rates between levels, the C7 level tended to have the highest union rate at 6 months (83.3%), which may be due to the larger lamina diameter when compared to the other levels.

This study showed that two of 68 levels (2.9%) had evidence of loosening or screw back-out but the maxillofacial titanium miniplate still provided sufficient stability to maintain canal expansion. This may have occurred due to the intact supraspinous and interspinous ligaments and because we applied plates at all levels. There was no study that mentioned the sufficient loads that were needed to maintain canal expansion, but fusion on the hinged side in laminoplasty did not need as much rigid fixation across the motion segments when using spinal fusion procedures.

The first advantage of the maxillofacial titanium miniplate over the commercial laminoplasty plate is the cost. The second advantage is that when cases have a bony anatomical variation or the open-door laminoplasty site does not match the commercial laminoplasty plate the maxillofacial titanium miniplate can be adjusted in length and bent in three dimensions to fit the contour of the abnormal anatomy on the open-door side (Figure 7).

A limitation of this study was the 6-month follow-up period. But Wang et al. [15] reported that reclosure of laminoplasty or the "spring-back" phenomenon usually occurs before six months. However a long-term follow-up is needed. Another limitation of this study included not comparing the union rate of the maxillofacial titanium miniplate to other surgical instruments.

## 5. Conclusions

Open-door laminoplasty using a maxillofacial titanium miniplate is a safe and simple fixation technique for the treatment of multiple levels of cervical myelopathy and OPLL. This technique can provide union rates that are comparable to other techniques. A maxillofacial titanium miniplate can maintain canal expansion without failures, dislodgements, or premature closures and is less expensive than the other new titanium miniplate.

## Conflict of Interests

The authors declare no conflict of interests.

## Acknowledgment

The research was supported by grant from Faculty of Medicine Prince of Songkla University.

## References

[1] K. Hirabayashi, J. Miyakawa, K. Satomi, T. Maruyama, and K. Wakano, "Operative results and postoperative progression of ossification among patients with ossification of cervical posterior longitudinal ligament," Spine, vol. 6, no. 4, pp. 354–364, 1981.

[2] T. Itoh and H. Tsuji, "Technical improvements and results of laminoplasty for compressive myelopathy in the cervical spine," Spine, vol. 10, no. 8, pp. 729–736, 1985.

[3] K. Satomi, J. Ogawa, Y. Ishii, and K. Hirabayashi, "Short-term complications and long-term results of expansive open-door laminoplasty for cervical stenotic myelopathy," Spine Journal, vol. 1, no. 1, pp. 26–30, 2001.

[4] M. Matsumoto, K. Watanabe, T. Tsuji et al., "Risk factors for closure of lamina after open-door laminoplasty: clinical article," Journal of Neurosurgery, vol. 9, no. 6, pp. 530–537, 2008.

[5] A. Ono, T. Yokoyama, T. Numasawa, K. Wada, and S. Toh, "Dural damage due to a loosened hydroxyapatite intraspinous spacer after spinous process-splitting laminoplasty. Report of two cases," Journal of Neurosurgery, vol. 7, no. 2, pp. 230–235, 2007.

[6] A. Kanemura, M. Doita, T. Iguchi, K. Kasahara, M. Kurosaka, and M. Sumi, "Delayed dural laceration by hydroxyapatite spacer causing tetraparesis following double-door laminoplasty," Journal of Neurosurgery, vol. 8, no. 2, pp. 121–128, 2008.

[7] A. E. Park and J. G. Heller, "Cervical laminoplasty: use of a novel titanium plate to maintain canal expansion-surgical technique," Journal of Spinal Disorders and Techniques, vol. 17, no. 4, pp. 265–271, 2004.

[8] M. F. O'Brien, D. Peterson, A. T. H. Casey, and H. A. Crockard, "A novel technique for laminoplasty augmentation of spinal canal area using titanium miniplate stabilization: a computerized morphometric analysis," Spine, vol. 21, no. 4, pp. 474–484, 1996.

[9] J. M. Rhee, B. Register, T. Hamasaki, and B. Franklin, "Plate-only open door laminoplasty maintains stable spinal canal expansion with high rates of hinge union and no plate failures," Spine, vol. 36, no. 1, pp. 9–14, 2011.

[10] N. Tanaka, K. Nakanishi, Y. Fujimoto et al., "Expansive laminoplasty for cervical myelopathy with interconnected porous calcium hydroxyapatite ceramic spacers: comparison with autogenous bone spacers," Journal of Spinal Disorders and Techniques, vol. 21, no. 8, pp. 547–552, 2008.

[11] J. L. Jiang, X. L. Li, X. G. Zhou, H. Lin, and J. Dong, "Plate-only open-door laminoplasty with fusion for treatment of multilevel degenerative cervical disease," Journal of Clinical Neuroscience, vol. 19, no. 6, pp. 804–809, 2012.

[12] K. L. Whitcroft, L. Massouh, R. Amirfeyz, and G. C. Bannister, "A comparison of neck movement in the soft cervical collar and rigid cervical brace in healthy subjects," *Journal of Manipulative and Physiological Therapeutics*, vol. 34, no. 2, pp. 119–122, 2011.

[13] S. Assano, Y. Nohara, T. Kiya et al., "Postoperative management without immobilization of the cervical spine in patients undergoing cervical laminoplasty: effects on clinical and radiological outcomes," in *Proceedings of the 27th Annual Meeting of the Cervical Spine Society*, Seattle, WA, December 1999.

[14] S. Kawai, K. Sunago, K. Doi, M. Saika, and T. Taguchi, "Cervical laminoplasty (Hattori's method). Procedure and follow-up results," *Spine*, vol. 13, no. 11, pp. 1245–1250, 1988.

[15] H. Q. Wang, K. C. Mak, D. Samartzis et al., "'Spring-back' closure associated with open-door cervical laminoplasty," *Spine Journal*, vol. 11, no. 9, pp. 832–838, 2011.

[16] J. G. Heller and A. A. Qureshi, "Open door laminoplasty: biomechanical comparison of current laminar stabilization methods to a novel laminoplasty plate," *Spine*, 2003.

[17] C. Boontangjai, T. Keereratnikom, and B. Tangtrakulwanich, "Operative results of laminoplasty in multilevel cervical spondylosis with myelopathy: a comparison of two surgical techniques," *Journal of the Medical Association of Thailand*, vol. 95, no. 3, pp. 378–382, 2012.

# 27

# Monoaxial Pedicle Screws Are Superior to Polyaxial Pedicle Screws and the Two Pin External Fixator for Subcutaneous Anterior Pelvic Fixation in a Biomechanical Analysis

**Rahul Vaidya, Ndidi Onwudiwe, Matthew Roth, and Anil Sethi**

*Detroit Medical Center, Orthopedics Department, Wayne State School of Medicine, 4D UHC, St. Antoine Street, 540 E Canfield Street, Detroit, MI 48201, USA*

Correspondence should be addressed to Rahul Vaidya; rvaidya@dmc.org

Academic Editor: Christian Bach

*Purpose.* Comparison of monoaxial and polyaxial screws with the use of subcutaneous anterior pelvic fixation. *Methods.* Four different groups each having 5 constructs were tested in distraction within the elastic range. Once that was completed, 3 components were tested in torsion within the elastic range, 2 to torsional failure and 3 in distraction until failure. *Results.* The pedicle screw systems showed higher stiffness ($4.008 \pm 0.113$ Nmm monoaxial, $3.638 \pm 0.108$ Nmm Click-x; $3.634 \pm 0.147$ Nmm Pangea) than the exfix system ($2.882 \pm 0.054$ Nmm) in distraction. In failure testing, monoaxial pedicle screw system was stronger (360 N) than exfixes (160 N) and polyaxial devices which failed if distracted greater than 4 cm (157 N Click-x or 138 N Pangea). The exfix had higher peak torque and torsional stiffness than all pedicle systems. In torsion, the yield strengths were the same for all constructs. *Conclusion.* The infix device constructed with polyaxial or monoaxial pedicle screws is stiffer than the 2 pin external fixator in distraction testing. In extreme cases, the use of reinforcement or monoaxial systems which do not fail even at 360 N is a better option. In torsional testing, the 2 pin external fixator is stiffer than the pedicle screw systems.

## 1. Introduction

A technique of subcutaneous anterior pelvic fixation for anterior pelvic ring fractures has been recently reported and has been termed "infix" [1]. It involves two supra-acetabular pins [2–5] and a subcutaneous rod, tunneled under the skin, at the top of the "bikini area" [6, 7]. In a multicenter study, infix has been shown to be effective in the treatment of pelvic fractures when combined with the appropriate posterior fixation. It has good patient tolerance, avoids the traditional complications of external fixation [8], and is useful to reduce pelvic injuries [9, 10]. When constructed with traditional polyaxial pedicle screws, infix is biomechanically as effective at posterior SI compression as a femoral distracter [11] and stiffer than a traditional 2 pin anterior external fixator in single stance gait testing in synthetic pelvic models [11, 12].

Pedicle screw implants use a rod screw construct which can be made with monoaxial screws where the head of the

pedicle screw is immobile or polyaxial screws where the head of the pedicle screw can rotate in several directions. Polyaxial screws allow surgeons maneuverability when applying these devices, so that the screw heads do not have to line up exactly to attach the rod. The maneuverability of these screws is at the expense of some strengths of the construct. We have used monoaxial screws to construct the infix device in extremely unstable situations such as APC3 injuries or used C-rings (Synthes Spine, USA) to reinforce polyaxial constructs with good success (Figure 1). However there have been reports of failures of the infix construct in 3 APC injuries in a the multicenter series requiring revision surgery [8] and in another case report [11] all using polyaxial screws.

The purpose of this study is to evaluate the stiffness, and strength to failure of a supra-acetabular internal fixation construct when constructed with either monoaxial or polyaxial screws and compare it with a standard two pin external fixation device. The constructs were tested in in polyethelene

(a)

(b)

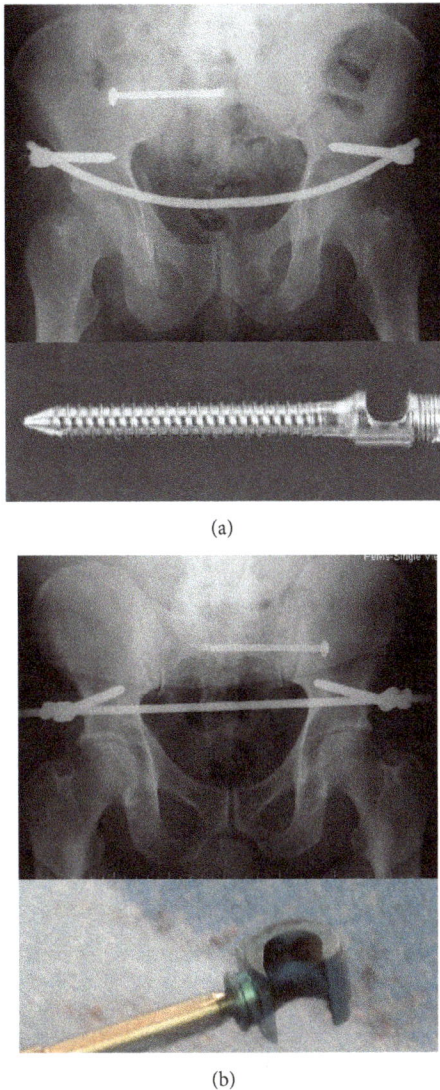

FIGURE 1: X-rays with an (infix) with (a) a monoaxial system and (b) a polyaxial system reinforced with C-rings.

blocks, as it was found that testing to failure in synthetic pelvic models or cadavers failed at the screw bone interface making it difficult to test the devices to extremes. This is the standard material that is used for pedicle screw construct testing in cyclic loading and failure for the US Food and Drug Administration.

## 2. Methods

Six millimeter Schanz screws, an 11 mm carbon fiber rod, and external fixation clamps were used for the two pin external fixator system (Synthes, USA). The pedicle screw systems employed 7 mm × 55 mm titanium screws and a 6 mm titanium rod (Synthes Spine, USA). These are the commercially available standard implants that can be used for each device. All screws were inserted into ultra-high molecular weight polyethylene (UHMWPE) blocks measuring 75 mm × 25 mm × 25 mm. (Figure 2). The dimensions were created to mimic the normal pelvis from CT evaluations of both devices in

human subjects [6] and previous biomechanical studies in a synthetic bone models [10, 11]. The constructs were assembled to have an active longitudinal length of 280 mm. For the pedicle screw systems, a gap of 15 mm was left between the screw head and test block, resulting in a construct moment arm of 75 mm. This is the distance that these screws would have to sit above the bone in a human case (Figure 3). The external fixator (exfix) constructs were assembled with a 145 mm construct moment arm. This included 60 mm in the block, 40 mm of soft tissue from the pelvic bone to the skin, and another 45 mm above the skin where the clamps would attach.

*2.1. Testing Procedures.* Four different constructs were tested in this study with each group having five constructs for a total of twenty that were tested. These included (1) Large External Fixation System (Synthes, West Chester, PA), (2) monoaxial pedicle screw system (Universal Spinal System, Synthes, West Chester, PA), (3) Polyaxial Pedicle Screw System 1 (Click-x Pedicle Screw System, Synthes, West Chester, PA), (4) Polyaxial Pedicle Screw System 2 (Pangea Pedicle Screw System, Synthes, West Chester, PA).

All four constructs with 5 samples each were tested first in distraction in the elastic range (20 mm of displacement). Once distraction testing was completed, all components were tested in torsion (Figure 4) within the elastic range (10°). Two components from each construct group were retested to torsional failure (or 60°). The remaining three components in each construct group were then retested in distraction until failure (or 75 mm).

Distraction was performed on an MTS RT/50 Electromechanical Test Frame (MTS Corp., Eden Prairie, MN). Standard clevis fixtures were rigidly attached to the load cell and lower platen of the test machine. Constructs were mounted to the clevis fixtures using 12.7 mm diameter steel hinge pins. An axial distraction load was applied to the construct at a test speed of 5 mm/min. Load-displacement curves were acquired for each construct and bending yield load, stiffness, and ultimate bending failure load were calculated, as applicable. Yield load calculations were based on 0.020 times the active length.

Torsional testing was performed on an MTS Bionix Electromechanical Torsion Test Frame (MTS Corp., Eden Prairie, MN). Clevis fixtures that prevented rotation of the test block were rigidly attached to the load cell and lower platen of the test machine. Constructs were mounted to the clevis fixtures using 12.7 mm diameter steel hinge pins. Spacers, that prevent test block rotations about the hinge pins, were manually set. Angular displacement was applied to the construct at a test speed of 60° per min, up to a maximum of 60°. Axial load was maintained at 0 N. Torque-angular displacement curves were acquired for each construct tested and torsional yield load, stiffness, and ultimate torque were calculated, if applicable. Yield torque was based on a 5° offset.

### 2.2. Statistics

*2.2.1. Methodology.* In this experiment, comparisons of different treatments to a single control (exfix) were desired.

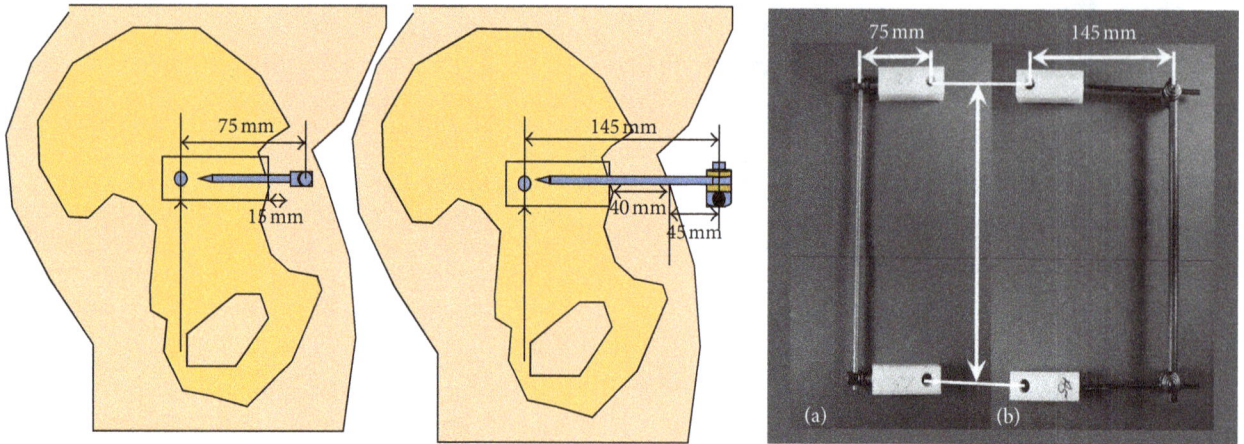

FIGURE 2: Measurements of the set-up for testing in polyethylene blocks.

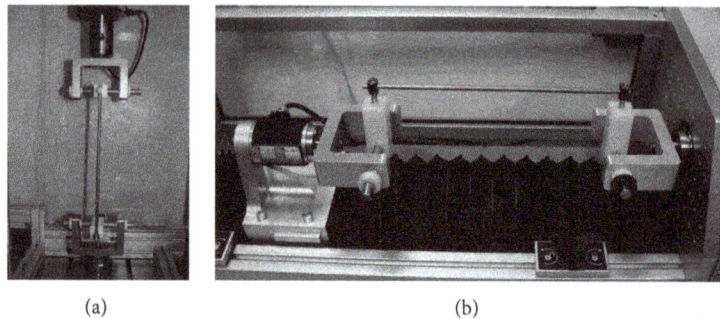

(a)

(b)

FIGURE 3: Set-up for testing. (a) Distraction MTS RT/50 Electromechanical Test. (b) Torsion MTS Bionix Electromechanical Torsion Test Frame (MTS Corp., Eden Prairie, MN).

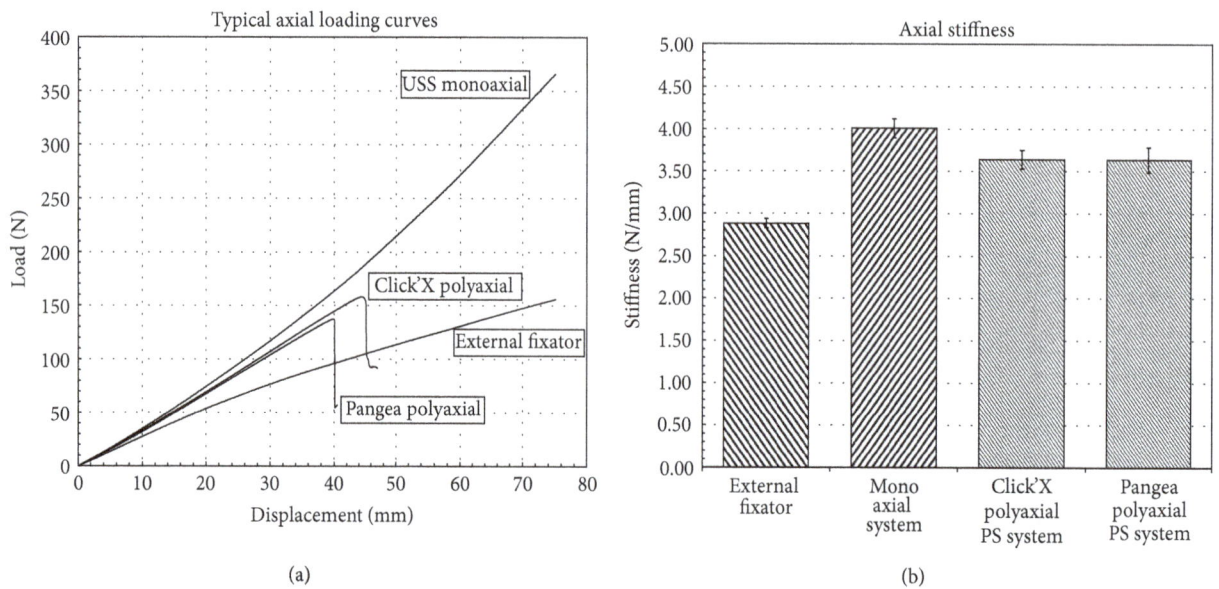

(a)

(b)

FIGURE 4: (a) Load displacement curves for axial testing which show that the polyaxial systems failed after 40 mm of displacement. (b) The polyaxial screws were slightly less stiff than the monoaxial system and all three-screw systems were stiffer than the external fixator.

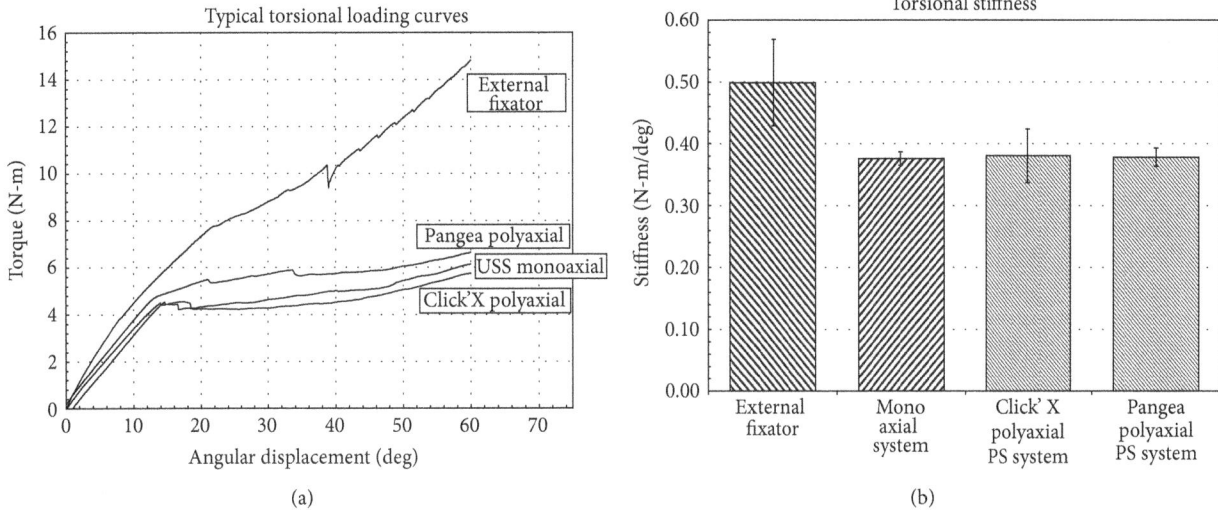

FIGURE 5: Typical torsion loading curves which show that the external fixator is stiffer than the pedicle screw systems.

Thus, there are only $a - 1$ comparisons to be made where $a - 1$ is the number of treatments (excluding the control). The appropriate statistical analysis in this case which controls the overall type I error rate, $a$, is Dunnett's Test [13, 14]. The hypotheses of interest are

$$H_0 : \mu_i = \mu_a, \qquad (1)$$
$$H_1 : \mu_i \neq \mu_a$$

for $i = 1, 2, 3, \ldots, a - 1$. Dunnett's procedure is a modification of the usual $t$-test. For each hypothesis, the observed differences were computed in the sample means and they reject the null hypothesis if

$$|\bar{y}_{i\cdot} - \bar{y}_{a\cdot}| > d_\alpha (a - 1, f) \sqrt{\text{MSE} \left( \frac{1}{n_i} + \frac{1}{n_a} \right)}, \qquad (2)$$

where MSE is the mean square error from a one-way ANOVA and the constant, $d_\alpha(a - 1, f)$, requires special tables and takes into account the degrees of freedom ($f$), number of treatments ($a - 1$), and the type I error rate, $\alpha$. The data was analyzed using Dunnett's Test using a type I error of $\alpha = 0.05$. Using (2), if the absolute value of any paired difference of means between a treatment and control exceeds 0.071 for torsion data or 0.181 for axial data, then the difference is significant.

## 3. Results

*3.1. Distraction Testing in the Elastic Range.* The monoaxial construct was significantly stiffer ($4.008 \pm 0.113$ Nmm) in distraction in the elastic range than the polyaxial systems (Click-x $3.638 \pm 0.108$ Nmm; Pangea Poly $3.634 \pm 0.147$ Nmm) and the external fixator ($2.882 \pm 0.054$ Nmm) ($P < .05$). Both polyaxial constructs were significantly stiffer in distraction in the elastic range than the external fixator ($P < .05$) (Figure 4).

*3.2. Distraction Testing to Failure.* No failures were observed in either the external fixator or monoaxial pedicle screw group when tested up to 75 mm of displacement. Therefore, when tested to failure, the peak loads reported correspond to the maximum load at that displacement which was 360 N for the monoaxial construct and 160 N for the external fixator (Figure 4). The polyaxial (Click-x and Pangea) systems both failed at 40–50 mm displacement. This was due to the rod slipping in the screw head. Yield loads were $157 \pm 4$ N at 45 mm for Click-x and $138 \pm 6$ N at 40 mm for Pangea poly.

*3.3. Torsion Testing.* The external fixator was significantly stiffer in torsion in the elastic range ($0.5 \pm 0.071$ N-m/deg) than the monoaxial ($0.376 \pm 0.011$ N-m/deg), Click-x ($0.382 \pm 0.045$ N-m/deg) or Pangea poly ($0.378 \pm 0.015$ N-m/deg) systems ($P < .05$) (Figure 4). Yield torques were similar for all constructs (Figure 5). The weak points in the constructs were the long Schanz pins that bent in the external fixator and the 6 mm rod and the screw-rod interface. The external fixator bent through the long schanz pins and the pedicle screw constructs moved through the 6 mm bar or the screw rod connector interface.

## 4. Discussion

Historically pelvic fractures have been treated by a variety of closed methods including slings and skeletal traction. With the advent of external fixation for the management of these injuries, improved functional outcomes have been achieved. The application of an external frame anteriorly restores stability in partially stable pelvic fractures [14]. Unstable fractures require anterior and posterior fixation [14, 15]. External fixation plays a role in the acute management of pelvic fractures. However, its role in the definitive management of these injuries is limited [14]. When used for definitive management, the fixator is retained for eight to twelve weeks which allows sufficient healing to occur.

Prolonged use of pelvic external fixation leads to higher incidence of complications. There are reports of a marked difference in the complication rate between temporary and definitive fixators (21% and 62%, resp.) [16].

Using the principles of external fixation, a construct was designed to be placed under the skin which minimizes the possibility of pin tract infection and loosening [1]. This frame (infix) allows patients to sit upright, turn over from side to side, and lie in the prone position [8]. Pedicle screw systems have been reported to be useful for posterior pelvic fixation in scoliosis surgery and in posterior fractures [17], but the ability to place constructs anteriorly required anatomic dissections, examining patients, a definition of the "Bikini Area" as an anatomically stable area in sitting and standing and ultrasound confirmation once placed in patients [6]. It also required the knowledge that pedicle screw fixators were comparable to the standard of care, the external fixator [11, 12]. Results from the present study show that the pedicle screw systems had significantly higher stiffness than the external fixator to counteract distraction, which is the main function of anterior external pelvic fixation. The monoaxial pedicle screw system proved to be superior to the polyaxial screw systems, when tested up to 75 mm of distraction. The use of monoaxial screws to the uninitiated surgeon who tries to use this construct may be challenging since precise placement of the screws is mandatory for positioning of the connecting rod. Conversely, polyaxial screws allow some room for inaccuracies in their placement. It was found that the polyaxial screw constructs tested were still stiffer than the external fixator in distraction up to 40 mm of displacement or $157 \pm 4$ N at 45 mm for Click-x and $138 \pm 6$ N at 40 mm for Pangea after which the rod slid in the screw head. It is rare that the constructs would experience this amount of displacement; however, it has been reported [13] and may be one of the reason that in APC3 injuries, some constructs have demonstrated slippage or failure [8]. We have used monoaxial screws in situations that require excessive tension or added C-rings (Synthes Spine) on the outside of the polyaxial screws where one might see excessive tension or on the inside for lateral compression injuries. This was performed in 2 cases where the construct failed, but the original belief was that the failure was due to cross threading the caps in excessively large individuals [8]. Owen et al. [13] have suggested using 2 infix devices for this type of problem. In these cases, we recommend using monoaxial screws or reinforcing c-rings with polyaxial screws, which are both cheaper than 2 infix devices. Perhaps new implants should be designed to counteract the forces seen in extreme cases and the standard polyaxial pedicle screw implants may be suboptimal in some APC3 injuries.

When tested in torsion, the external fixator showed significantly higher peak torque and torsional stiffness compared to both the monoaxial and polyaxial screw systems. Yield loads for torsion however were similar for all four constructs. Clinically, the vertical displacement of pelvic fractures is unable to be controlled with anterior external fixation alone and posterior fixation is what surgeons use to hold the pelvis in reduction [14].

We have used infix acutely in several damage control situations once we became comfortable with the technique. Monoaxial screws were generally used in these instances as the construct appeared to be superior to the 2 pin external fixator. The construct remained in place until the definitive procedure when we loosened the infix, used the screws to help reduce the posterior injury, fixed the posterior pelvis, and readjusted the infix. In order to consider this, one has to have a set readily available and be very familiar with the technique, otherwise, it is best to use equipment that the surgeon is familiar with.

This study was performed with ultra-high molecular weight polyethylene blocks and simulations of the motions that the constructs would have to resist and is thus limited. The goal was to compare the two pin external fixator verses the pedicle screw fixator construct and not so much the bone screw interface, which appears to have been eliminated by using polyethylene. The screws used for the internal fixation construct, USS monoaxial, Click-x polyaxial, and Pangea polyaxial have thread designs that are made to increase purchase in cancellous bone such as a vertebral body or pelvis. This may also increase the strength of these devices verses the standard Schanz pin thread for the external fixator.

## 5. Conclusion

The biomechanical stability of this novel supra-acetabular internal fixation technique when constructed with traditionally available spinal instrumentation is comparable in stiffness to a two pin external fixator in distraction but less so in torsion. In addition, polyaxial constructs behaved favorably in stiffness testing when compared to monoaxial constructs and the external fixator in distraction. Both of these internal fixation constructs were less stiff than the external fixator in torsional testing. Testing to failure found that polyaxial screws may slip after 4 cm of distraction when the monoaxial screws and external fixator do not. This may be clinically relevant in extreme cases, and the use of monoaxial pedicle screws or to reinforce the polyaxial construct with C-rings on either side is recommended to prevent this. The development of a specific implant for anterior subcutaneous internal fixation may prove beneficial especially one that is able to counteract torsional forces.

## Acknowledgments

The authors would like to thank David J. Svach, Ed McShane, and Michael Bushelow for all the help they provided. Funding was provided by Synthes Spine for this paper.

## References

[1] R. Vaidya, R. Colen, J. Vigdorchik, F. Tonnos, and A. Sethi, "Treatment of unstable pelvic ring injuries with an internal anterior fixator and posterior fixation: initial clinical series," *Journal of Orthopaedic Trauma*, vol. 26, no. 1, pp. 1–8, 2012.

[2] G. J. Haidukewych, S. Kumar, and B. Prpa, "Placement of half-pins for supra-acetabular external fixation: an anatomic study,"

*Clinical Orthopaedics and Related Research*, no. 411, pp. 269–273, 2003.

[3]  W.-Y. Kirn, T. C. Hearn, O. Seleem, E. Mahalingam, D. Stephen, and M. Tile, "Effect of pin location on stability of pelvic external fixation," *Clinical Orthopaedics and Related Research*, no. 361, pp. 237–244, 1999.

[4]  K. Abumi, M. Saita, T. Iida, and K. Kaneda, "Reduction and fixation of sacroiliac joint dislocation by the combined use of S1 pedicle screws and the Galveston technique," *Spine*, vol. 25, no. 15, pp. 1977–1983, 2000.

[5]  K.-J. Ponsen, P. Joosse, G. A. H. van Dijke, and C. J. Snijders, "External fixation of the pelvic ring: an experimental study on the role of pin diameter, pin position, and parasymphyseal fixator pins," *Acta Orthopaedica*, vol. 78, no. 5, pp. 648–653, 2007.

[6]  R. Vaidya, B. Oliphant, R. Jain et al., "The bikini area and bikini line as a location for anterior subcutaneous pelvic fixation: an anatomic and clinical investigation," *Clinical Anatomy*, vol. 26, no. 3, pp. 392–399, 2013.

[7]  D. J. Merriman, W. M. Ricci, C. M. McAndrew, and M. J. Gardner, "Is application of an internal anterior pelvic fixator anatomically feasible?" *Clinical Orthopaedics and Related Research*, vol. 470, no. 8, pp. 2111–2115, 2012.

[8]  R. Vaidya, E. N. Kubiak, P. F. Bergin et al., "Complications of anterior subcutaneous internal fixation for unstable pelvis fractures: a multicenter study," *Clinical Orthopaedics and Related Research*, vol. 470, no. 8, pp. 2124–2131, 2012.

[9]  M. J. Gardner, S. Mehta, A. Mirza, and W. M. Ricci, "Anterior pelvic reduction and fixation using a subcutaneous internal fixator," *Journal of Orthopaedic Trauma*, vol. 26, no. 5, pp. 314–321, 2012.

[10]  R. Vaidya, B. W. Oliphant, I. Hudson, M. Herrema, and D. Knesek, "Sequential reduction and fixation for windswept pelvic ring injuries (LC3) corrects the deformity until healed," *International Orthopaedics*, vol. 37, no. 8, pp. 1555–1560, 2013.

[11]  J. M. Vigdorchik, A. O. Esquivel, X. Jin, K. H. Yang, and R. Vaidya, "Anterior internal fixator versus a femoral distractor and external fixation for sacroiliac joint compression and single stance gait testing: a mechanical study in synthetic bone," *International Orthopaedics*, vol. 37, no. 7, pp. 1341–1346, 2013.

[12]  J. M. Vigdorchik, A. O. Esquivel, X. Jin, K. H. Yang, N. A. Onwudiwe, and R. Vaidya, "Biomechanical stability of a supra-acetabular pedicle screw Internal Fixation device (INFIX) vs External Fixation and plates for vertically unstable pelvic fractures," *Journal of Orthopaedic Surgery and Research*, vol. 7, no. 1, article 31, 2012.

[13]  M. T. Owen, B. Tinkler, and R. Stewart, "Failure and aalvage of "INFIX" instrumentation for pelvic ring disruption in a morbidly obese patient," *Journal of Orthopaedic Trauma*, vol. 27, no. 10, pp. e243–e246, 2013.

[14]  M. Tile, "The management unstable injuries of the pelvic ring," *Journal of Bone and Joint Surgery B*, vol. 81, no. 6, pp. 941–943, 1999.

[15]  E. W. Van den Bosch, R. van der Kleyn, M. Hogervorst, and A. B. van Vugt, "Functional outcome of internal fixation for pelvic ring fractures," *Journal of Trauma*, vol. 47, no. 2, pp. 365–371, 1999.

[16]  W. T. M. Mason, S. N. Khan, C. L. James, T. J. S. Chesser, and A. J. Ward, "Complications of temporary and definitive external fixation of pelvic ring injuries," *Injury*, vol. 36, no. 5, pp. 599–604, 2005.

[17]  K. Abumi, M. Saita, T. Iida, and K. Kaneda, "Reduction and fixation of sacroiliac joint dislocation by the combined use of S1 pedicle screws and the Galveston technique," *Spine*, vol. 25, no. 15, pp. 1977–1983, 2000.

# 28

# Achieving Accurate Ligament Balancing Using Robotic-Assisted Unicompartmental Knee Arthroplasty

**Johannes F. Plate,**[1] **Ali Mofidi,**[2] **Sandeep Mannava,**[1] **Beth P. Smith,**[1] **Jason E. Lang,**[1] **Gary G. Poehling,**[1] **Michael A. Conditt,**[3] **and Riyaz H. Jinnah**[1]

[1] *Department of Orthopaedic Surgery, Wake Forest School of Medicine, Medical Center Boulevard, Winston-Salem, NC 27157-1070, USA*

[2] *Morriston Hospital, Swansea SA6-6NL, UK*

[3] *MAKO Surgical Corp., 2555 Davie Road, Fort Lauderdale, FL 33317, USA*

Correspondence should be addressed to Riyaz H. Jinnah; rjinnah@wakehealth.edu

Academic Editor: William L. Bargar

Unicompartmental knee arthroplasty (UKA) allows replacement of a single compartment in patients with limited disease. However, UKA is technically challenging and relies on accurate component positioning and restoration of natural knee kinematics. This study examined the accuracy of dynamic, real-time ligament balancing using a robotic-assisted UKA system. Surgical data obtained from the computer system were prospectively collected from 51 patients (52 knees) undergoing robotic-assisted medial UKA by a single surgeon. Dynamic ligament balancing of the knee was obtained under valgus stress prior to component implantation and then compared to final ligament balance with the components in place. Ligament balancing was accurate up to 0.53 mm compared to the preoperative plan, with 83% of cases within 1 mm at 0°, 30°, 60°, 90°, and 110° of flexion. Ligamentous laxity of $1.31 \pm 0.13$ mm at 30° of flexion was corrected successfully to $0.78 \pm 0.17$ mm ($P < 0.05$). Robotic-assisted UKA allows accurate and precise reproduction of a surgical balance plan using dynamic, real-time soft-tissue balancing to help restore natural knee kinematics, potentially improving implant survival and functional outcomes.

## 1. Introduction

Unicompartmental knee arthroplasty (UKA) has seen resurgence in the past decade with approximately 51,300 cases performed in 2009 and an estimated growth of 32.5% annually [1–3]. Benefits of UKA compared to total knee arthroplasty include reduced blood loss, reduced perioperative morbidity, faster recovery, shorter rehabilitation, increased postoperative range of motion, and reduced surgical cost [4–9]. However, proper patient selection is vital and the procedure remains technically demanding as the minimally invasive procedure limits surgical exposure and impedes precise component alignment and fixation [3, 6, 10–14]. UKA failures have mainly been attributed to improper component alignment leading to altered knee biomechanics with accelerated polyethylene wear if deformity is undercorrected,

disease progression in other compartments if overcorrected, and anterior knee pain [6, 8, 15–17]. UKA component position and alignment are intricately associated with soft-tissue balancing during this procedure.

UKA allows for minimal disruption of the patient's native anatomy and is intended to restore the normal height of the affected compartment to produce normal ligament tension during the flexion-extension cycle. The success of UKA relies on proper soft-tissue tensioning to obtain a balanced flexion-extension gap and varus-valgus stability [14]. While advances in surgical instrumentation with improved alignment guides and cutting blocks for minimally invasive surgery and navigation systems have improved component positioning in UKA, soft-tissue tensioning is still dependent on surgeon ability and experience. Achieving proper ligament balance throughout the flexion-extension cycle and avoiding tightness or laxity

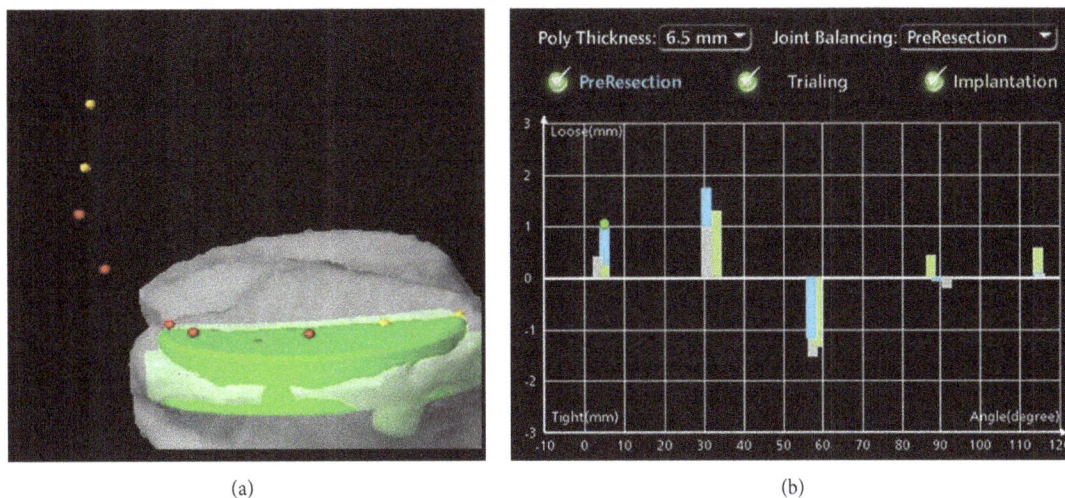

(a)                                                                                    (b)

Figure 1: Ligament balancing was measured throughout various angles during the flexion-extension cycle relative to tibia and mechanical axis. (a) The colored dots represent measurements during femoral range of motion. (b) Intraoperative screenshot of the robotic system showing ligament balance at 0°, 30°, 60°, 90°, and 110° of flexion before resection, with the trial component in place, and after implantation.

are complex and partly rely on component size and position [14, 18]. Increased soft-tissue tightness may decrease the range of motion and increase wear while increased laxity may lead to joint instability and knee pain.

Robotic-assisted UKA allows for improved component positioning [2, 3, 19] with the ability of real-time, dynamic ligament balancing intraoperatively. The robotic system uses optical motion capture technology that dynamically tracks intracortical markers fixed to the tibia and femur. The purpose of the current study was to describe the technique of soft-tissue tensioning and assess the accuracy of robotic-assisted ligament balancing based on an intraoperative balance plan during 52 consecutive medial robotic-assisted medial UKAs. We hypothesized that robotic-assisted UKA accurately produces ligament tension according to an intraoperative balance plan devised before component implantation.

## 2. Material and Methods

*2.1. Robotic-Assisted Ligament Balancing Technique for UKA.* While the surgical technique using a robotic-assisted UKA system has been described elsewhere in detail [6], this paper will focus on how to obtain accurate ligament balance for replacement of the medial compartment. Preoperative CT scans are used by the computer system to render a three-dimensional model of patient anatomy. Intraoperatively, anatomic landmarks are used to register the patient to the robot following intracortical placement of the femoral and tibial marker array. A minimally invasive medial joint incision is made, and medial osteophytes are resected. The knee is then ranged through a number of flexion-extension cycles. Valgus stress is then applied by the surgeon to open up the medial compartment and bring the knee into its "natural" alignment. The ligament balance is then analyzed and displayed by the computer system in real time as deviation from

the optimal tracking pattern of the prosthesis calculated by the computer in millimeters (mm) during numerous flexion-extension cycles at 0°, 30°, 60°, 90°, and 110° of flexion (Figure 1). Negative deviation depicts ligamentous tightness and positive values indicate ligamentous laxity.

The values obtained during the range of motion with valgus stress serve as the intraoperative balance plan for ligamentous tensioning. Using the computer system, component position or size can be altered, and the resulting changes in predicted ligament balance can be observed in real-time. If there is predicted laxity, component size and position can be changed to increase tightness, thereby programming the robot to alter bone cuts based on the preoperative CT scans and intraoperative findings. After the bone resections have been made using the robotic arm, the trial components are inserted and ligamentous tension is compared to the intraoperative balance plan. If proper balance is achieved with the trial components in place, the final components are inserted and cemented, and final ligamentous balance is obtained during range of motion.

*2.2. Assessment of Ligament Balancing Accuracy.* The intraoperative data from 51 consecutive patients (52 knees) who underwent robotic-assisted UKA (MAKOplasty, MAKO Surgical Corp.) of the medial compartment by a single surgeon (RHJ) were prospectively collected over a 6-month period. All patients received a fixed-bearing UKA with an onlay cemented tibial component and cemented femoral component. Following registration of the robotic system and prior to incision, the intraoperative balance plan for ligament tensioning was obtained under valgus stress. After implantation of the final components, dynamic measurements were repeated without valgus stress. Data was stored on the computer system (Figure 1), and the actual ligament balancing was compared to the intraoperative balance plan by subtracting the planned measurements at 0°, 30°, 60°, and 90° of flexion

TABLE 1: Comparison of the intra-operative balance plan and ligament balance measurements following component implantation. Data is expressed as mean ± standard error of the mean in millimeters.

| Flexion angle | Balance plan | After implantation | Change in balance | P value |
|---|---|---|---|---|
| 0° | 0.34 ± 0.12 | 0.08 ± 0.18 | −0.26 ± 0.17 | $P > 0.05$ |
| 30° | 1.31 ± 0.13 | 0.78 ± 0.17 | −0.53 ± 0.18 | $P < 0.05^*$ |
| 60° | −0.28 ± 0.11 | −0.33 ± 0.14 | −0.04 ± 0.15 | $P > 0.05$ |
| 90° | −0.49 ± 0.12 | −0.32 ± 0.13 | 0.16 ± 0.13 | $P > 0.05$ |
| 110° | 0.03 ± 0.16 | −0.07 ± 0.19 | −0.10 ± 0.14 | $P > 0.05$ |

*A $P$ value less than 0.05 was considered statistically significant.

from the actual postoperative measurements. Analysis of variance (ANOVA) was used to compare ligament balance at 0°, 30°, 60°, 90°, and 110° of flexion with Bonferroni post-hoc comparison with alpha 0.05. All data are presented as mean ± standard error of the mean (SEM).

## 3. Results

The mean age of patients in this study was 67 years (range, 50–90 years) with a mean body mass index of 31.4 kg/m$^2$ (range, 21.5–43.8 kg/m$^2$). The surgical indication in all patients was isolated osteoarthritis of the medial compartment of the knee. Intraoperative measurements under valgus stress before component implantation revealed that ligamentous balance significantly changed during the flexion-extension cycle (Figure 2, $P < 0.001$). At 0° (0.34 ± 0.12 mm) and 30° (1.31 ± 0.13 mm) of flexion, the ligaments were relatively loose, at 60° (−0.28 ± 0.11 mm) and 90° (−0.49 ± 0.12 mm) of knee flexion ligaments were relatively tight, and at 110° of flexion close to neutral (0.07 ± 0.15). Comparison of the intraoperative balance plan to measurements after component implantation revealed similar ligament balance at 0° (0.11±0.17 mm), 60° (0.78±0.18 mm), 90° (−0.28±0.13 mm), and 110° (−0.02 ± 0.19 mm) degrees of flexion ($P > 0.05$). Ligament balance at 30° of flexion was significantly reduced (0.88 ± 0.18 mm) after component implantation compared to the intraoperative balance plan indicating tighter ligament balance ($P < 0.05$).

Overall, the variation in ligament tensioning between the intraoperative balance plan and measurements after component implantation was less than 1 mm in 83% of the cases (Table 1 and Figure 3). At 0°, the mean change was −0.26 ± 0.17 mm (range, −4.40–2.20 mm), at 30° −0.53 ± 0.18 mm (range, −5.30–1.80 mm), at 60° −0.04 ± 0.15 mm (range, −3.10–2.30 mm), at 90° 0.16±0.13 mm (range, −2.70–2.00 mm), and at 110° −0.10 ± 0.14 mm (range, −2.2–2.0).

## 4. Discussion and Conclusion

Successful outcomes of UKA rely on the restoration of normal knee kinematics and muscle lever arms of the knee joint. Therefore, restoration of proper ligamentous length and tension is a vital component of the UKA surgical technique. Using a robotic-assisted UKA system, we showed that real-time, dynamic ligament balancing reproduced planned ligamentous balance and, when appropriate, was able to increase

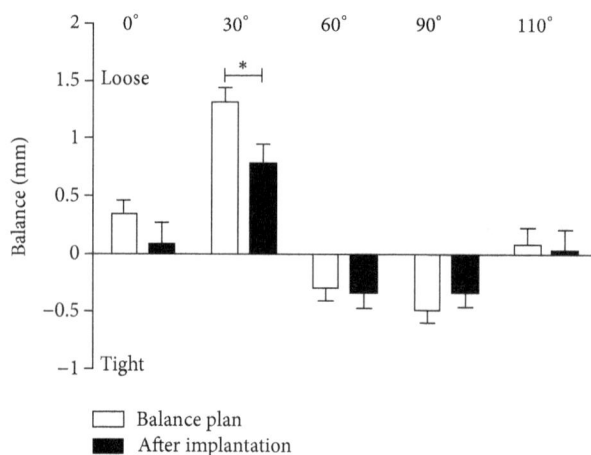

FIGURE 2: Analysis of ligament balance at various degrees of knee flexion. The intraoperative balance plan was similar measurements obtained after component implantation at 0°, 60°, 90°, and 110°. At 30°, ligament balance was relatively loose and surgically corrected, revealing a significant difference ($^*P < 0.05$) between the balance plan and measurements after component implantation.

ligament tightness when there was relative preoperative laxity.

Whiteside pointed out that proper ligament balance in combination with component alignment and fixation is vital for the success of UKA [14]. In a normal knee, the ligaments and menisci control anterior-posterior and varus-valgus movement between the femur and tibia. Medial compartment osteoarthritis with loss of cartilage and bone substance leads to a varus deformity and contracture of the medial capsule and ligaments [20]. The goal of medial UKA for a correctable varus deformity is to restore the normal height of the compartment, thereby achieving ligamentous balance and natural alignment of the joint. This "gap filling" procedure is in contrast to total knee arthroplasty in which bone cuts are made first and then soft-tissues are released to obtain a rectangular flexion-extension gap. Component malpositioning by only 2° during UKA can lead to failure [6, 9, 10, 13, 21], because normal joint biomechanics are altered without achieving proper ligamentous balance possibly leading to increased polyethylene wear and accelerated progression of degenerative disease in the uninvolved compartment [15–17].

During conventional UKA, soft-tissue balance is assessed with the trial components in place and with subjective varus-valgus stress testing, commonly at 0° and 90° [22].

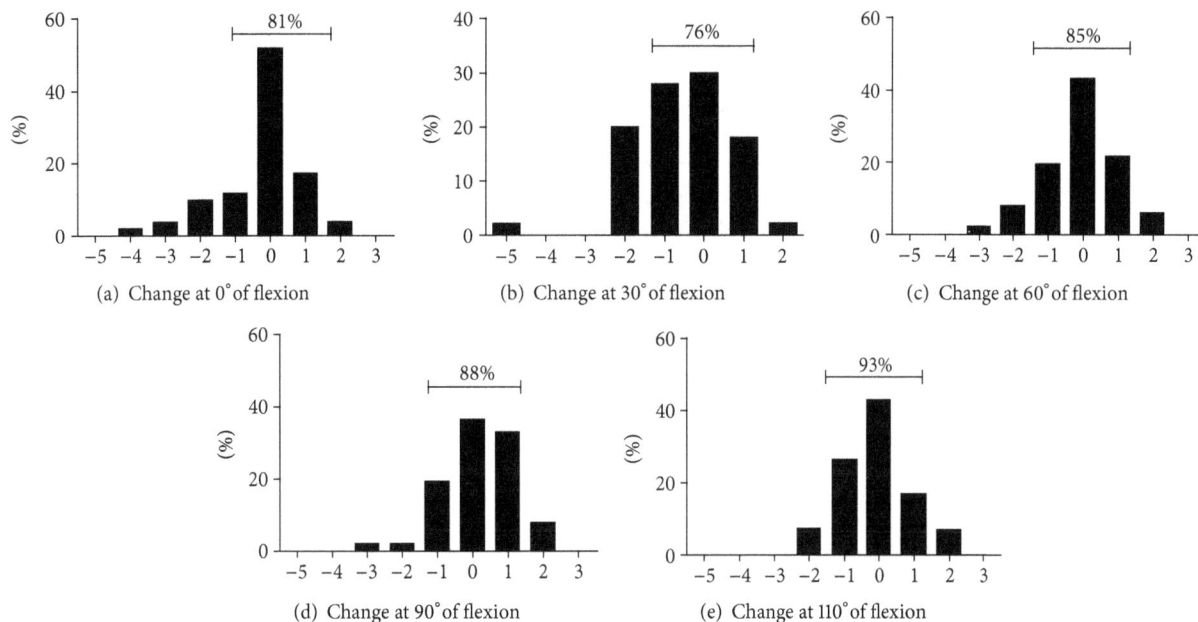

FIGURE 3: At 0° (a), 60° (c), 90° (d), and 110° (e), ligament balance between 1 mm and −1 mm was achieved in 81% to 93% of cases. At 30° (b), 76% of cases were balanced between 1 mm and −1 mm due to a necessary increase in ligament tightness.

The restoration of the normal height of the compartment is vital to achieve proper ligamentous balance. The appropriate ligament balance is left to surgeon's feel and has been described as an art that requires ability and experience [23]. While intraoperative measuring devices are available for total knee arthroplasty [23], their use remains ambiguous and there is currently no such device available for UKA. Navigation systems for UKA have become available to improve component positioning and alignment; however, these systems are incapable of assessing ligament balance. Robotic-assisted systems assess ligamentous balance dynamically and in real-time at various flexion angles. Placing a valgus stress on the knee after medial osteophytes have been removed opens the medial compartment and brings the knee into its natural alignment. These measurements enable the fine tuning of the planned component position to achieve optimal component height and orientation, and thereby ligamentous balance. Following bone resection using the high speed burr with haptic feedback, the femoral and tibial trial components are inserted, and balance measurements are repeated. If necessary, bone cuts can be adjusted for optimal implant orientation. Using a robotic-assisted UKA system, the surgeon has the ability to measure ligament tightness or laxity objectively during dynamic, real-time analysis by the computer system. Natural knee kinematics can be restored based on objective measurements, in addition to surgical acumen.

Specifically, fixed-bearing tibial components, such as the implants used in this study, rely on proper soft-tissue tensioning. There is low conformity between the femoral and tibial components with low contact areas allowing for unconstrained movements between the femur and tibia controlled only by the ligamentous apparatus [24]. Conversely, mobile-bearing UKA systems have high conformity of the tibial and femoral components to increase their contact areas and reduce contact stress. Mobile-bearing systems came in favor to reduce contact stress of the articulating surface thereby preventing polyethylene fatigue and failure [24]. With highly-crosslinked polyethylene components available that are more resistant to wear, Burton et al. and Taddei et al. showed decreased wear during *in vitro* testing with a fixed-bearing UKA compared to a mobile-bearing UKA [24, 25]. In a recent meta-analysis of clinical, radiological, and kinematic outcomes comparing fixed- to mobile-bearing UKA, Smith et al. showed similar improvements and outcomes between 146 mobile-bearing UKAs and 147 fixed-bearing UKAs at a mean 5.8 ± 3.1 years [26]. Despite the design of the prosthesis, proper ligament balance is essential for long-term survival and functional improvements.

There have been numerous advances in UKA instrumentation and cement or cementless fixation techniques that have led to an increase in the survivorship of UKA in the past decade [27, 28]. Minimal invasive instrumentation has become available for more precise component positioning, and improvements in polyethylene components have led to decreased wear. However, robotic-assisted UKA systems have been shown to increase the precision of component placement [2, 19, 29], and the opportunity for real-time, dynamic ligament balancing offers an additional advantage. Dunbar et al. assessed the accuracy of component placement in 20 patients who received postoperative CT scans [29]. In comparison to the preoperative plan, accuracy (root-mean-square error) for femoral and tibial component placement was within 1.6 mm and 3.0° in all directions [29]. Lonner et al. compared tibial component alignments between manual UKA and robotic-assisted UKA and found a greater variance in component position, increased tibial slope, and increased varus alignment when the tibia was prepared manually [19].

A major limitation of this study is the lack of clinical or functional outcomes in this patient cohort; the study was intended to assess the accuracy of ligament tensioning only based upon the intraoperative balance plan. There are currently no studies available on the clinical outcomes of robotic-assisted UKA due to the novelty of the device. Certainly, long-term studies on the outcomes of the robotic-assisted device compared to manual UKA are needed to delineate a possible advantage of the robot in light of the financial investment. However, based on the technical demands of UKA, we believe that improved component positioning and alignment in combination with dynamic, real-time assessment of ligament balance offered by the robotic-assisted system may improve outcomes.

To our knowledge, this is the first study assessing real-time dynamic ligament balancing with a robotic-assisted system for UKA. We conclude from our findings that robotic-assisted UKA can accurately and precisely reproduce intraoperatively planned ligamentous balance using real-time, dynamic measurements. In combination with high accuracy of component placement, robotic-assisted systems may improve functional outcomes and survivorship of UKA patients; however, further investigations into the benefits of robotic systems for UKA are needed.

## Acknowledgments

The authors J. F. Plate, A. Mofidi, S. Mannava, B. P. Smith, and J. E. Lang report no conflict of interests. The authors R. H. Jinnah, G. G. Poehling, and M. A. Conditt have received financial support from MAKO Surgical Corp., Fort Lauderdale, FL, USA. R. H. Jinnah and G. G. Poehling have received payment as consultants and are stock holders. M. A. Conditt receives compensation as Senior Director of Clinical Research. All authors certify that this investigation was performed in conformity with ethical principles of research. Institutional Review Board approval was obtained prior to the study.

## References

[1] M. Hoffman, "MAKO Robotics Yearly Numbers for Unicompartmenal Knee Arthroplasty," Fort Wayne, A. J. Floyd, E-mail, 2010.

[2] A. D. Pearle, P. F. O'Loughlin, and D. O. Kendoff, "Robot-assisted unicompartmental knee arthroplasty," *Journal of Arthroplasty*, vol. 25, no. 2, pp. 230–237, 2010.

[3] M. Roche, P. F. O'Loughlin, D. Kendoff, V. Musahl, and A. D. Pearle, "Robotic arm-assisted unicompartmental knee arthroplasty: preoperative planning and surgical technique," *American Journal of Orthopedics*, vol. 38, no. 2, supplement, pp. 10–15, 2009.

[4] J. M. Bert, "Unicompartmental knee replacement," *Orthopedic Clinics of North America*, vol. 36, no. 4, pp. 513–522, 2005.

[5] T. Borus and T. Thornhill, "Unicompartmental knee arthroplasty," *Journal of the American Academy of Orthopaedic Surgeons*, vol. 16, no. 1, pp. 9–18, 2008.

[6] M. A. Conditt and M. W. Roche, "Minimally invasive robotic-arm-guided unicompartmental knee arthroplasty," *Journal of Bone and Joint Surgery. American*, vol. 91, supplement 1, pp. 63–68, 2009.

[7] J. Y. Jenny, E. Ciobanu, and C. Boeri, "The rationale for navigated minimally invasive unicompartmental knee replacement," *Clinical Orthopaedics and Related Research*, no. 463, pp. 58–62, 2007.

[8] J. H. Lonner, "Indications for unicompartmental knee arthroplasty and rationale for robotic arm-assisted technology," *American Journal of Orthopedics*, vol. 38, no. 2, suplement, pp. 3–6, 2009.

[9] A. D. Pearle, D. Kendoff, and V. Musahl, "Perspectives on computer-assisted orthopaedic surgery: movement toward quantitative orthopaedic surgery," *Journal of Bone and Joint Surgery. American*, vol. 91, no. 1, pp. 7–12, 2009.

[10] S. A. Banks, M. K. Harman, and W. A. Hodge, "Mechanism of anterior impingement damage in total knee arthroplasty," *Journal of Bone and Joint Surgery. American*, vol. 84, no. 2, pp. 37–42, 2002.

[11] G. Li, R. Papannagari, E. Most et al., "Anterior tibial post impingement in a posterior stabilized total knee arthroplasty," *Journal of Orthopaedic Research*, vol. 23, no. 3, pp. 536–541, 2005.

[12] U. I. Maduekwe, M. G. Zywiel, P. M. Bonutti, A. J. Johnson, R. E. Delanois, and M. A. Mont, "Scientific evidence for the use of modern unicompartmental knee arthroplasty," *Expert Review of Medical Devices*, vol. 7, no. 2, pp. 219–239, 2010.

[13] E. M. Mariani, M. H. Bourne, R. T. Jackson, S. T. Jackson, and P. Jones, "Early failure of unicompartmental knee arthroplasty," *Journal of Arthroplasty*, vol. 22, no. 6, supplement, pp. 81–84, 2007.

[14] L. A. Whiteside, "Making your next unicompartmental knee arthroplasty last: three keys to success," *Journal of Arthroplasty*, vol. 20, supplement 3, pp. 2–3, 2005.

[15] M. B. Collier, T. H. Eickmann, F. Sukezaki, J. P. McAuley, and G. A. Engh, "Patient, implant, and alignment factors associated with revision of medial compartment unicondylar arthroplasty," *Journal of Arthroplasty*, vol. 21, no. 6, supplement, pp. 108–115, 2006.

[16] P. Hernigou and G. Deschamps, "Alignment influences wear in the knee after medial unicompartmental arthroplasty," *Clinical Orthopaedics and Related Research*, no. 423, pp. 161–165, 2004.

[17] S. R. Ridgeway, J. P. McAuley, D. J. Ammeen, and G. A. Engh, "The effect of alignment of the knee on the outcome of unicompartmental knee replacement," *Journal of Bone and Joint Surgery. American*, vol. 84, no. 3, pp. 351–355, 2002.

[18] R. H. Emerson, W. C. Head, and P. C. Peters, "Soft tissue balance and alignment in medical unicompartmental knee arthroplasty," *Journal of Bone and Joint Surgery. American*, vol. 74, no. 6, pp. 807–810, 1992.

[19] J. H. Lonner, T. K. John, and M. A. Conditt, "Robotic arm-assisted UKA improves tibial component alignment: a pilot study," *Clinical Orthopaedics and Related Research*, vol. 468, no. 1, pp. 141–146, 2010.

[20] A. Claus and H. P. Scharf, "Ligament balancing and varus deformity in total knee arthroplasty," *Orthopade*, vol. 36, no. 7, pp. 643–649, 2007.

[21] S. E. Park and C. T. Lee, "Comparison of robotic-assisted and conventional manual implantation of a primary total knee arthroplasty," *Journal of Arthroplasty*, vol. 22, no. 7, pp. 1054–1059, 2007.

[22] W. M. Mihalko, K. J. Saleh, K. A. Krackow, and L. A. Whiteside, "Soft-tissue balancing during total knee arthroplasty in the varus knee," *Journal of the American Academy of Orthopaedic Surgeons*, vol. 17, no. 12, pp. 766–774, 2009.

[23] D. D. D'Lima, S. Patil, N. Steklov, and C. W. Colwell, "An ABJS best paper: dynamic intraoperative ligament balancing for total knee arthroplasty," *Clinical Orthopaedics and Related Research*, no. 463, pp. 208–212, 2007.

[24] A. Burton, S. Williams, C. L. Brockett, and J. Fisher, "*In vitro* comparison of fixed- and mobile meniscal-bearing unicondylar knee arthroplasties. Effect of design, kinematics, and condylar liftoff," *Journal of Arthroplasty*, vol. 27, no. 8, pp. 1452–1459, 2012.

[25] P. Taddei, E. Modena, T. M. Grupp, and S. Affatato, "Mobile or fixed unicompartmental knee prostheses? *In-vitro* wear assessments to solve this dilemma," *Journal of the Mechanical Behavior of Biomedical Materials*, vol. 4, no. 8, pp. 1936–1946.

[26] T. O. Smith, C. B. Hing, L. Davies, and S. T. Donell, "Fixed versus mobile bearing unicompartmental knee replacement: a meta-analysis," *Orthopaedics and Traumatology*, vol. 95, no. 8, pp. 599–605, 2009.

[27] G. Labek, K. Sekyra, W. Pawelka, W. Janda, and B. Stöckl, "Outcome and reproducibility of data concerning the Oxford unicompartmental knee arthroplasty: a structured literature review including arthroplasty registry data," *Acta Orthopaedica*, vol. 82, no. 2, pp. 131–135, 2011.

[28] A. V. Lombardi, K. R. Berend, M. E. Berend et al., "Current controversies in partial knee arthroplasty," *Instructional Course Lectures*, vol. 61, pp. 347–381, 2012.

[29] N. J. Dunbar, M. W. Roche, B. H. Park, S. H. Branch, M. A. Conditt, and S. A. Banks, "Accuracy of dynamic tactile-guided unicompartmental knee arthroplasty," *Journal of Arthroplasty*, vol. 27, no. 5, pp. 803–808.e1, 2012.

# 29

# Dynamic Stabilisation in the Treatment of Degenerative Disc Disease with Modic Changes

**Olcay Eser,**[1] **Cengiz Gomleksiz,**[2] **Mehdi Sasani,**[3] **Tunc Oktenoglu,**[3] **Ahmet Levent Aydin,**[4] **Yaprak Ataker,**[5] **Tuncer Suzer,**[3] **and Ali Fahir Ozer**[6]

[1] *Department of Neurosurgery, School of Medicine, Afyon Kocatepe University, Afyonkarahisar, Turkey*
[2] *Department of Neurosurgery, Ordu Medical Park Hospital, Ordu, Turkey*
[3] *Department of Neurosurgery, American Hospital, Istanbul, Turkey*
[4] *Neurosurgery Department, Istanbul Physical Therapy and Rehabilitation Hospital, Istanbul, Turkey*
[5] *Physical Therapy and Rehabilitation Department, American Hospital, Istanbul, Turkey*
[6] *Department of Neurosurgery, School of Medicine, Koc University, Rumelifeneri Yolu Sarıyer, Istanbul 34450, Turkey*

Correspondence should be addressed to Ali Fahir Ozer; alifahirozer@gmail.com

Academic Editor: Deniz Erbulut

*Objective.* Posterior dynamic stabilization is an effective alternative to fusion in the treatment of chronic instability and degenerative disc disease (DDD) of the lumbar spine. This study was undertaken to investigate the efficacy of dynamic stabilization in chronic degenerative disc disease with Modic types 1 and 2. Modic types 1 and 2 degeneration can be painful. Classic approach in such cases is spine fusion. We operated 88 DDD patients with Modic types 1 and 2 via posterior dynamic stabilization. Good results were obtained after 2 years of followup. *Methods.* A total of 88 DDD patients with Modic types 1 and 2 were selected for this study. The patients were included in the study between 2004 and 2010. All of them were examined with lumbar anteroposterior (AP) and lateral X-rays. Lordosis of the lumbar spine, segmental lordosis, and ratio of the height of the intervertebral disc spaces (IVSs) were measured preoperatively and at 3, 12, and 24 months after surgery. Magnetic resonance imaging (MRI) analysis was carried out, and according to the data obtained, the grade of disc degeneration was classified. The quality of life and pain scores were evaluated by visual analog scale (VAS) score and Oswestry Disability Index (ODI) preoperatively and at 3, 12, and 24 months after surgery. Appropriate statistical method was chosen. *Results.* The mean 3- and 12-month postoperative IVS ratio was significantly greater than that of the preoperative group ($P < 0.001$). However, the mean 1 and 2 postoperative IVS ratio was not significantly different ($P > 0.05$). Furthermore, the mean preoperative and 1 and 2 postoperative angles of lumbar lordosis and segmental lordosis were not significantly different ($P > 0.05$). The mean VAS score and ODI, 3, 12, and 24 months after surgery, decreased significantly, when compared with the preoperative scores in the groups ($P = 0.000$). *Conclusion.* Dynamic stabilization in chronic degenerative disc disease with Modic types 1 and 2 was effective.

## 1. Introduction

Chronic low back pain (LBP) has been one of the most common causes of disability in adults and is a very important disease for early retirement in industrialized societies. Degenerative disc disease (DDD) is the most frequent problem in patients with LBP. The prevalence of Modic changes among patients with DDD of the lumbar spine varies between 19% and 59%. Type 1 and 2 Modic changes are more common than type 3 and mixed changes [1–13].

Degenerative vertebral endplate and subchondral bone marrow changes were first noted on magnetic resonance imaging (MRI) by Roos et al. in 1987 [1]. A formal classification was subsequently provided by Modic et al. in 1988, based on a study of 474 patients, most of whom had chronic LBP [2]. They were found to be associated with DD [1–3]. Three different types have been described [2, 3]. Type I lesions (low T1 and high T2 signals) are assumed to indicate an ongoing active degenerative process. Type II lesions (high T1 and T2 signals) are thought to manifest a more stable and chronic degeneration. Type III lesions (low T1 and T2 signals) are associated with subchondral bone sclerosis. Modic changes are interesting because an association between Modic changes and LBP symptoms has been shown recently in population-based cohorts [10, 12, 14].

Kjaer et al. suggested that Modic changes constitute the crucial element in the degenerative process around the disk in relation to LBP and clinical findings [14]. They demonstrated that DDD on its own was a fairly quiet disorder, whereas DDD with Modic changes was much more frequently associated with clinical symptoms. Most authors agree that among Modic changes, type 1 changes are those that are most strongly associated with symptomatic LBP [5, 7, 12, 13]. Braithwaite et al. suggested that vertebral endplate could be a possible source of discogenic LBP [4]. Therefore, Modic changes appear to be a relatively specific but insensitive sign of a painful lumbar disc in patients with discogenic LBP.

Buttermann et al. suggested that abnormal endplates associated with inflammation are a source of pain, and treating endplates directly with anterior fusion may be a preferred treatment for this subset of degenerative patients [15]. Chataigner et al. suggested that anterior fusion is effective for the treatment of LBP due to DDD when associated with vertebral plate changes [16]. Fritzell et al. reported that posterior lumbar fusion in patients with severe chronic LBP can diminish pain and decrease disability more efficiently than commonly used nonsurgical treatment, through a prospective multicenter randomized controlled trial from the Swedish Lumbar Spine Study Group [17]. Kwon et al. suggested that PLIF procedures in which TFC is used in patients with Modic types 1 and 2 showed an acceptably high success and fusion rate [18].

Segmental fusion operations are performed frequently as treatment for DDD with Modic types 1 and 2. Nevertheless, fusion also carries various risks such as adjacent segment degeneration, bone graft donor place pain, and pseudoarthrosis [19–22]. Dynamic stabilization controls abnormal movements in an unstable, painful segment and facilitates healthy load transfer, preventing degeneration of the adjacent segment [23]. Recently, several clinical studies reported that dynamic stabilization yielded good clinical results and represented a safe and effective alternative technique to spine arthrodesis in selected cases of degenerative lumbar spine instability [24–26].

The purpose of the current study was to assess the efficacy of dynamic stabilization in DDD with Modic types 1 and 2.

## 2. Materials and Methods

A total of 88 DDD patients with Modic types 1 and 2 were selected for this study. The patients were included in the study between 2004 and 2010. Among them, 70 patients showed Modic type 1 (80%) and 18 patients exhibited Modic type 2 (20%). The study patients consisted of 30 males and 58 females, with a mean age of 45 years (range: 25–65 years). All the patients received surgery, with 59 patients at L4-5 level (67%), 22 patients at L5-S1 level (25%), and 7 patients at L3-4

level (8%). Furthermore, 23 patients had (26 %) grade 3 and 65 patients had (74%) grade 4 disc degeneration.

Patients were informed about the operation. All the patients completed the consent forms. The patients had leg and/or chronic LBP, and those who had previously undergone spinal surgery were excluded. We also excluded patients with spinal tumor, infection, spondylolisthesis, traumatic vertebral fracture, scoliosis, and serious systemic disease. Patients were diagnosed to have DDD with Modic changes on MRI. All patients were examined with lumbar anteroposterior (A-P) and lateral X-rays. *Cosmic* (Ulrich GmbH & Co. KG, Ulm, Germany) and *Safinaz* (Medikon *AS*, Turkey) dynamic pedicle screws and rigid rod system were used together with the microdiscectomy procedure in all patients.

*2.1. Evaluation of Quality and Pain Scores.* The quality of life and pain scores were evaluated using visual analog scale (VAS) score (0, no pain; 10, worst pain) and Oswestry Disability Index (ODI) both preoperatively and at 3, 12, and 24 months after surgery (Table 2).

*2.2. Radiological Analysis.* The patients underwent preoperative MRI and/or computed tomography (CT). Furthermore, all patients had AP and lateral standing X-rays of the lumbar spine preoperatively and at 3 (1 postoperative), 12 (2 postoperative), and 24 months (3 postoperative) after surgery. Lordosis of the lumbar spine (L1-S1) was measured as the angle between the lines drawn on lateral standing X-rays from the lower endplate of L1 and upper endplate of S1. Segmental lordosis of the operative level (or levels) was measured as the angle between lines drawn from the upper and lower endplates of the vertebrae across which instrumentation spanned preoperatively as well as 3, 12, and 24 months after surgery. The ratio of the height of the intervertebral disc spaces (IVSs) to the vertebral body height was measured and compared preoperatively and postoperatively. The IVS ratio was calculated as the mean anterior and posterior intervertebral disc height divided by the vertebral height of the rostral vertebra of the motion segment.

*2.3. MRI Evaluation.* Lumber sagittal MRI was performed with a slice of 5 mm thickness. A T2-weighted image with a repetition of 2500 msec and an echo time of 90 msec of the lumbar spine was taken for all the participants. The signal intensity of nucleus pulposus of the discs L2-L3, L3-L4, L4-L5, and L5-S1 was evaluated independently by three radiologists. The grade of disc degeneration was determined according to Schneiderman's classification: Grade 1, normal signal intensity; Grade 2, heterogeneous decreased signal intensity; Grade 3, diffuse loss of signal; Grade 4, signal void. MRI analysis was carried out, and according to the data obtained, the grade of disc degeneration was classified as mild (Grades 1-2), and severe (Grades 3-4).

In this study, before surgery, endplate abnormalities were divided into Modic type 1 signals (low intensity on T1-weighted spin-echo images and high intensity on T2-weighted spin-echo images) and Modic type 2 signals (high intensity on both T1- and T2-weighted spin-echo images).

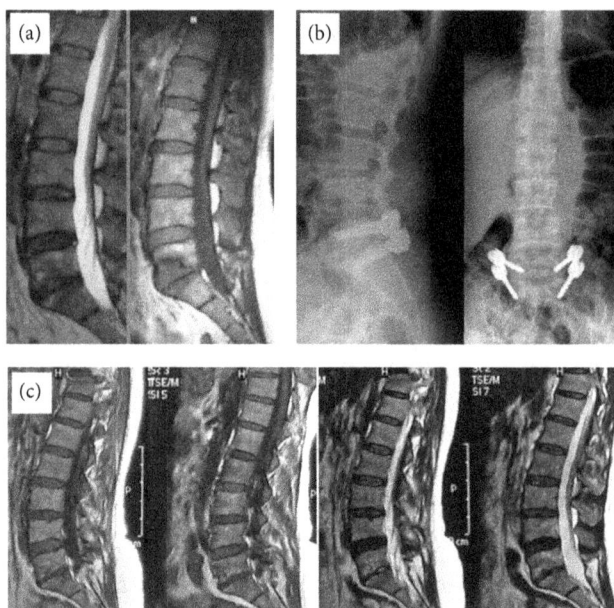

FIGURE 1: A 43-year-old female patient complained of severe back pain, particularly when standing or walking. (a) T1- and T2-weighted images showing hypointense corpus changes in upper and lower endplates. (b) Dynamic stabilization carried out with Safinaz screws. (c) T1- and T2-weighted MR images showing degenerative changes that shifted to Modic type 3, 2 years later.

*2.4. Operative Technique.* All patients were taken into the operating room under general anesthesia in the prone position. Prophylactic antibiotics were given to all of them before the operation. All operations were performed using operational microscopy and standard surgical technique. The level of operation was determined via intraoperative fluoroscopy. When the interlaminar level with disc herniation was approached from the medial aspect, laminotomy was widened with the help of a high-speed drill. After identifying the correct nerve root, free disc fragments under the nerve root and passageway were removed. Decompression was completed by performing the required laminotomy. After carrying out the microdecompression procedure, we also executed posterior dynamic transpedicular stabilization from the same incision with the help of lateral intraoperative fluoroscopy using Wiltse approach via inside lateral paravertebral muscle. The dynamic pedicle hinged screws used in our cases were Cosmic (Ulrich Gmbh & Co. KG, Ulm, Germany) and Safinaz (Medikon, Turkey), in combination with rigid rods (Figure 1).

*2.5. Statistical Methods.* Kolmogorov-Smirnov test was used for homogeneity of the groups to comply with the normal distribution test. Friedman and Wilcoxon test was used for statistical analysis.

## 3. Results

In Table 1, the median, minimum and maximum range, Lumbar lordosis, $\alpha$ angle, and IVS value are given. The mean 1, 2, and 3 postoperative IVS ratio was significantly greater than that of the preoperative group ($P < 0.001$, Table 1). However, the mean 1 and 2 postoperative IVS ratio was not significantly different ($P > 0.05$). The mean preoperative and 1, 2, and 3 postoperative angles of lumbar lordosis and segmental lordosis were not significantly different ($P > 0.05$). Furthermore, the mean lumbar lordosis preoperative and 1, 2, and 3 postoperative values were not significantly different ($P > 0.05$).

All cases of Modic type 1 degeneration upgraded to type 2 or 3 degeneration after 24 months without pain.

From Table 2, it can be noted that the mean VAS pain score and ODI score 3, 12, and 24 months after surgery decreased significantly, when compared with the preoperative scores in the groups ($P = 0.000$). Furthermore, 24 months after surgery, the mean VAS score and ODI score decreased significantly, when compared with preoperative scores and postoperative 3- and 12-month scores in the groups ($P = 0.000$).

## 4. Discussion

Abnormalities of the vertebral endplate and vertebral bone marrow were described by Modic et al. [2]. Abnormalities associated with decreased signal intensity on T1-weighted spin-echo images (Modic type 1) correlated with segmental hypermobility and LBP [3]. Fayad et al. found that patients with chronic LBP and predominantly type 1 inflammatory Modic changes had better short-term relief of symptoms following intradiscal steroid injection than those with predominantly type 2 changes, which further supports the inflammatory nature of Modic type 1 changes and the role of inflammation in the generation of LBP [27]. Two recent publications suggest a possible relationship between bone marrow abnormalities revealed by MRI and discogenic pain [4, 28]. In these studies, moderate and severe types 1 and 2 endplate abnormalities were considered abnormal, and all the tested discs caused concordant pain on provocation [6]. Ohtori et al. reported that endplate abnormalities in patients with discogenic pain are related to inflammation and axonal growth into the abnormal bone marrow induced by cytokines, such as tumor necrosis factor-$\alpha$ [29]. Thus, tumor necrosis factor-$\alpha$ expression and sensory nerve in-growth in abnormal endplates may be a cause of LBP [29].

It has been reported that Modic type 1 change is associated with pathology, including disruption and fissuring of the endplate with regions of degeneration and regeneration and vascular granulation tissue [2, 5]. In addition, an increased amount of reactive woven bone as well as prominent osteoclasts and osteoblasts has been observed [2]. It has been reported that there were increases in the amount of cytokines and the density of sensory nerve fibers in the endplate and bone marrow in Modic type 1 change, when compared with normal subjects, strongly suggesting that the endplates and vertebral bodies are the sources of pain [29, 30]. These reports suggest that Modic type 1 signal shows an active inflammatory stage [2, 5, 29, 30]. In contrast, type 2 changes were found to be associated with fatty degeneration of the red marrow and its replacement by yellow marrow. Thus, it

TABLE 1: Results of radiological lumbar lordosis, $\alpha$ angle, and intervertebral space (IVS).

|  | Preop | Postop (3 months) | Postop (12 months) | Postop (24 months) | P value |
|---|---|---|---|---|---|
| Lumbar lordosis (LL) |  |  |  |  |  |
| Median | 44.85 | 43.45 | 43.86 | 43.56 | 0.059 |
| Min–max | 14–72 | 18–70 | 18–71 | 17–69 |  |
| $\alpha$ angle |  |  |  |  |  |
| Median | 10.17 | 9.98 | 9.93 | 10.06 | 0.685 |
| Min–max | 1–30 | 0–33 | 0–31 | 2–32 |  |
| Intervertebral space (IVS) |  |  |  |  |  |
| Median | 0.28 | 0.27 | 0.28 | 0.28 | 0.029 |
| Min–max | 0-0 | 0-0 | 0-0 | 0-0 |  |

Friedman test (mean and $P$ value); Wilcoxon Signed Ranks Test IVS (preop 3 months: $P < 0.005$, preop 12 months: $P < 0.004$, and preop 24 months: $P < 0.005$).

TABLE 2: Comparison of the outcomes of visual analog scale (VAS) and Oswestry Disability Index (ODI) scores in the groups. Both groups exhibited significant reduction in pain over time.

|  | Mean | Comparison | | P value |
|---|---|---|---|---|
| Visual analog scale (VAS) | Preop: 7.20 3 months: 2.70 12 months: 1.53 24 months: 0.95 | Preop: 3 months Preop: 12 months Preop: 24 months 3–12 months | 3–24 months 12–24 months | 0.000 |
| Oswestry Disability Index (ODI) | Preop: 65.90 3 months: 22.80 12 months: 11.10 24 months: 4.94 | Preop: 3 months Preop: 12 months Preop: 24 months 3–12 months | 3–24 months 12–24 months | 0.000 |

Friedman test (mean and $P$ value); Wilcoxon Signed Ranks Test.

had been concluded that type 1 changes correspond to the inflammatory stage of DDD and indicate an ongoing active degenerative process, whereas type 2 changes represent the fatty stage of DDD and are related to a more stable and chronic process.

In the study by Toyone et al. [5], 70% of the patients with type 1 Modic changes and 16% of those with type 2 changes were found to have segmental hypermobility, defined as a sagittal translation of 3 mm or more on dynamic flexion-extension films [5]. In a study assessing osseous union following lumbar fusion in 33 patients, Lang et al. found that all 19 patients with solid fusion had type 2 Modic changes, whereas 10 of the 14 patients with nonunion had type 1 changes [31, 32]. They suggested that Modic type 1 in patients with unstable fusions might be related to reparative granulation tissue, inflammation, edema, and hyperemic changes. They concluded that the persistence of type 1 Modic changes after fusion suggests pseudoarthrosis. Similarly, Buttermann et al. observed that nonfusion was associated predominantly with the persistence of type 1 Modic changes [15]. There are patients having very low back pain Modic type 1 and in addition patients with unbearable pain will spend for the failed fusion surgery. For this reason, we performed dynamic stabilization in Modic type 1 and 2 patients.

Hinged screw systems have been used for posterior dynamic stabilization in the current series. The advantages of this system are as follows. (i) These systems stabilize the spine and restore the neutral zone [33–35]. (ii) They provide a simple surgery, when compared with anterior, posterior, or combined fusion surgery. (iii) These types of dynamic systems allow performing lumbar lordosis during the surgery. (iv) Pseudoarthrosis rate is high in cases with fusion surgery [16, 31]. (v) The clinical experience demonstrated good results in the literature [36, 37].

Chataigner et al. studied 56 patients who underwent anterior procedures with bone grafting for LBP [16]. Their best results were obtained in patients with Modic type 1 lesions. The results were poorer in patients who had black discs without endplate involvement or Modic type 2 lesions. Among five nonunions, three requiring posterior revision surgery were observed in Modic type 2 changes. Anterior surgery, with disc herniation associated with Modic type 1 or 2 as the basis for the implementation of changes, is difficult. Because these patients for the treatment of disc herniation and discectomy ago posterior made, then the patients given the same or a different session, the anterior position to apply the anterior fusion surgery. Anterior surgery is time consuming and is an intervention method with a high likelihood of complications. For these patients instead of an application, we propose a posterior dynamic stabilization.

Kwon et al. studied the long-term efficacy of PLIF with a threaded fusion cage based on vertebral endplate changes in DDD [18]. They found that the fusion rate was 80.8% for patients with Modic type 1 changes, 83.6% with Modic type 2 changes, and 54.5% with Modic type 3 changes. Furthermore, the nonfusion rate was 20%. This ratio is higher for patients with Modic type 1 as a high proportion of patients continue to complain about pain and do not see the benefits of treatment. Vital et al. assessed the clinical and radiological outcomes following instrumented posterolateral fusion in 17 patients with chronic LBP and type 1 Modic changes [32]. Six months later, all type 1 changes had converted, with 76.5% being converted to type 2 changes and 23.5% back to normal, and clinical improvement was seen in all patients. They concluded that fusion accelerates the course of type 1 Modic changes probably by correcting the mechanical instability, and that these changes appear to be a good indicator of satisfactory surgical outcome after arthrodesis.

The natural course of the signal anomalies reported by Modic et al. was subsequently followed up by the same authors [2]. Five of the six type 1 lesions were replaced by type 2 signal anomalies over 14–36 months. The type 2 lesions remained stable over 2-3 years of follow-up evaluation. Lang et al. showed that the persistence of Modic type 1 signal after arthrodesis suggests pseudoarthrosis [31]. Toyone et al. concluded that Modic type 1 signal is associated with instability, requiring arthrodesis more commonly than Modic type 2 change, which can accompany nerve-root compromise [5].

In brief, we can state that Modic type 1 changes are associated with instability and painful disorders connected with instability. In such cases, posterior dynamic stabilization could be an effective and alternative treatment modality.

# References

[1] A. de Roos, H. Kressel, C. Spritzer, and M. Dalinka, "MR imaging of marrow changes adjacent to end plates in degenerative lumbar disk disease," *The American Journal of Roentgenology*, vol. 149, no. 3, pp. 531–534, 1987.

[2] M. T. Modic, P. M. Steinberg, J. S. Ross, T. J. Masaryk, and J. R. Carter, "Degenerative disk disease: assessment of changes in vertebral body marrow with MR imaging," *Radiology*, vol. 166, no. 1, pp. 193–199, 1988.

[3] M. T. Modic, T. J. Masaryk, J. S. Ross, and J. R. Carter, "Imaging of degenerative disk disease," *Radiology*, vol. 168, no. 1, pp. 177–186, 1988.

[4] I. Braithwaite, J. White, A. Saifuddin, P. Renton, and B. A. Taylor, "Vertebral end-plate (Modic) changes on lumbar spine MRI: correlation with pain reproduction at lumbar discography," *European Spine Journal*, vol. 7, no. 5, pp. 363–368, 1998.

[5] T. Toyone, K. Takahashi, H. Kitahara, M. Yamagata, M. Murakami, and H. Moriya, "Vertebral bone-marrow changes in degenerative lumbar disc disease: an MRI study of 74 patients with low back pain," *Journal of Bone and Joint Surgery B*, vol. 76, no. 5, pp. 757–764, 1994.

[6] D. Weishaupt, M. Zanetti, J. Hodler et al., "Painful lumbar disk derangement: relevance of endplate abnormalities at MR imaging," *Radiology*, vol. 218, no. 2, pp. 420–427, 2001.

[7] D. Mitra, V. N. Cassar-Pullicino, and I. W. Mccall, "Longitudinal study of vertebral type-1 end-plate changes on MR of the lumbar spine," *European Radiology*, vol. 14, no. 9, pp. 1574–1581, 2004.

[8] G. Schmid, A. Witteler, R. Willburger, C. Kuhnen, M. Jergas, and O. Koester, "Lumbar disk herniation: correlatlon of histologic findings with marrow signal intensity changes in vertebral endplates at MR imaging," *Radiology*, vol. 231, no. 2, pp. 352–358, 2004.

[9] M. Karchevsky, M. E. Schweitzer, J. A. Carrino, A. Zoga, D. Montgomery, and L. Parker, "Reactive endplate marrow changes: a systematic morphologic and epidemiologic evaluation," *Skeletal Radiology*, vol. 34, no. 3, pp. 125–129, 2005.

[10] P. Kjaer, C. Leboeuf-Yde, L. Korsholm, J. S. Sorensen, and T. Bendix, "Magnetic resonance imaging and low back pain in adults: a diagnostic imaging study of 40-year-old men and women," *Spine*, vol. 30, no. 10, pp. 1173–1180, 2005.

[11] M. Kuisma, J. Karppinen, J. Niinimäki et al., "A three-year follow-up of lumbar spine endplate (Modic) changes," *Spine*, vol. 31, no. 15, pp. 1714–1718, 2006.

[12] M. Kuisma, J. Karppinen, J. Niinimäki et al., "Modic changes in endplates of lumbar vertebral bodies: prevalence and association with low back and sciatic pain among middle-aged male workers," *Spine*, vol. 32, no. 10, pp. 1116–1122, 2007.

[13] H. B. Albert and C. Manniche, "Modic changes following lumbar disc herniation," *European Spine Journal*, vol. 16, no. 7, pp. 977–982, 2007.

[14] P. Kjaer, L. Korsholm, T. Bendix, J. S. Sorensen, and C. Leboeuf-Yde, "Modic changes and their associations with clinical findings," *European Spine Journal*, vol. 15, no. 9, pp. 1312–1319, 2006.

[15] G. R. Buttermann, K. B. Heithoff, J. W. Ogilvie, E. E. Transfeldt, and M. Cohen, "Vertebral body MRI related to lumbar fusion results," *European Spine Journal*, vol. 6, no. 2, pp. 115–120, 1997.

[16] H. Chataigner, M. Onimus, and A. Polette, "Surgery for degenerative lumbar disc disease. Should the black disc be grafted?" *Revue de Chirurgie Orthopedique et Reparatrice de l'Appareil Moteur*, vol. 84, no. 7, pp. 583–589, 1998.

[17] P. Fritzell, O. Hägg, P. Wessberg, and A. Nordwall, "2001 Volvo award winner in clinical studies: lumbar fusion versus nonsurgical treatment for chronic low back pain. A multicenter randomized controlled trial from the Swedish lumbar spine study group," *Spine*, vol. 26, no. 23, pp. 2521–2534, 2001.

[18] Y. M. Kwon, D. K. Chin, B. H. Jin, K. S. Kim, Y. E. Cho, and S. U. Kuh, "Long term efficacy of posterior lumbar interbody fusion with standard cages alone in lumbar disc diseases combined with modic changes," *Journal of Korean Neurosurgical Society*, vol. 46, no. 4, pp. 322–327, 2009.

[19] M. D. Rahm and B. B. Hall, "Adjacent-segment degeneration after lumbar fusion with instrumentation: a retrospective study," *Journal of Spinal Disorders*, vol. 9, no. 5, pp. 392–400, 1996.

[20] J. Zucherman, K. Hsu, G. Picetti, A. White, G. Wynne, and L. Taylor, "Clinical efficacy of spinal instrumentation in lumbar degenerative disc disease," *Spine*, vol. 17, no. 7, pp. 834–837, 1992.

[21] M. Putzier, S. V. Schneider, J. F. Funk, S. W. Tohtz, and C. Perka, "The surgical treatment of the lumbar disc prolapse: nucleotomy with additional transpedicular dynamic stabilization versus nucleotomy alone," *Spine*, vol. 30, no. 5, pp. E109–E114, 2005.

[22] J. C. Banwart, M. A. Asher, and R. S. Hassanein, "Iliac crest bone graft harvest donor site morbidity: a statistical evaluation," *Spine*, vol. 20, no. 9, pp. 1055–1060, 1995.

[23] D. K. Sengupta, "Dynamic stabilization devices in the treatment of low back pain," *Neurology India*, vol. 53, no. 4, pp. 466–474, 2005.

[24] T. Kaner, M. Sasani, T. Oktenoglu, M. Cosar, and A. F. Ozer, "Utilizing dynamic rods with dynamic screws in the surgical treatment of chronic instability: a prospective clinical study," *Turkish Neurosurgery*, vol. 19, no. 4, pp. 319–326, 2009.

[25] G. S. Sapkas, G. S. Themistocleous, A. F. Mavrogenis, I. S. Benetos, N. Metaxas, and P. J. Papagelopoulos, "Stabilization of the lumbar spine using the dynamic neutralization system," *Orthopedics*, vol. 30, no. 10, pp. 859–865, 2007.

[26] O. Ricart and J. M. Serwier, "Dynamic stabilisation and compression without fusion using Dynesys for the treatment of degenerative lumbar spondylolisthesis: a prospective series of 25 cases," *Revue de Chirurgie Orthopedique et Reparatrice de l'Appareil Moteur*, vol. 94, no. 7, pp. 619–627, 2008.

[27] F. Fayad, M. M. Lefevre-Colau, F. Rannou et al., "Relation of inflammatory modic changes to intradiscal steroid injection outcome in chronic low back pain," *European Spine Journal*, vol. 16, no. 7, pp. 925–931, 2007.

[28] H. S. Sandhu, L. P. Sanchez-Caso, H. K. Parvataneni, F. P. Cammisa, F. P. Girardi, and B. Ghelman, "Association between findings of provocative discography and vertebral endplate signal changes as seen on MRI," *Journal of Spinal Disorders*, vol. 13, no. 5, pp. 438–443, 2000.

[29] S. Ohtori, G. Inoue, T. Ito et al., "Tumor necrosis factor-immunoreactive cells and PGP 9.5-immunoreactive nerve fibers in vertebral endplates of patients with discogenic low back pain and modic type 1 or type 2 changes on MRI," *Spine*, vol. 31, no. 9, pp. 1026–1031, 2006.

[30] M. F. Brown, M. V. J. Hukkanen, I. D. McCarthy et al., "Sensory and sympathetic innervation of the vertebral endplate in patients with degenerative disc disease," *Journal of Bone and Joint Surgery B*, vol. 79, no. 1, pp. 147–153, 1997.

[31] P. Lang, N. Chafetz, H. K. Genant, and J. M. Morris, "Lumbar spine fusion: assessment of functional stability with magnetic resonance imaging," *Spine*, vol. 15, no. 6, pp. 581–588, 1990.

[32] J. M. Vital, O. Gille, V. Pointillart et al., "Course of Modic 1 six months after lumbar posterior osteosynthesis," *Spine*, vol. 28, no. 7, pp. 715–720, 2003.

[33] C. Schilling, S. Krüger, T. M. Grupp, G. N. Duda, W. Blömer, and A. Rohlmann, "The effect of design parameters of dynamic pedicle screw systems on kinematics and load bearing: an in vitro study," *European Spine Journal*, vol. 20, no. 2, pp. 297–307, 2011.

[34] W. Schmoelz, J. F. Huber, T. Nydegger, Dipl-Ing, L. Claes, and H. J. Wilke, "Dynamic stabilization of the lumbar spine and its effects on adjacent segments: an in vitro experiment," *Journal of Spinal Disorders and Techniques*, vol. 16, no. 4, pp. 418–423, 2003.

[35] H. Bozkuş, M. Şenoğlu, S. Baek et al., "Dynamic lumbar pedicle screw-rod stabilization: in vitro biomechanical comparison with standard rigid pedicle screw-rod stabilization—laboratory investigation," *Journal of Neurosurgery: Spine*, vol. 12, no. 2, pp. 183–189, 2010.

[36] A. F. Ozer, N. R. Crawford, M. Sasani et al., "Dynamic lumbar pedicle screw-rod stabilization: two year follow-up and comparison with fusion," *Open Orthopaedics*, vol. 4, pp. 137–141, 2010.

[37] T. Oktenoglu, A. F. Ozer, M. Sasani et al., "Posterior dynamic stabilization in the treatment of lumbar degenerative disc disease: 2-year follow-up," *Minimally Invasive Neurosurgery*, vol. 53, no. 3, pp. 112–116, 2010.

# 30

# A Longitudinal Low Dose $\mu$CT Analysis of Bone Healing in Mice: A Pilot Study

**Lu-Zhao Di,**[1] **Vanessa Couture,**[1] **Élisabeth Leblanc,**[1,2] **Yasaman Alinejad,**[1]
**Jean-François Beaudoin,**[1,3] **Roger Lecomte,**[1,3,4] **François Berthod,**[5,6] **Nathalie Faucheux,**[1,7]
**Frédéric Balg,**[1,2] **and Guillaume Grenier**[1,2]

[1] *Research Center of CHUS (CRCHUS), 3001, 12th Avenue North, Sherbrooke, QC, Canada J1H 5N4*

[2] *Department of Orthopedic Surgery, Faculty of Medicine and Health Sciences, University of Sherbrooke, 3001, 12th Avenue North, Sherbrooke, QC, Canada J1H 5N4*

[3] *Sherbrooke Molecular Imaging Centre (CIMS), CRCHUS, 3001, 12th Avenue North, Sherbrooke, QC, Canada J1H 5N4*

[4] *Department of Nuclear Medicine and Radiobiology, Faculty of Medicine and Health Sciences, University of Sherbrooke, 3001, 12th Avenue North, Sherbrooke, QC, Canada J1H 5N4*

[5] *Laboratoire d'Organogénèse Expérimentale (LOEX), Research Center of CHUQ, Enfant-Jésus Hospital, 1401, 18th Street, Quebec City, QC, Canada G1J 1Z4*

[6] *Department of Surgery, Faculty of Medicine, Laval University, 2325 Université Street, Quebec City, QC, Canada G1V 0A6*

[7] *Department of Chemical and Biotechnological Engineering, Faculty of Engineering, University of Sherbrooke, 2500 Université Boulevard, Sherbrooke, QC, Canada J1K 2R1*

Correspondence should be addressed to Guillaume Grenier; guillaume.grenier@usherbrooke.ca

Academic Editor: Panagiotis Korovessis

Low dose microcomputed tomography ($\mu$CT) is a recently matured technique that enables the study of longitudinal bone healing and the testing of experimental treatments for bone repair. This imaging technique has been used for studying craniofacial repair in mice but not in an orthopedic context. This is mainly due to the size of the defects (approximately 1.0 mm) in long bone, which heal rapidly and may thus negatively impact the assessment of the effectiveness of experimental treatments. We developed a longitudinal low dose $\mu$CT scan analysis method combined with a new image segmentation and extraction software using Hounsfield unit (HU) scores to quantitatively monitor bone healing in small femoral cortical defects in live mice. We were able to reproducibly quantify bone healing longitudinally over time with three observers. We used high speed intramedullary reaming to prolong healing in order to circumvent the rapid healing typical of small defects. Bone healing prolongation combined with $\mu$CT imaging to study small bone defects in live mice thus shows potential as a promising tool for future preclinical research on bone healing.

## 1. Introduction

Bone healing is a constantly growing field of research with important clinical implications. Precise and effective monitoring of bone healing is thus essential. Histological preparations are traditionally used to assess tissue composition and bone repair processes. However, they are limited to two-dimensional analyses of three-dimensional (3D) structures and semiquantitative scoring systems. Biomechanical testing is also a reliable quantitative method for assessing bone repair but is limited to endpoint analyses, as are histological preparations [1]. Because of high inter- and intrasubject variability, such studies involving several time points require large numbers of animals, which increases the cost of labor-intensive experiments [2].

The use of $\mu$CT in experimental medicine has increased exponentially over the past few years because this imaging technique provides reliable and highly reproducible results [3]. $\mu$CT imaging enables both noninvasive, tissue-preserving imaging and quantitative 3D morphometry of bone structures, notably of woven bone [4, 5], and has thus rapidly evolved to become the gold standard for microarchitecture

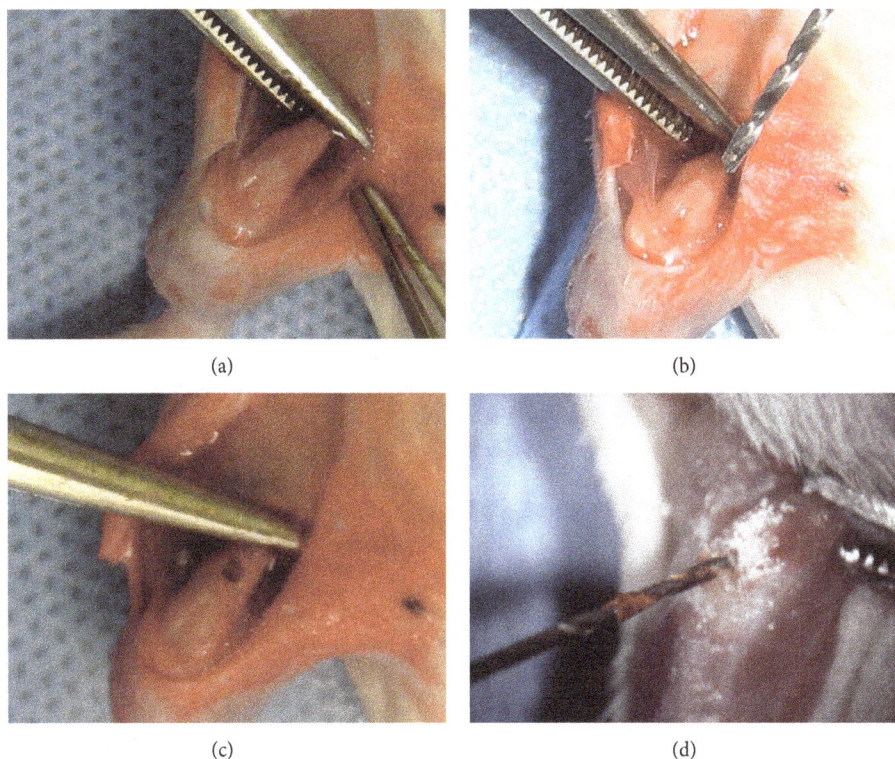

(a)

(b)

(c)

(d)

FIGURE 1: Surgical procedure for creating diaphyseal femoral cortical defects and intramedullary reaming. The femur was exposed (a) and the quadriceps was reclined by everting the patella (b). A cortical defect was created in the distal midshaft portion of the femur using a drill bit (c). Reaming was performed by drilling through the intercondylar notch of the femur (d).

analyses [6, 7]. Longitudinal low dose μCT analyses have been used to study treatments for enhancing the healing of calvarial defects in murine models [8–11] and to quantify tumor-induced osteolysis [12]. However, μCT data collection often requires *ex vivo* specimens, meaning that the animals have to be sacrificed [6]. While a few investigators have reported using low dose μCT to study bone architecture *in vivo* [13–15], none has used longitudinal μCT scans to evaluate the healing of drill hole cortical defects in mice, mainly because spontaneous healing occurs quickly, making it difficult to assess the effect of treatments on bone healing [16]. To slow down spontaneous bone healing, Gao et al. irradiated the limbs of mice to reduce the contribution of endogenous cells to bone healing [17], while effective irradiation impairs nonstem cell therapies, such as growth factors that stimulate the recruitment and differentiation of the endogenous progenitors required for bone repair.

In the present study, we used low dose μCT imaging to perform longitudinal quantitative analyses of bone healing of femoral cortical defects in mice. To assess bone healing, we performed longitudinal μCT scans of live animals using a dedicated small-animal low dose μCT scanner and analyzed the images using custom semiautomated segmentation and coregistration software. Despite creating noncritical size femoral defects, our results enabled us to show that intramedullary reaming is effective in slowing down spontaneous bone healing and significantly increasing the time required for the defect to heal. In summary, the combination

of low dose μCT scan imaging of live animals and bone reaming appears to be a valuable tool for evaluating the kinetics of long bone healing following treatments with drugs, biomaterials, and/or cells in mice.

## 2. Materials and Methods

*2.1. Animals.* Skeletally mature 12- to 16-week-old male CD1 (Charles River, Saint-Constant, QC, Canada) mice were used. This study was carried out in strict accordance with the recommendations in the Guide for the Care and Use of Laboratory Animals of the National Institutes of Health. The protocol was approved by the Committee on the Ethics of Animal Experiments of the University of Sherbrooke (Permit Number 141-11B). Prior to surgery, the mice received a narcotic (Buprenorphine; 0.05–0.1 mg/kg) to control pain as well as a preventive dose of antibiotic (penicillin G; 60,000 U).

*2.2. Surgical Procedure for Creating Femoral Cortical Defects and Reaming the Medullar Cavity.* A diaphyseal cortical defect of the anterodistal femur was created using a modified drill hole technique [18, 19] with or without intramedullary reaming as shown in Figure 1. Briefly, the mice were anesthetized (isoflurane), their limbs were shaved, and the skin was disinfected using a 0.5% chlorhexidine solution (Dexidin 0.5; Atlas Laboratory, Montreal, QC, Canada). A skin incision was made to expose the medial quadriceps and knee. A medial parapatellar approach was then made to the knee and was extended proximally through the quadriceps to expose the distal femur by lateral patellar eversion. A 3/64″ drill bit (Model 865; Dremel, Mount Prospect, IL, USA) was used to create a 1.1 mm-diameter circular defect in the anterior cortex of both femurs 4 mm above the femoral condyles. The defects were irrigated with normal saline to remove bone residues. Intramedullary reaming was performed on one femur by drilling a 1/32″-hole through the intercondylar notch and then reaming the full length of the medullary cavity. The reamer was kept in the medullary cavity at high speed for 10 s.

The defects were then covered by reclining the quadriceps back to its original position and repositioning the patella. The incision was closed using nonabsorbable sutures. The surgery was performed by an orthopedic surgeon using sterile materials in aseptic conditions. The mice were used for live $\mu$CT imaging and/or were euthanized for histological examinations.

*2.3. Low Dose Microcomputed Tomography ($\mu$CT) Scan Imaging.* Low dose $\mu$CT scan imaging was performed using a Gamma Medica Triumph X-O small-animal CT scanner composed of a 40 W X-ray tube with a 75 $\mu$m focal spot diameter and a 2240 × 2368 CsI flat panel X-ray detector. The detector pixel size was 50 $\mu$m, and a 2 × 2 pixel binning scheme was used. Scans were performed at 60 kVp and 230 $\mu$A using 512 projections in fly mode to reduce exposure with a 59.20 mm FOV. Images were reconstructed using the general purpose reconstruction FBP kernel from the Gamma Medica software over an isotropic 116 $\mu$m voxel spacing grid providing a voxel volume of $1.56 \times 10^{-3}$ mm$^3$. Air and water phantoms (15 mL Falcon tubes) were scanned for each imaging session to allow normalization in HU. The live mice were scanned once prior to surgery as a control and then at days 0 (immediately after surgery), 7, 14, 21, 30, 35, 44, 57, and 78 after surgery. To minimize movement, the mice were isoflurane-sedated during the $\mu$CT imaging. The dose of radiation administered was 11.7 cGy per scan, as measured by dosimeter.

*2.4. Software to Quantify Bone Healing.* Custom software was written to automatically calculate the size of the cortical defects. The $\mu$CT scans consisted of 512 individual image slices stacked in a RAW file and converted to the NIFTI format using Fiji freeware (ImageJ, Version 1.42q; National Institutes of Health, USA) [20]. ITK-SNAP freeware (http://www.itksnap.org) was used to segment structures [21] and manually delineate 3D ROI on the cortical defects in the postsurgery (day 0) scans. Tracing an irregular anatomic contour adjacent to the cortical surface was deemed the best approach to create the 3D ROI. We used software provided by the Image Analysis and Visualization Platform (PAVI, Sherbrooke, QC) to virtually extract, align, and save images of each mouse femur to smaller volumes. The virtually extracted femurs were then registered to the day 0 postsurgery reference femur using FSL Flirt [22, 23]. Since we did not want the spatial information of the bones to be lost, we parameterized Flirt to use a rigid body transformation with 6 degrees of freedom. After registration, a linear transformation was applied to the voxel signal intensities to convert them to the HU [24] scale using water for calibration. This allowed the signals from different scans made at different time points to be calibrated. The HU scale makes it possible to conduct analyses of absolute voxel signal intensities in order to determine the material density in each voxel (bone, muscle, water, etc.). We then calculated the kinetics of cortical defect healing using the previously determined 3D ROI, which became relevant for each time point after registration. The volumes and sizes of the cortical defects in treated and control femurs for each mouse were then quantified over time as were their densities based on the HU scale. The HU ranges for empty or soft tissue reaction (e.g., hematoma) ($-1000$ to $+800$ HU), woven bone ($+1200$ to $+1900$ HU), and compact bone ($>2700$ HU; comparable to intact bone) were based on published results from other groups [25–27] as well as on results from specific anatomical sites with known tissue compositions.

*2.5. Statistics.* To calculate the sample size required, we used the following repeated sample size estimation formula, ($n = 2 + C(s/d)^2$), where $s$ is the standard deviation and $d$ is the difference measured, with a $C$ of 7.85, a power of 80%, and an alpha of 0.05. The difference $d$ was measured between the volumes of the cortical deficits in the left and right femurs on postoperative day 29 when the dissimilarity between the two femurs was the most marked. The standard deviation was also calculated using the results on postoperative day 29. The standard deviation was 0.255, and the measured difference was 0.36. The sample size required for a significant result was thus at least 6 mice.

One outcome of the study was the assessment of the agreement among three observers with respect to their 3D ROI determinations for the same $\mu$CT scan. This was represented by a Bland-Altman plot [28]. Graphically, the mean differences and the 95% confidence intervals (CI) were represented. An intraclass coefficient (ICC) was also used to assess their reliability and validity. The ICC for the interobserver agreement was obtained by comparing blind measurements of the three observers. For clinical studies, a Cronbach alpha value over 0.85 is considered very good, while a value over 0.9 is considered "ideal" [29].

The main outcome of the present study was to assess the differences in 3D ROI voxel HU cortical defect volumes between the reamed and unreamed femurs relative to the respective postoperative day 0 volumes. The comparison of means between reamed and unreamed samples at the same time point was analyzed using two-way ANOVA and Sidak's multiple comparisons test. $P$ values less than 0.05 were considered significant.

Statistical analyses were performed using SPSS v20.0.0, and the results were graphed using Prism v5.0.

## 3. Results

*3.1. 3D ROI: Analysis of Interobserver Agreement.* Since initial 3D ROI segmentation may be subjective and thus overestimate or underestimate healing, we verified the interobserver

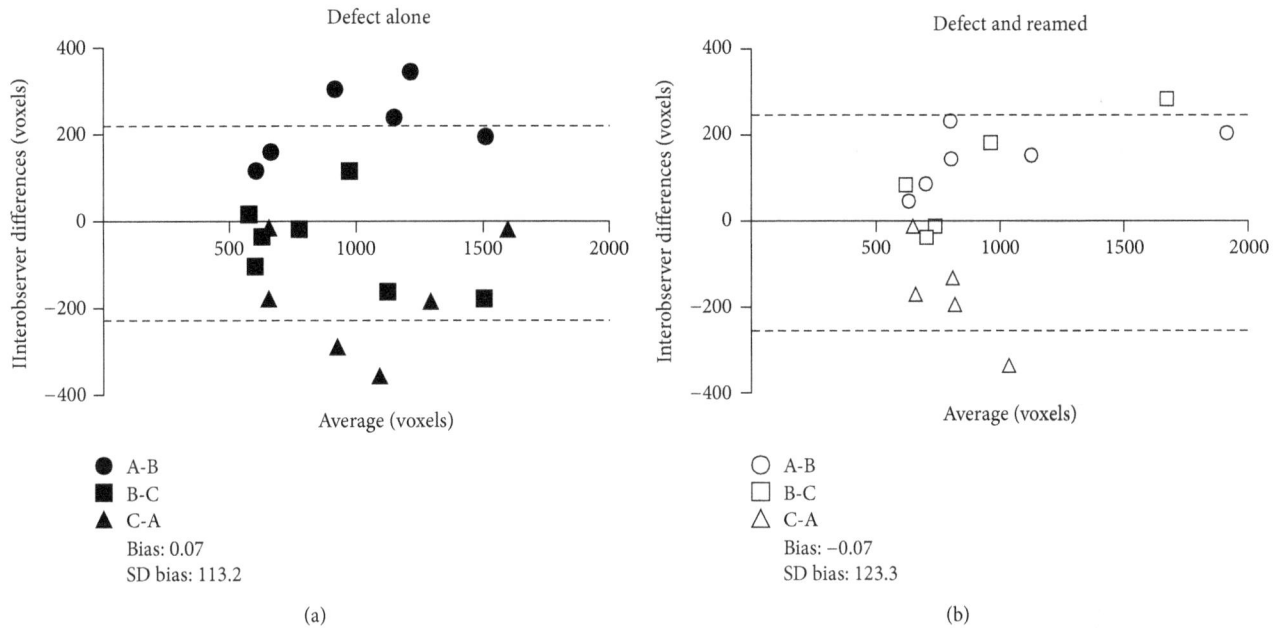

FIGURE 2: Interobserver agreement in the determination of 3D ROI. A Bland-Altman plot was used to graph differences in the absolute number of voxels per 3D ROI as a function of the average size of the defect. This made it possible to assess the agreement between three observers in the determination of the 3D ROI. Eighteen μCT images from (a) unreamed femurs with a defect and (b) reamed femurs with a defect were blindly analyzed. The two-by-two comparison of the three observers (A-B, B-C, and C-A) showed a 95% confidence interval from −226.5 to +226.4 and from −245.9 to +247.1 for unreamed femurs with a defect and reamed femurs with a defect, respectively. An interclass correlation (ICC) was used to compare interobserver variability. The ICC scores were 0.864 (very good, $P < 0.0001$) and 0.905 (ideal, $P < 0.0001$) for the unreamed femurs with a defect and the reamed femurs with a defect, respectively.

agreement, which was represented using Bland-Altman plots (Figure 2). We used three observers (A-B-C) to blindly determine the 3D ROI of the defects. The results are presented as the difference in the absolute number of voxels per 3D ROI as a function of the average size of the defect. Of the 36 scans, 18 were of femurs with a defect but no reaming (Figure 2(a)) and 18 were of femurs with a defect and reaming (Figure 2(b)). The two-by-two comparison of the three observers (A-B, B-C, and C-A) showed that the 95% confidence interval of the evaluations of the observers ranged from −226.5 to +226.4 (21.9% ± 5.0) and from −245.9 to +247.1 (20.1% ± 3.2) for defects without reaming and defects with reaming, respectively.

To determine whether the interobserver agreement was significant, we calculated an interclass correlation (ICC), which allowed us to compare interobserver variability for a given sample. The ICC was 0.864 (very good, $P < 0.0001$) for the defect without reaming and 0.905 (ideal, $P < 0.0001$) for the defect with reaming, indicating very good interobserver agreement. In addition, there was no significant difference between the 3D ROI of the defect without reaming and the defect with reaming.

*3.2. Longitudinal Low Dose μCT Analysis of Bone Healing.* We determined the difference in the kinetics of bone healing between reamed and unreamed femurs by calculating the number of voxels in nonorganized substrate, woven bone, and compact bone. Figure 3(a) shows reconstructed images

of anteroposterior views of the femurs with their defects on days 0 and 21 as well as on day 57 after surgery, when the most significant variations in tissue composition of the reamed and unreamed femurs were observed. In addition to visualizing the registration of the femurs at different times, it is possible to identify the position of the 3D ROIs overlaid on the defects along different views (Figure 3(b)). Cross-sectional views of the femurs can also be seen in which the 3D ROI is apparent (Figure 3(c)). In both representations, the voxels of the 3D ROI are color-coded to differentiate between the various components in the defect, that is, empty/soft tissue reaction (red), woven bone (blue), and compact bone comparable to intact bone (green). Figures 3(b) and 3(c) show that woven bone and compact bone formation is delayed in the reamed preparation compared to the unreamed preparation.

We used our custom software to verify the filling kinetics of the defects (Figure 4(a)). Graphing the percentage of voxels in the −1000 to +800 HU range within the 3D ROI over time revealed that reaming caused a significant delay in healing. It took 11 and 16 days after surgery for 50% healing to occur in the unreamed and reamed femurs, respectively, while 75% healing took approximately 16 and 36 days, respectively. By day 57, there was no significant difference in healing between the two surgical procedures.

We also assessed the formation of woven bone by graphing the percentage of voxels in the +1200 to +1900 HU range within the 3D ROI as a function of time (Figure 4(b)). The percentage of voxels related to woven bone was significantly

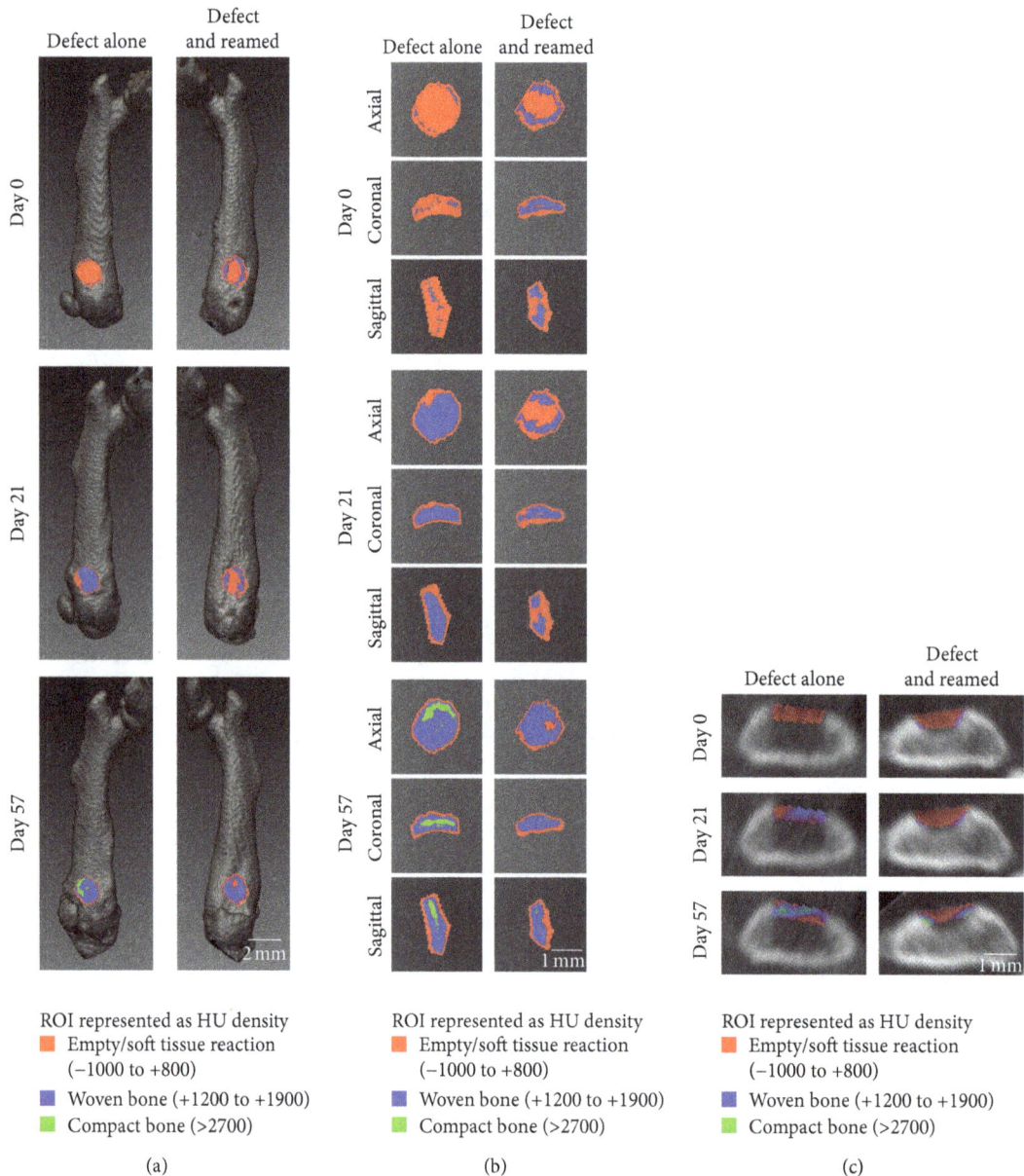

FIGURE 3: Bone healing monitoring as a function of time using low dose $\mu$CT scans of live mice. (a) Representative views of 3D $\mu$CT reconstructed images of femurs on days 0, 21, and 57 after surgery. Variations in the density of the 3D ROI (determined at day 0 after surgery) make it possible to estimate the tissue composition. (b) 3D ROI can also be observed in axial, coronal, and sagittal views. (c) Representative cross-sectional views of the femur in which the 3D ROI is apparent in one image (slice). The colored voxels make it possible to see changes in defect composition as a function of time where most of the voxels were red on day 0 and blue on day 28, with an increasing proportion of green on day 57. Nonorganized substrate (red: −1000 to +800 HU), woven bone (blue: +1200 to +1900 HU), and compact bone (green; >2700 HU).

higher in the unreamed preparations, with the percentage reaching a plateau around day 29 of 40% and 29% for the unreamed and reamed preparations, respectively. Interestingly, the percentages decreased to 20% by day 57, when no significant difference between the preparations was observed.

We investigated the formation of compact bone by graphing the percentage of voxels in the 3D ROI with >2700 HU

as a function of time (Figure 4(c)). The percentage of voxels related to dense bone increased significantly faster in the unreamed femurs than in the reamed femurs. This difference was observed by day 35, when the percentage reached 30% for the unreamed femurs but only 8% for the reamed femurs. The percentage increased until day 57, reaching nearly 40% for the unreamed femurs and nearly 22% for the reamed femurs.

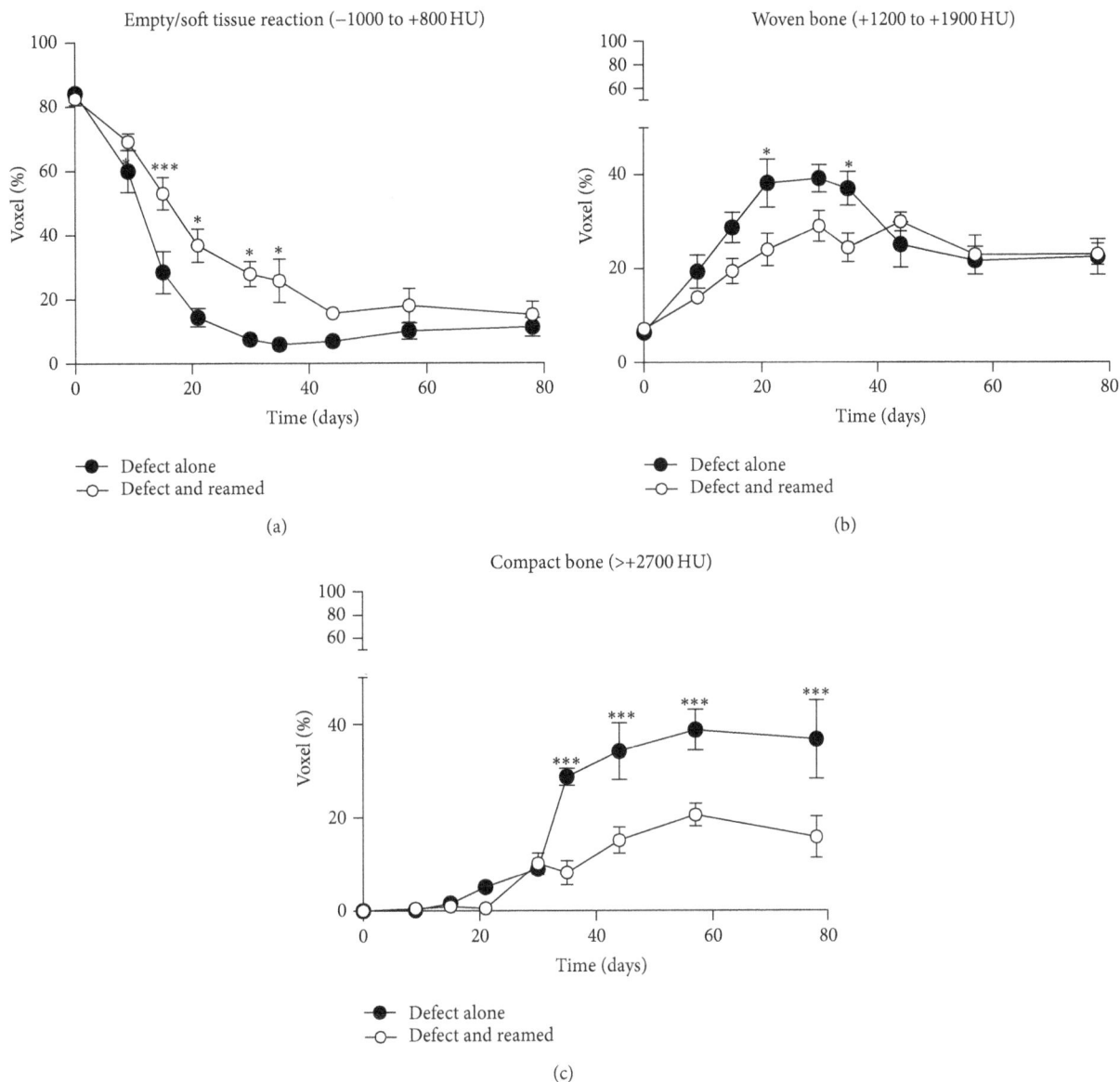

(a)

(b)

(c)

FIGURE 4: Bone healing as a function of time for a defect without reaming and a defect with reaming. (a) The results were quantified and plotted as a percentage of voxels representing nonorganized material as a function of time for unreamed femurs with a defect and reamed femurs with a defect. The percentages of (b) woven and (c) dense bone formation as a function of time were also graphed. The results were obtained from nine mice ($n = 9$; $^*P < 0.05$, $^{***}P < 0.0001$).

## 4. Discussion

μCT is a precise tool for bone imaging, and in recent decades it has been shown to be the gold standard for studying bone structure [30]. It has been shown to be a relevant tool for craniofacial studies in small rodents, in which it is possible to create critical size bone or nonhealing defects [8–11]. Unfortunately, such critical size defects cannot be created in the long bones of mice without using nails or other materials that can impair μCT imaging [31, 32]. On the other hand, small noncritical size bone defects heal spontaneously and rapidly, which may hinder the effectiveness of experimental treatments [16]. To widen this "therapeutical" window, we reamed the endosteum of the medullar region of the bone.

The aim of our study was to evaluate the utility of using longitudinal low dose μCT scans to assess the healing of noncritical size defects (1 mm) in long bones in mice and to investigate the effect of intramedullary reaming on healing times.

Longitudinal studies of small cortical defects using low dose μCT scan are challenging for many reasons. First, bone defects created using small drill bits are subject to operator bias due to differences in the angle at which the drill bit enters the femur and due to micromovements once the bit is fully introduced. This bias must be taken into account given the size of the defects (1 mm), which are much smaller than calvarial defects, which can be up to 5 mm in diameter in mice [8]. Second, small defects are assessed using multiple scans of the animals, which, while immobilized, are not in exactly the same position, which in turn increases the risk of miscalculations. To circumvent these experimental biases, the corresponding femur of each animal was first rigorously aligned in space, making it possible to exactly superpose the 3D ROI. The 3D ROIs at day 0 (after operation) were then set and their coordinates were applied to all time points. The results of each time point were relativized to the initial 3D ROI at day 0 (before and after operation). By applying this procedure, we were able to assess callus formation and mineralization over time by using calibrated voxels expressed in HU that were applied to different tissue composition categories, that is, empty or soft tissue reaction (e.g., hematoma), woven bone, and mineralized compact bone. More importantly, the bone healing process over time described in the present study matched that of previous $\mu$CT and histological studies [33–35].

In addition, our results showed that the healing of cortical defects is significantly affected by the endosteal reaming procedure. This was shown by the significant delay in defect filling and the formation of woven and compact bone over time. In terms of compositional analyses, Hayward et al. suggested that the use of contrast-enhanced $\mu$CT scans may improve the evaluation of nonmineralized (e.g., cartilage) and mineralized tissues in fracture calluses [36]. From our experience, we had no difficulty in distinguishing between these tissues. This may be due to the ranges of HU that we used to categorize the tissues and the use of the 3D ROI at day 0 (prior to surgery) as a reference. Our software made it possible to follow changes in the tissue density of a healing region as small as 1 mm$^3$. Low dose $\mu$CT analyses may thus provide a reasonable estimate of the tissue mineralization of healing bone based on HU.

Our study also showed that appropriate analysis software and suitable image resolution limit observer variability. Since our software relies on manual tracings of an initial volume of interest (3D ROI) on native $\mu$CT scans, interobserver differences may occur given that the exact delineation of cortical defects depends partly on the judgment of the observers. We hypothesized that the greatest interobserver variability is caused by the semisubjective delineation of the initial cortical defect, which is a bias that may be compounded. However, our ICC interobserver analysis showed that this bias is small for experienced observers and does not affect the results. Alternatives include global and local threshold segmentation, but since our 3D ROI was relatively small and well delineated, we judged that manual tracing segmentation would be the most convenient. This finding also implied that, depending on the type of experiment, investigators should choose the appropriate $\mu$CT resolution to maintain an acceptable level of precision.

While low dose $\mu$CT scans have limited resolution compared to high dose scans, our study showed that the resolution is sufficient and, importantly, low dose scans avoid the biological risk associated with repeated radiation exposure [37–40]. Laperre et al. reported that they observed no hematological toxicity or radiotoxic effect on bone microarchitecture with triple radiation doses of 43.4 cGy per scan [39], which

correspond to a cumulative dose of 130 cGy. In our study, the cumulative dose was under 120 cGy, which is far less than 200 cGy, the dose at which the tumor risk increases in mice, thus making any radiation-induced effect on bone healing unlikely [41].

The creation of defects by drilling a hole in the bone cortex is a widely used and effective model for studying bone healing [16, 35], and it is well known that it leads to spontaneous healing [16, 42]. Many reasons could explain the healing delay observed in the reamed preparations. Previous studies have shown that vascular compromise can induce a significant healing delay or even nonunion in rodent fracture models [43, 44]. Since medullar vascularization accounts for about two-thirds of total bone vascularization [45], it is reasonable to think that its disruption could increase healing time. In addition, a loss of medullar substance and endosteum may also contribute to the delay in healing since they contain progenitor cells that contribute to bone healing [35, 46]. Other groups have used different approaches to slow down spontaneous bone healing. To assess how transplanted MSC contribute to healing cortical bone defects, Gao et al. sublethally irradiated the hindlimbs of mice in order to prevent endogenous MSC from participating in the cortical healing process [17]. Prolonging bone healing by medullar reaming may be a useful and simple procedure for limiting spontaneous healing and widening the window for studying the effect of compounds and exogenous stem cells.

## 5. Conclusion

We showed that low dose $\mu$CT scans can be used to quantify and characterize bone healing in live mice. Using 3D ROI coordinates determined immediately following surgery, it was possible to evaluate variations in tissue density within the 3D ROI and show that reaming delays the healing of cortical defects in mice. The proposed experimental approach reduces the number of animals needed, provides quantitative longitudinal results, and is reproducible between different observers. Bone healing prolongation combined with $\mu$CT imaging to study small bone defects in live mice thus shows potential as a promising tool for future preclinical research on bone healing.

## Conflict of Interests

The authors declare that there is no conflict of interests regarding the publication of this paper.

## Acknowledgments

The authors are grateful to Dr. David Alcoloumbre, Dr. Otman Sarrhini, and Geneviève Drouin for their assistance and Drs. Maxime Descoteaux, Matthieu Dumont, and Félix C. Morency from PAVI. Lu-Zhao Di is the recipient of a scholarship from the Canadian Institutes of Health Research (CIHR). Élisabeth Leblanc is the recipient of scholarships from the Fondation pour la Recherche et l'Enseignement en Orthopédie de Sherbrooke (FREOS) and CIHR. Guillaume Grenier holds a New Investigator Award from the Fonds de Recherche du Québec-Santé (FRQS). This work was supported by grants from CIHR, the National Science and Engineering Research Council of Canada (NSERC), the Canada Foundation for Innovation (CFI), and the Réseau de Thérapie Cellulaire du FRQS (ThéCell). The Centre d'imagerie moléculaire de Sherbrooke is part of the FRQS-funded CRCHUS.

# References

[1] A. M. Parfitt, M. K. Drezner, F. H. Glorieux et al., "Bone histomorphometry: standardization of nomenclature, symbols, and units. Report of the ASBMR Histomorphometry Nomenclature Committee," *Journal of Bone and Mineral Research*, vol. 2, no. 6, pp. 595–610, 1987.

[2] M. E. Oetgen, G. A. Merrell, N. W. Troiano, M. C. Horowitz, and M. A. Kacena, "Development of a femoral non-union model in the mouse," *Injury*, vol. 39, no. 10, pp. 1119–1126, 2008.

[3] J. F. Griffith and H. K. Genant, "Bone mass and architecture determination: state of the art," *Best Practice & Research: Clinical Endocrinology & Metabolism*, vol. 22, no. 5, pp. 737–764, 2008.

[4] L. A. Feldkamp, S. A. Goldstein, A. M. Parfitt, G. Jesion, and M. Kleerekoper, "The direct examination of three-dimensional bone architecture in vitro by computed tomography," *Journal of Bone and Mineral Research*, vol. 4, no. 1, pp. 3–11, 1989.

[5] J. H. Kinney, N. E. Lane, and D. L. Haupt, "In vivo, three-dimensional microscopy of trabecular bone," *Journal of Bone and Mineral Research*, vol. 10, no. 2, pp. 264–270, 1995.

[6] M. L. Bouxsein, S. K. Boyd, B. A. Christiansen, R. E. Guldberg, K. J. Jepsen, and R. Müller, "Guidelines for assessment of bone microstructure in rodents using micro-computed tomography," *Journal of Bone and Mineral Research*, vol. 25, no. 7, pp. 1468–1486, 2010.

[7] A. C. Jones, C. H. Arns, A. P. Sheppard, D. W. Hutmacher, B. K. Milthorpe, and M. A. Knackstedt, "Assessment of bone ingrowth into porous biomaterials using MICRO-CT," *Biomaterials*, vol. 28, no. 15, pp. 2491–2504, 2007.

[8] C. M. Cowan, Y.-Y. Shi, O. O. Aalami et al., "Adipose-derived adult stromal cells heal critical-size mouse calvarial defects," *Nature Biotechnology*, vol. 22, no. 5, pp. 560–567, 2004.

[9] C. M. Cowan, T. Aghaloo, Y.-F. Chou et al., "MicroCT evaluation of three-dimensional mineralization in response to BMP-2 doses in vitro and in critical sized rat calvarial defects," *Tissue Engineering*, vol. 13, no. 3, pp. 501–512, 2007.

[10] T. Aghaloo, C. M. Cowan, Y.-F. Chou et al., "Nell-1-induced bone regeneration in calvarial defects," *The American Journal of Pathology*, vol. 169, no. 3, pp. 903–915, 2006.

[11] S.-Y. Park, K.-H. Kim, K.-T. Koo et al., "The evaluation of the correlation between histomorphometric analysis and micro-computed tomography analysis in AdBMP-2 induced bone regeneration in rat calvarial defects," *Journal of Periodontal and Implant Science*, vol. 41, no. 5, pp. 218–226, 2011.

[12] L. C. Johnson, R. W. Johnson, S. A. Munoz, G. R. Mundy, T. E. Peterson, and J. A. Sterling, "Longitudinal live animal micro-CT allows for quantitative analysis of tumor-induced bone destruction," *Bone*, vol. 48, no. 1, pp. 141–151, 2011.

[13] J. H. Waarsing, J. S. Day, and H. Weinans, "An improved segmentation method for in vivo μCT imaging," *Journal of Bone and Mineral Research*, vol. 19, no. 10, pp. 1640–1650, 2004.

[14] J. H. Waarsing, J. S. Day, J. C. van Der Linden et al., "Detecting and tracking local changes in the tibiae of individual rats: a novel method to analyse longitudinal in vivo micro-CT data," *Bone*, vol. 34, no. 1, pp. 163–169, 2004.

[15] V. David, N. Laroche, B. Boudignon et al., "Noninvasive in vivo monitoring of bone architecture alterations in hindlimb-unloaded female rats using novel three-dimensional microcomputed tomography," *Journal of Bone and Mineral Research*, vol. 18, no. 9, pp. 1622–1631, 2003.

[16] J. E. Henderson, C. Gao, and E. J. Harvey, "Skeletal phenotyping in rodents: tissue isolation and manipulation," in *Osteoporosis Research*, G. Duque and K. Watanabe, Eds., Springer, London, UK, 2011.

[17] C. Gao, J. Seuntjens, G. N. Kaufman et al., "Mesenchymal stem cell transplantation to promote bone healing," *Journal of Orthopaedic Research*, vol. 30, no. 8, pp. 1183–1189, 2012.

[18] Y.-X. He, G. Zhang, X.-H. Pan et al., "Impaired bone healing pattern in mice with ovariectomy-induced osteoporosis: a drill-hole defect model," *Bone*, vol. 48, no. 6, pp. 1388–1400, 2011.

[19] M. Nagashima, A. Sakai, S. Uchida, S. Tanaka, M. Tanaka, and T. Nakamura, "Bisphosphonate (YM529) delays the repair of cortical bone defect after drill-hole injury by reducing terminal differentiation of osteoblasts in the mouse femur," *Bone*, vol. 36, no. 3, pp. 502–511, 2005.

[20] M. D. Abramoff, P. J. Magelhaes, and S. J. Ram, "Image processing with imageJ," *Biophotonics International*, vol. 11, no. 7, pp. 36–42, 2004.

[21] P. A. Yushkevich, J. Piven, H. C. Hazlett et al., "User-guided 3D active contour segmentation of anatomical structures: significantly improved efficiency and reliability," *NeuroImage*, vol. 31, no. 3, pp. 1116–1128, 2006.

[22] D. N. Greve and B. Fischl, "Accurate and robust brain image alignment using boundary-based registration," *NeuroImage*, vol. 48, no. 1, pp. 63–72, 2009.

[23] M. Jenkinson, P. Bannister, M. Brady, and S. Smith, "Improved optimization for the robust and accurate linear registration and motion correction of brain images," *NeuroImage*, vol. 17, no. 2, pp. 825–841, 2002.

[24] G. N. Hounsfield, "Computed medical imaging," *Science*, vol. 210, no. 4465, pp. 22–28, 1980.

[25] A. Katsumata, A. Hirukawa, S. Okumura et al., "Effects of image artifacts on gray-value density in limited-volume cone-beam computerized tomography," *Oral Surgery, Oral Medicine, Oral Pathology, Oral Radiology and Endodontology*, vol. 104, no. 6, pp. 829–836, 2007.

[26] P. Mah, T. E. Reeves, and W. D. McDavid, "Deriving Hounsfield units using grey levels in cone beam computed tomography," *Dentomaxillofacial Radiology*, vol. 39, no. 6, pp. 323–335, 2010.

[27] A. Donneys, N. S. Nelson, S. S. Deshpande et al., "Quantifying mineralization using bone mineral density distribution in the mandible," *Journal of Craniofacial Surgery*, vol. 23, no. 5, pp. 1502–1506, 2012.

[28] J. M. Bland and D. G. Altman, "Applying the right statistics: analyses of measurement studies," *Ultrasound in Obstetrics & Gynecology*, vol. 22, no. 1, pp. 85–93, 2003.

[29] J. M. Bland and D. G. Altman, "Cronbach's alpha," *The British Medical Journal*, vol. 314, no. 7080, article 572, 1997.

[30] J. L. Tremoleda, M. Khalil, L. L. Gompels, M. Wylezinska-Arridge, T. Vincent, and W. Gsell, "Imaging technologies for preclinical models of bone and joint disorders," *EJNMMI Research*, vol. 1, no. 1, pp. 1–14, 2011.

[31] B. De Man, J. Nuyts, P. Dupont, G. Marchal, and P. Suetens, "Metal streak artifacts in X-ray computed tomography: a simulation study," *IEEE Transactions on Nuclear Science*, vol. 46, no. 3, pp. 464–472, 1999.

[32] S. D. Cook, L. P. Patron, S. L. Salkeld, K. E. Smith, B. Whiting, and R. L. Barrack, "Correlation of computed tomography with histology in the assessment of periprosthetic defect healing," *Clinical Orthopaedics and Related Research*, vol. 467, no. 12, pp. 3213–3220, 2009.

[33] H. Uusitalo, J. Rantakokko, M. Ahonen et al., "A metaphyseal defect model of the femur for studies of murine bone healing," *Bone*, vol. 28, no. 4, pp. 423–429, 2001.

[34] T. M. Campbell, W. T. Wong, and E. J. Mackie, "Establishment of a model of cortical bone repair in mice," *Calcified Tissue International*, vol. 73, no. 1, pp. 49–55, 2003.

[35] L. Monfoulet, B. Rabier, O. Chassande, and J.-C. Fricain, "Drilled hole defects in mouse femur as models of intramembranous cortical and cancellous bone regeneration," *Calcified Tissue International*, vol. 86, no. 1, pp. 72–81, 2010.

[36] L. N. M. Hayward, C. M. J. De Bakker, L. C. Gerstenfeld, M. W. Grinstaff, and E. F. Morgan, "Assessment of contrast-enhanced computed tomography for imaging of cartilage during fracture healing," *Journal of Orthopaedic Research*, vol. 31, no. 4, pp. 567–573, 2013.

[37] L. Yu, X. Liu, S. Leng et al., "Radiation dose reduction in computed tomography: techniques and future perspective," *Imaging in Medicine*, vol. 1, pp. 65–84, 2009.

[38] R. Duran-Struuck and R. C. Dysko, "Principles of bone marrow transplantation (BMT): providing optimal veterinary and husbandry care to irradiated mice in BMT studies," *Journal of the American Association for Laboratory Animal Science*, vol. 48, no. 1, pp. 11–22, 2009.

[39] K. Laperre, M. Depypere, N. van Gastel et al., "Development of micro-CT protocols for in vivo follow-up of mouse bone architecture without major radiation side effects," *Bone*, vol. 49, no. 4, pp. 613–622, 2011.

[40] R. J. Klinck, G. M. Campbell, and S. K. Boyd, "Radiation effects on bone architecture in mice and rats resulting from in vivo micro-computed tomography scanning," *Medical Engineering and Physics*, vol. 30, no. 7, pp. 888–895, 2008.

[41] K. S. Crump, P. Duport, H. Jiang, N. S. Shilnikova, D. Krewski, and J. M. Zielinski, "A meta-analysis of evidence for hormesis in animal radiation carcinogenesis, including a discussion of potential pitfalls in statistical analyses to detect hormesis," *Journal of Toxicology and Environmental Health Part B: Critical Reviews*, vol. 15, no. 3, pp. 210–231, 2012.

[42] C. Bosch, B. Melsen, and K. Vargervik, "Importance of the critical-size bone defect in testing bone-regenerating materials," *The Journal of Craniofacial Surgery*, vol. 9, no. 4, pp. 310–316, 1998.

[43] K. Hietaniemi, J. Peltonen, and P. Paavolainen, "An experimental model for non-union in rats," *Injury*, vol. 26, no. 10, pp. 681–686, 1995.

[44] C. Lu, T. Miclau, D. Hu, and R. S. Marcucio, "Ischemia leads to delayed union during fracture healing: a mouse model," *Journal of Orthopaedic Research*, vol. 25, no. 1, pp. 51–61, 2007.

[45] F. W. Rhinelander, "Thevascular response of bone to internal fixation," in *The Science and Practice of Intramedullary Nailing*, C. C. Edwards, Ed., pp. 25–29, Lea & Febiger, Philadelphia, Pa, USA, 1987.

[46] C. Colnot, "Skeletal cell fate decisions within periosteum and bone marrow during bone regeneration," *Journal of Bone and Mineral Research*, vol. 24, no. 2, pp. 274–282, 2009.

# 31

# Hindfoot Valgus following Interlocking Nail Treatment for Tibial Diaphysis Fractures: Can the Fibula Be Neglected?

**Metin Uzun,**[1] **Adnan Kara,**[2] **Müjdat Adaş,**[3] **Bülent Karslioğlu,**[4]
**Murat Bülbül,**[5] **and Burak Beksaç**[6]

[1]*Orthopaedic Department, Acıbadem Maslak Hospital, Darüşşafaka Street, Büyükdere Street No. 40, Maslak, Sarıyer, Istanbul, Turkey*
[2]*Orthopaedic Department, Şişli Etfal Training and Education Hospital, Şişli, Istanbul, Turkey*
[3]*Okmeydani Education and Training Hospital, Okmeydani, Istanbul, Turkey*
[4]*Orthopaedic Department, Kasımpaşa Military Hospital, Istanbul, Turkey*
[5]*Orthopaedic Department, Medipol University, Istanbul, Turkey*
[6]*Orthopaedic Department, Acıbadem University, Darüşşafaka Street, Büyükdere Street No. 40, Maslak, Sarıyer, Istanbul, Turkey*

Correspondence should be addressed to Metin Uzun; drmetinuzun@gmail.com

Academic Editor: Allen L. Carl

*Purpose.* We evaluated whether intramedullary nail fixation for tibial diaphysis fractures with concomitant fibula fractures (except at the distal one-third level) managed conservatively with an associated fibula fracture resulted in ankle deformity and assessed the impact of the ankle deformity on lower extremity function. *Methods.* Sixty middle one-third tibial shaft fractures with associated fibular fractures, except the distal one-third level, were included in this study. All tibial shaft fractures were anatomically reduced and fixed with interlocking intramedullary nails. Fibular fractures were managed conservatively. Hindfoot alignment was assessed clinically. Tibia and fibular lengths were compared to contralateral measurements using radiographs. Functional results were evaluated using the Knee Injury and Osteoarthritis Outcome Score (KOOS) and the Foot and Ankle Disability Index Score (FADI). *Results.* Anatomic union, defined as equal length in operative and contralateral tibias, was achieved in 60 fractures (100%). Fibular shortening was identified in 42 fractures (68%). Mean fibular shortening was 1.2 cm (range, 0.5–2 cm). Clinical exams showed increased hindfoot valgus in 42 fractures (68%). The mean KOOS was 88.4, and the mean FADI score was 90. *Conclusion.* Fibular fractures in the middle or proximal one-third may need to be stabilized at the time of tibial intramedullary nail fixation to prevent development of hindfoot valgus due to fibular shortening.

## 1. Introduction

Diaphyseal tibial fractures are generally treated surgically and are frequently accompanied by fibular fractures [1–3]. The usual treatment for a concomitant fibular fracture in the distal one-third is surgical fixation, but if it occurs in the middle or proximal one-third, it is typically treated symptomatically [1–3]. Ankle alignment and functional results in patients symptomatically treated for fibular fractures are unclear [1, 2, 4, 5].

We evaluated whether conservative treatment for these concomitant-associated fibular fractures leads to ankle deformity and assessed the functional results of an ankle deformity, if present.

## 2. Materials and Methods

The study included 60 consecutive patients with unilateral middle one-third tibial fractures treated by anatomic reduction and interlocking intramedullary nail fixation and who had been managed conservatively for a proximal to middle one-third (except distal one-third level) fibular fracture. Three surgeons performed the surgeries at three different centers. All fractures were closed. Patients who had tibial union complications and/or who had undergone a second surgery were excluded. The mean follow-up period was 20 months (range, 12–36 months) (Figure 1).

Hindfoot alignment was evaluated clinically with a goniometer at the follow-up assessment, in the manner described

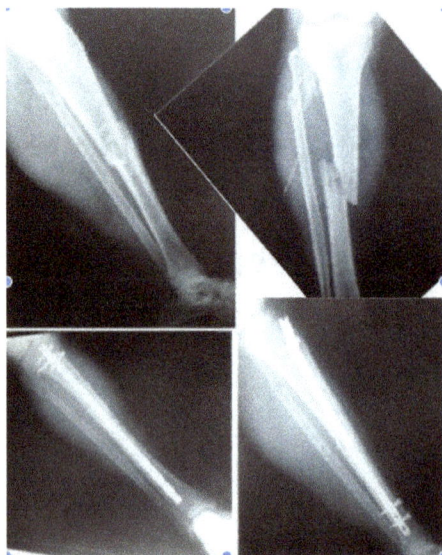

FIGURE 1: Anteroposterior and lateral X-ray images showing a middle one-third tibial shaft fracture with an associated fibular fracture and a healed tibial fracture treated with intramedullary nailing.

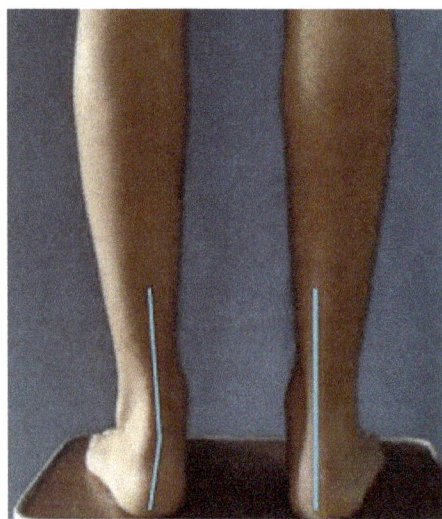

FIGURE 2: Stance position. Solid lines were marked on the skin, and dashed lines have been added to the photograph to identify the tibial angle and the calcaneal stance.

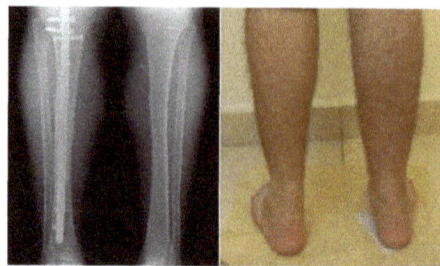

FIGURE 3: Clinical images showing the crus heel relationship.

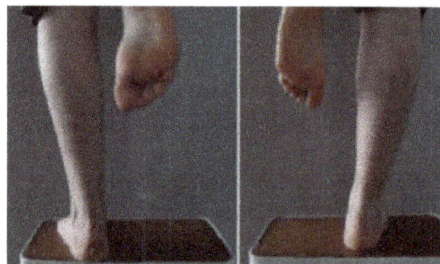

FIGURE 4: Clinical images showing differences in opposite extremities due to weight-bearing.

by Astrom and Arvidson [6] (Figure 2). Full-length anteroposterior and lateral radiographs of the tibia and fibula were obtained for both lower extremities at the same distance and used to compare tibial and fibular lengths for the injured and contralateral limbs [6]. Lengthening was measured with a computer digital system. Functional outcome scores were determined for each patient using the Knee Injury and Osteoarthritis Outcome Score (KOOS) and the Foot and Ankle Disability Index Score (FADI) [7, 8].

This study was approved by the authors' Institutional Review Board. All authors certify that their institution has approved the reporting of this case series and that all investigations conformed with the ethical principles of research.

## 3. Results

All patients demonstrated radiographic union of both the tibia and fibula. Anatomic union occurred in 60 cases (100%) and was defined for tibia with an equal length to the contralateral limb (Figure 1). Fibular shortening was identified in 42 cases (68%). Mean fibular shortening was 1.2 cm (range, 0.5–2 cm) (Figure 3). The increase in calcaneal valgus on the clinical hindfoot examination was a mean of 5° compared to that of the other extremity (Figures 3 and 4). The mean KOOS score was 88.4, and the mean FADI score was 90.

## 4. Discussion

Tibial fractures are one of the most frequent orthopedic problems [1, 3]. Treatment remains controversial due to the variety of fracture patterns and soft tissue problems associated with these injuries.

Successful results have been reported for tibial intramedullary nailing in cases with associated proximal and middle one-third fibular fractures, as in the current study [9–11]. Although associated distal one-third fibular fractures are less commonly present with tibial diaphysis fractures, the accepted treatment for these cases is surgical fixation of the fibula. Associated distal one-third fibular fractures were excluded from our study, but we evaluated outcomes from nonsurgical management for more proximal fibular fractures associated with tibial shaft fractures treated with intramedullary fixation. Complications have been reported following both surgical and conservative treatment of tibial fractures, including lower extremity angulation, rotational deformity, and ankle malalignment [12, 13]. Although these complications may compromise lower extremity function and result in knee or ankle pain, impaired tibial alignment was noted, but no complications related to the ankle were reported in a study by Pobłocki et al. [14]. In contrast to those results, a previous study on patients with tibial fractures found that a delayed diagnosis was associated with a Maisonneuve, syndesmotic, or posterior or medial malleolar fracture at a rate of 20.1% [10]. A tibial alignment disorder may be a rather common complication for distal or proximal fractures, and functional impairment is expected due to the long-term effects of an alignment disorder, but a hindfoot deformity usually does not occur following a middiaphyseal fracture.

Although fibular fractures may lead to fibular shortening, Hooper et al. [2] reported successful results after conservatively treating isolated diaphyseal fibular fractures. No complications related to the ankle occurred but no information was provided about bone shortening. In the present study, fibular shortening was common, and a valgus calcaneal deformity was noted after bone healing from a tibial shaft fracture. Fibular length was measured and compared to a healthy fibula using the same exposure time, position, and distance on X-rays. Although computed tomography is the best method for measuring fibular length, it was not available to us. A hindfoot assessment must be done in a standing, weight-bearing position. We used the goniometer method described by Astrom and Arvidson [6]. Coronal plane alignment can be assessed using X-rays as described by Saltzman [15] or on a long axial view under weight-bearing. We did not use these techniques, as X-ray quality depends on the technician [15, 16]. A hindfoot alignment disorder is dynamic; thus, hindfoot cases must be evaluated in the weight-bearing position both clinically and radiologically.

Whorton and Henley [11] showed that fixing the fibula in patients with open tibial and fibular shaft fractures has no effect on bone healing or alignment of the tibia. However, some studies have reported that fixing the fibula in patients with distal tibial or fibular fractures increases fracture stability up to week 12 after surgery [16–18]. Biomechanical results have shown that fixing the fibula may help prevent loss of alignment in distal tibial fractures repaired with either intramedullary nailing or plate fixation methods [16, 19].

## 5. Conclusion

Shortening the fibula in patients with upper level fibular fractures associated with tibial fractures treated with intramedullary nailing may cause a dynamic hindfoot valgus deformity. All hindfoot cases must be evaluated in the weight-bearing position both clinically and radiologically. Additional study is needed to determine if long-term functional outcomes in patients treated with tibial nailing can be improved by surgical reduction and fixation of associated suprasyndesmotic fibular fractures.

## Conflict of Interests

All authors certify that they have no commercial associations (e.g., consultancy, stock ownership, equity interest, or patent/licensing arrangement) that would pose a conflict of interests in connection with the submitted paper.

## Acknowledgments

The English in this document has been checked by at least two professional editors, both native speakers of English. For a certificate, please see http://www.textcheck.com/certificate/1cVSx3.

## References

[1] J. G. Garrick, R. S. Riggins, R. K. Requa, and P. R. Lipscomb, "Fracture of the mid-shaft of the tibia and fibula. A survey of treatment," *Clinical Orthopaedics and Related Research*, vol. 88, pp. 131–137, 1972.

[2] G. Hooper, R. A. Buxton, and W. J. Gillespie, "Isolated fractures of the shaft of the tibia," *Injury*, vol. 12, no. 4, pp. 283–287, 1981.

[3] J. F. Keating, R. S. Kuo, and C. M. Court-Brown, "Bifocal fractures of the tibia and fibula. Incidence, classification and treatment," *Journal of Bone and Joint Surgery*, vol. 76, no. 3, pp. 395–400, 1994.

[4] K. Weise, H. Hermichen, and S. Weller, "Significance of the fibula in tibial fractures and pseudarthroses," *Aktuelle Traumatologie*, vol. 15, no. 5, pp. 195–204, 1985.

[5] T. C. Merchant and F. R. Dietz, "Long-term follow-up after fractures of the tibial and fibular shafts," *The Journal of Bone and Joint Surgery—Series A*, vol. 71, no. 4, pp. 599–606, 1989.

[6] M. Astrom and T. Arvidson, "Alignment and joint motion in the normal foot," *Journal of Orthopaedic & Sports Physical Therapy*, vol. 22, no. 5, pp. 216–222, 1995.

[7] E. M. Roos, H. P. Roos, L. S. Lohmander, C. Ekdahl, and B. D. Beynnon, "Knee injury and osteoarthritis outcome score (KOOS)—development of a self-administered outcome measure," *Journal of Orthopaedic & Sports Physical Therapy*, vol. 28, no. 2, pp. 88–96, 1998.

[8] R. L. Martin, R. G. Burdett, and J. J. Irrgang, "Development of the foot and ankle disability index (FADI)," *Journal of Orthopaedic & Sports Physical Therapy*, vol. 29, pp. A32–A33, 1999.

[9] A. H. Schmidt, C. G. Finkemeier, and P. Tornetta III, "Treatment of closed tibial fractures," *Instructional Course Lectures*, vol. 52, pp. 607–622, 2003.

[10] E. K. Stuermer and K. M. Stuermer, "Tibial shaft fracture and ankle joint injury," *Journal of Orthopaedic Trauma*, vol. 22, no. 2, pp. 107–112, 2008.

[11] A. M. Whorton and M. B. Henley, "The role of fixation of the fibula in open fractures of the tibial shaft with fractures of the ipsilateral fibula: Indications and outcomes," *Orthopedics*, vol. 21, no. 10, pp. 1101–1105, 1998.

[12] H. A. Vallier, B. A. Cureton, and B. M. Patterson, "Factors influencing functional outcomes after distal tibia shaft fractures," *Journal of Orthopaedic Trauma*, vol. 26, no. 3, pp. 178–183, 2012.

[13] L. K. Cannada, J. O. Anglen, M. T. Archdeacon, D. Herscovici Jr., and R. F. Ostrum, "Avoiding complications in the care of fractures of the tibia," *Instructional Course Lectures*, vol. 58, pp. 27–36, 2009.

[14] K. Pobłocki, M. Domaradzki, J. Gawdzik, P. Prochacki, and R. Rajewski, "Complications after intramedullary nailing of the tibia," *Chirurgia Narządów Ruchu i Ortopedia Polska*, vol. 76, no. 5, pp. 274–277, 2011.

[15] C. L. Saltzman and G. Y. El-Khoury, "The hindfoot alignment view," *Foot & Ankle International*, vol. 16, no. 9, pp. 572–576, 1995.

[16] E. J. Strauss, D. Alfonso, F. J. Kummer, K. A. Egol, and N. C. Tejwani, "The effect of concurrent fibular fracture on the fixation of distal tibia fractures: a laboratory comparison of intramedullary nails with locked plates," *Journal of Orthopaedic Trauma*, vol. 21, no. 3, pp. 172–177, 2007.

[17] A. Kumar, S. J. Charlebois, E. L. Cain, R. A. Smith, A. U. Daniels, and J. M. Crates, "Effect of fibular plate fixation on rotational stability of simulated distal tibiae fractures treated with intramedullary nailing," *Journal of Bone and Joint Surgery—Series A*, vol. 85, no. 4, pp. 604–608, 2003.

[18] K. A. Egol, R. Weisz, R. Hiebert, N. C. Tejwani, K. J. Koval, and R. W. Sanders, "Does fibular plating improve alignment after intramedullary nailing of distal metaphyseal tibia fractures?" *Journal of Orthopaedic Trauma*, vol. 20, no. 2, pp. 94–103, 2006.

[19] S. A. Stufkens, C. J. van Bergen, L. Blankevoort, C. N. van Dijk, B. Hintermann, and M. Knupp, "The role of the fibula in varus and valgus deformity of the tibia: a biomechanical study," *Journal of Bone and Joint Surgery*, vol. 93, no. 9, pp. 1232–1239, 2011.

# 32

# Outcomes of Geriatric Hip Fractures Treated with AFFIXUS Hip Fracture Nail

**Ahmed Mabrouk,**[1] **Mysore Madhusudan,**[2] **Mohammed Waseem,**[2] **Steven Kershaw,**[2] **and Jochen Fischer**[2]

[1]*ST2 Plastic Surgery, St. Andrews Centre for Plastic Surgery and Burns, Broomfield Hospital, Chelmsford, Essex CM1 7ET, UK*
[2]*Macclesfield Hospital, Victoria Road, Macclesfield, Cheshire SK10 3BL, UK*

Correspondence should be addressed to Ahmed Mabrouk; nabilangel2010@yahoo.com

Academic Editor: Boris Zelle

Geriatric hip fractures are one of the commonest fractures worldwide. The purpose of this study was to report the outcomes of a series of unstable geriatric hip fractures treated with AFFIXUS hip fracture nail. A retrospective study of 100 unstable geriatric hip fractures treated with AFFIXUS hip fracture nail is presented. The mean follow-up duration was 8 months (range 3–32). Of the patients 83% were female. The average age was 85 years. The fracture was treated by closed reduction and intramedullary fixation. The mean acute hospital stay was 17.6 days. Systemic complications occurred in 29 patients (29%) and local complications in 3 patients (3%) including lag screw cutout in one patient (1%), lag screw backout in one patient (1%), and deep infection in one patient (1%). Mechanical failures and periprosthetic fractures were not observed in our series. Fractures united in all patients. Preinjury activity level was recovered in 78% of the patients. The results of AFFIXUS hip fracture nail were satisfactory in most elderly patients. The unique design of the lag screw and its thread spacing had effectively reduced cut-out rate.

## 1. Introduction

The incidence of hip fractures has been rising in geriatric population in many parts of the world, and the number of hip fractures is expected to reach 512,000 in 2040 [1]. The aim of surgery is to allow early mobilization and prompt return to prefracture activity level [2]. The demand for prompt mobilization with full loading of the affected limb, combined with a desire for the most gentle treatment, becomes increasingly difficult to meet in an ageing patient with advanced osteoporosis [3].

Several clinical and biomechanical studies have analyzed the results of different implants such as the dynamic hip screw (Synthes, USA), the gamma nail (Stryker, Germany), and the proximal femoral nail (Synthes, USA). Those devices have suffered cutout, implant breakage, femoral shaft fracture, and subsequent loss of reduction in the clinical practice [4–8]. AFFIXUS hip fracture nail is a new device introduced in 2011 by DePuy Orthopaedics, Inc., USA. It combines the principle

of the compression hip screw with the biomechanical advantages of an intramedullary nail. The major development is the unique design and thread spacing of the lag screw which provides better resistance to cutout.

To our knowledge, there are no studies on the AFFIXUS nail in the literature. The purpose of this study was to report initial results of the AFFIXUS nail in the treatment of geriatric hip fractures.

## 2. Patients and Methods

With approval from our clinical effectiveness department, we conducted a retrospective review of 104 consecutive unstable geriatric hip fractures, treated with AFFIXUS hip fracture nail, at our institution from July 2011 to December 2013. Inclusion criteria were patients aged 60 and above with proximal femur fracture (AO/OTA classification [9] types: 31-A2, 31-A3, 32-A2, and 32-A3). We excluded patients younger than 60 years old with pathological hip fractures and

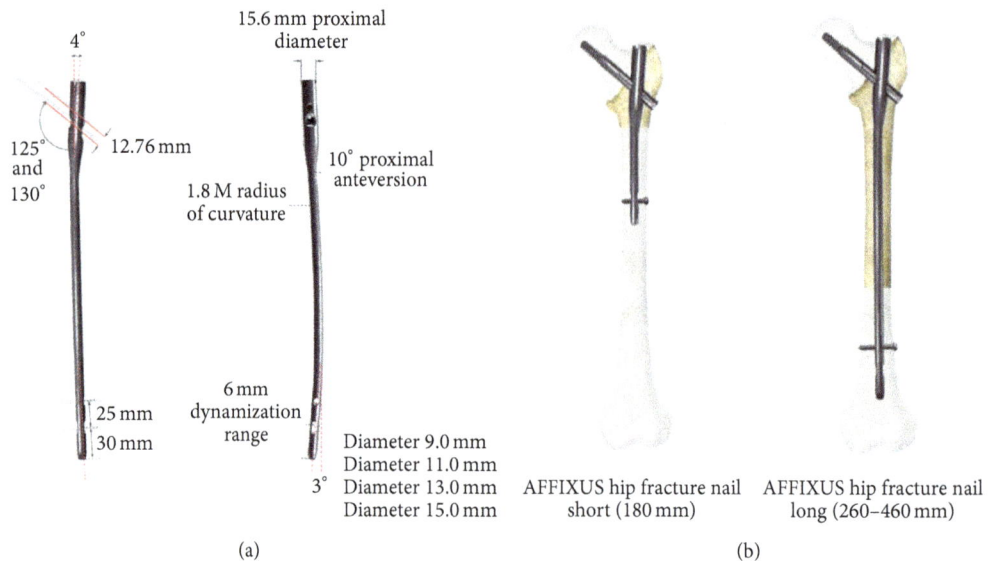

FIGURE 1: (a) AFFIXUS nail diagram. (b) Short and long AFFIXUS nails.

TABLE 1: Preoperative variables.

| Variable | Value |
| --- | --- |
| Mean age (Y) | 85 (62–102) |
| Sex (male : female) | (1 : 4) |
| Side (R : L) | (1 : 1) |
| Fracture classification (AO/OTA) | |
|   31-A2 | 50 |
|   31-A3 | 46 |
|   32-A2 | 3 |
|   32-A3 | 1 |
| Mechanism of injury | |
|   Fracture following a mechanical fall | 98 |
|   Healing insufficiency fracture | 1 |
|   DHS revision into a nail | 1 |
| ASA classification | |
|   1 | 1 |
|   2 | 18 |
|   3 | 41 |
|   4 | 39 |

periprosthetic hip fractures. A total of 100 patients were available for outcome analysis in this study. Preoperative variables are listed in Table 1.

AFFIXUS nail is available in 2 sizes, short (180 mm) and long (260–460 mm) (Figure 1); the unique thread spacing and lag screw design help to resist displacement and cutout. There is 10° of proximal anteversion built into the nail. The cannulated lag screw measures 10.5 mm in diameter for bone preservation. There is a choice of 125° and 130° neck angles to provide a range of anatomical options. The chamfer on the front distal tip facilitates insertion and decreases risk of stress on the anterior cortex in the distal femur. The 3° distal bend facilitates ease of insertion through the proximal intertrochanteric/subtrochanteric region. There is a preloaded set screw for ease of use and a 5.0 mm antirotation (AR) screw for rotational control. The shouldered lag screw and AR screw help preventing medial screw disengagement.

All surgeries were performed within 48 hours of admission [10]. All fractures were treated by closed reduction under C-arm fluoroscopy control. All operations were performed or supervised by experienced consultant orthopedic surgeon. Any postoperative blood transfusion was recorded. The reduction of head and neck fragment was evaluated by Garden alignment index (GAI) and lag screw position was evaluated by tip apex distance (TAD) [11, 12].

In all cases, antithrombotic prophylaxis was given using low molecular weight heparin and antibiotic prophylaxis was provided. The medical care and rehabilitation protocol was identical, all patients were reviewed by an orthogeriatrician within 48 hours of admission, and patients were mobilized on the first postoperative day. Partial weight bearing as tolerated or restricted weight bearing was allowed according to the surgeon's recommendation on the following day.

The average follow-up period was 8 months (range 3–32 months) with SD (standard deviation) of 7. Clinical and radiographic examinations were performed at the time of admission and at two, four, and eight months postoperatively. We noted any change in the position of the implants and the progress of fracture union. Garden alignment index (GAI) and tip apex distance (TAD) were recorded. Radiographic measurements were performed manually, by two independent observers (Ahmed Mabrouk and Mysore Madhusudan) using a protractor and a ruler to provide values for GAI and TAD.

## 3. Results

The average age of the patients was 85 years (SD 8.1), of which 83% were female. According to AO/OTA classification

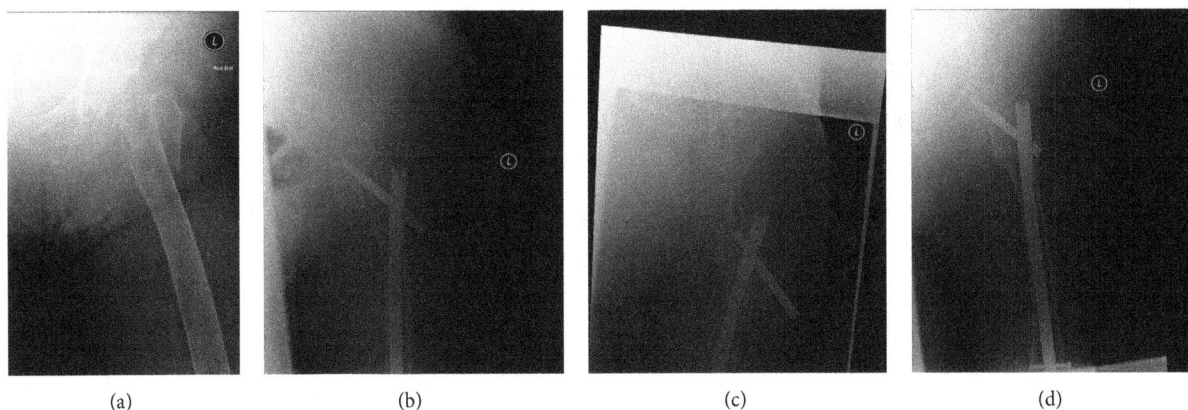

FIGURE 2: (a) 83-year-old female with proximal femoral fracture (AO/OTA type 31-A3). (b) Immediate postoperative radiograph. (c) Radiograph 15 months after surgery showing the backout. (d) Radiograph after revision of the lag screw.

system [9], 50 cases were type 31-A2 (50%), 46 cases were type 31-A3 (46%), 3 cases were type 32-A2 (3%), and 1 case was type 32-A3 (1%). The long nail (260–460 mm length) was used in 61 cases (61%) and short nail was used in 39 cases (39%). The favored length of the lag screw was 90–105 mm. All distal locking was performed statically by means of one 5 mm screw.

According to Garden alignment index, postoperative X-rays showed a near-anatomical fracture reduction in almost all cases. Implant positioning with a mean TAD 24.9 mm (SD 1.8) was performed in 99 cases (99%). In 95 cases, placement of the lag screw was perceived as "ideal," in the lower half more to the centre of the femoral neck. Lag screw was placed in the lower third of the femoral neck in 4 cases and in the upper third of the femoral neck in one case.

The mean acute hospital stay was 17.6 days (SD 6.6). Additionally, 27 patients had a rehabilitation period with a mean of 44.2 days (SD 27). During the postoperative period, systemic complications occurred in 29 patients including 11 pneumonia, 8 urinary tract infections, 3 myocardial ischemia, 1 heart failure, 4 postoperative anemia requiring transfusion, 1 hypoproteinaemia, and 1 pulmonary embolism. There were three local complications as reflected in Table 2. We had one deep wound infection that required incision and drainage. Any haematomata of the surgical wound resolved satisfactorily. Superficial infections also resolved favourably once the appropriate antibiotic treatment was instituted.

Any haematomata of the surgical wound resolved satisfactorily. Cases of superficial infection also resolved favourably once the appropriate antibiotic treatment was instituted. Mechanical failures such as bending or breaking of the implant were not seen. Backout was seen in one case, 5 months after surgery for which the lag screw was revised (Figure 2). One case of cutout was observed 15 months after surgery when the fracture had united and AFFIXUS nail was removed (Figure 3). In our series we had one case of on-table revision of DHS into a short AFFIXUS nail (Figure 4), which showed the versatility of AFFIXUS nail indications.

## 4. Discussion

In this study, although the follow-up period was not adequate to measure long-term outcomes, the average 8-month results

TABLE 2: Postoperative complications.

| Complications | Number of cases |
|---|---|
| Systemic complications | |
| Pneumonia | 11 |
| Myocardial infarction | 3 |
| Cardiac failure | 1 |
| Urinary tract infection | 8 |
| Hypoproteinaemia | 1 |
| Deep venous thrombosis | 0 |
| Pulmonary embolism | 1 |
| Postoperative anaemia required transfusion | 4 |
| Local complications | |
| Deep infection | 1 |
| Lag screw cutout | 1 |
| Lag screw back out | 1 |

of AFFIXUS nail fixations were satisfactory. The results showed that AFFIXUS nail provided reliable fixation of hip fractures in elderly patients. The operative procedure for AFFIXUS nail was easily performed, thus reducing blood loss and operative time. In our study, intraoperative variables and systemic complications were similar to those encountered by other authors for different implants in different institutions. However, our local complication rate was much better than those recorded by other authors [5, 13–15]. The overall complication rate requiring further surgery was 3%. The cut-out rate was 1%. The backout rate was 1%. Fracture healing was achieved in all patients. No cases of implant breakage and fatigue were seen during the follow-up period.

Hrubina et al. [13] recorded a total of 39 (11%) specific complications of the dynamic hip screw system in their series. Of these, 44% were intraoperative complications including insufficient reduction, broken tip of a K-wire, faulty technical procedure, and fracture of the distal fragment during surgery, in addition to postoperative complications including "cut-out" phenomenon, avascular necrosis of the femoral head,

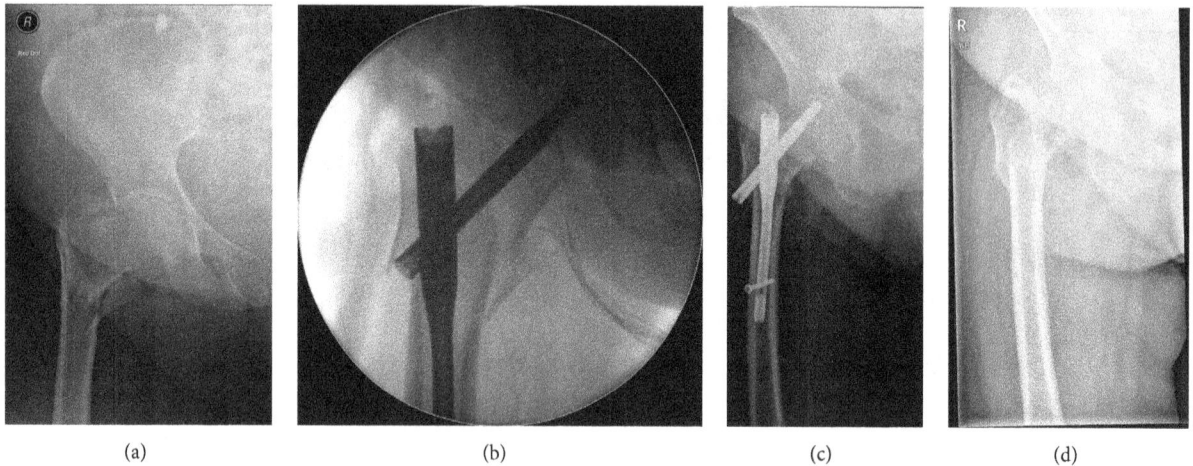

FIGURE 3: (a) 90-year-old female with proximal femoral fracture (AO/OTA type 31-A2). (b) Intraoperative radiograph anteroposterior view. (c) 5 months after surgery showing the cutout. (d) Immediately after removal of the nail.

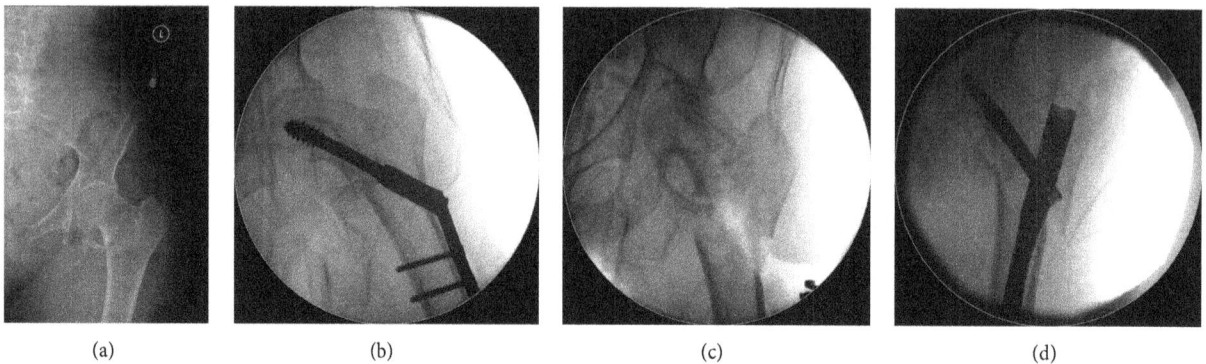

FIGURE 4: (a) 95-year-old female with proximal femoral fracture (AO/OTA type 31-A3). (b) Intraoperative radiograph showing the DHS. (c) Intraoperative radiograph after removal of the DHS. (d) Intraoperative radiograph showing the revision with AFFIXUS nail.

progression of coxarthrosis, screw breakage, femoral fracture under the plate, pseudarthrosis, and late infection. Hesse and Gächter [5] reported 8% of implant related complications in a series of trochanteric fractures treated with gamma nails. These complications included the following: a short gamma nail needed a conversion to a long gamma nail due to pseudarthrosis or femur fracture at the distal interlocking bolt. Other complications included distal femur fracture through the distal bolt, necessitating a plate osteosynthesis.

In our series, the choice of short and long AFFIXUS nails using a single set of user-friendly instruments made the operative procedure straight forward without intraoperative complications. AFFIXUS nail chamfer on the front distal tip facilitates insertion and decreases risk of stress on the anterior cortex of the distal femur, which reduced the risk of periprosthetic fractures. The design of the lag screw and its thread spacing reduced the incidence of screw cutout. The 2 failure cases included a lag screw backout, which was likely due to inherent instability caused by the Z effect for a proximal femur fracture [16]. The other short AFFIXUS used cutout because the orientation and placement of the lag screw were too superior and TAD was 38 mm.

Baumgaertner et al. [11] described a lower complication rate for implant tips placed close to the subchondral bone

of the femoral head as none of the screws with a tip-apex distance of twenty-five millimeters or less cutout, but there was a very strong statistical relationship between an increasing tip-apex distance and cut-out rate, regardless of all other variables related to the fracture. This is similar to our series, as all the lag screws had a mean TAD of twenty-five millimeters. The cut-out case had a TAD of 38 mm.

In conclusion, the results of AFFIXUS hip fracture nail were satisfactory in most elderly patients. The unique design of the lag screw and its thread spacing had effectively reduced the cut-out rate. No mechanical failure was observed in our series.

## Conflict of Interests

The authors declare that there is no conflict of interests regarding the publication of this paper.

## References

[1] X. Huang, F. Leung, Z. Xiang et al., "Proximal femoral nail versus dynamic hip screw fixation for trochanteric fractures: A meta-analysis of randomized controlled trials," *The Scientific World Journal*, vol. 2013, Article ID 805805, 8 pages, 2013.

[2]  J.-S. Pu, L. Liu, G.-L. Wang, Y. Fang, and T.-F. Yang, "Results of the proximal femoral nail anti-rotation (PFNA) in elderly Chinese patients," *International Orthopaedics*, vol. 33, no. 5, pp. 1441–1444, 2009.

[3]  F. Bonnaire, H. Zenker, C. Lill, A. T. Weber, and B. Linke, "Treatment strategies for proximal femur fractures in osteoporotic patients," *Osteoporosis International*, vol. 16, no. 2, pp. S93–S102, 2005.

[4]  A. Appelt, N. Suhm, M. Baier, and P.-J. Meeder, "Complications after intramedullary stabilization of proximal femur fractures: a retrospective analysis of 178 patients," *European Journal of Trauma and Emergency Surgery*, vol. 33, no. 3, pp. 262–267, 2007.

[5]  B. Hesse and A. Gächter, "Complications following the treatment of trochanteric fractures with the gamma nail," *Archives of Orthopaedic and Trauma Surgery*, vol. 124, no. 10, pp. 692–698, 2004.

[6]  L. J. Domingo, D. Cecilia, A. Herrera, and C. Resines, "Trochanteric fractures treated with a proximal femoral nail," *International Orthopaedics*, vol. 25, no. 5, pp. 298–301, 2001.

[7]  S. Papasimos, C. M. Koutsojannis, A. Panagopoulos, P. Megas, and E. Lambiris, "A randomised comparison of AMBI, TGN and PFN for treatment of unstable trochanteric fractures," *Archives of Orthopaedic and Trauma Surgery*, vol. 125, no. 7, pp. 462–468, 2005.

[8]  I. B. Schipper, E. W. Steyerberg, R. M. Castelein et al., "Treatment of unstable trochanteric fractures: randomised comparison of the gamma nail and the proximal femoral nail," *Journal of Bone and Joint Surgery*, vol. 86, no. 1, pp. 86–94, 2004.

[9]  M. E. Müller, S. Nazarian, P. Koch, and J. Schatzker, *The Comprehensive Classification of Fractures of Long Bones*, Springer, Berlin, Germany, 1990.

[10]  R. Griffiths, J. Alper, A. Beckingsale et al., "Management of proximal femoral fractures 2011: Association of Anaesthetists of Great Britain and Ireland," *Anaesthesia*, vol. 67, no. 1, pp. 85–98, 2012.

[11]  M. R. Baumgaertner, S. L. Curtin, D. M. Lindskog, and J. M. Keggi, "The value of the tip-apex distance in predicting failure of fixation of peritrochanteric fractures of the hip," *Journal of Bone and Joint Surgery—Series A*, vol. 77, no. 7, pp. 1058–1064, 1995.

[12]  R. Clifford, "Garden's Alignment Index," 2014, http://www.wheelessonline.com.

[13]  M. Hrubina, M. Skoták, and J. Běkhoune, "Complications of dynamic hip screw treatment for proximal femoral fractures," *Acta Chirurgiae Orthopaedicae et Traumatologiae Cechoslovaca*, vol. 77, no. 5, pp. 395–401, 2010.

[14]  J. Windolf, D. A. Hollander, M. Hakimi, and W. Linhart, "Pitfalls and complications in the use of the proximal femoral nail," *Langenbeck's Archives of Surgery*, vol. 390, no. 1, pp. 59–65, 2005.

[15]  T. Pavelka, J. Matejka, and H. Cervenková, "Complications of internal fixation by a short proximal femoral nail," *Acta Chirurgiae Orthopaedicae et Traumatologiae Cechoslovaca*, vol. 72, no. 6, pp. 344–354, 2005.

[16]  R. E. Santos Pires, E. O. Santana, L. E. Nascimento Santos, V. Giordano, D. Balbachevsky, and F. B. dos Reis, "Failure of fixation of trochanteric femur fractures: clinical recommendations for avoiding Z-effect and reverse Z-effect type complications," *Patient Safety in Surgery*, vol. 5, p. 17, 2011.

# 33

# Posterior Transpedicular Dynamic Stabilization versus Total Disc Replacement in the Treatment of Lumbar Painful Degenerative Disc Disease: A Comparison of Clinical Results

**Tunc Oktenoglu,[1] Ali Fahir Ozer,[2] Mehdi Sasani,[1] Yaprak Ataker,[3] Cengiz Gomleksiz,[4] and Irfan Celebi[5]**

[1] Neurosurgery Department, American Hospital, 34365 Istanbul, Turkey
[2] Neurosurgery Department, Koc University School of Medicine, 34450 Istanbul, Turkey
[3] Physical Therapy and Rehabilitation Department, American Hospital, 34365 Istanbul, Turkey
[4] Neurosurgery Department, Mengücek Gazi Training and Research Hospital, School of Medicine, Erzincan University, 2400 Erzincan, Turkey
[5] Radiology Department, Sisli Etfal Hospital, 34360 Istanbul, Turkey

Correspondence should be addressed to Ali Fahir Ozer; alifahirozer@gmail.com

Academic Editor: Deniz Erbulut

*Study Design.* Prospective clinical study. *Objective.* This study compares the clinical results of anterior lumbar total disc replacement and posterior transpedicular dynamic stabilization in the treatment of degenerative disc disease. *Summary and Background Data.* Over the last two decades, both techniques have emerged as alternative treatment options to fusion surgery. *Methods.* This study was conducted between 2004 and 2010 with a total of 50 patients (25 in each group). The mean age of the patients in total disc prosthesis group was 37,32 years. The mean age of the patients in posterior dynamic transpedicular stabilization was 43,08. Clinical (VAS and Oswestry) and radiological evaluations (lumbar lordosis and segmental lordosis angles) of the patients were carried out prior to the operation and 3, 12, and 24 months after the operation. We compared the average duration of surgery, blood loss during the surgery and the length of hospital stay of both groups. *Results.* Both techniques offered significant improvements in clinical parameters. There was no significant change in radiologic evaluations after the surgery for both techniques. *Conclusion.* Both dynamic systems provided spine stability. However, the posterior dynamic system had a slight advantage over anterior disc prosthesis because of its convenient application and fewer possible complications.

## 1. Introduction

Currently, one of the most important causes of chronic low back pain is thought to be a painful disc [1–3]. Some biomechanical and biochemical changes play a role in intervertebral disc degeneration; on the other hand intrinsic, extrinsic, and genetic factors are also important. Compression of the spine, torsional injuries, overload, and congenital anomalies have been shown to contribute to disc degeneration with applying excessive pressure onto intervertebral discs [4–10]. Despite numerous research studies, the etiology and physiopathology of disc degeneration remain unknown [2]. Annular tears resulting from degeneration of the annulus fibrosis, that contains pain receptors and internal disc ruptures, are the most common cause of pain [11–13]. Today, it is believed that degenerative disc disease (DDD) might cause instability in spine segments, and it is widely accepted that progressive back pain results due to this instability [14–16]. In fact, segmental instability begins when disc height deterioration is initiated by the progression of intervertebral disc degeneration. Instability as a consequence of disc degeneration has been described by Frymoyer [14, 15] as primary segmental instability and by Kirkaldy-Willis and Farfan [2] as the discogenic pain and instability stage in the overall process of degeneration. Benzel [16] included degenerative disc disease among the chronic instabilities and described the disease as "dysfunctional segmental motion" and "torsional instability." Fusion is the standard surgical treatment option for painful lumbar degenerative disc disease that is unresponsive to conservative treatment modalities. Nonetheless, the side effects of fusion (pseudarthrosis, adjacent segment disease, and the donor site morbidity) and suboptimal clinical satisfaction rates, which have been reported even in patients with radiologically observed fusion, have led to a search for alternative treatments [17–22].

Numerous dynamic techniques were developed over the last two decades. Recently, these devices were classified as total disc replacement (TDR) and posterior transpedicular dynamic systems (PTDS) [23]. Both PTDS and TDR have been widely used in surgical treatment of degenerative disc diseases of the lumbar spine. Numerous studies showed promising clinical results [24–35]. However, there is no study that compares the TDR and PTDS techniques in the treatment of DDD.

In this prospective study, we evaluated and compared the clinic and radiologic outcome of TDR and PTDS in patients with painful lumbar degenerative disc disease through an extensive literature review.

## 2. Material and Methods

*2.1. Total Disc Replacement Group.* We performed TDR on 25 patients (14 females and 11 males). The mean age of the patients was 37.32 (with a range from 25 to 50), and the mean follow-up period was 29.16 months (with a range from 24 to 42 months).

A lumbar total disc replacement (Maverick, Medtronic Sofamor Danek, Memphis, TN, USA) was placed into the intervertebral disc space with open window laparotomy technique [36].

All patients in the TDR group had a lumbar single-level painful disc. 15 patients showed L4-L5 DDD, and 10 patients showed L5-S1 DDD (Figure 1). All of the patients were informed about the surgery, and they signed a written, informed consent form. The inclusion criteria for TDR surgery included a complaint of lower back pain that had duration of at least 12 months and at least six months of conservative treatment without satisfactory results. Other inclusion criteria were that the patients must be less than 50 years old and have no signs of lumbar degenerative spondylolisthesis or osteoarthritis in their facet joints, which was confirmed with computerized tomography (CT) and dynamic plain radiographs. The patients also had to have symptomatic lumbar degenerative disc disease that was visible in magnetic resonance imaging (MRI) as a blackened disc as well as a confirmation of the diagnosis by displaying pain behaviors during discography.

*2.2. Posterior Dynamic Transpedicular Stabilization Group.* We performed posterior dynamic transpedicular stabilization on 25 patients (13 females and 12 males). The mean age of the patients was 43.08 years (with a range from 24 to 55 years),

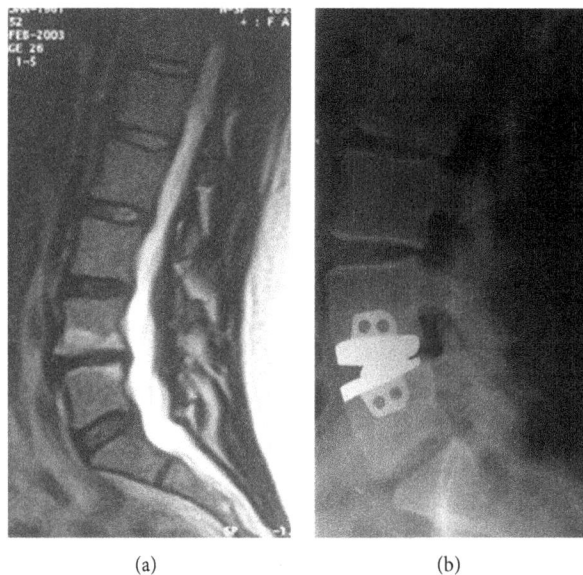

(a)　　　　　　　　　　(b)

FIGURE 1: A 30-year-old woman complained of severe back pain attacks. She had no neurological deficits. (a) T2-weighted MRI scans showed advanced degeneration with Modic changes in the L4-L5 disc. (b) Maverick disc prosthesis was applied.

and the mean follow-up period was 36.48 months (with a range from 24 to 48 months).

Patients in the dynamic posterior stabilization group were operated with the Cosmic (Ulrich GmbH & Co. KG, Ulm, Germany) posterior dynamic transpedicular stabilization system (hinged screw-rigid rod) through transmuscular approach [35].

All cases in the PTDS group had one-level painful disc disease. The operated discs were L4-L5 region (16 cases) and L5-S1 region (9 cases) (Figure 2).

Similar to the patients in the TDR group, the inclusion criteria included a confirmed diagnosis of symptomatic lumbar degenerative disc disease through MRI and positive discography, a complaint of lower back pain that had a duration of at least 12 months, at least 6 months of conservative treatment without satisfactory results, and the absence of apparent instability confirmed with lumbosacral dynamic X-rays.

*2.3. Clinical Evaluation.* We evaluated and compared the average surgical time, blood loss during the surgery, and the length of the stay in hospital for both groups of patients (Table 1). The visual analog scale (VAS) and the Oswestry Disability Index (ODI) were used for the clinical evaluations and follow-up examinations. Clinical evaluations of the patients were carried out in the data at preoperative period and 3, 12, and 24 months after the surgery (Tables 2 and 3).

*2.4. Radiological Evaluation.* To diagnose lumbar disc disease, an MRI examination of each patient was performed and a black disc was observed. Pain symptoms were confirmed with the detection of provocative pain through a discography

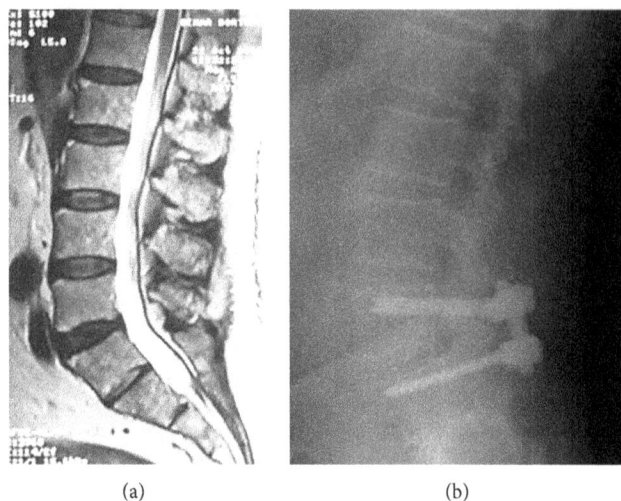

(a)　　　　　　　　　　　　　　(b)

FIGURE 2: (a) A 50-year-old male complained of severe back pain attacks. (a) T2-weighted MRI scans showed degeneration of the disc at L4-L5 lumbar disc (L5- S1 considered as sacralization). (b) Following posterior transpedicular dynamic stabilization with the Cosmic system.

TABLE 1: Comparison of TDR and PTDS groups.

|  |  | TDR ($n = 25$) | PTDS ($n = 25$) | $P$ |
|---|---|---|---|---|
| Age | Min–Max | 25–50 | 24–55 | $0.018^{*}$ |
|  | Mean ± SD | 37.32 ± 6.62 | 43.08 ± 9.65 |  |
| Followup (month) | Min–Max | 24–42 | 24–48 | $0.001^{**}$ |
|  | Mean ± SD | 29.16 ± 4.77 | 36.48 ± 6.72 |  |
| Length of hospital stay (day) | Min–Max | 3–5 | 2–5 | $0.022^{*}$ |
|  | Mean ± SD | 3.56 ± 0.58 | 3.04 ± 0.93 |  |
| Operation time (minute) | Min–Max | 120–260 | 40–70 | $0.001^{**}$ |
|  | Mean ± SD | 181.20 ± 39.40 | 52.40 ± 7.79 |  |
| Blood loss (mL.) | Min–Max | 300–600 | 75–175 | $0.001^{**}$ |
|  | Mean ± SD | 402.00 ± 91.83 | 103.00 ± 22.03 |  |

Student's $t$-test, $^{*}P < 0.05$, $^{**}P < 0.01$.

which was applied to the black disc. Lumbosacral plain and dynamic (hyperflexion and hyperextension) X-rays and CT examinations of the patients were carried out by independent radiology experts in preoperative. Follow-up plain X-Ray studies were obtained 3, 12, and 24 months after the surgery. Control CT study was performed in postoperative 24 months. Loose screws as well as broken screws, instrument migration, subsidence, and spontaneous fusion were evaluated. Additionally lumbar lordosis angle (LL) and segmental lordosis angle ($\alpha$) data was obtained (Tables 4 and 5) (Figure 3).

2.5. Statistical Analysis. The Number Cruncher Statistical System (NCSS) 2007 and 2008 PASS Statistical Software (Utah, USA) were used for statistical analysis of the data. In addition to descriptive statistical methods (e.g., mean, standard deviation), Student's $t$-test was used to compare the normally distributed parameters between the two groups. The Mann-Whitney $U$ test was used for the comparison of parameters with nonnormal distribution. Bonferroni test was used to compare the follow-up data with normal distribution,

and paired sample $t$-test was used for dual comparison. In nonnormal distribution group, the follow-up data compared with Friedman test and Wilcoxon test was used for dual comparison. The significance level was $P < 0.05$.

## 3. Results

There was statistically significant difference observed between the mean ages and follow-up periods of the groups ($P < 0.05$) (Table 1). The PTDS applied to significantly older patients was compared to TDR group.

There was a statistically significant difference ($P < 0.01$) between the level of blood loss in the two groups. The level of blood loss was significantly higher in the TDR group compared to the PTDS group (Table 1, Figure 4).

The operation time was significantly longer ($P < 0.01$) in the TDR group compared to the posterior dynamic stabilization group (Table 1, Figure 5).

There was significant difference in the length of the hospital stay between the two groups ($P < 0.05$) (Table 1).

TABLE 2: (a) The comparison of VAS scores. (b) The comparison of decrease % in follow-up VAS data.

(a)

| VAS | | TDR ($n = 25$) | PTDS ($n = 25$) | $^aP$ |
|---|---|---|---|---|
| Preop VAS | Min–Max | 6–10 | 6–9 | 0.219 |
| | Mean ± SD | 8.24 ± 1.09[8] | 7.96 ± 0.79 [8] | |
| VAS (3 months) | Min–Max | 0–5 | 1–5 | 0.588 |
| | Mean ± SD | 2.44 ± 1.16 [2]$^{\ddagger}$ | 2.64 ± 0.91 [2]$^{\ddagger}$ | |
| VAS (12 months) | Min–Max | 0–3 | 0–4 | 0.087 |
| | Mean ± SD | 1.68 ± 0.85 [2]$^{\ddagger}$ | 1.28 ± 0.94 [1]$^{\ddagger}$ | |
| VAS (24 months) | Min–Max | 0–2 | 0–3 | 0.240 |
| | Mean ± SD | 0.84 ± 0.69 [1]$^{\ddagger}$ | 0.68 ± 0.85 [1]$^{\ddagger}$ | |
| $^bP$ | | 0.001$^{**}$ | 0.001$^{**}$ | |

$^a$Mann-Whitney $U$ test, $^b$Friedman test.
$^{\ddagger}$Wilcoxon signed-rank test $P < 0.001$.
$^{**}P < 0.01$.

(b)

| VAS (decrease %) | TDR ($n = 25$) Mean ± SD | PTDS ($n = 25$) Mean ± SD | $P$ |
|---|---|---|---|
| Preop * VAS (3 months) | 70.18 ± 14.14 | 66.18 ± 13.57 | 0.374 |
| Preop * VAS (12 months) | 79.91 ± 10.00 | 83.71 ± 12.08 | 0.214 |
| Preop * VAS (24 months) | 89.86 ± 8.41 | 91.30 ± 10.78 | 0.519 |

Mann-Whitney $U$ test.

TABLE 3: (a) The comparison of ODI scores. (b) The comparison of decrease % in follow-up OSW data.

(a)

| ODI | | TDR ($n = 25$) | PTDS ($n = 25$) | $^aP$ |
|---|---|---|---|---|
| Preop ODI | Min–Max | 40–100 | 46–98 | 0.847 |
| | Mean ± SD | 67.20 ± 20.79 | 66.16 ± 16.82 | |
| ODI (3 months) | Min–Max | 12–56 | 12–38 | 0.069 |
| | Mean ± SD | 32.32 ± 10.87$^{\ddagger}$ | 27.16 ± 8.63$^{\ddagger}$ | |
| ODI (12 months) | Min–Max | 4–34 | 2–26 | 0.010$^{*}$ |
| | Mean ± SD | 18.00 ± 7.64$^{\ddagger}$ | 12.88 ± 5.75$^{\ddagger}$ | |
| ODI (24 months) | Min–Max | 2–20 | 2–18 | 0.408 |
| | Mean ± SD | 9.12 ± 4.28$^{\ddagger}$ | 8.04 ± 4.53$^{\ddagger}$ | |
| $^bP$ | | 0.001$^{**}$ | 0.001$^{**}$ | |

$^a$Student's $t$-test, $^b$repeated measures test.
$^{\ddagger}$Adjustment for multiple comparisons: Bonferroni $P < 0.01$.
$^{*}P < 0.05$, $^{**}P < 0.01$.

(b)

| ODI (decrease %) | TDR ($n = 25$) Mean ± SD | PTDS ($n = 25$) Mean ± SD | $P$ |
|---|---|---|---|
| Preop * ODI (3 months) | 49.96 ± 16.46 | 54.91 ± 20.00 | 0.669 |
| Preop * ODI (12 months) | 72.80 ± 9.33 | 78.22 ± 11.68 | 0.093 |
| Preop * ODI (24 months) | 86.15 ± 6.15 | 86.33 ± 8.92 | 0.808 |

Mann-Whitney $U$ test.

Preoperative VAS and ODI levels were not significantly ($P > 0.05$ and $P > 0.05$) different between the groups (Tables 2 and 3).

In both groups the clinical parameters (VAS and ODI) showed significant improvement in all postoperative time periods when compared to preoperative data (Tables 2 and 3, $P < 0.01$). There were no statistically significant differences observed between the groups for the each follow-up VAS ($P < 0.05$, Table 2). The ODI data showed significant difference only in postop 12 months. The PTDS group had significantly

TABLE 4: The comparison of LL angles.

| LL | | TDR ($n = 25$) | PTDS ($n = 25$) | $^{a}P$ |
|---|---|---|---|---|
| Preop LL | Min–Max | 25–65 | 34–72 | 0.948 |
| | Mean ± SD | 49.60 ± 10.46 | 49.80 ± 11.26 | |
| LL (3 months) | Min–Max | 26–65 | 34–69 | 0.747 |
| | Mean ± SD | 49.52 ± 9.51 | 48.60 ± 10.52 | |
| LL (12 months) | Min–Max | 24–64 | 30–67 | 0.764 |
| | Mean ± SD | 49.60 ± 10.15 | 48.72 ± 10.50 | |
| LL (24 months) | Min–Max | 22–65 | 35–65 | 0.786 |
| | Mean ± SD | 49.56 ± 10.38 | 48.80 ± 9.30 | |
| | $^{b}P$ | 0.998 | 0.890 | |

$^{a}$Student's $t$-test, $^{b}$repeated measures test.
LL: lumbar lordosis.

TABLE 5: The comparison of SL ($\alpha$) angles.

| ALPHA | | TDR ($n = 25$) | PTDS ($n = 25$) | $^{a}P$ |
|---|---|---|---|---|
| Preop ALPHA | Min–Max | 4–17 | 4–30 | 0.274 |
| | Mean ± SD | 10.32 ± 3.06 | 11.68 ± 5.33 | |
| ALPHA (3 months) | Min–Max | 3–19 | 3–33 | 0.566 |
| | Mean ± SD | 10.40 ± 3.70 | 11.20 ± 5.84 | |
| ALPHA (12 months) | Min–Max | 4–16 | 2–31 | 0.392 |
| | Mean ± SD | 10.36 ± 2.90 | 11.52 ± 6.05 | |
| ALPHA (24 months) | Min–Max | 5–14 | 3–30 | 0.248 |
| | Mean ± SD | 10.32 ± 2.28 | 11.56 ± 4.79 | |
| | $^{b}P$ | 0.989 | 0.858 | |

$^{a}$Student's $t$-test, $^{b}$repeated measures test.
SL: segmental lordosis.

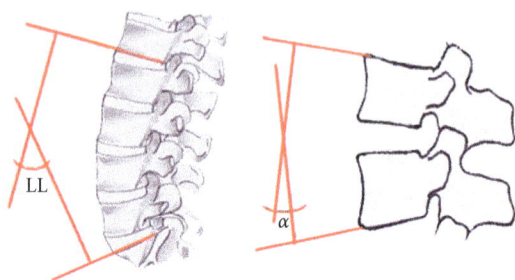

FIGURE 3: Lordosis of the lumbar spine (L1-S1) was measured via the angle between the lines drawn from the lower endplate of L1 and the upper endplate of S1 (LL). Additionally segmental lordosis ($\alpha$) at the operation level was measured via the angle between the lines drawn from the upper and lower endplates of the vertebrae that form the operation segments.

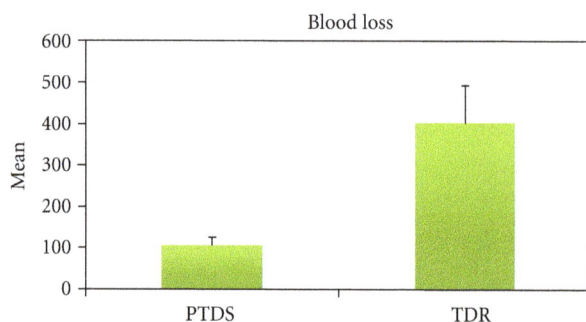

FIGURE 4: The data of blood loss in surgery for both groups.

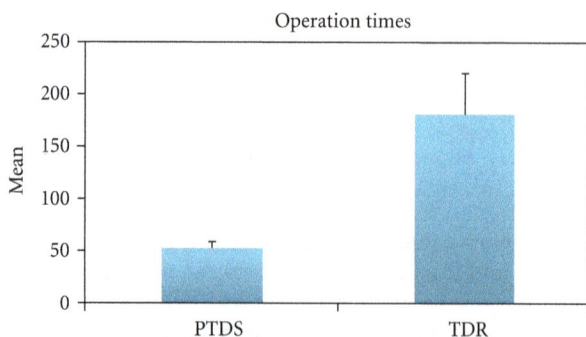

FIGURE 5: The data of operation times for both groups.

better outcome in this time period. However this advantage did not persist. There was no significant difference in 24-month scores ($P > 0.05$, Table 3) (Figures 6 and 7).

There were no significant differences observed between the preoperative and postoperative lumbar (LL) and segmental lordosis (alpha) evaluations for both techniques ($P > 0.05$) (Tables 4 and 5).

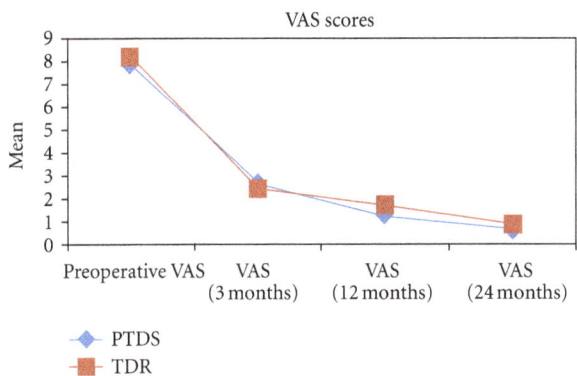

FIGURE 6: The distribution of VAS scores for both groups.

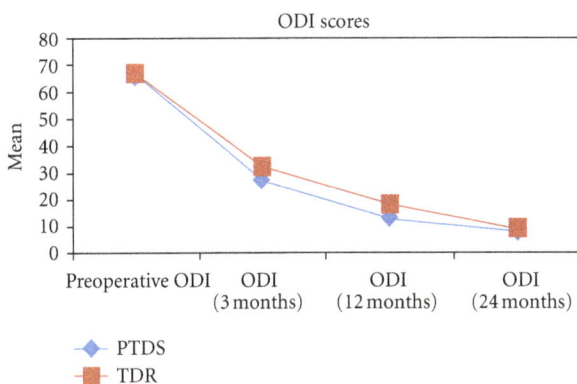

FIGURE 7: The distribution of ODI scores for both groups.

No surgical morbidity and/or complications observed in the group treated with PTDS. There were two iliac vein injuries that occurred in two patients in the TDR group. These injuries were sutured in the operation with no mortality and residual morbidity.

## 4. Discussion

Fusion has been widely used as a surgical treatment for painful disc disease. Fusion eliminates the abnormal movements and offers satisfactory outcome. On the other hand, even in patients with 100% fusion achieved with applying 360° fusion method, the satisfaction rate is not necessary optimal and might be low as 30% [19–21, 23, 24]. Donor site problems have also been a significant complication in fusion surgery [20]. Therefore, alternative treatment techniques were developed in an attempt to prevent side effects that are commonly observed after fusion surgery and to improve the patient satisfaction rate. In recent years, dynamic systems that provide spine mobility have been developed to avoid the well-known side effects of fusion technique. Today indications and contraindications of TDR and PTDS are well known [23]. Both techniques can be used for the same indications. A painful black disc can be treated with application of either technique.

TDR was developed over the past ten years as a promising surgery that was preferable over fusion surgery because the proponents of TDR claimed that the procedure preserves mobility and reduces the risk of adjacent segment disease. After a ten-year effort by Büttner-Janz et al., TDR was announced as a new solution method for painful disc disease [37]. Numerous TDR systems were developed and offered for clinical application [29, 32, 38]. Biomechanical studies showed that the TDR prosthesis stabilizes the spine while providing nearly intact segmental motion [29, 32, 39]. Early clinical results of TDR in the treatment of DDD showed promising outcomes [37, 40–46].

The patients treated with TDR usually have short recuperation times and less postoperative pain compared to fusion procedure. On the other hand, TDR application has several significant limitations including; (a) the patient should be between 30 and 50 years old, (b) there should not be any posterior column disruption, (c) intervertebral disc height should be ≥4 mm, and (d) single-level DDD is more appropriate to apply TDR. Beside these limitations TDR is an anterior approach which has its inherent risks such as injury to intra-abdominal organs and vascular structures. Additionally, the lesions in the peritoneal cavity caused by abrasion, ischemia, desiccation, infection, thermal injury, and foreign bodies can result in adhesion formation [47].

TDR is used extensively around the world; however severe complications have been associated with the technique [48, 49]. In this study we observed mild iliac vein injuries during the placement of the lumbar disc prosthesis in the two patients within the TDR group. Other possible disadvantages of TDR technique are as follows: revision surgery is quite difficult, biomechanically the L5-S1 level had no normal segmental motion, and results of two-level TDR use were not considered to be satisfactory according to patients [50]. Putzier et al. [51] concluded that the long-term results of a study by Charité were not satisfactory and they concluded their article yearning to fusion technique.

Guyer et al. [52] published the results of a 5-year study showing that TDR was not superior to fusion. The authors concluded that there was no strong evidence that TDR was superior to fusion, and they suggested that high-quality, randomized controlled trials with relevant control groups and a long-term followup were needed to evaluate the effectiveness and safety of TDR [53].

Posterior dynamic stabilization systems are designed to increase the success of spinal surgery and to eliminate the complications of fusion with rigid instrumentation such as adjacent segment disease (12.2–18.5%) [54] due to the stress-shielding properties (2–3% per year after stabilization) [55], pseudarthrosis (3–55%) [18, 56, 57], device-related osteopenia [58], and loss of motion in fused spinal segments. Besides these side effects of fusion, clinical healing might be suboptimal in cases even with satisfactory radiological results [22, 59]. Therefore, the use of posterior dynamic stabilization in the surgical treatment of DDD may provide greater patient satisfaction, resulting from shorter hospital stays, less recuperation time, and none of the disadvantages related to fusion, which requires more invasive procedures.

Numerous biomechanical studies proved that hinged screw stabilization can stabilize the spine almost as well as the rigid screw stabilization used in fusion surgery in the treatment of chronic lumbar instability [60, 61]. There are no randomized controlled studies in the literature because PTDS is a new technique. However, there are many retrospective studies that are precursors for future randomized studies. Recently, studies on PTDS have shown very encouraging clinical results and demonstrated that these systems provide stabilization that is similar to the posterior rigid stabilization obtained with fusion surgery [23–28, 30, 31, 34, 35, 60, 62, 63].There are few studies which concluded that dynamic stabilization is not superior to rigid stabilization [63–66]. Although these results showed that there was no advantage of PTDS over fusion surgery in clinical outcome, on the other hand these studies also showed that PTDS is superior to fusion due to the simplicity of the procedure, low morbidity, and reduced hospitalization time to achieve similar satisfactory outcome as fusion. Similarly numerous studies have shown that posterior dynamic transpedicular stabilization caused less intraoperative blood loss and had a shorter operating time [25, 28, 31, 35]. Furthermore, several studies reported that PTDS slows down intervertebral disc degeneration by removing the load from the degenerative disc tissue and providing better load distribution which is an important advantage of this technique [25, 27, 30].

Based on previous studies, if a disc is in the beginning stage of degeneration and if there is only posterior annulus defect, the disc might repair itself after PTDS. On the other hand, if the disc has advanced degeneration including decreased disc height, significant dehydration, and/or slight bulging, fusion might occur slowly after PTDS. However, in both of these scenarios, the patient would be pain-free. In cases of advanced disc degeneration, the fusion results are satisfactory because fusion occurs easily. If PTDS is applied to advanced disc degeneration cases, the segments might fuse and the results will be the same. Therefore in regard of motion preservation, TDR may be a superior treatment in this group of patients if they have intact facet joints.

Huang et al. [67] reported the advantages and disadvantages of nonfusion technology in spinal surgery. Some of the potential benefits of nonfusion implants were the elimination of possible complications due to bone grafts and pseudarthrosis as well as a reduction in the surgical morbidity and the incidence of adjacent level degeneration. The potential risks of nonfusion implants included mechanical failure, dissolution and migration, subsidence, and same-level degeneration.

Previous studies suggested that lumbar total disc prosthesis would reduce the stress on the adjacent disc, after sagittal balance is restored. Harrop et al. [68] reviewed the literature on lumbar adjacent segment degeneration after fusion and TDR. They concluded that adjacent segment disease had a stronger relationship with fusion than arthroplasty. Stoll et al. [34] reported symptomatic adjacent segment disease in 9% of their posterior dynamic transpedicular stabilization patients after a 38-month follow-up period. Cakir et al. [63] reported their results after performing PTDS with Dynesys and TDR with ProDisc (Synthes-Spine Solutions, New York, NY). They suggested that both dynamic systems were promising alternative options compared to fusion for patients with different pathologies because of reduced morbidity. Cakir et al. [63]

obtained good clinical results with both systems. Both TDR and PTDS result in less adjacent segment disease. Although a reduced incidence of adjacent segment degeneration appears to be the most important advantage of nonfusion systems, this advantage has not been proven.

Considering all of the features of both techniques, PTDS is a less invasive surgery compared to fusion and TDR techniques. Additionally, PTDS has no age limitation and does not require intact posterior spinal column as TDR technique. Finally, anterior lumbar disc prosthesis requires transperitoneal or retroperitoneal intervention and usually requires a multidisciplinary approach (general surgeon, cardiovascular surgeon, and spinal surgeon). Naturally, the complication rate decreases with a conventional surgical approach and increases when complex anatomical structures are involved in the surgery.

## 5. Conclusion

In this study, we observed that both dynamic techniques TDR and PTDS offered satisfactory outcome in the surgical treatment of lumbar DDD. However, in this limited study, PTDS had several advantages over TDR such as (a) less invasive technique, (b) shorter operation time, (c) less intraoperative bleeding, and (d) lower complication rates. Further prospective, randomized clinical studies with a larger number of patients and with a longer follow-up period are needed to support our findings.

## References

[1] N. Bogduk, "The innervation of the lumbar spine," *Spine*, vol. 8, no. 3, pp. 286–293, 1983.

[2] W. H. Kirkaldy-Willis and H. F. Farfan, "Instability of the lumbar spine," *Clinical Orthopaedics and Related Research*, vol. 165, pp. 110–123, 1982.

[3] F. P. Morgan and T. King, "Primary instability of lumbar vertebrae as a common cause of low back pain," *Journal of Bone and Joint Surgery (British Volume)*, vol. 39, no. 1, pp. 6–22, 1957.

[4] J. MALINSKY, "The ontogenetic development of nerve terminations in the intervertebral discs of man," *Acta Anatomica*, vol. 38, pp. 96–113, 1959.

[5] M. C. Battié, T. Videman, and E. Parent, "Lumbar disc degeneration: epidemiology and genetic influences," *Spine*, vol. 29, no. 23, pp. 2679–2690, 2004.

[6] A. Ong, J. Anderson, and J. Roche, "A pilot study of the prevalence of lumbar disc degeneration in elite athletes with lower back pain at the Sydney 2000 Olympic Games," *British Journal of Sports Medicine*, vol. 37, no. 3, pp. 263–266, 2003.

[7] T. Videman, S. Sarna, M. C. Battie et al., "The long-term effects of physical loading and exercise lifestyles on back- related symptoms, disability, and spinal pathology among men," *Spine*, vol. 20, no. 6, pp. 699–709, 1995.

[8] C. J. Wallach, L. G. Gilbertson, and J. D. Kang, "Gene therapy applications for intervertebral disc degeneration," *Spine*, vol. 28, no. 15, supplement, pp. S93–S98, 2003.

[9] H. A. Horner and J. P. G. Urban, "2001 Volvo award winner in basic science studies: effect of nutrient supply on the viability of cells from the nucleus pulposus of the intervertebral disc," *Spine*, vol. 26, no. 23, pp. 2543–2549, 2001.

[10] L. Ala-Kokko, "Genetic risk factors for lumbar disc disease," *Annals of Medicine*, vol. 34, no. 1, pp. 42–47, 2002.

[11] M. A. Edgar and J. A. Ghadially, "Innervation of the lumbar spine," *Clinical Orthopaedics and Related Research*, vol. 115, pp. 35–41, 1976.

[12] M. Grönblad, J. Virri, S. Rönkkö et al., "A controlled biochemical and immunohistochemical study of human synovial-type (group II) phospholipase A2 and inflammatory cells in macroscopically normal, degenerated, and herniated human lumbar disc tissues," *Spine*, vol. 21, no. 22, pp. 2531–2538, 1996.

[13] H. V. Crock, "Internal disc disruption. A challenge to disc prolapse fifty years on," *Spine*, vol. 11, no. 6, pp. 650–653, 1986.

[14] J. W. Frymoyer, "Segmental instability," in *The Adult Spine*, J. W. Frymoyer, Ed., pp. 1873–1891, Raven Press, New York, NY, USA, 1991.

[15] J. W. Frymoyer and D. K. Selby, "Segmental instability: rationale for treatment," *Spine*, vol. 10, no. 3, pp. 280–286, 1985.

[16] E. C. Benzel, "Stability and instability of the spine," in *Biomechanics of Spine Stabilization*, E. C. Benzel, Ed., pp. 29–43, Thime, New York, NY, USA, 2001.

[17] S. J. Suratwala, M. R. Pinto, T. J. Gilbert, R. B. Winter, and J. M. Wroblewski, "Functional and radiological outcomes of 360° fusion of three or more motion levels in the lumbar spine for degenerative disc disease," *Spine*, vol. 34, no. 10, pp. E351–E358, 2009.

[18] A. A. Faundez, J. D. Schwender, Y. Safriel et al., "Clinical and radiological outcome of anterior-posterior fusion versus transforaminal lumbar interbody fusion for symptomatic disc degeneration: a retrospective comparative study of 133 patients," *European Spine Journal*, vol. 18, no. 2, pp. 203–211, 2009.

[19] B. I. Martin, S. K. Mirza, B. A. Comstock, D. T. Gray, W. Kreuter, and R. A. Deyo, "Reoperation rates following lumbar spine surgery and the influence of spinal fusion procedures," *Spine*, vol. 32, no. 3, pp. 382–387, 2007.

[20] J. C. Banwart, M. A. Asher, and R. S. Hassanein, "Iliac crest bone graft harvest donor site morbidity: a statistical evaluation," *Spine*, vol. 20, no. 9, pp. 1055–1060, 1995.

[21] T. R. Lehmann, K. F. Spratt, and J. E. Tozzi, "Long-term follow-up of lower lumbar fusion patients," *Spine*, vol. 12, no. 2, pp. 97–104, 1987.

[22] P. Fritzell, O. Hägg, and A. Nordwall, "Complications in lumbar fusion surgery for chronic low back pain: comparison of three surgical techniques used in a prospective randomized study. A report from the Swedish lumbar spine study group," *European Spine Journal*, vol. 12, no. 2, pp. 178–189, 2003.

[23] T. Kaner, M. Sasani, T. Oktenoglu, and A. F. Ozer, "Dynamic stabilization of the spine: a new classification system," *Turkish Neurosurgery*, vol. 20, no. 2, pp. 205–215, 2010.

[24] T. Kaner, M. Sasani, T. Oktenoglu, M. Cosar, and A. F. Ozer, "Utilizing dynamic rods with dynamic screws in the surgical treatment of chronic instability: a prospective clinical study," *Turkish Neurosurgery*, vol. 19, no. 4, pp. 319–326, 2009.

[25] T. Kaner, S. Dalbayrak, T. Oktenoglu, M. Sasani, A. L. Aydin, and F. O. Ozer, "Comparison of posterior dynamic and posterior rigid transpedicular stabilization with fusion to treat degenerative spondylolisthesis," *Orthopedics*, vol. 33, no. 5, 2010.

[26] T. Kaner, M. Sasani, T. Oktenoglu et al., "Minimum two-year follow-up of cases with recurrent disc herniation treated with microdiscectomy and posterior dynamic transpedicular stabilisation," *Open Orthopaedics*, vol. 4, pp. 120–125, 2010.

[27] T. Kaner, M. Sasani, T. Oktenoglu, M. Cosar, and A. F. Ozer, "Clinical outcomes after posterior dynamic transpedicular stabilization with limited lumbar discectomy: carragee classification system for lumbar disc herniations," *SAS Journal*, vol. 4, no. 3, pp. 92–97, 2010.

[28] A. F. Ozer, N. R. Crawford, M. Sasani et al., "Dynamic lumbar pedicle screw-rod stabilization: two year follow-up and comparison with fusion," *Open Orthopaedics*, vol. 4, pp. 137–141, 2010.

[29] M. Sasani, T. Öktenoğlu, K. Tuncay, N. Canbulat, S. Carilli, and F. A. Özer, "Total disc replacement in the treatment of lumbar discogenic pain with disc herniation: a prospective clinical study," *Turkish Neurosurgery*, vol. 19, no. 2, pp. 127–134, 2009.

[30] M. Putzier, S. V. Schneider, J. F. Funk, S. W. Tohtz, and C. Perka, "The surgical treatment of the lumbar disc prolapse: nucleotomy with additional transpedicular dynamic stabilization versus nucleotomy alone," *Spine*, vol. 30, no. 5, pp. E109–E114, 2005.

[31] A. Von Strempel, D. Moosmann, C. Stoss et al., "Stabilization of the degenerated lumbar spine in the nonfusion technique with cosmic posterior dynamic system," *The Wall Street Journal*, vol. 1, pp. 40–47, 2006.

[32] J. C. Le Huec, H. Mathews, Y. Basso et al., "Clinical results of Maverick lumbar total disc replacement: two-year prospective follow-up," *Orthopedic Clinics of North America*, vol. 36, no. 3, pp. 315–322, 2005.

[33] M. Kanayama, T. Hashimoto, K. Shigenobu et al., "Adjacent-segment morbidity after Graf ligamentoplasty compared with posterolateral lumbar fusion," *Journal of Neurosurgery*, vol. 95, no. 1, pp. 5–10, 2001.

[34] T. M. Stoll, G. Dubois, and O. Schwarzenbach, "The dynamic neutralization system for the spine: a multi-center study of a novel non-fusion system," *European Spine Journal*, vol. 11, no. 2, supplement, pp. S170–S178, 2002.

[35] T. Oktenoglu, A. F. Ozer, M. Sasani et al., "Posterior dynamic stabilization in the treatment of lumbar degenerative disc disease: 2-year follow-up," *Minimally Invasive Neurosurgery*, vol. 53, no. 3, pp. 112–116, 2010.

[36] S. Carilli, T. Oktenoglu, and A. F. Ozer, "Open-window laparotomy during a transperitoneal approach to the lower lumbar vertebrae: new method for reducing complications," *Minimally Invasive Neurosurgery*, vol. 49, no. 4, pp. 227–229, 2006.

[37] K. Büttner-Janz, K. Schelnack, and Zippel H, "An alternative teratment strategy for lumbar disc damage using the SB Charité modular disc prosthesis," *Zeitschrift fur Orthopadie und Ihre Grenzgebiete*, vol. 125, no. 1, pp. 1–6, 1987.

[38] T. Marnay, *ProDisc Retrospective Clinical Study: 7–11 Year Follow Up*, Spine Solutions, New York, NY, USA, 2002.

[39] T. J. Errico, "Lumbar disc arthroplasty," *Clinical Orthopaedics and Related Research*, no. 435, pp. 106–117, 2005.

[40] S. Blumenthal, P. C. McAfee, R. D. Guyer et al., "A prospective, randomized, multicenter food and drug administration investigational device exemptions study of lumbar total disc replacement with the CHARITÉ artificial disc versus lumbar fusion—part I: evaluation of clinical outcomes," *Spine*, vol. 30, no. 14, pp. 1565–1575, 2005.

[41] J. Zigler, R. Delamarter, J. M. Spivak et al., "Results of the prospective, randomized, multicenter food and drug administration investigational device exemption study of the ProDisc-L total disc replacement versus circumferential fusion for the treatment of 1-level degenerative disc disease," *Spine*, vol. 32, no. 11, pp. 1155–1162, 2007.

[42] S. H. Hochschuler, D. D. Ohnmeiss, R. D. Guyer, and S. L. Blumenthal, "Artificial disc: preliminary results of a prospective study in the United States," *European Spine Journal*, vol. 11, no. 2, supplement, pp. S106–S110, 2002.

[43] H. Mayer, K. Wiechert, A. Korge, and I. Qose, "Minimally invasive total disc replacement: surgical technique and preliminary clinical results," *European Spine Journal*, vol. 11, no. 2, supplement, pp. S124–S130, 2002.

[44] R. Bertagnoli and S. Kumar, "Indications for full prosthetic disc arthroplasty: a correlation of clinical outcome against a variety of indications," *European Spine Journal*, vol. 11, no. 2, supplement, pp. S131–S136, 2002.

[45] P. C. McAfee, B. Cunningham, G. Holsapple et al., "A prospective, randomized, multicenter food and drug administration investigational device exemption study of lumbar total disc replacement with the CHARITÉtrade; artificial disc versus lumbar fusion—part II: evaluation of radiographic outcomes and correlation of surgical technique accuracy with clinical outcomes," *Spine*, vol. 30, no. 14, pp. 1576–1583, 2005.

[46] T. David, "Charité artifi cial disc long term results of one level (10 year)," *Spine*, vol. 32, no. 6, pp. 661–666, 2007.

[47] F. H. Geisler, S. L. Blumenthal, R. D. Guyer et al., "Neurological complications of lumbar artificial disc replacement and comparison of clinical results with those related to lumbar arthrodesis in the literature: results of a multicenter, prospective, randomized investigational device exemption study of Charité intervertebral disc. Invited submission from the Joint section meeting on disorders of the spine and peripheral nerves, March 2004," *Journal of Neurosurgery: Spine*, vol. 1, no. 2, pp. 143–154, 2004.

[48] C. Rosen, P. D. Kiester, and T. Q. Lee, "Lumbar disk replacement failures: review of 29 patients and rationale for revision," *Orthopedics*, vol. 32, no. 8, article 562, 2009.

[49] A. van Ooij, F. Cumhur Oner, and A. J. Verbout, "Complications of artificial disc replacement: a report of 27 patients with the SB Charité disc," *Journal of Spinal Disorders and Techniques*, vol. 16, no. 4, pp. 369–383, 2003.

[50] C. J. Siepe, H. M. Mayer, K. Wiechert, and A. Korge, "Clinical results of total lumbar disc replacement with ProDisc II: three-year results for different indications," *Spine*, vol. 31, no. 17, pp. 1923–1932, 2006.

[51] M. Putzier, J. F. Funk, S. V. Schneider et al., "Charité total disc replacement—clinical and radiographical results after an average follow-up of 17 years," *European Spine Journal*, vol. 15, no. 2, pp. 183–195, 2006.

[52] R. D. Guyer, P. C. McAfee, R. J. Banco et al., "Prospective, randomized, multicenter food and drug administration investigational device exemption study of lumbar total disc replacement with the CHARITÉ artificial disc versus lumbar fusion: five-year follow-up," *Spine Journal*, vol. 9, no. 5, pp. 374–386, 2009.

[53] K. D. van den Eerenbeemt, R. W. Ostelo, B. J. van Royen, W. C. Peul, and M. W. van Tulder, "Total disc replacement surgery for symptomatic degenerative lumbar disc disease: a systematic review of the literature," *European Spine Journal*, vol. 19, no. 8, pp. 1262–1280, 2010.

[54] P. Park, H. J. Garton, V. C. Gala, J. T. Hoff, and J. E. McGillicuddy, "Adjacent segment disease after lumbar or lumbosacral fusion: review of the literature," *Spine*, vol. 29, no. 17, pp. 1938–1944, 2004.

[55] V. K. Goel, T. H. Lim, J. Gwon et al., "Effects of rigidity of an internal fixation device: a comprehensive biomechanical investigation," *Spine*, vol. 16, no. 3, pp. S155–S161, 1991.

[56] S. M. Juratli, G. M. Franklin, S. K. Mirza, T. M. Wickizer, and D. Fulton-Kehoe, "Lumbar fusion outcomes in Washington State workers' compensation," *Spine*, vol. 31, no. 23, pp. 2715–2723, 2006.

[57] A. Waguespack, J. Schofferman, P. Slosar, and J. Reynolds, "Etiology of long-term failures of lumbar spine surgery," *Pain Medicine*, vol. 3, no. 1, pp. 18–22, 2002.

[58] P. C. McAfee, I. D. Farey, C. E. Sutterlin, K. R. Gurr, K. E. Warden, and B. W. Cunningham, "The effect of spinal implant rigidity on vertebral bone density: a canine model," *Spine*, vol. 16, no. 6, supplement, pp. S190–S197, 1991.

[59] N. Boos and J. K. Webb, "Pedicle screw fixation in spinal disorders: a European view," *European Spine Journal*, vol. 6, no. 1, pp. 2–18, 1997.

[60] H. Bozkuş, M. Şenoğlu, S. Baek et al., "Dynamic lumbar pedicle screw-rod stabilization: in vitro biomechanical comparison with standard rigid pedicle screw-rod stabilization—laboratory investigation," *Journal of Neurosurgery: Spine*, vol. 12, no. 2, pp. 183–189, 2010.

[61] W. Schmoelz, U. Onder, A. Martin, and A. Von Strempel, "Non-fusion instrumentation of the lumbar spine with a hinged pedicle screw rod system: an in vitro experiment," *European Spine Journal*, vol. 18, no. 10, pp. 1478–1485, 2009.

[62] V. K. Goel, R. J. Konz, H. T. Chang et al., "Hinged-dynamic posterior device permits greater loads on the graft and similar stability as compared with its equivalent rigid device: a three-dimensional finite element assessment," *Journal of Prosthetics and Orthotics*, vol. 13, no. 1, pp. 17–20, 2001.

[63] B. Cakir, M. Richter, K. Huch, W. Puhl, and R. Schmidt, "Dynamic stabilization of the lumbar spine," *Orthopedics*, vol. 29, no. 8, pp. 716–722, 2006.

[64] D. Grob, A. Benini, A. Junge, and A. F. Mannion, "Clinical experience with the dynesys semirigid fixation system for the lumbar spine: surgical and patient-oriented outcome in 50 cases after an average of 2 years," *Spine*, vol. 30, no. 3, pp. 324–331, 2005.

[65] P. Korovessis, Z. Papazisis, G. Koureas, and E. Lambiris, "Rigid, semirigid versus dynamic instrumentation for degenerative lumbar spinal stenosis: a correlative radiological and clinical analysis of short-term results," *Spine*, vol. 29, no. 7, pp. 735–742, 2004.

[66] C. C. Würgler-Hauri, A. Kalbarczyk, M. Wiesli, H. Landolt, and J. Fandino, "Dynamic neutralization of the lumbar spine after microsurgical decompression in acquired lumbar spinal stenosis and segmental instability," *Spine*, vol. 33, no. 3, pp. E66–E72, 2008.

[67] R. C. Huang, F. P. Girardi, M. R. Lim, and F. P. Cammisa, "Advantages and disadvantages of nonfusion technology in spine surgery," *Orthopedic Clinics of North America*, vol. 36, no. 3, pp. 263–269, 2005.

[68] J. S. Harrop, J. A. Youssef, M. Maltenfort et al., "Lumbar adjacent segment degeneration and disease after arthrodesis and total disc arthroplasty," *Spine*, vol. 33, no. 15, pp. 1701–1707, 2008.

# 34

# Outcome and Structural Integrity of Rotator Cuff after Arthroscopic Treatment of Large and Massive Tears with Double Row Technique: A 2-Year Followup

**Ignacio Carbonel,**[1] **Angel A. Martínez,**[1] **Elisa Aldea,**[2] **Jorge Ripalda,**[1] **and Antonio Herrera**[3]

[1] *Shoulder and Elbow Unit, Department of Orthopaedic and Trauma Surgery, Miguel Servet University Hospital, Zaragoza, Spain*
[2] *Emergency Department, Royo Villanova Hospital, Zaragoza, Spain*
[3] *Department of Orthopaedic and Trauma Surgery, Miguel Servet University Hospital and Department of Orthopaedic Surgery, School of Medicine, University of Zaragoza, Zaragoza, Spain*

Correspondence should be addressed to Antonio Herrera; aherrera@salud.aragon.es

Academic Editor: Masato Takao

*Purpose.* The purpose of this study was to evaluate the functional outcome and the tendon healing after arthroscopic double row rotator cuff repair of large and massive rotator cuff tears. *Methods.* 82 patients with a full-thickness large and massive rotator cuff tear underwent arthroscopic repair with double row technique. Results were evaluated by use of the UCLA, ASES, and Constant questionnaires, the Shoulder Strength Index (SSI), and range of motion. Follow-up time was 2 years. Magnetic resonance imaging (MRI) studies were performed on each shoulder preoperatively and 2 years after repair. *Results.* 100% of the patients were followed up. UCLA, ASES, and Constant questionnaires showed significant improvement compared with preoperatively ($P < 0.001$). Range of motion and SSI in flexion, abduction, and internal and external rotation also showed significant improvement ($P < 0.001$). MRI studies showed 24 cases of tear after repair (29%). Only 8 cases were a full-thickness tear. *Conclusions.* At two years of followup, in large and massive rotator cuff tears, an arthroscopic double row rotator cuff repair technique produces an excellent functional outcome and structural integrity.

## 1. Introduction

Maximizing tendon healing is the primary goal of rotator cuff repair surgery. Tendon healing has been shown to improve active motion, strength, and patient self-assessed function after rotator cuff repair [1, 2].

Whereas small and medium sized rotator cuff tears are successfully managed with any surgical repair in the vast majority of cases, the optimal management of big and massive rotator cuff tears has been controversial and continues to evolve. Tendon retraction, adhesions, and poor tissue quality common in these tears make repair one of the most technically complex procedures in the shoulder.

Arthroscopic techniques and instrumentations are improving rapidly, and arthroscopic rotator cuff repair has gained popularity. Double row of anchors technique is reported to reestablish the normal rotator cuff footprint and increase the contact area for healing [3, 4] so anatomical and biomechanical are better than with the single row technique [4–8].

The purpose of this study was to evaluate the functional outcome and the tendon healing after arthroscopic double row rotator cuff repair of large and massive rotator cuff tears.

## 2. Materials and Methods

*2.1. Patient Selection.* Patients were recruited among those referred by primary care doctors because of symptoms of rotator cuff tears and were enrolled in the study by the senior surgeons of the Shoulder and Elbow unit at the Miguel Servet University Hospital in Zaragoza, Spain.

Recruitment started in January 2008 and was completed in January 2010. 82 patients were eligible. All patients received the allocated treatment.

Of 82 patients recruited, 2-year results were available for all of them.

Inclusion criteria included the following: (1) rotator cuff tear, clinically confirmed, in a sane patient with complete passive range of motion with inability to perform activities of daily living, (2) full-thickness tears bigger than 30 mm with MRI evidence, (3) older than 18, (4) no tendinous surgery in the shoulder, (5) healthy contralateral shoulder, and (6) informed consent for the surgery.

Exclusion criteria included the following: (1) glenohumeral osteoarthritis, (2) ipsilateral shoulder pathology, (3) previous rotator cuff surgery on the affected shoulder, (4) contralateral shoulder pathology, (5) fatty degeneration grade 4 of Fuchs, (7) the active use of steroids, and (8) inability to complete questionnaires or to complete the rehabilitation treatment.

*2.2. Clinical Evaluation.* Preoperative and postoperative clinical evaluations were performed on all patients preoperatively and 2 years postoperatively. Data were collected to allow a determination of the University of California, Los Angeles (UCLA) score [9], Constant-Murley score [10], and the shoulder index of the American Shoulder and Elbow Surgeons (ASES) [11]. The range of motion was evaluated with a goniometer in flexion, abduction, internal rotation, and external rotation. Muscle strength was tested using a spring-scale myometer (Manley 2012 spring-scale; Manley Tool and Machine, Independence, MO). Flexion, abduction, internal rotation, and external rotation muscle power were evaluated. We compared muscle strength using a new evaluation method, the Shoulder Strength Index (SSI). Instead of using the absolute value of the muscle strength, we used relative muscle strength of the affected shoulder compared with the muscle strength of the contralateral shoulder. Because normal muscle strength for each patient is totally different from that of others, comparison of the absolute values is meaningless. To calculate the SSI, muscle strength of the affected shoulder is divided by the muscle strength of the contralateral shoulder. The strength of the muscle power of both shoulders should be evaluated consecutively to ensure reproducibility and reliability.

*2.3. Imaging.* All patients received a standard preoperative assessment using standard radiographs: anteroposterior projections; neutral, external, and internal rotation; and an axillary view.

Nonarthrographic MRI studies were performed on all patients preoperatively and 2 years after repair. This has been shown to be a reliable method of evaluating the repaired rotator cuff [12–14]. The following sequences were performed: coronal and sagittal T1-weighted with TR 500/TE 15, coronal and sagittal FSE T2-weighted with fat saturation 4500/60, and axial FSE proton density with fat saturation 2500/12.

All scans were read by a musculoskeletal specialty. Size of the tear in the anteroposterior dimension, retraction of the tendon medially, and fatty degeneration were recorded in preoperative scans. Postoperative scans divided the rotator cuff in three groups: (1) full-thickness tear, defined as fluid signal and/or absence of visible tendon fibers extending across the entire tendon from inferior to superior, (2) partial-thickness tear defined as a partial tendon defect, and (3) cuff integrity when appeared to have sufficient thickness compared with normal cuff with homogenously low intensity on each image.

*2.4. Surgical Technique.* All the operations were performed in a standardized manner. Patients underwent brachial plexus block associated with general anesthesia and were placed in a lateral decubitus position. The arm was suspended at approximately 30°–45° of abduction and 20° of forward flexion. Distraction of the shoulder joint was accomplished with 4 kg of traction. To control bleeding we used radiofrequency, adrenalin admixture for the irrigation fluid and asked the anesthesiologist to lower the systolic blood pressure to 90 mm Hg if possible. We worked with an arthroscopic pump maintained fluid pressure at 50 mm Hg, increasing it temporally on demand up to 75 mm Hg.

Standard anterior and posterior portals were produced, and the arthroscope was inserted into the glenohumeral joint through the posterior portal. A diagnostic arthroscopy was then performed to evaluate the extent of the rotator cuff tear, any lesions of the biceps tendon, and other associated lesions. The arthroscope was then removed from the glenohumeral joint and redirected into the subacromial space. After complete bursectomy was performed, arthroscopic subacromial decompression was performed to create a flat acromial undersurface in all patients. Osteophytes in the inferior part of the acromioclavicular joint were also removed, because not only an anterolateral subacromial spur but also medial subacromial spur and inferior clavicular spur were suspected as a cause of subacromial impingement. Tear size, pattern, and mobility of the torn cuff were evaluated. The edges of the tendon were debrided until strong healthy tissues were secured. For reattachment of the rotator cuff tendons, a cancellous bone bed was prepared in the footprint of the greater tuberosity with a bur until bleeding occurred. If mobility of a tendon was insufficient for repair, procedures to mobilize the tendon, such as release of the coracohumeral ligament and detachment of the rotator cuff from the bursal and articular sides, were performed.

The standard operating portals included the lateral portal for instrumentation, an accessory superior portal for anchor placement, and the previously established anterior and posterior portals. Frequently anterolateral and posterolateral portals are used.

The anchors used were Bio-corkscrew double loaded with number 2 FiberWire sutures (Arthrex, Naples, FL). These anchors were used by the 3 surgeons in both techniques.

For double row repairs, 1 row of anchors was placed in the medial aspect of the footprint, just lateral to the articular surface of the humeral head. Both sutures were passed through the tendon in a mattress fashion. A lateral row of anchors was then placed in the lateral aspect of the footprint, slightly proximal to the greater tuberosity. The lateral row sutures were passed in a simple suture fashion. Just 1 of the 2 sutures was passed through the tendon. When sutures had been placed, they were sequentially tied using a locking, sliding knot with back-up half-hitches. In all cases it was able to reestablish the anatomical footprint.

The L-shaped and U-shaped tears were first repaired with a side-to-side suture, providing margin convergence of the 2 edges of the cuff, before the fixation of the cuff to the bone.

*2.5. Postoperative Management.* The postoperative protocol was the same for the 82 cases. The arm was supported using a sling with an abduction pillow. Active elbow and wrist flexion and extension movements and pendular movements of the shoulder were initiated on the day after surgery. After 3 weeks, passive and assisted-active exercises were initiating. At 6 weeks, the sling was removed and the patient began active movements and strengthening exercises of the rotator cuff and scapular stabilizers progressively. Rehabilitation was consistently performed with the assistance of physical therapists. Full return to sports and heavy labor were allowed after 6 months according to individual functional recovery.

*2.6. Statistical Methods.* A statistical consultant recommended comparative tests based on the distribution of the data. Prerepair and postrepair comparisons were made using paired $t$-tests when data were normally distributed. For data that were not normally distributed, the Mann Whitney rank sum test was used. The significance level was set at $P = 0.05$.

All statistical analyses were performed by an independent statistician using the SPSS statistical package version 11.0.

## 3. Results

This study includes 82 patients, 36 males and 46 females. The mean ages of patients were $58.33 \pm 5.2$. The mean area of rotator cuff tear was $43 \pm 6.1$ mm$^2$.

The mean number of anchors used in double row repair technique was $3.28 \pm 0.6$ (Table 1).

*3.1. Patient Functional Assessment.* UCLA postoperative score was $27.6 \pm 1.7$; ASES index was $82.7 \pm 3.1$; and Constant score was $76.1 \pm 2.3$. The scores showed a significant improvement compared with preoperative status ($P < 0.001$) (Table 2).

*3.2. Range of Motion.* Patients' active flexion increased significantly from 92° to 145° ($P < 0.001$). Active abduction increased significantly from 90° to 125° ($P < 0.001$). Active external rotation increased significantly from 44° to 56° ($P < 0.001$). Active internal rotation increased significantly from 40° to 52° ($P < 0.001$) (Table 3).

*3.3. Strength Measurements: SSI.* All the measurements of strength (flexion, abduction, and internal and external rotation) showed a significant improvement in postoperatively results (Table 4).

TABLE 1: Tear description.

| | |
|---|---|
| Mean age (years) | $58.33 \pm 5.2$ |
| Gender | |
| Male | 36 |
| Female | 46 |
| Mean area (mm$^2$) | $43 \pm 6.1$ |
| Number of anchors | $3.28 \pm 0.6$ |

TABLE 2: Functional assessment.

| | Media ± DS | | $P$ |
|---|---|---|---|
| | Preop | Postop | |
| UCLA (0–35) | $11.6 \pm 1.6$ | $27.6 \pm 1.7$ | <0.001 |
| Constant (0–100) | $42.2 \pm 5.1$ | $76.1 \pm 2.3$ | <0.001 |
| ASES (0–100) | $41.3 \pm 4.2$ | $82.7 \pm 3.1$ | <0.001 |

TABLE 3: Range of motion.

| | Media ± DS | | $P$ |
|---|---|---|---|
| | Preop | Postop | |
| External rotation, deg | $44.2 \pm 4.1$ | $56.1 \pm 3.2$ | <0.001 |
| Internal rotation, deg | $40.3 \pm 4.3$ | $52.8 \pm 2.9$ | <0.001 |
| Flexion, deg | $92.7 \pm 10.6$ | $145.2 \pm 6.7$ | <0.001 |
| Abduction, deg | $90.1 \pm 9.8$ | $125.6 \pm 7.6$ | <0.001 |

TABLE 4: Strength measurements: SSI.

| | Media ± DS | | $P$ |
|---|---|---|---|
| | Preop | Postop | |
| Flexion SSI | $0.50 \pm 0.05$ | $0.74 \pm 0.03$ | <0.001 |
| Abduction SSI | $0.52 \pm 0.06$ | $0.72 \pm 0.03$ | <0.001 |
| Internal rotation SSI | $0.61 \pm 0.03$ | $0.72 \pm 0.03$ | <0.001 |
| External rotation SSI | $0.65 \pm 0.03$ | $0.78 \pm 0.02$ | <0.001 |

TABLE 5: Imaging.

| MRI | Intact | Partial-thickness defect | Full-thickness defect |
|---|---|---|---|
| Double row | 58 | 16 | 8 |

*3.4. Structural Integrity by MRI.* MRI studies at final followup showed an intact rotator cuff in 58 patients, partial-thickness defects in 16 patients, and full-thickness defects in 8 patients (Table 5).

Range of motion and patient functional assessment showed difference between cases of intact repair and retear (Table 6).

## 4. Discussion

Recent arthroscopic repair techniques for rotator cuff tears have emphasized the potential for a double row repair to add strength to the repair and hopefully decrease the anatomic failure rate [15–20]. Several studies have indicated that results in cases of anatomic failure, although clinically improved, are not as good as those that are anatomically intact, especially

TABLE 6

| Rotator cuff repair | Intact | Partial-thickness defect | Full-thickness defect | $P$ |
|---|---|---|---|---|
| External rotation, deg | 61.3 ± 3.1 | 52.1 ± 2.9 | 45.2 ± 3.3 | <0.001 |
| Internal rotation, deg | 58.1 ± 2.2 | 50.6 ± 3.5 | 39.5 ± 4.1 | <0.001 |
| Flexion, deg | 151.3 ± 5.2 | 140.1 ± 4.7 | 115.8 ± 7.2 | <0.001 |
| Abduction, deg | 135.4 ± 4.7 | 120.5 ± 5.2 | 102.3 ± 5.2 | <0.001 |
| UCLA | 28.9 ± 2.1 | 26.8 ± 1.9 | 24.7 ± 2.5 | <0.001 |
| Constant | 80.3 ± 3.9 | 74.1 ± 4.3 | 63.2 ± 4.7 | <0.001 |
| ASES | 85.0 ± 4.3 | 79.7 ± 5.1 | 71.9 ± 4.1 | <0.001 |

if strength measurements are made [15, 21, 22]. Therefore, trying to achieve and maintain an intact cuff is a paramount goal in cuff repair. Biomechanical studies have emphasized the potential improvement of outcomes by double row repair technique [23–28]. Some clinical studies have already validated this idea in large and massive rotator cuff tears [29].

Park et al. [29] recently conducted a study in which 40 consecutive patients were treated with 1 row technique and the following 38 with double row technique. At 2 years after surgery, ASES, Constant, and SSI were significantly better in both groups but no significant improvements were found between both groups. When the comparison was made to the size of the rupture, functional assessment was significantly better with the double row in large and massive tears (>3 cm) ($P < 0.05$). The authors concluded that the repair with the double row technique has a greater role in the treatment of large and massive tears.

Also Denard et al. [30] concluded that double row repair was 4.9 times more likely to lead to a good or excellent long-term functional outcome after repair of massive rotator cuff tears.

Lafosse et al. [18] evaluated 105 patients undergoing arthroscopic double row repair of rotator cuff tears, enjoying positive results functionally and structurally. The improvement in the Constant scale was 43.2 ± 15.1 preoperatively to 80.1 ± 11.1 after a mean of 23 months. Assessment by MRI and arthroTC revealed a total of 12 failures (11%), a lower rate than previously collected with other techniques of repair with tears comparable in size and shape. In shoulders with an intact cuff at followup was also observed a better clinical outcome. The only category in which they found a statistically significant difference was the assessment of pain ($P < 0.0001$).

Anderson et al. [15] published a series of 48 patients (52 shoulders) who underwent doublerow repair in full thickness rotator cuff tears. The average size of the tear was of 2.47 cm. Postoperative followup included functional assessment, physical examination, ultrasound, and tests of strength. With a mean followup of 30 months, ultrasound showed a 17% of tears. The L'Insalata scale ($P < 0.001$), mobility ($P < 0.001$), and strength (antepulsion, $P < 0.001$, external rotation, $P < 0.001$; internal rotation, $P < 0.033$) were statistically significant improvements with respect to preoperative values. Patients with an intact rotator cuff showed a significant improvement in antepulsion ($P = 0.006$) and external rotation ($P = 0.001$).

Huijsmans et al. [17] presented the results of 238 patients undergoing repair with a new doublerow suture technique. 90% of patients had a performance status of good to excellent, and 82.9% remained intact after the repair with ultrasound control.

A new evaluation method, the SSI, only used in Park et al.'s article [29], was introduced and reflects patients subjective judgement about the operation as well as their rehabilitation status. Because patients will always compare the operated shoulder with the unaffected shoulder, the only standard function of the shoulder will be that of the unaffected shoulder. Using the SSI, clinicians can more easily explain the goals of surgery and rehabilitation to the patient. In addition, data from the SSI indicate that arthroscopic rotator cuff repair will restore about 80% of muscle power to the unaffected shoulder. These data could be used to counsel patients before surgery.

Follow-up time is also an important aspect for evaluation of these results but it is a fact that there is no clear consensus. Some studies say that the failures appear late in large and massive tears [3], while in the open repair technique, improvements appear overtime. In other studies, these failures appear in very early stages after repair [31] while others appear in later stages of evolution [32], In our study we followed up for 24 months because we have observed that it is long enough to assess the functional recovery of the shoulder and problems with the surgery appear early after surgery.

The failure rate in most of the other studies is around 15–20% [19, 29, 31, 33]. Our results are higher (29%) but our study only included large and massive tears. There are few studies that showed results in large and massive tears and results are variable, from 17% to 44% retear rates [17–20].

An area of inconsistency within the literature is whether the presence of a defect after rotator cuff repair necessarily affects functional outcome. In our study we detected differences in strength in full thickness defects but in partial thickness defects these differences were less significative. Klepps et al. [34], as well as Knudsen et al. [35], detected no significant effect of repair integrity on functional outcome. Harryman et al. [2] had similar results except with those who had a large recurrent defect. However, Gazielly et al. [1] found a close correlation between the functional score and the anatomical condition of the rotator cuff.

Radiologic method of pre- and postoperative evaluation may also account for some of the variability of failure results. We used noncontrast magnetic resonance imaging to evaluate postoperative rotator cuff repair integrity. It is approved as a proper imaging test for this purpose and the most commonly used in these studies but it has somewhat limited ability in differentiating scar tissue from healed rotator cuff. High resolution shoulder ultrasonography has been evaluated and found to have an extremely high sensitivity (91%), specificity (86%), and accuracy (89%) in correctly identifying rotator cuff integrity postoperative [36]. Ultrasonography also provides dynamic evaluation of the rotator cuff, improving the ability to differentiate scar from healed cuff, although the results are highly operator dependent, and at our institution there are no musculoskeletal radiologists with extensive ultrasound experience and we achieve better results with noncontrast magnetic resonance imaging.

## 5. Conclusion

At two years of follow-up, in large and massive rotator cuff tears, an arthroscopic double row rotator cuff repair technique produces an excellent functional outcome and structural integrity.

## References

[1] D. F. Gazielly, P. Gleyze, and C. Montagnon, "Functional and anatomical results after rotator cuff repair," Clinical Orthopaedics and Related Research, no. 304, pp. 43–53, 1994.

[2] D. T. Harryman II, L. A. Mack, K. Y. Wang, S. E. Jackins, M. L. Richardson, and F. A. Matsen III, "Repairs of the rotator cuff: correlation of functional results with integrity of the cuff," Journal of Bone and Joint Surgery A, vol. 73, no. 7, pp. 982–989, 1991.

[3] L. M. Galatz, C. M. Ball, S. A. Teefey, W. D. Middleton, and K. Yamaguchi, "The outcome and repair integrity of completely arthroscopically repaired large and massive rotator cuff tears," Journal of Bone and Joint Surgery A, vol. 86, no. 2, pp. 219–224, 2004.

[4] I. K. Y. Lo and S. S. Burkhart, "Double-row arthroscopic rotator cuff repair: re-establishing the footprint of the rotator cuff," Arthroscopy, vol. 19, no. 9, pp. 1035–1042, 2003.

[5] P. C. Brady, P. Arrigoni, and S. S. Burkhart, "Evaluation of residual rotator cuff defects after in vivo single- versus double-row rotator cuff repairs," Arthroscopy, vol. 22, no. 10, pp. 1070–1075, 2006.

[6] A. S. Curtis, K. M. Burbank, J. J. Tierney, A. D. Scheller, and A. R. Cunan, "The insertional footprint of the rotator cuff: an anatomic study," Arthroscopy, vol. 22, no. 6, pp. 603–609, 2006.

[7] M. C. Park, N. S. ElAttrache, J. E. Tibone, C. S. Ahmad, B. J. Jun, and T. Q. Lee, "Part I: footprint contact characteristics for a transosseous-equivalent rotator cuff repair technique compared with a double-row repair technique," Journal of Shoulder and Elbow Surgery, vol. 16, no. 4, pp. 461–468, 2007.

[8] R. L. Waltrip, N. Zheng, J. R. Dugas, and J. R. Andrews, "Rotator cuff repair: a biomechanical comparison of three techniques," American Journal of Sports Medicine, vol. 31, no. 4, pp. 493–497, 2003.

[9] H. Ellman, G. Hanker, and M. Bayer, "Repair of the rotator cuff: end-result study of factors influencing reconstruction," Journal of Bone and Joint Surgery A, vol. 68, no. 8, pp. 1136–1144, 1986.

[10] C. R. Constant and A. H. G. Murley, "A clinical method of functional assessment of the shoulder," Clinical Orthopaedics and Related Research, vol. 214, pp. 160–164, 1987.

[11] R. R. Richards, K. N. An, L. U. Bigliani et al., "A standardized method for the assessment of shoulder function," Journal of Shoulder and Elbow Surgery, vol. 3, pp. 347–352, 1994.

[12] B. Fuchs, M. K. Gilbart, J. Hodler, and C. Gerber, "Clinical and structural results of open repair of an isolated one-tendon tear of the rotator cuff," Journal of Bone and Joint Surgery A, vol. 88, no. 2, pp. 309–316, 2006.

[13] B. Jost, C. W. A. Pfirrmann, C. Gerber, and Z. Switzerland, "Clinical outcome after structural failure of rotator cuff repairs," Journal of Bone and Joint Surgery A, vol. 82, no. 3, pp. 304–314, 2000.

[14] S. A. Teefey, D. A. Rubin, W. D. Middleton, C. F. Hildebolt, R. A. Leibold, and K. Yamaguchi, "Detection and quantification of rotator cuff tears: comparison of ultrasonographic, magnetic resonance imaging, and arthroscopic findings in seventy-one consecutive cases," Journal of Bone and Joint Surgery A, vol. 86, no. 4, pp. 708–716, 2004.

[15] K. Anderson, M. Boothby, D. Aschenbrener, and M. Van Holsbeeck, "Outcome and structural integrity after arthroscopic rotator cuff repair using 2 rows of fixation: minimum 2-year follow-up," American Journal of Sports Medicine, vol. 34, no. 12, pp. 1899–1905, 2006.

[16] M. Apreleva, M. Özbaydar, P. G. Fitzgibbons, and J. J. P. Warner, "Rotator cuff tears: the effect of the reconstruction method on three-dimensional repair site area," Arthroscopy, vol. 18, no. 5, pp. 519–526, 2002.

[17] P. E. Huijsmans, M. P. Pritchard, B. M. Berghs, K. S. Van Rooyen, A. L. Wallace, and J. F. De Beer, "Arthroscopic rotator cuff repair with double-row fixation," Journal of Bone and Joint Surgery A, vol. 89, no. 6, pp. 1248–1257, 2007.

[18] L. Lafosse, R. Brozska, B. Toussaint, and R. Gobezie, "The outcome and structural integrity of arthroscopic rotator cuff repair with use of the double-row suture anchor technique," Journal of Bone and Joint Surgery A, vol. 89, no. 7, pp. 1533–1541, 2007.

[19] H. Sugaya, K. Maeda, K. Matsuki, and J. Moriishi, "Repair integrity and functional outcome after arthroscopic double-row rotator cuff repair: a prospective outcome study," Journal of Bone and Joint Surgery A, vol. 89, no. 5, pp. 953–960, 2007.

[20] H. Sugaya, K. Maeda, K. Matsuki, and J. Moriishi, "Functional and structural outcome after arthroscopic full-thickness rotator cuff repair: single-row versus dual-row fixation," Arthroscopy, vol. 21, no. 11, pp. 1307–1316, 2005.

[21] J. Bishop, S. Klepps, I. K. Lo, J. Bird, J. N. Gladstone, and E. L. Flatow, "Cuff integrity after arthroscopic versus open rotator cuff repair: a prospective study," Journal of Shoulder and Elbow Surgery, vol. 15, no. 3, pp. 290–299, 2006.

[22] P. Boileau, N. Brassart, D. J. Watkinson, M. Carles, A. M. Hatzidakis, and S. G. Krishnan, "Arthroscopic repair of full-thickness tears of the supraspinatus: does the tendon really heal?" Journal of Bone and Joint Surgery A, vol. 87, no. 6, pp. 1229–1240, 2005.

[23] D. H. Kim, N. S. ElAttrache, J. E. Tibone et al., "Biomechanical comparison of a single-row versus double-row suture anchor technique for rotator cuff repair," American Journal of Sports Medicine, vol. 34, no. 3, pp. 407–414, 2006.

[24] C. B. Ma, L. Comerford, J. Wilson, and C. M. Puttlitz, "Biomechanical evaluation of arthroscopic rotator cuff repairs: double-row compared with single-row fixation," *Journal of Bone and Joint Surgery A*, vol. 88, no. 2, pp. 403–410, 2006.

[25] S. W. Meier and J. D. Meier, "The effect of double-row fixation on initial repair strength in rotator cuff repair: A Biomechanical Study," *Arthroscopy*, vol. 22, no. 11, pp. 1168–1173, 2006.

[26] S. W. Meier and J. D. Meier, "Rotator cuff repair: the effect of double-row fixation on three-dimensional repair site," *Journal of Shoulder and Elbow Surgery*, vol. 15, no. 6, pp. 691–696, 2006.

[27] C. D. Smith, S. Alexander, A. M. Hill et al., "A biomechanical comparison of single and double-row fixation in arthroscopic rotator cuff repair," *Journal of Bone and Joint Surgery A*, vol. 88, no. 11, pp. 2425–2431, 2006.

[28] Y. Tuoheti, E. Itoi, N. Yamamoto et al., "Contact area, contact pressure, and pressure patterns of the tendon-bone interface after rotator cuff repair," *American Journal of Sports Medicine*, vol. 33, no. 12, pp. 1869–1874, 2005.

[29] J. Y. Park, S. H. Lhee, J. H. Choi, H. K. Park, J. W. Yu, and J. B. Seo, "Comparison of the clinical outcomes of single- and double-row repairs in rotator cuff tears," *American Journal of Sports Medicine*, vol. 36, no. 7, pp. 1310–1316, 2008.

[30] P. J. Denard, A. Z. Jiwani, A. Ladermann, and S. S. Burkhart, "Long-term outcome of arthroscopic massive rotator cuff repair: the importance of double-row fixation," *Arthroscopy*, vol. 28, no. 7, pp. 909–915, 2012.

[31] C. Gerber, B. Fuchs, and J. Hodler, "The results of repair of massive tears of the rotator cuff," *Journal of Bone and Joint Surgery A*, vol. 82, no. 4, pp. 505–515, 2000.

[32] R. T. Burks, J. Crim, N. Brown, B. Fink, and P. E. Greis, "A prospective randomized clinical trial comparing arthroscopic single- and double-row rotator cuff repair: magnetic resonance imaging and early clinical evaluation," *American Journal of Sports Medicine*, vol. 37, no. 4, pp. 674–682, 2009.

[33] A. Grasso, G. Milano, M. Salvatore, G. Falcone, L. Deriu, and C. Fabbriciani, "Single-row versus double-row arthroscopic rotator cuff repair: A Prospective Randomized Clinical Study," *Arthroscopy*, vol. 25, no. 1, pp. 4–12, 2009.

[34] S. Klepps, J. Bishop, J. Lin et al., "Prospective evaluation of the effect of rotator cuff integrity on the outcome of open rotator cuff repairs," *American Journal of Sports Medicine*, vol. 32, no. 7, pp. 1716–1722, 2004.

[35] H. B. Knudsen, J. Gelineck, J. O. Søjbjerg, B. S. Olsen, H. V. Johannsen, and O. Sneppen, "Functional and magnetic resonance imaging evaluation after single-tendon rotator cuff reconstruction," *Journal of Shoulder and Elbow Surgery*, vol. 8, no. 3, pp. 242–246, 1999.

[36] W. D. Prickett, S. A. Teefey, L. M. Galatz, R. P. Calfee, W. D. Middleton, and K. Yamaguchi, "Accuracy of ultrasound imaging of the rotator cuff in shoulders that are painful postoperatively," *Journal of Bone and Joint Surgery A*, vol. 85, no. 6, pp. 1084–1089, 2003.

# 35

# Early Clinical and Radiographic Results of Minimally Invasive Anterior Approach Hip Arthroplasty

**Tamara Alexandrov,[1] Elke R. Ahlmann,[2] and Lawrence R. Menendez[3]**

[1] Department of Orthopaedics, Los Angeles County-University of Southern California Medical Center, 1200 N. State Street, GNH 3900, Los Angeles, CA 90033, USA

[2] University of Southern California, Keck School of Medicine, Los Angeles County-University of Southern California Medical Center, 1200 N. State Street, GNH 3900, Los Angeles, CA 90033, USA

[3] University of Southern California, Keck School of Medicine, USC University Hospital, 1510 San Pablo Street, Suite 634, Los Angeles, CA 90033-4608, USA

Correspondence should be addressed to Elke R. Ahlmann; ahlmann2002@yahoo.com

Academic Editor: Christian Bach

We present a retrospective review of the early results and complications in a series of 35 consecutive patients with 43 total hip arthroplasties performed through an anterior muscle sparing minimally invasive approach. We found the early complication rates and radiographic outcomes comparable to those reported from arthroplasties performed via traditional approaches. Complications included dislocation (2%), femur fracture (2%), greater trochanteric fracture (12%), postoperative periprosthetic intertrochanteric fracture (2%), femoral nerve palsy (5%), hematoma (2%), and postoperative iliopsoas avulsion (2%). Radiographic analysis revealed average cup anteversion of $19.6° \pm 6.6$, average cup abduction angle of $48.4° \pm 7$, stem varus of $0.9° \pm 2$, and a mean leg length discrepancy of 0.7 mm. The anterior approach to the hip is an attractive alternative to the more traditional approaches. Acceptable component placement with comparable complication rates is possible using a muscle sparing technique which may lead to faster overall recovery.

## 1. Introduction

Despite advances in implants and greater understanding of hip biomechanics, complications such as dislocation, abductor weakness, leg length discrepancy, and component malpositioning continue to plague recipients of total hip arthroplasties [1–14]. In attempts to circumvent these complications many investigators have recently turned to the anterior approach first described by J. Judet and R. Judet in 1950 [15–21]. It has been referred to as a minimally invasive technique that allows exposure of the proximal femur and acetabulum through a small incision without the need to cut muscles or perform osteotomies. Theoretically, this should lead to shorter recovery time and fewer major complications that have been associated with the more traditional approaches.

Minimally invasive total hip arthroplasty has recently become popular in attempts to decrease recovery time and improve cosmesis. Shorter operative times and faster return to normal gait have been noted in some studies [22–24]; however, others found no difference in functional outcome scores, early function, hospital stay, and intraoperative blood loss [23–27]. Another concern involves accurate component placement as the smaller incision lends itself to poor visualization and cemented stems placed through a minimally invasive incision may have a propensity for varus positioning and a higher incidence of acetabular component malposition [25, 27].

The purpose of this study was to evaluate our early intraoperative and postoperative experience with the anterior minimally invasive approach to total hip arthroplasty and to compare the clinical results to those reported for traditional approaches. Postoperative radiographs were also reviewed to determine whether accurate component placement and leg length equality can be achieved with this technique.

## 2. Materials and Methods

We performed a retrospective review of the first 43 consecutive primary hip arthroplasties in 35 patients performed by a single surgeon via the anterior minimally invasive approach at our institution between 2002 and 2008. We began performing the anterior approach in 2002 and have since then exclusively used this technique for all primary total hip procedures. Eight of these patients underwent bilateral total hip arthroplasties, and, of these, five patients had both hips operated on the same day. There were 14 male and 29 female patients with a mean age of 62 years (range, 39 to 83). Twenty-four of the arthroplasties performed were on the left hip and 19 were performed on the right one. The average body mass index (BMI) was 26 (range, 18 to 37). Patients had an average of 2 (range, 0 to 4) reported medical problems, among the most common being hypertension and hypothyroidism. The etiology of the hip disease was degenerative arthritis in 29 hips, avascular necrosis in eight hips, and rheumatoid arthritis in six hips. One of the patients with degenerative joint disease had a previously undiagnosed femoral neck fracture on presentation and one had a history of pigmented villonodular synovitis. Two of the patients with rheumatoid arthritis had large benign cystic masses in their hips that were resected at the time of surgery. The average length of followup was 16.8 months (range, 12 to 60.7 months).

All operations were performed by the senior author (LRM). The surgical technique utilized is similar to other published reports [18, 19]. The Stryker MIS system (Stryker, Rutherford, NJ, USA) was used in the first 18 patients and the Corail system (DePuy Orthopaedics, Warsaw, IN, USA) was used in the last 25.

The patient was placed in supine position on the PROfx table (Mizuho OSI, Union City, CA, USA) and the operative extremity draped such that the limb could be manipulated freely. An incision 8 cm in length was made beginning at a point 1 cm distal and 2 cm lateral to the anterior superior iliac spine and heading in a longitudinal/oblique direction towards the greater trochanter. Once the skin incision had been made and the fascia over the tensor fascia lata reached, full thickness flaps were elevated. A self-retaining Dexterity Protractor retractor sleeve (Dexterity Surgical Inc., Roswell, GA, USA), as has been popularized in abdominal surgery, [28] was inserted within the incision to allow for maximal retraction without damaging the surrounding skin (Figure 1). The fascia overlying the tensor fascia lata was incised in line with the skin incision, taking great care to protect the lateral femoral cutaneous nerve. The interval between the tensor fascia lata muscle and the sartorius was then identified and bluntly developed, as was the deeper interval between the gluteus medius and the rectus femoris. The ascending branch of the lateral femoral circumflex artery found in the distal portion of this interval was ligated. The reflected head of the rectus femoris muscle was then identified and divided from

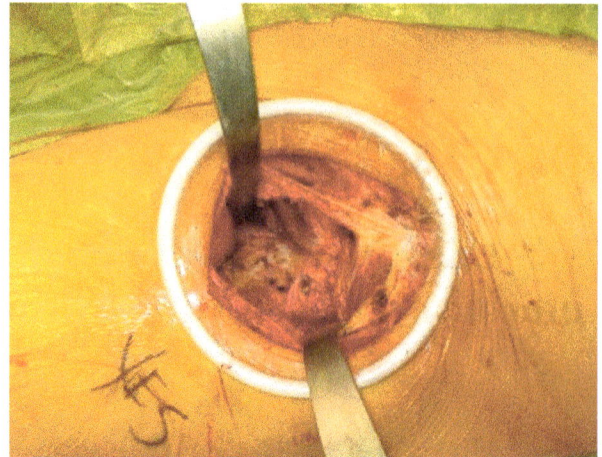

FIGURE 1: Exposure of the joint capsule seen through the Dexterity Protractor ring (Dexterity Surgical Inc., Roswell, GA, USA) which self-retracts and protects the skin and soft tissues.

the superior lip of the acetabulum. The anterior joint capsule was then visualized.

An anterior capsulectomy was performed to access the hip joint. We have found capsulectomy to be preferable to capsulotomy as the divided capsule otherwise interferes with visualization and cup placement. Once the capsule was incised, the femoral head and neck were exposed by two Hohmann retractors placed on either side of the neck. In order to aid with removal of the head, the hip was first partially dislocated to loosen soft tissue attachments. This was done by placing manual traction and externally rotating the leg spar. After this, traction was then released, and the neck cut was made with an oscillating saw. A corkscrew instrument was then placed into the femoral head and the head was removed with the use of a skid. Long curved scissors were used to divide the ligamentum teres.

After the head was removed, attention was turned to the acetabulum. The Hohmann retractors were placed over the anterior and posterior rims of the acetabulum for exposure. The labrum was cleared from the edges of the acetabulum as were any overriding osteophytes and excess tissue. After visualization was achieved the acetabulum was reamed to the appropriate size. At this time intraoperative fluoroscopic imaging was used to confirm appropriate placement of the reamers and trials (Figure 2). Our goal for acetabular component placement was abduction of 40–45 degrees and anteversion of 15–20 degrees. The live components were then placed in the acetabulum. In this series, 41 acetabular cups were press fit and two were cemented. Nineteen of the press fit cups were additionally fixated with screws.

Attention was then directed towards the femur, where the femoral hook attachment was placed around the proximal femur. The hook attachment allowed the femur to be delivered anteriorly and was controlled by a jack at the head of the table (Figure 3). Excessive anterior force must be avoided as this risks fracture of the greater trochanter. The leg was then externally rotated, extended, and adducted to gain maximal exposure of the proximal femur. The lateral gutter

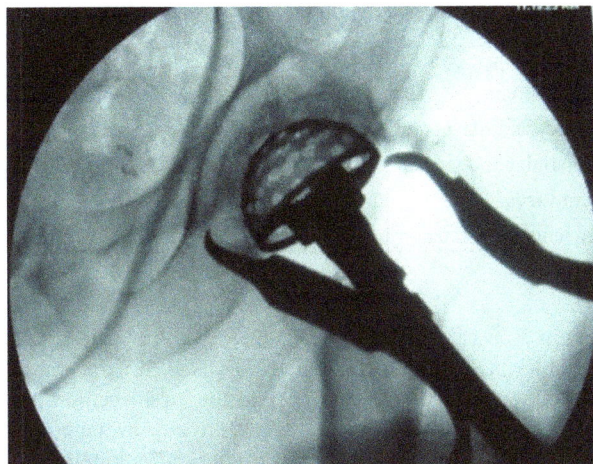

FIGURE 2: Preparation of the acetabulum with reamers is performed under fluoroscopic guidance.

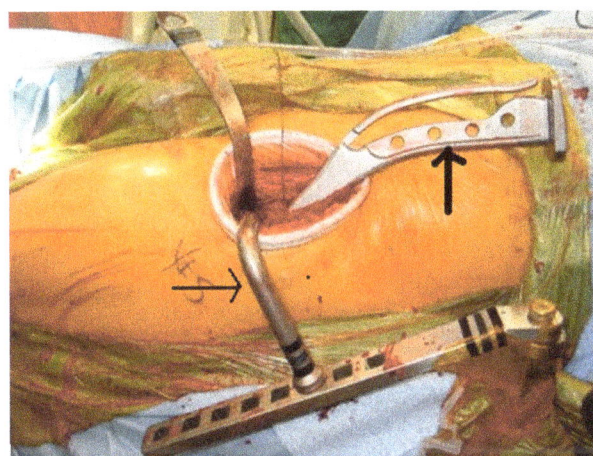

FIGURE 3: Intraoperative photograph illustrating the use of the femoral hook attachment (thin arrow) and curved broach handle (thick arrow), used to prepare the femur.

of the femur was cleared of excess tissue to allow component placement without varus. Specially shaped broach handles were used to gain exposure to the intramedullary canal and the femur was broached to the appropriate size. Fluoroscopy was again used to confirm trial component placement. Once the femoral component was inserted the trial femoral head was placed. In order to locate the hip, the femoral hook was lowered and the leg brought into traction and internal rotation using the leg spar. Stability was then assessed by placing the leg in a neutral position and slowly rotating it to 90 degrees of external rotation. If stable, the hip should remain reduced when the femur is pulled laterally with a hook placed around the neck of the femoral component. Leg length discrepancy was also determined by performing an AP of the pelvis with fluoroscopy and comparing the positions of the lesser trochanters.

After live component placement, all wounds were closed in the usual manner and a suction drain was inserted in the hip joint. The patients received antibiotics until the drain was

removed once the output had decreased to <50 mL/day, and all patients were placed on pharmacologic DVT prophylaxis for six weeks postoperatively. Patients were seen by the physical therapist on the first postoperative day and encouraged to ambulate with full weight without the use of a brace. Patients were restricted only to anterior hip precautions which consisted of no external rotation with the hip in full extension. They were otherwise given no other restrictions as to motion or activities. Patients were discharged from the hospital when becoming medically stable. Routine followup occurred postoperatively at 6 weeks, 3 months, 6 months, 1 year, and annually thereafter.

The patients' clinical records were reviewed for operative time, intraoperative complications, estimated blood loss, surgical technique, length of admission, postoperative course, and complications. The findings were compared to historical controls from the existing literature.

Postoperative radiographs were reviewed to determine acetabular anteversion, acetabular cup abduction, femoral stem varus positioning, and leg length discrepancy. Acetabular component anteversion was calculated as the arcsin of the short axis of the ellipse formed by the cup divided by the longer axis [29, 30]. Acetabular inclination was taken as the angle between a line drawn between the teardrops and the long axis of the acetabular ellipse [29, 31–33]. The distance between a point chosen on the lesser trochanters and a line drawn between the ischial tuberosities was used to determine leg length discrepancy. All calculations and measurements were performed by a single orthopaedic surgeon (TA).

## 3. Results

Operation time averaged 146 minutes (range, 100 to 245) for unilateral hips, 278 minutes (range, 205 to 352) for bilateral hips, and 176 minutes (range, 110 to 352) for all hips combined. The mean intraoperative blood loss was 1157 mL (range, 410 to 2600), and patients received an average of 2 units (range, 0 to 4) of packed red blood cells intraoperatively. Postoperatively they received a mean of 1 unit (range, 0 to 3) in addition to that given during surgery. The average hospital stay for unilateral hips was 5.3 days (range, 2 to 8 days) and 8.4 days (range, 3 to 14 days) for bilateral hips. When comparing the data from our first ten cases to our last ten cases we found an improvement in surgical time and intraoperative blood loss, indicating that these parameters improve with surgeon experience (Table 1).

Intraoperative complications included two fractures (5%, 2/43) (Table 2). One femoral shaft fracture occurred which was stabilized with cables as well as one greater trochanteric fracture that was fixed with cerclage wires. The femoral fracture occurred in a patient with severe osteopenia and avascular necrosis of the proximal femur. When the contralateral hip arthroplasty was performed at a later time, the femoral shaft was prophylactically secured with cables to prevent a similar occurrence.

Six fractures were reported in the postoperative period (14%, 6/43). Five minimally displaced fractures of the greater trochanter were noted during postoperative followup. All were amenable to nonoperative treatment. One patient

TABLE 1: Comparison of intraoperative and postoperative data for first ten unilateral versus last ten unilateral hip cases.

|  | First 10 cases | Last 10 cases |
|---|---|---|
| Surgical time (average minutes) | 229.5 (range, 165–315) | 139 (range, 100–170) |
| Intraoperative blood loss (average milliliters) | 2180 (range, 600–2600) | 500 (range, 250–900) |
| Hospital stay (average days) | 4.5 (range, 2–8) | 4.4 (range, 3–9) |
| Complications | 4 | 3 |

TABLE 2: Intraoperative and postoperative complications following anterior approach total hip arthroplasty.

| Complication | Number of hips | Complication rate |
|---|---|---|
| Intraoperative |  |  |
| Femoral fracture | 1 | 2.3% |
| Greater trochanter fracture | 1 | 2.3% |
| Postoperative |  |  |
| Greater trochanter fracture | 5 | 11.6% |
| Femoral nerve palsy | 2 | 4.6% |
| Intertrochanteric fracture | 1 | 2.3% |
| Iliopsoas avulsion | 1 | 2.3% |
| Dislocation | 1 | 2.3% |
| Hematoma | 1 | 2.3% |

TABLE 3: Postoperative radiographic measurements.

| Radiographic measurement | Average value | Range |
|---|---|---|
| Acetabular anteversion | $19.6° \pm 6.6°$ | 5° to 30° |
| Acetabular abduction | $48.4° \pm 7°$ | 34° to 70° |
| Stem varus | $0.9° \pm 2°$ | −4° to 6° |
| Leg length discrepancy | 7 mm | 3 to 14 mm |

version was calculated on the AP of the hip when it was available. Otherwise, the AP pelvis was used. Since acetabular anteversion appears smaller on radiographs centered on the pubis [35], this may have caused our average to be underestimated. The average acetabular cup abduction was found to be $48.4° \pm 7°$ (range, 34° to 70°). Fifteen hips had abduction of greater than 50 degrees. The mean stem varus was found to be $0.9° \pm 2°$ (range, −4° to 6°). The average leg length discrepancy was 7 mm (range, 3 to 14 mm).

## 4. Discussion

The main benefits of the anterior approach are fast recovery and improved early patient function. In our experience, almost all patients achieve full weight bearing by the first postoperative day, and most are able to ambulate without the use of crutches by the time of their hospital discharge. None of the patients in this series ambulated with a postoperative limp or had any evidence of muscle weakness often seen with the posterior and lateral approaches to the hip where the incidence of limp has been documented in up to 20% of patients [1, 2]. This is primarily attributable to the fact that no muscles are cut or sustain extensive damage during the anterior approach [36].

Dislocation rates for total hip arthroplasty range from 0.3% to 11% [1–10, 37, 38]. Rates of dislocation with the posterior hip approach are higher than those reported for lateral and anterolateral approaches [6, 7, 13]. This may be due to several factors including violation of the posterior capsule, division of the short external hip rotators, and component positioning. A study comparing the dislocation rate between capsulectomy and capsular repair with a posterolateral approach reported 2.8% dislocations with capsulotomy, while repair of the capsule resulted in a significantly lower rate of 0.6% dislocations [3]. Previous studies on the anterior hip approach have reported a dislocation rate ranging between 0% and 2% [18, 19, 21, 39, 40]. Our dislocation rate of 2% falls within this range.

Another factor associated with dislocation may be component malpositioning [4, 5, 37, 38]. The more common surgical approaches require that the patient be positioned in the lateral decubitus position which may result in tilting of the pelvis anteriorly during surgery [11, 12]. This anterior pelvic tilt if unrecognized intraoperatively may result in placement of the acetabular cup with inadequate anteversion, thus predisposing to posterior dislocation. This may be avoided with the anterior approach which appears to allow for reproducible and accurate component placement. In a

returned to the operating room postoperatively for internal fixation of a periprosthetic intertrochanteric fracture.

There were no infections or wound dehiscences in this series. One patient developed a deep hematoma that was surgically evacuated one week after the primary procedure. This patient had been treated with anticoagulants prior to surgery for a remote history of pulmonary embolism.

Two documented femoral nerve palsies were noted during the follow-up period, both of which were confirmed with EMG. All symptoms resolved in both patients within three months of surgery. In addition, one postoperative iliopsoas avulsion was diagnosed clinically and treated with physical therapy with subsequent improvement of symptoms.

One hip dislocation occurred in this series six weeks after surgery (2%, 1/43) after a fall. A successful closed reduction was performed and the patient was placed in a hip abduction brace for six weeks. Upon 17 months of followup the patient has not had any recurrent episodes of instability.

Acetabular and femoral component placement with the anterior approach was measured on plain radiographs (Table 3). Of the 43 hips operated, 41 had radiographs available for review. The average acetabular anteversion was $19.6° \pm 6.6°$ (range, 5° to 30°). When both AP pelvis and AP hip radiographs were available (31 hips), anteversion was confirmed by comparing the two [29, 30, 34]. In the cases where only one of the two views was available (10 hips), anteversion was assumed. The acetabular component

study of 100 cadavers, the average acetabular anteversion was found to be 19.9° ± 6.6 [41]. Our calculated cup anteversion of 19.6° ± 6.6 is well within the recommended "safe zone" of 5 to 25 degrees [4] and is comparable to physiologic measurements [32, 42–45]. For our calculations we used two separate methods to calculate the angle of anteversion [29, 30, 43] and both methods independently obtained a value of 19.6° ± 6.6. We therefore believe that our results are as accurate as possible and are comparable to the only other previous study reporting cup anteversion values of 19.4° ± 5.2 [18]. Our mean cup abduction angle of 48.4° ± 7, leg length discrepancy of 7 mm, and stem varus of 0.9° ± 2 are all within recommended guidelines [4, 41] and are similar to those findings reported by other investigators with this technique [18–20].

Another notable complication in our series was a 14% (6/43) rate of greater trochanteric fracture, which is similar to that reported in a large multicenter study of 1,152 patients in which 12% sustained greater trochanter fractures. Of the fractures in our series, one occurred intraoperatively and was secured with cables, and 5 were noted postoperatively. The 5 postoperative fractures, none of which required surgery, represented either small avulsions or were nondisplaced. We believe that these fractures may have occurred either during elevation of the femoral hook component of the table when excessive anteriorly directed force may have caused avulsion or fracture of the greater trochanter in osteoporotic patients or during the reduction maneuver required to relocate the hip during trialing and final hip relocation. During broaching the femur is in a shortened, adducted, extended, and externally rotated position. When the hip is then reduced, if abduction is performed prior to traction, internal rotation, and flexion, the greater trochanter abuts the ilium and may easily fracture. This was observed intraoperatively in the one case requiring cable fixation. It is the recommendation that the reduction maneuver be performed initially with traction, internal rotation, flexion back to neutral, and lastly abduction, and this must be emphasized to the assistant in control of the leg spars. The ankle injuries apparently caused by intraoperative traction reported in previous studies [18, 21] were not encountered in our series.

Two femoral nerve palsies occurred in our series, both of which resolved within three months postoperatively. We believe that these may have occurred when the hip was placed in a hyperextended position using the leg spar of the table during femoral canal preparation. The femoral nerve is susceptible to traction injury during this time if the hip is placed in excessive extension. Studies have shown that extensive hip abduction and external rotation may also be associated with femoral nerve traction injury [40, 46, 47]. Care must be taken when performing the anterior approach to assure that the hip is not in a position of excessive abduction and extension placing excessive tension and traction on the femoral nerve.

There does appear to be a rather steep learning curve when performing this procedure as our operative time and our blood loss significantly improved with time and additional surgeon experience as seen when comparing our first ten to our last ten cases. This was also found in a large multicenter observational study, where surgeons who

had performed less than 100 cases were twofold more likely to have complications in their patients [48]. Another series defined the learning curve to be around 40 cases, or 6 months in a high volume hip arthroplasty center, after which operating time and blood loss stabilize, and approach-related complications can be avoided [49].

The anterior minimally invasive muscle sparing approach to the hip is an attractive alternative to the more traditional posterior, lateral, and anterolateral approaches. From our early results we can conclude that the incidence of early dislocation is not increased and that accurate reproducible component placement is possible. As with any new technique, a period of trial and error is necessary to identify weaknesses in the approach and to develop new technical advances. In this series of our first 43 cases, we have demonstrated that there is a learning curve with this procedure and care must be taken to avoid certain pitfalls and complications which are specific to the instrumentation and technique of the anterior approach. Further studies are necessary to objectively examine whether the anterior minimally invasive approach provides advantages in terms of recovery time and long-term functional outcome in comparison to other approaches. We believe that as it gains popularity, this could become a superior approach with advantages for both surgeon and patient.

## Conflict of Interests

The authors disclose that they have no potential conflict of interests that may bias the work.

## References

[1] H. A. Demos, C. H. Rorabeck, R. B. Bourne, S. J. MacDonald, and R. W. McCalden, "Instability in primary total hip arthroplasty with the direct lateral approach," *Clinical Orthopaedics and Related Research*, no. 393, pp. 168–180, 2001.

[2] J. L. Masonis and R. B. Bourne, "Surgical approach, abductor function, and total hip arthroplasty dislocation," *Clinical Orthopaedics and Related Research*, no. 405, pp. 46–53, 2002.

[3] W. M. Goldstein, T. F. Gleason, M. Kopplin, and J. J. Branson, "Prevalence of dislocation after total hip arthroplasty through a posterolateral approach with partial capsulotomy and capsulorrhaphy," *Journal of Bone and Joint Surgery A*, vol. 83, supplement 2, pp. 2–7, 2001.

[4] G. E. Lewinnek, J. L. Lewis, and R. Tarr, "Dislocations after total hip-replacement arthroplasties," *Journal of Bone and Joint Surgery A*, vol. 60, no. 2, pp. 217–220, 1978.

[5] D. E. McCollum and W. J. Gray, "Dislocation after total hip arthroplasty: causes and prevention," *Clinical Orthopaedics and Related Research*, no. 261, pp. 159–170, 1990.

[6] M. A. Ritter, L. D. Harty, M. E. Keating, P. M. Faris, and J. B. Meding, "A clinical comparison of the anterolateral and posterolateral approaches to the hip," *Clinical Orthopaedics and Related Research*, no. 385, pp. 95–99, 2001.

[7] J. M. Roberts, F. H. Fu, E. J. McClain, and A. B. Ferguson Jr., "A comparison of the posterolateral and anterolateral approaches to total hip arthroplasty," *Clinical Orthopaedics and Related Research*, vol. 187, pp. 205–210, 1984.

[8] G. M. van Stralen, P. J. Struben, and C. J. van Loon, "The incidence of dislocation after primary total hip arthroplasty using posterior approach with posterior soft-tissue repair," *Archives of Orthopaedic and Trauma Surgery*, vol. 123, no. 5, pp. 219–222, 2003.

[9] P. A. Frndak, T. H. Mallory, and A. V. Lombardi Jr., "Translateral surgical approach to the hip: the abductor muscle 'split'," *Clinical Orthopaedics and Related Research*, no. 295, pp. 135–141, 1993.

[10] T. H. Mallory, A. V. Lombardi Jr., R. A. Fada, S. M. Herrington, and R. W. Eberle, "Dislocation after total hip arthroplasty using the anterolateral abductor split approach," *Clinical Orthopaedics and Related Research*, no. 358, pp. 166–172, 1999.

[11] I. Asayama, Y. Akiyoshi, M. Naito, and M. Ezoe, "Intraoperative pelvic motion in total hip arthroplasty," *The Journal of Arthroplasty*, vol. 19, no. 8, pp. 992–997, 2004.

[12] M. Ezoe, M. Naito, I. Asayama, T. Ishiko, and M. Fujisawa, "Pelvic motion during total hip arthroplasty with translateral and posterolateral approaches," *Journal of Orthopaedic Science*, vol. 10, no. 2, pp. 167–172, 2005.

[13] A. J. Vicar and C. R. Coleman, "A comparison of the anterolateral, transtrochanteric, and posterior surgical approaches in primary total hip arthroplasty," *Clinical Orthopaedics and Related Research*, vol. 188, pp. 152–159, 1984.

[14] B. S. Bal, P. Kazmier, T. Burd, and T. Aleto, "Anterior trochanteric slide osteotomy for primary total hip arthroplasty. Review of nonunion and complications," *Journal of Arthroplasty*, vol. 21, no. 1, pp. 59–63, 2006.

[15] J. Judet and R. Judet, "The use of an artificial femoral head for arthroplasty of the hip joint," *The Journal of Bone and Joint Surgery*, vol. 32, no. 2, pp. 166–173, 1950.

[16] M. N. Smith-Petersen, "Approach to and exposure of the hip joint for mold arthroplasty," *The Journal of Bone & Joint Surgery A*, vol. 31, no. 1, pp. 40–46, 1949.

[17] R. E. Kennon, J. M. Keggi, R. S. Wetmore, L. E. Zatorski, M. H. Huo, and K. J. Keggi, "Total hip arthroplasty through a minimally invasive anterior surgical approach," *Journal of Bone and Joint Surgery A*, vol. 85, supplement 4, pp. 39–48, 2003.

[18] J. M. Matta, C. Shahrdar, and T. Ferguson, "Single-incision anterior approach for total hip arthroplasty on an orthopaedic table," *Clinical Orthopaedics and Related Research*, no. 441, pp. 115–124, 2005.

[19] P. Paillard, "Hip replacement by a minimal anterior approach," *International Orthopaedics*, vol. 31, supplement 1, pp. S13–S15, 2007.

[20] F. Rachbauer, "Minimally invasive total hip arthroplasty via direct anterior approach," *Orthopade*, vol. 34, no. 11, pp. 1103–1110, 2005.

[21] T. Siguier, M. Siguier, and B. Brumpt, "Mini-incision anterior approach does not increase dislocation rate: a study of 1037 total hip replacements," *Clinical Orthopaedics and Related Research*, no. 426, pp. 164–173, 2004.

[22] Y. Inaba, L. D. Dorr, Z. Wan, L. Sirianni, and M. Boutary, "Operative and patient care techniques for posterior mini-incision total hip arthroplasty," *Clinical Orthopaedics and Related Research*, no. 441, pp. 104–114, 2005.

[23] L. Ogonda, R. Wilson, P. Archbold et al., "A minimal-incision technique in total hip arthroplasty does not improve early postoperative outcomes: a prospective, randomized, controlled trial," *Journal of Bone and Joint Surgery A*, vol. 87, no. 4, pp. 701–710, 2005.

[24] T. P. Sculco, "Minimally invasive total hip arthroplasty: in the affirmative," *Journal of Arthroplasty*, vol. 19, no. 4, pp. 78–80, 2004.

[25] S. T. Woolson, C. S. Mow, J. F. Syquia, J. V. Lannin, and D. J. Schurman, "Comparison of primary total hip replacements performed with a standard incision or a mini-incision," *Journal of Bone and Joint Surgery A*, vol. 86, no. 7, pp. 1353–1358, 2004.

[26] F. Bottner, S. Delgado, and T. P. Sculco, "Minimally invasive total hip replacement: the posterolateral approach," *American Journal of Orthopedics*, vol. 35, no. 5, pp. 218–224, 2006.

[27] J. S. Teet, H. B. Skinner, and L. Khoury, "The effect of the "Mini" incision in total hip arthroplasty on component position," *Journal of Arthroplasty*, vol. 21, no. 4, pp. 503–507, 2006.

[28] M. A. Pelosi II and M. A. Pelosi III, "Self-retaining abdominal retractor for minilaparotomy," *Obstetrics and Gynecology*, vol. 96, no. 5, pp. 775–778, 2000.

[29] R. H. McLaren, "Prosthetic hip angulation," *Radiology*, vol. 107, no. 3, pp. 705–706, 1973.

[30] H. Seradge, K. R. Nagle, and R. J. Miller, "Analysis of version in the acetabular cup," *Clinical Orthopaedics and Related Research*, vol. 166, pp. 152–157, 1982.

[31] O. Müller, P. Reize, D. Trappmann, and N. Wülker, "Measuring anatomical acetabular cup orientation with a new X-ray technique," *Computer Aided Surgery*, vol. 11, no. 2, pp. 69–75, 2006.

[32] O. Müller, B. Lembeck, P. Reize, and N. Wülker, "Quantification and visualization of the influence of pelvic tilt upon measurement of acetabular inclination and anteversion," *Zeitschrift fur Orthopadie und Ihre Grenzgebiete*, vol. 143, no. 1, pp. 72–78, 2005.

[33] D. W. Murray, "The definition and measurement of acetabular orientation," *Journal of Bone and Joint Surgery B*, vol. 75, no. 2, pp. 228–232, 1993.

[34] R. Pradhan, "Planar anteversion of the acetabular cup as determined from plain anteroposterior radiographs," *Journal of Bone and Joint Surgery B*, vol. 81, no. 3, pp. 431–435, 1999.

[35] T. G. Goergen and D. Resnick, "Evaluation of acetabular anteversion following total hip arthroplasty: necessity of proper centring," *British Journal of Radiology*, vol. 48, no. 568, pp. 259–260, 1975.

[36] R. M. Meneghini, M. W. Pagnano, R. T. Trousdale, and W. J. Hozack, "Muscle damage during MIS total hip arthroplasty: Smith-peterson versus posterior approach," *Clinical Orthopaedics and Related Research*, no. 453, pp. 293–298, 2006.

[37] D. J. Berry, M. von Knoch, C. D. Schleck, and W. S. Harmsen, "The cumulative long-term risk of dislocation after primary charnley total hip arthroplasty," *Journal of Bone and Joint Surgery A*, vol. 86, no. 1, pp. 9–14, 2004.

[38] C. D. Fackler and R. Poss, "Dislocation in total hip arthroplasties," *Clinical Orthopaedics and Related Research*, no. 151, pp. 169–178, 1980.

[39] E. Sariali, P. Leonard, and P. Mamoudy, "Dislocation after total hip arthroplasty using hueter anterior approach," *Journal of Arthroplasty*, vol. 23, no. 2, pp. 266–272, 2008.

[40] M. K. Ackland, W. B. Bourne, and H. K. Uhthoff, "Anteversion of the acetabular cup. Measurement of angle after total hip replacement," *Journal of Bone and Joint Surgery B*, vol. 68, no. 3, pp. 409–413, 1986.

[41] T. R. Light and K. J. Keggi, "Anterior approach to hip arthroplasty," *Clinical Orthopaedics and Related Research*, vol. 152, pp. 255–260, 1980.

[42] M. Maruyama, J. R. Feinberg, W. N. Capello, and J. A. D'Antonio, "Morphologic features of the acetabulum and femur: anteversion angle and implant positioning," *Clinical Orthopaedics and Related Research*, no. 393, pp. 52–65, 2001.

[43] T. Kalteis, M. Handel, T. Herold, L. Perlick, C. Paetzel, and J. Grifka, "Position of the acetabular cup—accuracy of radiographic calculation compared to CT-based measurement," *European Journal of Radiology*, vol. 58, no. 2, pp. 294–300, 2006.

[44] K. H. Widmer, "A simplified method to determine acetabular cup anteversion from plain radiographs," *Journal of Arthroplasty*, vol. 19, no. 3, pp. 387–390, 2004.

[45] D. M. Hassan, G. H. F. Johnston, W. N. C. Dust, G. Watson, and D. Cassidy, "Radiographic calculation of anteversion in acetabular prostheses," *Journal of Arthroplasty*, vol. 10, no. 3, pp. 369–372, 1995.

[46] M. Al Hakim and M. B. Katirji, "Femoral mononeuropathy induced by the lithotomy position: a report of 5 cases with a review of literature," *Muscle and Nerve*, vol. 16, no. 9, pp. 891–895, 1993.

[47] L. J. Kuo, I.-W. Penn, S. F. Feng, and C. M. Chen, "Femoral neuropathy after pelvic surgery," *Journal of the Chinese Medical Association*, vol. 67, no. 12, pp. 644–646, 2004.

[48] Anterior Total Hip Arthroplasty Collaborative (ATHAC) Investigators, M. Bhandari, J. M. Matta et al., "Outcomes following the single-incision anterior approach to total hip arthroplasty: a multicenter observational study," *Orthopedic Clinics of North America*, vol. 40, no. 3, pp. 329–342, 2009.

[49] B. E. Seng, K. R. Berend, A. F. Ajluni, and A. V. Lombardi Jr., "Anterior-supine minimally invasive total hip arthroplasty: defining the learning curve," *Orthopedic Clinics of North America*, vol. 40, no. 3, pp. 343–350, 2009.

# 36

# Accuracy of Implant Placement Utilizing Customized Patient Instrumentation in Total Knee Arthroplasty

**William D. Bugbee,**[1] **Hideki Mizu-uchi,**[2] **Shantanu Patil,**[2] **and Darryl D'Lima**[2]

[1] Division of Orthopaedic Surgery, Scripps Clinic, 10666 North Torrey Pines Road, MS116, La Jolla, CA 92037, USA
[2] Shiley Center for Orthopaedic Research & Education at Scripps Clinic, 11025 North Torrey Pines Road, Suite 200, La Jolla, CA 92037, USA

Correspondence should be addressed to William D. Bugbee; bugbee.william@scrippshealth.org

Academic Editor: Masato Takao

Customized patient instrumentation (CPI) combines preoperative planning with customized cutting jigs to position and align implants during total knee arthroplasty (TKA). We compared postoperative implant alignment of patients undergoing surgery with CPI to traditional TKA instrumentation for accuracy of implant placement. Twenty-five consecutive TKAs using CPI were analyzed. Preoperative CT scans of the lower extremities were segmented using a computer program. Limb alignment and mechanical axis were computed. Virtual implantation of computer-aided design models was done. Postoperative coronal and sagittal view radiographs were obtained. Using 3D image-matching software, relative positions of femoral and tibial implants were determined. Twenty-five TKAs implanted using traditional instrumentation were also analyzed. For CPI, difference in alignment from the preoperative plan was calculated. In the CPI group, the mean absolute difference between the planned and actual femoral placements was $0.67°$ in the coronal plane and $1.2°$ in the sagittal plane. For tibial alignment, the mean absolute difference was $0.9°$ in the coronal plane and $1.3°$ in the sagittal plane. For traditional instrumentation, difference from ideal placement for the femur was $1.5°$ in the coronal plane and $2.3°$ in the sagittal plane. For the tibia, the difference was $1.8°$ in the coronal plane. CPI achieved accurate implant positioning and was superior to traditional TKA instrumentation.

## 1. Introduction

Accurate alignment and positioning of implants in total knee arthroplasty (TKA) is an important goal of the procedure. Numerous studies have demonstrated a high frequency of implant malalignment in TKA, regardless of the surgical techniques utilized [1–7]. The innovation cycle of TKA has mirrored this fundamental concept. Initially, free-hand surgical cuts were performed prior to the placement of implant components. Subsequently, mechanical alignment guides were devised based on bony or external landmarks, and predetermined angular or measured resections were performed. More recently, image-guided or imageless computer navigation systems have been developed to guide the surgical procedure and ultimate component alignment. The most recent innovation in TKA is customized patient instrumentation (CPI), which has been introduced as a next generation technology in an effort to further improve the accuracy and precision of surgical technique, implant placement, and alignment. The concept of CPI revolves around the use of preoperatively obtained imaging studies such as plain radiographs, magnetic resonance imaging (MRI), or computed tomography (CT) scans that are then manipulated in software programs to generate three-dimensional models of an individual patient's knee anatomy and limb alignment. This model is utilized to create a customized surgical plan, which defines the surgical cuts of the tibia and femur. This surgical plan is used to create customized cutting jigs that uniquely fit the individual patient's anatomy.

The purpose of this study was to determine if a CT-based customized patient instrumentation system resulted in accurate implantation of tibial and femoral components in TKA and to compare the CPI protocol to standard mechanical alignment guides used in traditional TKA with respect to femoral and tibial component alignment.

## 2. Materials and Methods

*2.1. Patients.* With the approval of our institutional review board, we retrospectively analyzed 25 consecutive patients who underwent TKA using CT-based CPI (TruMatch, Depuy, Warsaw, Indiana). Preoperative CT scans were obtained per the device manufacturer's protocol and were used to generate a surgical plan based on predefined surgeon preferences as well as restoration of ideal mechanical alignment (Figure 1). Customized cutting guides were then made and delivered sterile to the operating room (Figure 2). Standard TKA was performed utilizing custom cutting blocks rather than traditional mechanical jigs (Figures 3(a) and 3(b)).

A second cohort of matched patients who underwent TKA using traditional instrumentation was analyzed for comparison. In the traditional TKA cohort, the targeted ideal placement was defined as 90° to the mechanical axis in the coronal and sagittal views for the femur and 90° in the coronal view for tibia. All patients underwent a standard postoperative rehabilitation protocol and were followed at 3 months, 6 months, and 1 year postoperatively. At the time of the latest clinical followup, postoperative radiographs (coronal and sagittal views) were obtained.

*2.2. Accuracy of Implant Placement.* Preoperative CT scans of the patient's lower extremity were segmented using MIMICS 13.0 (Materialise, Belgium) (Figure 4). Three-dimensional (3D) models of the knee joint and the bones were created from which limb alignment and mechanical axis were computed for each joint. The mechanical axis of the unoperated limb was calculated by a line joining the center of the femoral head to the middle of the talar dome. The models were then imported into a modeling and design software Rhino (McNeel North America, Seattle, WA). Based on the preoperative planning protocol, virtual implantation of the TKA computer-aided design (CAD) models was performed using Rhino (Figure 5). This constituted the "ideal" planned position of the femoral and tibial components.

The digitized postoperative knee radiographs were analyzed to determine the final placement of the actual implants. To convert the two-dimensional radiographs to 3D, an open source image matching software JointTrack (University of Florida) was used. The relative positions of the femoral and tibial implant were thus obtained from the radiographs. This data was then imported into Rhino to accurately determine the position of implanted components. This position was compared with the virtual surgical placement. The difference in planned and actual placement of the implants was calculated in the sagittal and coronal planes for the CPI group (Figure 6). In the traditional TKA group, the targeted alignment was 90° in both planes for femur and 90° in coronal plane for the tibia in sagittal view. In the traditional TKA

group, implant positions were calculated in the same manner as for the CPI group.

*2.3. Statistics.* Statistical analysis included *t*-test for equality of means and was determined using SPSS 13 (IBM software, Armonk, NY).

## 3. Results

In the CPI group, the mean absolute difference from the planned femoral placement was 0.8° (±0.6°) in the coronal plane and was 1.2° (±0.9°) in the sagittal plane (Table 1). The single outlier in this group (−4.4° difference) was a patient with posttraumatic femoral deformity, which necessitated a deviation from the planned protocol intraoperatively. In the traditional TKA group, this difference from ideal placement was 1.5° (±1.6°) in the coronal plane and 2.3° (±1.3°) in the sagittal plane. For the tibial tray, the difference from planned placement was 1.0° (±1.0°, range, −1.6° to 1.7°) in the coronal plane for the CPI group, while in the traditional TKA group, the difference from ideal placement was 1.8° (±1.6°, range, −3° to 6.4°) in the coronal plane. The comparison between the CPI and the traditional TKA group was statistically significant for femoral implant positioning ($P < 0.01$) but not for the tibial implant positioning. More outliers (±3°) occurred in the traditional TKA group.

## 4. Discussion

Interest in custom or patient-specific cutting guides is increasing. The potential for improved surgical efficiency with decreased operative times using fewer instruments and the possibility of improvements in surgical accuracy compared to conventional mechanical instruments are attractive features. Although computer-assisted techniques have demonstrated improved component alignment in TKA, the relative cost and increased operative time has led to resistance in the widespread adoption of this technique during TKA surgery [7, 8].

Few published clinical studies are available analyzing CT-based CPI for TKA. The results of our study validates the concept that using a CT-based protocol to create a three-dimensional model and subsequent cutting guides resulted in accurate surgical positioning of the TKA implants. The second question we asked was whether customized patient instrumentation was more accurate than traditional mechanical instrumentation utilizing intramedullary femoral alignment guides and extramedullary tibial guides. In our study, the CPI was more accurate than mechanical instrumentation on the femoral side and equal on the tibial side. CPI was associated with fewer outliers. A number of clinical studies have evaluated TKA alignment utilizing similar MRI-based patient-specific guides. Nunley et al. [9] evaluated 150 primary TKA using either conventional instrumentation, mechanical-axis-based patient-specific instrumentation, or kinematic-based patient-specific instrumentation. They found that these MR-based systems had a similar number of mechanical outliers as mechanical instruments

TABLE 1: Mean absolute difference between the planned (CPI) and ideal (traditional TKA) placement of the femoral and tibial components. Asterisk denote statistical significance (paired *t*-test two tailed).

| | CPI cohort<br>Mean (SD, range) | Traditional TKA cohort<br>Mean (SD, range) | P value |
|---|---|---|---|
| Femur | | | |
| Coronal* | 0.8° (±0.6°; −1.0° to 1.5°) | 1.5° (±1.6°; −3.9° to 2.9°) | $P < 0.01$ |
| Sagittal* | 1.2° (±0.9°; −4.4° to 2.4°) | 2.3° (±1.3°; −2.5° to 4.7°) | $P < 0.001$ |
| Tibia | | | |
| Coronal | 1.0° (±1.0°; −1.6° to 1.7°) | 1.8° (±1.6°; −3° to 6.4°) | |

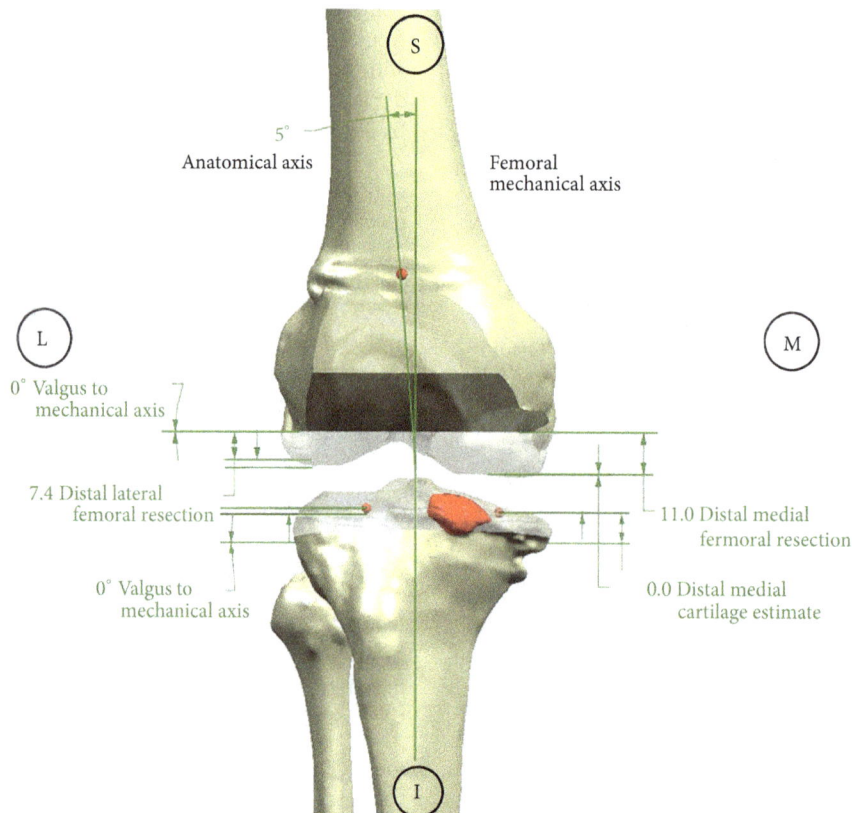

FIGURE 1: Portion of the surgical plan generated from preoperative CT scanning.

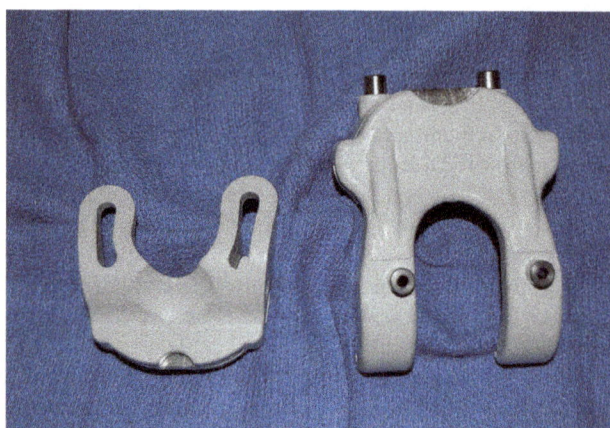

FIGURE 2: Tibial (left) and femoral (right) customized cutting guides.

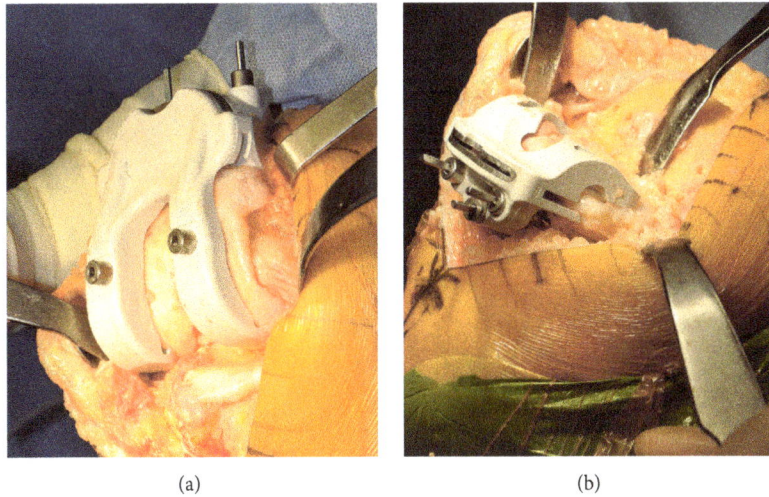

FIGURE 3: (a) Femoral cutting guide after placement on the distal femur. (b) Tibial cutting guide after placement on the proximal tibia.

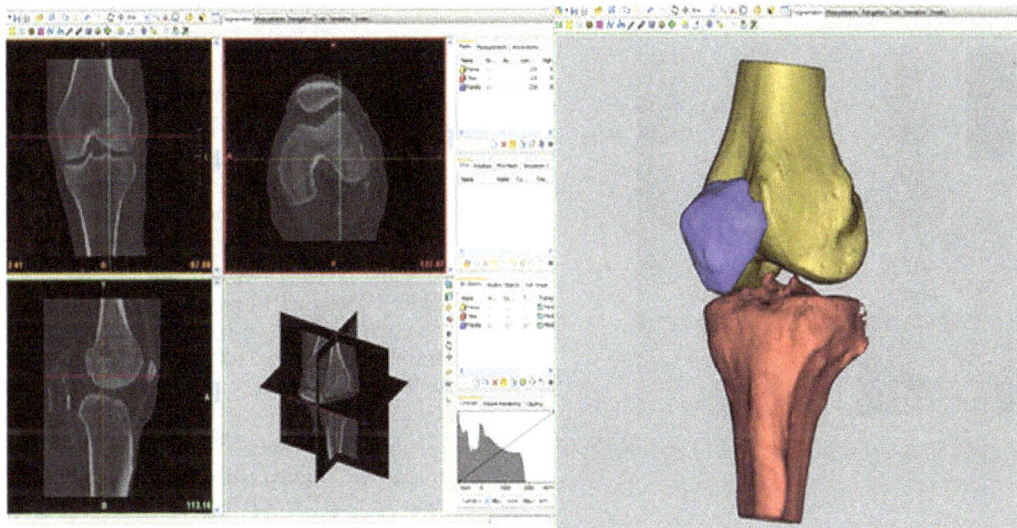

FIGURE 4: Segmenting process rendering CT scan into 3D model of the knee.

and, therefore, questioned their clinical utility. Ng et al. [10] reviewed 569 TKA performed with an MRI-based patient-specific instrumentation system and found slightly better mechanical alignment and fewer outliers than in a matched group of 155 conventionally instrumented TKAs.

The question of whether a CT-based or MR-based system is superior is not yet fully clarified. The relative advantage of a CT-based system is better bony landmark resolution than MR [11] and the ability to determine limb mechanical axis. Lower cost and shorter acquisition times are also potential advantages with CT. Relative disadvantages include the use of ionizing radiation.

Certain limitations of this study should be discussed. We did not attempt to measure clinical outcome. To date, no conclusive evidence has demonstrated that either computer navigation or customized patient instrumentation leads to improved clinical outcome or implant longevity. However,

many authors have demonstrated a correlation between coronal alignment and TKA failure [12, 13]. The clinical value of custom patient instrumentation has yet to be conclusively determined. Another limitation of the current study is the postoperative analysis using plain radiographs rather than CT scans. In this study, the precision of the data analysis would have been improved if patients underwent both preoperative and postoperative CT scans to obtain more accurate 2D to 3D modeling of the knee and limb.

Ongoing advances in CT-based bone modeling protocols and subsequent manufacture of customized cutting blocks should lead to further improvements in surgical precision and accuracy. Additionally, the analytical methodology used in this study may be valuable in validating the accuracy of other implant alignment systems or image-based CPI protocols and devices [14, 15]. In conclusion, CPI is a novel technique that offers the potential of increased accuracy and

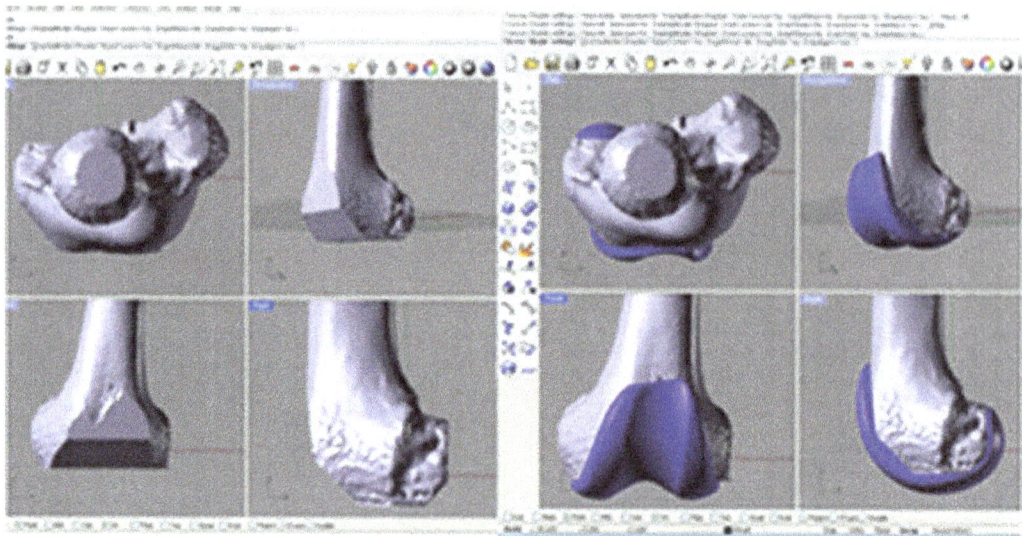

FIGURE 5: Virtual implantation of TKA based on ideal planned component position.

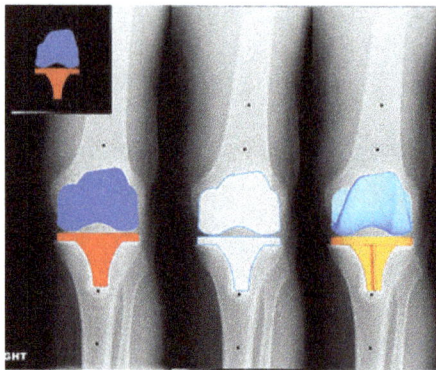

FIGURE 6: Comparison of actual versus planned surgical implantation.

efficiency in TKA. The CT-based CPI used in this study (Tru Match, DePuy, Warsaw, Indiana) accurately positioned implants relative to the preoperative plan and achieved overall implant alignment better than traditional mechanical instrumentation, with fewer outliers.

## References

[1] K. E. Teter, D. Bregman, and C. W. Colwell Jr., "The efficacy of intramedullary femoral alignment in total knee replacement," *Clinical Orthopaedics and Related Research*, no. 321, pp. 117–121, 1995.

[2] S. Patil, D. D. D'Lima, J. M. Fait, and C. W. Colwell Jr., "Improving tibial component coronal alignment during total knee arthroplasty with use of a tibial planing device," *Journal of Bone and Joint Surgery A*, vol. 89, no. 2, pp. 381–387, 2007.

[3] H. Mizu-uchi, S. Matsuda, H. Miura, H. Higaki, K. Okazaki, and Y. Iwamoto, "The effect of ankle rotation on cutting of the tibia in total knee arthroplasty," *Journal of Bone and Joint Surgery A*, vol. 88, no. 12, pp. 2632–2636, 2006.

[4] M. R. Reed, W. Bliss, J. L. Sher, K. P. Emmerson, S. M. G. Jones, and P. F. Partington, "Extramedullary or intramedullary tibial alignment guides: a randomized, prospective trial of radiological alignment," *Journal of Bone and Joint Surgery B*, vol. 84, no. 6, pp. 858–860, 2002.

[5] H. E. Cates, M. A. Ritter, E. M. Keating, and P. M. Faris, "Intramedullary versus extramedullary femoral alignment systems in total knee replacement," *Clinical Orthopaedics and Related Research*, no. 286, pp. 32–39, 1993.

[6] J. Y. Jenny, U. Clemens, S. Kohler, H. Kiefer, W. Konermann, and R. K. Miehlke, "Consistency of implantation of a total knee arthroplasty with a non-image-based navigation system: a case-control study of 235 cases compared with 235 conventionally implanted prostheses," *Journal of Arthroplasty*, vol. 20, no. 7, pp. 832–839, 2005.

[7] G. Matziolis, D. Krocker, U. Weiss, S. Tohtz, and C. Perka, "A prospective, randomized study of computer-assisted and conventional total knee arthroplasty: three-dimensional evaluation of implant alignment and rotation," *Journal of Bone and Joint Surgery A*, vol. 89, no. 2, pp. 236–243, 2007.

[8] W. G. Blakeney, R. J. K. Khan, and S. J. Wall, "Computer-assisted techniques versus conventional guides for component alignment in total knee arthroplasty: a randomized controlled trial," *Journal of Bone and Joint Surgery A*, vol. 93, no. 15, pp. 1377–1384, 2011.

[9] R. M. Nunley, B. S. Ellison, J. Zhu, E. L. Ruh, S. M. Howell, and R. L. Barrack, "Do patient-specific guides improve coronal alignment in total knee arthroplasty?" *Clinical Orthopaedics and Related Research*, vol. 470, no. 3, pp. 895–902, 2012.

[10] V. Y. Ng, J. H. DeClaire, K. R. Berend, B. C. Gulick, and A. V. Lombardi Jr., "Improved accuracy of alignment with patient-specific positioning guides compared with manual instrumentation in TKA," *Clinical Orthopaedics and Related Research*, vol. 470, no. 1, pp. 99–107, 2012.

[11] D. White, K. L. Chelule, and B. B. Seedhom, "Accuracy of MRI vs CT imaging with particular reference to patient specific templates for total knee replacement surgery," *International Journal of Medical Robotics and Computer Assisted Surgery*, vol. 4, no. 3, pp. 224–231, 2008.

[12] M. A. Ritter, P. M. Faris, E. M. Keating, and J. B. Meding, "Postoperative alignment of total knee replacement: its effect on

survival," *Clinical Orthopaedics and Related Research*, no. 299, pp. 153–156, 1994.

[13] M. E. Berend, M. A. Ritter, J. B. Meding et al., "Tibial component failure mechanisms in total knee arthroplasty," *Clinical Orthopaedics and Related Research*, no. 428, pp. 26–34, 2004.

[14] H. Mizu-uchi, S. Matsuda, H. Miura, K. Okazaki, Y. Akasaki, and Y. Iwamoto, "The evaluation of post-operative alignment in total knee replacement using a CT-based navigation system," *Journal of Bone and Joint Surgery B*, vol. 90, no. 8, pp. 1025–1031, 2008.

[15] H. Mizu-uchi, C. W. Colwell Jr., S. Matsuda, C. Flores-Hernandez, Y. Iwamoto, and D. D. D'Lima, "Effect of total knee arthroplasty implant position on flexion angle before implant-bone impingement," *Journal of Arthroplasty*, vol. 26, no. 5, pp. 721–727, 2011.

# 37

# Retrospective Review of Pectoralis Major Ruptures in Rodeo Steer Wrestlers

**Breda H. F. Lau,[1] Dale J. Butterwick,[2] Mark R. Lafave,[1] and Nicholas G. Mohtadi[3]**

[1] *Department of Physical Education and Recreational Studies, Mount Royal University, 4825 Mount Royal Gate SW, Calgary, AB, Canada T3E 6K6*
[2] *Faculty of Kinesiology, University of Calgary, 2500 University Dr NW, Calgary, AB, Canada T2N 1N4*
[3] *Faculty of Medicine, Health Sciences Centre, Foothills Campus, University of Calgary, 3330 Hospital Drive NW, Calgary, AB, Canada T2N 4N1*

Correspondence should be addressed to Breda H. F. Lau; blau@mtroyal.ca

Academic Editor: Elizaveta Kon

*Background.* Pectoralis major tendon ruptures have been reported in the literature as occupational injuries, accidental injuries, and sporting activities. Few cases have been reported with respect to rodeo activities. *Purpose.* To describe a series of PM tendon ruptures in professional steer wrestlers. *Study Design.* Case series, level of evidence, 4. *Methods.* A retrospective analysis of PM ruptures in a steer wrestling cohort was performed. Injury data between 1992 and 2008 were reviewed using medical records from the University of Calgary Sport Medicine Center. *Results.* Nine cases of pectoralis major ruptures in professional steer wrestlers were identified. Injuries occurred during the throwing phase of the steer or while breaking a fall. All athletes reported unexpected or abnormal behavior of the steer that contributed to the mechanism of injury. Seven cases were surgically repaired, while two cases opted for nonsurgical intervention. Eight cases reported successful return to competition following the injury. *Conclusion.* Steer wrestlers represent a unique cohort of PM rupture case studies. Steer wrestling is a demanding sport that involves throwing maneuvers that may predispose the muscle to rupture. All cases demonstrated good functional outcomes regardless of surgical or non-surgical treatment.

## 1. Introduction

Pectoralis major (PM) tendon ruptures have been reported in the literature. These ruptures present as occupational injuries [1, 2], accidental injuries [3], and sporting activities [4–7] primarily in weight lifting. Ruptures have also been reported in elderly patients during procedures for transferring, positioning, and dressing the patients [8–10]. Ruptures of the muscle belly typically present as the result of direct trauma or traction injuries. Falls onto outstretched arms often result in ruptures at the musculotendinous junction, whereas excessive tension on a maximally contracted muscle often results in ruptures of the tendinous insertion from the humerus [6, 8]. Sport-related PM ruptures usually result from activities requiring a large amount of upper body strength. Two articles have reported PM ruptures resulting from a rodeo event: one reported a professional bull rider who tore his left PM during a bull riding [11]; the other reported three cases of

PM ruptures during steer wrestling but failed to describe the events surrounding the injuries [12]. These three cases are included in this study and reported in further detail. The purpose of this paper is to describe a series of PM ruptures in professional rodeo steer wrestlers in order to expand upon and understand the nature of this injury behind this particular cohort of athletes. Therefore, descriptive information was gathered about the sport to identify prevalence, characterize PM ruptures, and determine mechanism of injury affecting rupture type and location.

Each year professional rodeo contestants compete during the rodeo season in an attempt to qualify for the national championship rodeo in Canada, the Canadian Finals Rodeo. Steer wrestling is one of the seven events at these finals. Steer wrestling is a rodeo event that requires considerable strength in addition to timing and coordination. The event consists of a 450 to 750 lb steer and two mounted cowboys: the contestant and the hazer. The steer is placed into a chute, with the contestant and the hazer on either side of the chute. The contestant waits behind a rope fastened to a string that is attached to the chute. When the contestant is ready, he calls for the steer, and the chute opens. The steer is given a head start, and the contestant must catch up to the steer. The job of the hazer is to mimic the pathway of the contestant on the opposite side of the steer relative to the contestant, in an effort to keep the steer running as straight as possible. The goal of the contestant is to wrestle the steer to the ground in a timely fashion.

There are three phases to steer wrestling: (1) the dismount: when the cowboy transfers from his horse to the steer; (2) the slide: when the cowboy positions himself for the throw; and (3) the throw: when the steer is wrestled to the ground with all four legs and head facing in the same direction [13]. The cowboy must position himself in a manner that allows his right arm to reach under the steer's right horn and his left hand to grab the top of the steer's left horn. As the cowboy dismounts from his horse, he uses his legs to brace against the ground, generating a large deceleration force. He must then lower his center of gravity and sit back. Finally, the cowboy must flex, adduct, internally rotate, and concentrically contract his right arm, while internally rotating the steer's right horn in an attempt to turn and tackle the steer down onto its left side.

## 2. Materials and Methods

Patient records from the University of Calgary Sport Medicine Center were retrospectively reviewed from 1992 to 2008. Patients were identified through diagnostic codes searching for PM injuries. To ensure that cases were not overlooked, cases were also searched using anatomical location (i.e., shoulder). Cases were also identified from caregivers of the Canadian Pro Rodeo Sport Medicine Team (CPRSMT). All patients diagnosed with a PM injury were reviewed. Clinical assessments were confirmed by a sport medicine physician, orthopaedic surgeon, or athletic therapist. Patient medical records and retrospective interview were used to collect the following information: patient demographics, previous medical history, mechanism of injury, physical findings, diagnostic imaging, treatment, and treatment outcome. This project was approved by the University of Calgary Conjoint Health Research Ethics Board.

## 3. Results

During the years 1992 to 2008, a total of 34 patients with a PM muscle injury were treated at the University of Calgary Sport Medicine Center. Six PM ruptures were reported in rodeo athletes, five of which were in steer wrestlers. Four additional cases of PM ruptures not treated at the center were identified by caregivers of the CPRSMT. In total, there were nine professional male steer wrestlers identified with PM ruptures of the right arm at the distal insertion of the PM into the humerus between 1992 and 2008. A complete tear of the PM was determined upon clinical examination of the injury presenting with discontinuity of the tendon at the musculotendinous junction or near insertion into the humerus and loss of muscular contour. The patient's ages ranged from 30 to 51 years (mean: $35 \pm 7$ years). Incomplete ruptures of the PM were also identified but were not included in this study. All cases occurred during rodeo competition participating at Canadian Professional Rodeo Association sanctioned rodeos.

Four of nine cases (44.4%, 95% CI: 12.0–76.9%) had a previous history of the right shoulder injury including rotator cuff tendinopathy, glenohumeral dislocation, and biceps brachii strain. Four cases (44.4%, 95% CI: 12.0–76.9%) reported previous PM strains. Three cases did not have previous injuries to either the right shoulder or PM (33.3%, 95% CI: 2.5–64.1%).

*3.1. Mechanism of Injury.* In seven of nine cases (77.8%, 95% CI: 50.6–104.9%) the PM was injured during the attempted throwing phase of the steer. For the other two cases (22.2%, 95% CI: −4.9–49.4%), injuries resulted when the contestant was forced to break his fall on the ground with his arm abducted and extended out to one side.

Table 1 presents trends surrounding events leading up to the incident that may have contributed to the mechanism of injury during the steer wrestling activity (e.g., steer behavior, horse behavior, hazer error). In all nine cases, unexpected or abnormal behavior of the steer was identified as a potential risk factor. In four cases (44.4%, 95% CI: 12.0–76.9%), the steer stopped prematurely during the chase. In three cases, both the steer and the hazer veered wide (33.3%, 95% CI: 2.5–64.1%). In two cases (22.2%, 95% CI: −4.9–49.4%), the mechanism of injury was due to unexpected movement of the steer as it failed to set up properly either by slowing down or bucking upwards.

*3.2. Physical Examination and Imaging.* Clinical examination revealed that eight of nine cases (88.9%, 95% CI: 68.3–109.4%) presented with full range of motion in the shoulder. One case was limited in external rotation and abduction but had sustained previous partial ruptures ($n = 2$) to the same PM. One case reported transient numbness in the hand distal to the injury site. The cases presented with physical findings including pain, swelling, ecchymosis, obvious defect due to muscle retraction, and weakness in resisted internal rotation, adduction, and horizontal flexion of the shoulder. Plain radiographs were ordered in three cases (33.3%, 95% CI: 2.5–64.1%), and one case received both ultrasound and magnetic resonance imaging.

*3.3. Operative versus Nonoperative Treatment.* Of nine cases, only two cases (22.2%, 95% CI: −4.9–49.4%) elected nonsurgical treatment with conservative progressive rehabilitative exercises. Eight of nine cases (88.9%, 95% CI: 68.3–109.4%) were able to successfully return to participation in professional steer wrestling. Both surgical and nonsurgical patients received physician directed rehabilitation and return to play guidelines. Rehabilitation included progressive exercises focusing on improving range of motion, strength, and endurance. One patient subsequently won the Canadian Finals Rodeo.

TABLE 1: Demographic data for all nine injured steer wrestlers.

| Case | Age | Prior shoulder injury | Prior PM* injury | Mechanism | Source of error |
|------|-----|-----------------------|------------------|-----------|-----------------|
| 1 | 30 | No | No | Throw | Steer bucked upwards unexpectedly |
| 2 | 30 | Bicep brachii strain | No | Fall | Hazer and steer veered wide |
| 3 | 31 | No | Yes | Fall | Steer stopped |
| 4 | 32 | GH** dislocation | No | Throw | Steer veered wide |
| 5 | 33 | RC tendinopathy | Yes | Throw | Steer and hazer veered wide |
| 6 | 33 | No | No | Throw | Steer stopped |
| 7 | 33 | No | No | Throw | Steer stopped |
| 8 | 48 | RC+ tendinopathy | Yes | Throw | Steer stopped |
| 9 | 50 | No | Yes | Throw | Steer slowed down |

*PM: pectoralis major; **GH: glenohumeral; +RC: rotator cuff.

## 4. Discussion

The first documented PM rupture case dates back to 1822, and since then, there have been more than 200 cases reported in the literature [14]. This report presents the largest series of ruptured PM tendons reported during steer wrestling. A five-year epidemiological study of injuries in Canadian professional rodeo indicated that steer wrestlers sustained 9.2 injuries/1000 steer wrestling exposures [15]. In the same study, the shoulder complex was the second most frequently injured body part when considering all rodeo events as a whole. Complete ruptures of muscles, tendons, or ligaments constituted 7% of all injuries. Rodeo caregivers found that distal biceps tendon ruptures in bull riders and some bareback riders, as well as complete ruptures of the PM [16] or latissimus dorsi [17, 18], were significant career interrupting events for these athletes.

The physical findings from these cases support diagnostic findings in the literature. Patients often experience a tearing sensation presenting with a large hematoma noted on acute evaluation. This is accompanied by limited shoulder motion secondary to pain and weakness on manual muscle testing for resistance to adduction or internal rotation [19]. All nine cases presented with a combination of the following signs or symptoms: tearing sensation, palpable or visible defect against isometric resistance, ecchymosis, swelling, pain, weakness, decreased range of motion, and decreased strength.

Two patients continued to steer wrestle without surgical intervention and one continued to steer wrestle during a national finals rodeo for six steer wrestling attempts after which surgical repair was completed. Although other internal rotators and adductors of the shoulder can apply forces to these movements, we found no reports of isokinetic or eccentric testing of these movements following PM rupture. Despite other muscles compensating, it is unlikely that there were no overall strength deficits.

The PM is a powerful adductor and internal rotator of the arm. Additionally, it contributes to forward flexion when the arm is in the extended or neutral position and backward extension when the arm is in the forward flexed position. The clavicular portion of the muscle serves primarily to forward flex and adduct the arm, whereas the sternocostal portion serves primarily to internally rotate and adduct the arm. The PM is at risk during any activity in which the arm is extended

and externally rotated while under maximal contraction [20]. For example, when PM injuries occur during weight training, the typical mechanism of injury is excessive tension from acute overload of an eccentrically loaded tendon. Fibers originating from the sternal head are maximally stretched when the weight is eccentrically lowered to the chest during bench press. During the deceleration and early lift phase of this exercise, the fibers can be overstretched, leading to failure of the viscoelastic force and rupture [11].

During the throwing phase in steer wrestling, the PM concentrically contracts to adduct the shoulder across the body in an attempt to throw the steer to the ground. Several steer wrestlers indicated that the steer stopped, veered away from the athlete, or bucked upwards. These unexpected steer movements instead resulted in a sudden, powerful eccentric load on the PM causing seven cases of complete ruptures of the PM at the humeral insertion of the right arm. It is not surprising that all PM ruptures occurred to the right arm as this is the arm that all steer wrestlers use to catch the horn of the steer in order to lever the steer to the ground.

Further risk factors to tendon rupture include muscle fatigue and microtrauma [20]. Six of nine cases in this study suffered previous injuries to the right shoulder or arm.

Steer wrestling is a demanding sport that involves a throwing maneuver that places the PM in an unusually heavy and eccentric load which may predispose the PM to rupture. It is acknowledged that independent, nomadic lifestyles of professional rodeo athletes present challenges to injury management, treatment, and prevention. For instance, only four contestants reported maintaining a structured strength training and flexibility program prior to injury. One study has suggested that tendons may not be able to adjust to increasing muscle mass and decreased flexibility associated with weight training [21]. This case series review illustrates that there may be advantages for structured, prospective study of PM ruptures in steer wrestling.

## 5. Conclusions

Canadian steer wrestlers present a unique cohort of PM ruptures. These cases demonstrate functional successful outcome with a variety of treatments. Treatment and rehabilitation decisions appear to lack evidence-based decision making. Rodeo is a popular international sport that takes place in countries such as the United States of America, Brazil, and Australia. We suspect that this particular injury is not unique to Canadian steer wrestlers. Therefore, this case series may serve as a future stimulus for an international structured approach examining prevention, treatment, rehabilitation, and return to participation.

# References

[1] K. Bak, E. A. Cameron, and I. J. P. Henderson, "Rupture of the pectoralis major: a meta-analysis of 112 cases," *Knee Surgery, Sports Traumatology, Arthroscopy*, vol. 8, no. 2, pp. 113–119, 2000.

[2] P. R. Catterson and R. D. Jarman, "Rupture of pectoralis major: an occupational injury," *Emergency Medicine Journal*, vol. 24, no. 11, article 799, 2007.

[3] B. K. Potter, R. A. Lehman Jr., and W. C. Doukas, "Simultaneous bilateral rupture of the pectoralis major tendon: a case report," *Journal of Bone and Joint Surgery A*, vol. 86, no. 7, pp. 1519–1521, 2004.

[4] P. J. Carek and A. L. Hawkins, "Rupture of pectoralis major during parallel bar dips: case report and review," *Medicine and Science in Sports and Exercise*, vol. 30, no. 3, pp. 335–338, 1998.

[5] H. P. Delport and M. S. Piper, "Pectoralis major rupture in athletes," *Archives of Orthopaedic and Traumatic Surgery*, vol. 100, no. 2, pp. 135–137, 1982.

[6] S. D. Dodds and S. W. Wolfe, "Injuries to the pectoralis major," *Sports Medicine*, vol. 32, no. 14, pp. 945–952, 2002.

[7] N. R. Dunkelman, F. Collier, J. L. Rook, W. Nagler, and M. J. Brennan, "Pectoralis major muscle rupture in windsurfing," *Archives of Physical Medicine and Rehabilitation*, vol. 75, no. 7, pp. 819–821, 1994.

[8] Y. Beloosesky, J. Grinblat, D. Hendel, and R. Sommer, "Pectoralis major rupture in a 97-year-old woman," *Journal of the American Geriatrics Society*, vol. 50, no. 8, pp. 1465–1467, 2002.

[9] Y. Beloosesky, J. Grinblat, M. Katz, D. Hendel, and R. Sommer, "Pectoralis major rupture in the elderly: clinical and sonographic findings," *Clinical Imaging*, vol. 27, no. 4, pp. 261–264, 2003.

[10] Y. Beloosesky, J. Grinblat, A. Weiss, P. H. Rosenberg, M. Weisbort, and D. Hendel, "Pectoralis major rupture in elderly patients: a clinical study of 13 patients," *Clinical Orthopaedics and Related Research*, no. 413, pp. 164–169, 2003.

[11] S. W. Wolfe, T. L. Wickiewicz, J. T. Cavanaugh, and P. Shirley, "Ruptures of the pectoralis major muscle. An anatomic and clinical analysis," *American Journal of Sports Medicine*, vol. 20, no. 5, pp. 587–593, 1992.

[12] R. G. Kakwani, J. J. Matthews, K. M. Kumar, A. Pimpalnerkar, and N. Mohtadi, "Rupture of the pectoralis major muscle: surgical treatment in athletes," *International Orthopaedics*, vol. 31, no. 2, pp. 159–163, 2007.

[13] C. Harris, M. DeBeliso, K. J. Adams, and M. Curtin, "Steer wrestling—event analysis and conditioning model," *Strength and Conditioning Journal*, vol. 26, no. 1, pp. 8–13, 2004.

[14] V. Äärimaa, J. Rantanen, J. Heikkilä, I. Helttula, and S. Orava, "Rupture of the pectoralis major muscle," *American Journal of Sports Medicine*, vol. 32, no. 5, pp. 1256–1262, 2004.

[15] D. J. Butterwick, B. Hagel, D. S. Nelson, M. R. LeFave, and W. H. Meeuwisse, "Epidemiologic analysis of injury in five years of Canadian Professional Rodeo," *American Journal of Sports Medicine*, vol. 30, no. 2, pp. 193–198, 2002.

[16] B. H. Lau, D. J. Butterwick, N. G. Mohtadi, and J. R. McAllister, "Pectoralis major ruptures in Canadian professional rodeo steer wrestlers," *Clinical Journal of Sport Medicine*, vol. 19, no. 3, article 260, 2009.

[17] D. J. Butterwick, N. G. Mohtadi, W. H. Meeuwisse, and J. B. Frizzell, "Rupture of latissimus dorsi in an athlete," *Clinical Journal of Sport Medicine*, vol. 13, no. 3, pp. 189–191, 2003.

[18] L. A. Hiemstra, D. Butterwick, M. Cooke, and R. E. A. Walker, "Surgical management of latissimus dorsi rupture in a steer wrestler," *Clinical Journal of Sport Medicine*, vol. 17, no. 4, pp. 316–318, 2007.

[19] R. C. Reut, B. R. Bach Jr., and C. Johnson, "Pectoralis major rupture: diagnosing and treating a weight-training injury," *Physician and Sportsmedicine*, vol. 19, no. 3, pp. 89–95, 1991.

[20] M. T. Provencher, K. Handfield, N. T. Boniquit, S. N. Reiff, J. K. Sekiya, and A. A. Romeo, "Injuries to the pectoralis major muscle: diagnosis and management," *American Journal of Sports Medicine*, vol. 38, no. 8, pp. 1693–1705, 2010.

[21] W. J. Rijnberg and B. Van Linge, "Rupture of the pectoralis major muscle in body-builders," *Archives of Orthopaedic and Trauma Surgery*, vol. 112, no. 2, pp. 104–105, 1993.

# 38

# The Use of an Intra-Articular Depth Guide in the Measurement of Partial Thickness Rotator Cuff Tears

**Michael J. Carroll,[1] Kristie D. More,[2] Stephen Sohmer,[3] Atiba A. Nelson,[2] Paul Sciore,[1] Richard Boorman,[1,2] Robert Hollinshead,[1,2] and Ian K. Y. Lo[1,2]**

[1] Section of Orthopedic Surgery, Department of Surgery, University of Calgary, 3280 Hospital Drive, Calgary, AB, Canada T2N 4Z6
[2] Sport Medicine Centre, University of Calgary, 2500 University Drive NW, Calgary, AB, Canada T2N 1N4
[3] University of British Columbia, 301-909 Island Highway, Campbell River, BC, Canada V9W 2C2

Correspondence should be addressed to Ian K. Y. Lo; ikylo@ucalgary.ca

Academic Editor: Robert Gillespie

*Purpose.* The purpose of this study was to compare the accuracy of the conventional method for determining the percentage of partial thickness rotator cuff tears to a method using an intra-articular depth guide. The clinical utility of the intra-articular depth guide was also examined. *Methods.* Partial rotator cuff tears were created in cadaveric shoulders. Exposed footprint, total tendon thickness, and percentage of tendon thickness torn were determined using both techniques. The results from the conventional and intra-articular depth guide methods were correlated with the true anatomic measurements. Thirty-two patients were evaluated in the clinical study. *Results.* Estimates of total tendon thickness ($r = 0.41$, $P = 0.31$) or percentage of thickness tears ($r = 0.67$, $P = 0.07$) using the conventional method did not correlate well with true tendon thickness. Using the intra-articular depth guide, estimates of exposed footprint ($r = 0.92$, $P = 0.001$), total tendon thickness ($r = 0.96$, $P = 0.0001$), and percentage of tendon thickness torn ($r = 0.88$, $P = 0.004$) correlated with true anatomic measurements. Seven of 32 patients had their treatment plan altered based on the measurements made by the intra-articular depth guide. *Conclusions.* The intra-articular depth guide appeared to better correlate with true anatomic measurements. It may be useful during the evaluation and development of treatment plans for partial thickness articular surface rotator cuff tears.

## 1. Introduction

Rotator cuff tears are a common cause of pain and disability in the adult shoulder [1], and surgery for the rotator cuff is one of the most common procedures performed in the shoulder. Rotator cuff tears may be divided into partial thickness tears and full thickness tears. Full-thickness tears involve complete disruption of the tendon thickness and are commonly treated with open or arthroscopic rotator cuff repair [1].

In clinical and cadaveric studies, partial thickness tears are approximately twice as common (6–39% incidence) as full-thickness tears [2–5]. These tears involve only partial disruption of the tendon thickness, and a portion of the tendon insertion remains intact on its footprint. Codman [3] first described partial thickness tears over seventy-five years ago. However, it was not until the development of arthroscopy

that partial thickness tears became a commonly diagnosed and treated condition [2, 4, 5].

It is generally believed that the extent of partial thickness tearing correlates with the severity of symptoms [3, 5]. Articular surface tears are commonly agerelated and may be due to degeneration, while bursal surface tears are felt to be secondary to extrinsic impingement. Furthermore, several authors have recommended different treatment regimens for partial-thickness rotator cuff tears based on the tendon thickness involved. For example, Weber [6, 7] has recommended that partial-thickness rotator cuff tears involving >50% of the tendon thickness should be repaired. While this recommendation has become the standard of care [2, 4, 5], determining the extent of partial thickness rotator cuff tears remains difficult and imprecise. Weber in his study [7] noted that "objective means of assessing the depth of tear have

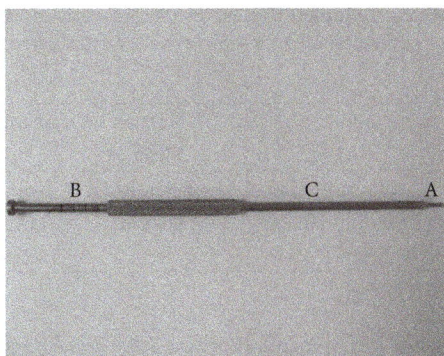

FIGURE 1: The assembled intra-articular depth guide. A: needle-tipped inner metallic probe used to penetrate the rotator cuff and measure the exposed bone bed. B: the distal end of the inner metallic probe is marked with numbers to measure total tendon thickness. C: outer metallic sleeve slides freely over the inner metallic probe.

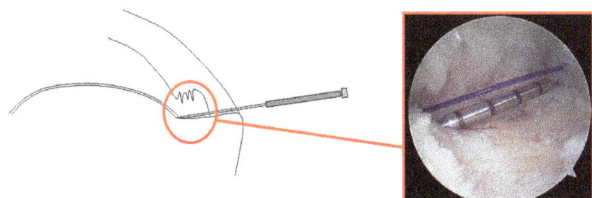

FIGURE 2: Schematic diagram and corresponding arthroscopic photo (of a right shoulder from a posterior glenohumeral portal) demonstrating the inner metallic sleeve penetrating the intact portion of the rotator cuff laterally at the area of greatest tendon involvement. The "needle tipped" portion of the intra-articular depth guide is inserted tangential to the bone bed and placed adjacent to the articular cartilage. (Note: all arthroscopic photos are oriented in the beach chair position).

proved elusive" and further Ruotolo and colleagues [8] in 2004 stated that "..., to date, no technique to accurately measure the thickness of a supraspinatus partial-thickness rotator cuff tear has been described."

A conventional method may be employed to determine the percentage of partial thickness tear. It begins with an estimate of the amount of exposed bone in the rotator cuff footprint based on relative shaver diameter. This information is then related to historic anatomic data as well as clinical (e.g., gender, stature) and radiographic data to determine a percentage thickness tear [8, 9]. Considering the variability of footprint anatomy [8], this technique may lead to imprecise estimations of partial thickness rotator cuff tears and potentially incorrect treatment. Since partial thickness tears are so common, a simple and accurate method of measuring tendon thickness is required. The purpose of this study was to compare the accuracy of the conventional method of determining the percentage of partial thickness rotator cuff tears to a new method using an intra-articular depth guide in a cadaveric model. We also characterize and describe utility of the intra-articular depth guide in a clinical setting.

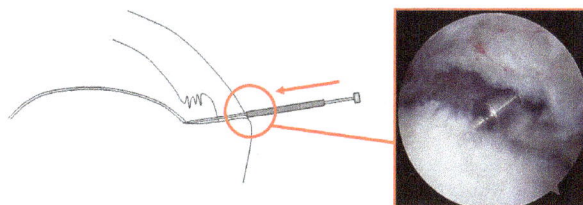

FIGURE 3: Schematic diagram and corresponding arthroscopic photo (of a right shoulder from a posterior subacromial portal) demonstrating advancement of the outer metallic sleeve to the bursal surface of the rotator cuff. The position of the outer sleeve on the inner metallic rod corresponds to the total tendon thickness.

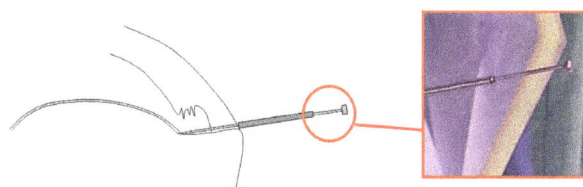

FIGURE 4: Schematic diagram and corresponding photo demonstrating that total tendon thickness can be read off the numbers on the distal portion of the inner metallic rod extracorporeally.

## 2. Methods

2.1. The Intra-Articular Depth Guide. The intra-articular depth guide (Arthrex, Inc., Naples, FL) is a simple tool used to quantify the percentage of tendon involved in partial thickness rotator cuff tears. This tool can be used to measure both bursal surface and articular surface tears. This study is limited to articular surface tears of the supraspinatus tendon.

The depth guide is designed and used similar to a standard depth gauge. It is a two-piece device with an inner "needle-tipped" metallic probe and an outer metallic sleeve, which slides freely over top (Figure 1). The inner probe measures the exposed footprint, while the outer sleeve determines the total tendon thickness.

To obtain an accurate measurement, the partial tear is first debrided on its articular surface. The tip of the inner metallic probe is then advanced through the remaining intact portion of the rotator cuff (Figure 2). Care is taken to ensure the depth guide is introduced tangential to the greater tuberosity with the tip of the inner metallic tube placed at the margin of the articular cartilage. The tip is marked by 3 mm lines and allows direct measurement of the exposed tendon footprint.

The outer metallic sleeve is then advanced through the deltoid until it is flush with the bursal surface of the rotator cuff tendon (Figure 3). The arthroscope may be placed in the subacromial space to ensure there is no interposed soft tissue between the tendon and guide. The total tendon thickness can then be read directly on the guide (Figure 4).

2.2. Cadaveric Study Design. The purpose of this study was to compare the accuracy of the conventional method of estimating the percentage of partial thickness rotator cuff tears to an intra-articular depth guide in a cadaveric model. The

TABLE 1: Measurements of the exposed footprint, total tendon thickness, and percentage of tendon thickness torn in cadaveric shoulders with simulated partial thickness articular surface rotator cuff tears using the methods of comparison to a known size, the intra-articular depth guide, and true anatomic measures.

| | Conventional technique | | Depth guide | | True anatomic measure | |
|---|---|---|---|---|---|---|
| | Mean | Range | Mean | Range | Mean | Range |
| Exposed footprint | 5.5 mm | 4 mm–8 mm | 6.8 mm | 5 mm–10 mm | 6.9 mm | 5 mm–10 mm |
| Total tendon thickness | 14.5 mm | 10 mm–18 mm | 13.5 mm | 11 mm–20 mm | 13.6 mm | 11 mm–22 mm |
| Percentage of thickness torn | 39% | 22%–50% | 52% | 30%–76% | 54% | 27%–72% |

design was reviewed and approved by the institutions ethics committee. The conventional method and the technique of the intra-articular depth guide are described above.

Twelve fresh frozen, unpaired cadaveric shoulders were identified for use in this study. In keeping with the scope of the study, specimens with full thickness rotator cuff tears were excluded. As such, four shoulders were removed from analysis. Cadavers with partial thickness articular surface tears of the rotator cuff were included. The mean age of the cadavers used was 71 years (range: 42–86); there were 6 female and 2 male patients.

Cadavers were mounted in the beach-chair position, and standard anterior and posterior glenohumeral portals were created with the pump maintaining pressure at 70 mmHg. In eight fresh frozen cadaveric shoulders, partial thickness articular surface tears of various amounts were created in the supraspinatus tendon with 5.5 mm shaver (Conmed Linvatec, Largo, FL). Existing partial tears underwent further debridement if required; the goal was to create tears involving approximately 33–67% of the total tendon thickness.

Each of the eight shoulders then underwent arthroscopic evaluation by two fellowship trained arthroscopic surgeons who were familiar with the depth guide. The extent of the partial thickness tear was estimated using the two techniques described. The shoulders were then dissected and a digital caliper (Mitutoyo, Japan) was used to determine the true amount of exposed footprint and total tendon thickness.

*2.3. Clinical Study Design.* The purpose of the clinical study was to characterize and describe the utility of the intra-articular depth guide in a clinical setting. From the period of January 2005–March 2006, all patients with partial thickness articular surface tears of the rotator cuff were evaluated.

All partial thickness articular surface tears were evaluated arthroscopically using both the conventional and intra-articular depth guide techniques.

*2.4. Statistical Analysis.* Absolute values for amount of footprint exposed and total tendon thickness were collected from (1) the conventional method, (2) intra-articular depth guide, and (3) true anatomic dissection in 8 shoulders.

The percentage of tendon thickness torn was determined for each group. It was calculated using the formula:

$$\text{Percentage of tendon thickness tear} = \frac{\text{Exposed footprint}}{\text{Total tendon thickness}} \times 100\%. \quad (1)$$

Mean amount of footprint exposed, total tendon thickness, and the percentage of thickness torn from the conventional method and intra-articular depth guide were compared to the true anatomic dissections using the Pearson correlation coefficient ($r$).

The mean difference in the percentage of tendon thickness torn using the two methods was also evaluated using a paired $t$-test. A $P$ value $< 0.05$ was considered statistically significant.

## 3. Results

*3.1. Cadaveric Study.* In the cadaveric study, the mean true amount of footprint exposed was 6.9 mm (range: 5–10 mm), the mean true total tendon thickness was 13.6 mm (range: 11 mm–22 mm), and the mean true percentage of tendon thickness torn was 54% (range: 27–72%). The results for the two methods of measurement as well as the true anatomic measures are summarized in Table 1.

Using the conventional method, the amount of exposed footprint correlated well with the true exposed footprint ($r = 0.83$, $P = 0.01$). However, total tendon thickness ($r = 0.41$, $P = 0.31$) and percentage of thickness torn ($r = 0.67$, $P = 0.07$) did not significantly correlate with the true anatomic measurements.

The intra-articular depth guide and true anatomical measurements correlated well in all categories. Statistical significance was achieved with the amount of exposed footprint ($r = 0.92$, $P = 0.001$), total tendon thickness ($r = 0.96$, $P = 0.0001$), and percentage of tendon thickness torn ($r = 0.88$, $P = 0.004$).

The difference in mean percentage of tendon thickness torn between the conventional method and true anatomic measurement was 15%± 12% (range: 2%–27%). The difference between the intra-articular depth guide and true anatomic measurement was 7%± 4% (range: 3%–13%). There was no statistically significant difference between the conventional method and intra-articular depth guide ($P = 0.09$).

*3.2. Clinical Study.* From January 2005 to March 2006, 32 patients with partial thickness tears of the supraspinatus tendon were evaluated both using the conventional method and the intra-articular depth guide. Inclusion criteria were male and female patients with partial thickness articular surface tears involving the supraspinatus tendon. The mean age of the patients was 50 ± 9.4 years with 9 female and 23 male patients involving 4 nondominant and 28 dominant shoulders. In 27 patients the primary diagnosis was a partial thickness tear of the rotator cuff, 3 patients had superior labral tears, 1 had adhesive capsulitis, and in 1 patient the primary diagnosis was osteoarthritis.

Using the conventional method, the amount of footprint exposed was estimated relative to shaver diameter. The mean exposed footprint was 5.1 mm (range: 0–18 mm). The surgeon estimated the total tendon thickness by taking a number of factors into consideration. Using known historical data in conjunction with the results of preoperative imaging (e.g., ultrasound, MRI, MRI arthrogram), clinical features (e.g., male/female, size of patient), and intraoperative findings (e.g., comparison to a known size instrument), an estimate was made. The mean total tendon thickness was 13.7 mm (range: 10–20 mm), and the mean percentage of thickness torn was 36.8% (0–90%).

Using the intra-articular depth guide, the mean footprint exposed was 6.2 mm (0–17 mm), the mean total tendon thickness was 16.4 mm (range: 13–22 mm), and the mean percentage of thickness torn was 38.1% (range: 0%–94%). The mean difference between the two methods for percentage of thickness torn was 6.8% (range: 0–26%).

The difference was significant enough clinically to alter the treatment decision for 7 patients when using 50% of the tendon thickness torn as a guide. In 4 cases, when using the intra-articular depth guide the tendon was determined to be <50% torn and was debrided instead of repaired; in 3 cases the tendon was found to be >50% torn and was repaired instead of undergoing debridement. Repairs were performed using a transtendon technique as previously described [10]. In brief, anchors were inserted transtendon along the medial margin of the footprint, and sutures were passed through the intact rotator cuff tendon using a mattress configuration. Sutures were then tied in the subacromial space to compress the tendon against the medial aspect of the footprint.

## 4. Discussion

This study describes a new method to quantify percentage of partial thickness rotator cuff tendon tears using an intra-articular depth guide. The guide enables the surgeon to accurately determine the amount of exposed footprint and the total tendon thickness. The technique is relatively simple and to our knowledge is the only method to directly measure the total tendon thickness and determine the percentage of thickness tears arthroscopically.

Measuring the amount of exposed footprint may be determined relatively accurately using both the conventional method or intra-articular guide. As compared to the conventional method of quantifying percentage of partial thickness tears (i.e., estimating amount of exposed footprint with reference to a shaver of known size), the intra-articular depth guide appeared to better correlate to true anatomic measurements. This finding is largely related to the accuracy in which the depth guide can determine total tendon thickness.

The significance of this finding relates to the fact that treatment decisions tend to be based on the percentage of tendon that is torn. Though controversial, there is a general consensus that partial thickness tears involving >50% of the tendon thickness should be repaired [2, 4–8]. Despite this, the percentage of partial thickness tears is inferred since no alternative method of quantifying them has been described. The conventional method relies on estimating the amount of footprint exposed and incorporating historical anatomic data. We have shown that it may be prone to error and may not correlate well with true anatomic measurements.

The current standard of treatment (using 6 mm of exposed bone bed) arbitrarily compares the amount of exposed bone in the rotator cuff footprint, to historical anatomical data to determine the percentage of tendon involvement. Recently, Ruotolo et al. [8] demonstrated that the mean medial to lateral thickness of the supraspinatus tendon insertion was approximately 12 mm and recommended that all tears with more than 7 mm of exposed bone lateral to the articular surface (i.e., 6 mm of exposed footprint) representing ">50% of the tendon substance" should be repaired.

Although this method may be applied in general, the medial to lateral thickness of the tendon in Nottage's study was remarkably variable and ranged from 8 to 15 mm [8]. This means that the 6 mm of exposed footprint recommendation may represent anywhere from 37 to 69% of the tendon thickness. Curtis and Tierney [9] provide further support and demonstrated in another cadaveric study that the supraspinatus tendon footprint was also quite variable in size. The average width was 16 mm, yet the tendon thickness ranged from 12 mm to 22 mm. Therefore, 6 mm of exposed bone bed could represent 27–50% of the total tendon thickness.

The intra-articular depth guide provides an accurate method of determining the amount of footprint exposed, total tendon thickness, and percentage of partial thickness tears. This information was utilized in our clinical series when 7 of 32 patients (22%) had their treatment plan modified based on measurements taken using the intra-articular depth guide when compared to the conventional method. Larger clinical studies in which treatment plans are designed using both techniques will provide additional information on the utility of the intra-articular depth gauge.

We acknowledge certain limitations to our study. While we acknowledge the sample size was small in both the cadaveric and clinical studies in the purpose of the study was to determine the accuracy of the intra-articular depth guide and we believe the results are significant and relevant. Furthermore, the inter- and intraobserver reliability of the intra-articular depth guide was not determined. We also described the clinical application of the intra-articular depth gauge in a small cohort of patients. In the description of patients, the true anatomic measurements were unknown. While confirming with open repair or dissection to determine the "true" percentage of the partial thickness tearing would have provided additional information, this would subject patient to unnecessary morbidity.

## 5. Conclusion

As compared to the conventional method of quantifying the percentage of partial thickness tears, the intra-articular depth guide appeared to better correlate to true anatomic measurements. This method may be useful during the evaluation and development of treatment plans for partial thickness articular surface rotator cuff tears. Larger clinical studies looking at patient outcomes are required to better characterize the utility of the intra-articular depth gauge in formulating treatment plans.

## Disclosures

Dr. Lo is a consultant with Arthrex, Inc.

## References

[1] R. H. Cofield, "Current concepts review. Rotator cuff disease of the shoulder," *Journal of Bone and Joint Surgery A*, vol. 67, no. 6, pp. 974–979, 1985.

[2] N. M. Breazeale and E. V. Craig, "Partial-thickness rotator cuff tears: pathogenesis and treatment," *Orthopedic Clinics of North America*, vol. 28, no. 2, pp. 145–155, 1997.

[3] E. Codman, *The Shoulder*, Thomas Todd, Boston, Mass, USA, 1934.

[4] H. Fukuda, "Partial-thickness rotator cuff tears: a modern view on Codman's classic," *Journal of Shoulder and Elbow Surgery*, vol. 9, no. 2, pp. 163–168, 2000.

[5] O. R. McConville and J. P. Iannotti, "Partial-thickness tears of the rotator cuff: evaluation and management.," *The Journal of the American Academy of Orthopaedic Surgeons*, vol. 7, no. 1, pp. 32–43, 1999.

[6] S. C. Weber, "Arthroscopic debridement and acromioplasty versus mini-open repair in the management of significant partial-thickness tears of the rotator cuff," *Orthopedic Clinics of North America*, vol. 28, no. 1, pp. 79–82, 1997.

[7] S. C. Weber, "Arthroscopic debridement and acromioplasty versus mini-open repair in the treatment of significant partial-thickness rotator cuff tears," *Arthroscopy*, vol. 15, no. 2, pp. 126–131, 1999.

[8] C. Ruotolo, J. E. Fow, and W. M. Nottage, "The supraspinatus footprint: an anatomic study of the supraspinatus tendon insertion," *Arthroscopy*, vol. 20, no. 3, pp. 246–249, 2004.

[9] A. Curtis and J. Tierney, "The footprint of the rotator cuff," in *Proceedings of the American Academy of Orthopaedic Surgeons Annual Meeting*, 1999.

[10] I. K. Y. Lo and S. S. Burkhart, "Transtendon arthroscopic repair of partial-thickness articular surface tears of the rotator cuff," *Arthroscopy*, vol. 20, no. 2, pp. 214–220, 2004.

# 39

# Assessment of Patients with a DePuy ASR Metal-on-Metal Hip Replacement: Results of Applying the Guidelines of the Spanish Society of Hip Surgery in a Tertiary Referral Hospital

**Jenaro Fernández-Valencia, Xavier Gallart, Guillem Bori, Sebastián Garcia Ramiro, Andrés Combalía, and Josep Riba**

*Hip Unit, Department of Orthopaedic Surgery and Traumatology, Hospital Clínic, Universitat de Barcelona, C/Villarroel 170, 08036 Barcelona, Spain*

Correspondence should be addressed to Jenaro Fernández-Valencia; jenarovalencia@gmail.com

Academic Editor: Panagiotis Korovessis

The prognosis associated with the DePuy ASR hip cup is poor and varies according to the series. This implant was withdrawn from use in 2010 and all patients needed to be assessed. We present the results of the assessment of our patients treated with this device, according to the Spanish Society of Hip Surgery (SECCA) algorithm published in 2011. This retrospective study evaluates 83 consecutive ASR cups, followed up at a mean of 2.9 years. Serum levels of chromium and cobalt, as well as the acetabular abduction angle, were determined in order to assess their possible correlation with failure, defined as the need for revision surgery. The mean Harris Hip Score was 83.2 (range 42–97). Eight arthroplasties (13.3%) required revision due to persistent pain and/or elevated serum levels of chromium/cobalt. All the cups had a correct abduction angle, and there was no correlation between elevated serum levels of metal ions and implant failure. Since two previous ASR implants were exchanged previously to the recall, the revision rate for ASR cups in our centre is 18.2% at 2.9 years.

## 1. Introduction

In September 2010, the Spanish Agency of Medicines and Medical Devices issued an alert calling for the withdrawal from use and recall of the ASR Hip Resurfacing System and ASR XL Acetabular System total hip replacement, both manufactured by DePuy International Ltd. The basis for the recall was a higher-than-normal failure rate and the possibility of metal debris (cobalt-chromium alloy) being deposited in the surrounding tissues and with possible toxic implications related to cobalt release. The Spanish Society of Hip Surgery (SECCA) published an algorithm for the assessment of patients who had been treated with one of these devices [1]. This paper reports the results obtained in a series of patients who were evaluated with this algorithm as a response to the recall.

## 2. Material and Method

In December 2010, a letter was sent out to all patients who had undergone a hip arthroplasty at the Hospital Clinic in Barcelona and who had been fitted with a DePuy ASR cup. This involved a total of 92 cups in 83 patients (10 women and 73 men), with a mean age of 51 years (range 24–66, SD 10). Nine of these patients had received a bilateral implant. Their mean body mass index was 28 kg/m$^2$ (range 21.1–36.2).

Five patients did not respond to the letter, and three had died for reasons unrelated to the hip surgery. This left a total of 83 DePuy ASR cups, 60 of which corresponded to resurfacing and 23 to the use of the short-stem Proxima implant. Mean time at follow-up was 2.9 years (range 0.9–5.5, SD 1.05). In the original indications for surgery, patients with chronic renal insufficiency, women of a fertile age, and patients with a known allergy to metals were all excluded.

All the surgical interventions used the modified Hardinge (lateral) approach [2], with the patient in the lateral decubitus position. A complete anterior capsulectomy was performed prior to dislocation of the femoral head. The acetabulum and femur were prepared in accordance with the standard technique. As part of our routine protocol for hip arthroplasty, all the patients received 1.5 g cefuroxime at induction of anaesthesia, with a further dose two hours later if required by the duration of surgery. Low molecular weight heparin was used for antithrombotic prophylaxis. For all the revised hips, at least one tissue sample was submitted for histological study. Two cases were metal-stained at some degree. All of the tissues were fixed in 10% formalin immediately after removal. Samples were examined by two different pathologists and were assessed for lymphocytes, macrophages, plasma cells, giant cells, necrosis, and metal wear particles.

During the follow-up assessment visit, all patients provided informed consent for their case to be studied. In all cases, the Harris Hip Score [3] was obtained, and radiology and laboratory tests were performed, including determination of serum chromium (Cr) and cobalt (Co) levels. The latter were measured by means of mass spectrometry (Perkin Elmer AA600 graphite furnace atomic absorption spectrometer), with the following being considered as elevated levels: >5 $\mu$g/L for Co and >2 $\mu$g/L for Cr. The Harris Hip Score was categorized using the criteria described by Marchetti et al. [4]: <70, poor; 70–79, fair; 80–89, good; and 90–100, excellent.

The standardized anterior-posterior radiographs of the pelvis were taken (with the foot internally rotated) before and after surgery. All radiographs were assessed to check that the hip presented a similar degree of rotation: this was done by noting the appearance of the lesser trochanter in the preoperative radiograph and searching for the best correspondence among the available postoperative radiographs. The acetabular abduction angle, as well as the presence of osteolysis or signs of loosening, was determined. The acetabular angle was measured as the angle between the horizontal tear drop line and the axis of the acetabular component [5].

In 13 patients, computed tomography (CT) was performed as a complementary evaluation to the above exams. This was done in the Department of Radiology using a Somatom Plus IV scanner (Siemens, Erlangen, Germany), with CT parameters being optimized using Siemens' own software. Images were obtained of the whole prosthesis, from the upper part of the acetabulum to the lower part of the femoral implant, using helical acquisition with the following parameters: kV = 120, mAs = 200, slice thickness = 3 mm, pitch = 1.5, and reconstruction space = 3 mm. A bone reconstruction algorithm and wide window were used to accentuate the border of bone structures, the aim being to minimize artefacts due to the metal prosthesis. The images were also reconstructed using a soft tissue algorithm.

Data were analysed using the statistical software IBM SPSS Statistics version 20. In addition to evaluating whether Cr and Co levels increased over time, a Spearman test was used to assess the possible relationship between the acetabular abduction angle and levels of these two metal ions.

The group of patients who underwent revision surgery was also compared with the group who did not in terms of sex, age, Cr and Co levels, acetabular abduction angle, cup size, and time since primary surgery. The chi-squared test was used to assess differences by sex, while the Mann-Whitney $U$ test was applied for the remaining variables. The level of statistical significance was set at $P \leq 0.05$.

## 3. Results

The mean Harris Hip Score (83.2, range 42–97) was regarded as good. The mean acetabular abduction angle was 39.8° (range 15–52, SD 5.5), and there were no cases of loosening or osteolysis.

Serum cobalt levels were elevated ($\geq$5 $\mu$g/L) in 10 patients (1 bilateral), with a mean in this subgroup of 12.3 $\mu$g/L (range 5–56, SD 14.2). Serum chromium levels were high ($\geq$2 $\mu$g/L) in 14 patients (4 bilateral), with a mean in this subgroup of 7.3 $\mu$g/L (range 2.1–40, SD 9.4).

The CT images obtained from 13 patients revealed no relevant findings, except for 2 patients with trochanteric bursitis, 1 with excess fluid in the iliopsoas bursa, 1 with a fluid collection anterior to the femoral neck, and 1 with fluid/swelling around the greater trochanter.

Cr and Co levels did not vary significantly over time ($P = 0.396$), and no relationship was observed between these levels and the acetabular abduction angle ($P > 0.05$). There were no differences between patients who underwent revision surgery and those who did not in terms of sex ($P = 0.653$), age ($P = 0.790$), levels of Cr ($P = 0.727$) and Co ($P = 0.447$), acetabular abduction angle ($P = 0.259$), cup size ($P = 0.087$), or time since primary surgery ($P = 0.819$).

Eight resurfacing implants required revision due to the presence of pain and/or elevated serum levels of chromium/cobalt. The intraoperative findings were of no relevance in six cases; in one case a solid pseudotumour was identified, while another patient presented with metallosis and a fluid-filled pseudotumour (Figure 1). The histology of the case of the pseudotumour showed lymphoplasmacellular infiltration and presence of macrophages and multinucleated giant cells depicting a foreign body reaction. There was also presence of polymorphonuclear cells at low ratio (less that 5 per wide microscopic field (×40)). The histology of the metallosis and fluid-filled pseudotumour showed severe pigmentary histiocytic reaction. Two other samples without the clinical appearance of fluid-filled pseudotumour showed also severe pigmentary histiocytic reaction. For the rest of the histologies, moderate to low rate of inflammatory cells was observed without signs of metallosis.

Added to these eight revisions after the recall, two previous ASR implants were exchanged previously to the recall: as a result, the revision rate for ASR cups in our centre is 18.2% at 2.9 years.

## 4. Discussion

Since the original findings of the Australian National Joint Replacement Registry [6], more recent series [7, 8] have

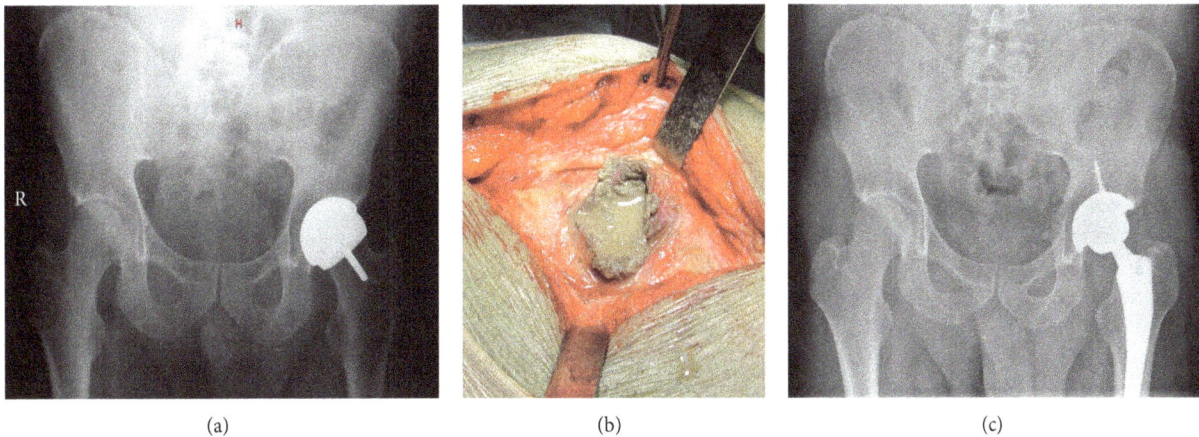

FIGURE 1: (a) Anterior-posterior radiograph of the pelvis prior to revision surgery, showing no relevant radiological findings related to the implant; (b) intraoperative appearance of the pseudotumour during revision surgery; and (c) radiograph of the same patient 6 months after revision.

confirmed the elevated failure rates associated with the DePuy metal-on-metal ASR system, both in the case of the resurfacing and in the case of the large-diameter prosthesis. This failure rate, followed by the subsequent recall of the implant, has received considerable attention in the literature [9]. One of the main concerns relates to the possible effects of the deposition of Cr and Co debris, both locally and in the bloodstream, there being three reported cases of cobalt toxicity associated with this prosthesis [10, 11].

The revision rate in our centre was found to be 18.2% at a mean follow-up of 2.9 years. In their review of the Australian National Registry, De Steiger et al. found that the cumulative revision rate at five years for arthroplasties involving the ASR Hip Resurfacing System was 10.9% (95% CI, 8.7% to 13.6%), compared with 4% (95% CI, 3.7% to 4.5%) for all other resurfacing prostheses [6]. Although this rate is high in itself, more recent series have reported results similar to our own, that is, even higher rates at shorter follow-up. For example, Bernthal et al. reported a revision rate at three years of 17.1% [8]. In their series, 12 implants that functioned correctly during the first postoperative year subsequently failed within 3 years, due to pain (7 cases), loosening (3 cases), and squeaking (2 cases). The remainder presented persistent pain without radiological evidence of loosening. The radiographs of patients in our series revealed no relevant findings, and the main cause of revision was the presence of persistent pain.

There is currently no consensus regarding what constitutes acceptable or clearly toxic levels of metal ions in the bloodstream of patients fitted with orthopaedic implants, although it has been suggested that below 2 $\mu$g/L is acceptable in the case of Co [12]. In fact, all implants may release these ions regardless of the friction pair. For example, a study of 41 knee arthroplasties found levels of Cr and Co to be 0.92 and 3.28 $\mu$g/L, respectively, in unilateral prostheses, and 0.98 and 4.28, respectively, in bilateral implants [13]. A case of cobalt intoxication has also been reported in a patient who did not originally have a metal-on-metal implant [14].

Reported levels of Co and Cr ions vary depending on the series. One multicentre study involving a 24-month follow-up of 77 patients implanted with a unilateral resurfacing prosthesis found that ion levels were generally low and had stabilized by 3 months [15]. Six patients had abnormally high metal ion levels, and all of them also had a cup abduction angle above 55°. In another study, Desy et al. reported that a smaller ASR cup diameter was associated with higher levels of Cr and Co, as well as with larger acetabular inclination [16]. Randelli et al. also found that a cup inclination angle greater than 50° led to increased concentrations of metal ions, although this angle was only present in three of their patients [17]. The study by de Haan et al. similarly observed a greater release of metal ions with abduction angles above 55° [18]. Langton et al. compared the metal ion concentrations associated with two kinds of resurfacing device, the ASR (DePuy) and the BHR (Smith & Nephew), and again found that concentrations were higher with larger inclination angles, although this was only the case for implants with a smaller cup diameter [19]. In our series, the acetabular abduction angle never exceeded 55°, and yet there were 10 cases of elevated Co levels and 14 cases of high Cr levels. This illustrates how it is not only the cup position which is important, but also the design and characteristics of the implant.

Our patients who required prosthesis revision showed no radiological signs of osteolysis or loosening, and their implants were correctly positioned. In one case a solid pseudotumour was observed, while another patient presented with metallosis and a fluid-filled pseudotumour. The failure of ASR prostheses has been attributed to their design, specifically to the increased risk of edge loading [18, 19], a problem that particularly affects smaller-diameter components [20]. Implant failure in the absence of radiological changes may be explained by soft tissue lesions secondary to the release of metal ions, a phenomenon that has been termed "adverse reaction to metal debris" (ARMD) and which includes various changes such as pseudotumours [21], aseptic lymphocyte-dominated vasculitis-associated lesions (ALVAL) [22], and metallosis [23]. AMRD is not considered to correlate to the amount of wear [24] and may be linked to a type IV hypersensitivity reaction [12].

## 5. Conclusions

Although we agree that it is important that acetabular abduction does not exceed 55°, this does not appear to have been a key factor in the failure of our ASR prostheses, since none of the patients in this series had an implant over that angle. The survival rate of the ASR cup at a mean of 2.9 years was 100% among patients with a short-stem Proxima implant and 82.8% in those with a resurfacing prosthesis.

## Conflict of Interests

The authors declare that there is no conflict of interests regarding the publication of this paper.

## References

[1] X. Gallart and O. Marín, "Information and advice for orthopedic surgeons: a decision tree to a patient with prosthesis with metal-metal friction pair," *Revista Espanola de Cirugia Ortopedica y Traumatologia*, vol. 55, no. 1, pp. 67–69, 2011.

[2] K. Hardinge, "The direct lateral approach to the hip," *Journal of Bone and Joint Surgery—Series B*, vol. 64, no. 1, pp. 17–19, 1982.

[3] W. H. Harris, "Traumatic arthritis of the hip after dislocation and acetabular fractures: treatment by mold arthroplasty. An end-result study using a new method of result evaluation," *Journal of Bone and Joint Surgery—Series A*, vol. 51, no. 4, pp. 737–755, 1969.

[4] P. Marchetti, R. Binazzi, V. Vaccari et al., "Long-term results with cementless Fitek (or Fitmore) cups," *Journal of Arthroplasty*, vol. 20, no. 6, pp. 730–737, 2005.

[5] M. Tannast, U. Langlotz, K.-A. Siebenrock, M. Wiese, K. Bernsmann, and F. Langlotz, "Anatomic referencing of cup orientation in total hip arthroplasty," *Clinical Orthopaedics and Related Research*, no. 436, pp. 144–150, 2005.

[6] R. N. De Steiger, J. R. Hang, L. N. Miller, S. E. Graves, and D. C. Davidson, "Five-year results of the ASR XL acetabular system and the ASR hip resurfacing system: an analysis from the Australian Orthopaedic Association National Joint Replacement Registry," *Journal of Bone and Joint Surgery A*, vol. 93, no. 24, pp. 2287–2293, 2011.

[7] D. J. Langton, S. S. Jameson, T. J. Joyce et al., "Accelerating failure rate of the ASR total hip replacement," *Journal of Bone and Joint Surgery—Series B*, vol. 93, no. 8, pp. 1011–1016, 2011.

[8] N. M. Bernthal, P. C. Celestre, A. I. Stavrakis, J. C. Ludington, and D. A. Oakes, "Disappointing short-term results with the DePuy ASR XL metal-on-metal total hip arthroplasty," *The Journal of Arthroplasty*, vol. 27, no. 4, pp. 539–544, 2012.

[9] D. Cohen, "How safe are metal-on-metal hip implants?" *BMJ*, vol. 344, no. 7846, Article ID e1410, pp. 1–6, 2012.

[10] S. S. Tower, "Arthroprosthetic cobaltism: Neurological and cardiac manifestations in two patients with metal-on-metal arthroplasty: a case report," *Journal of Bone and Joint Surgery A*, vol. 92, no. 17, pp. 2847–2851, 2010.

[11] X. Mao, A. A. Wong, and R. W. Crawford, "Cobalt toxicity—an emerging clinical problem in patients with metal-on-metal hip prostheses?" *The Medical Journal of Australia*, vol. 194, no. 12, pp. 649–651, 2011.

[12] C. Delaunay, I. Petit, I. D. Learmonth, P. Oger, and P. A. Vendittoli, "Metal-on-metal bearings total hip arthroplasty: the cobalt and chromium ions release concern," *Orthopaedics and Traumatology: Surgery and Research*, vol. 96, no. 8, pp. 894–904, 2010.

[13] J. Luetzner, F. Krummenauer, A. M. Lengel, J. Ziegler, and W.-C. Witzleb, "Serum metal ion exposure after total knee arthroplasty," *Clinical Orthopaedics and Related Research*, no. 461, pp. 136–142, 2007.

[14] D. Pelclova, M. Sklensky, P. Janicek, and K. Lach, "Severe cobalt intoxication following hip replacement revision: clinical features and outcome," *Clinical Toxicology*, vol. 50, no. 4, pp. 262–265, 2012.

[15] G. H. Isaac, T. Siebel, R. D. Oakeshott et al., "Changes in whole blood metal ion levels following resurfacing: serial measurements in a multi-centre study," *HIP International*, vol. 19, no. 4, pp. 330–337, 2009.

[16] N. M. Desy, S. G. Bergeron, A. Petit, O. L. Huk, and J. Antoniou, "Surgical variables influence metal ion levels after hip resurfacing," *Clinical Orthopaedics and Related Research*, vol. 469, no. 6, pp. 1635–1641, 2011.

[17] F. Randelli, L. Banci, S. Favilla, D. Maglione, and A. Aliprandi, "Radiographically undetectable periprosthetic osteolysis with asr implants: the implication of blood metal ions," *Journal of Arthroplasty*, vol. 28, no. 8, pp. 1259–1264, 2013.

[18] R. de Haan, C. Pattyn, H. S. Gill, D. W. Murray, P. A. Campbell, and K. de Smet, "Correlation between inclination of the acetabular component and metal ion levels in metal-on-metal hip resurfacing replacement," *Journal of Bone and Joint Surgery B*, vol. 90, no. 10, pp. 1291–1297, 2008.

[19] D. J. Langton, A. P. Sprowson, T. J. Joyce et al., "Blood metal ion concentrations after hip resurfacing arthroplasty: a comparative study of articular surface replacement and Birmingham hip resurfacing arthroplasties," *Journal of Bone and Joint Surgery Series B*, vol. 91, no. 10, pp. 1287–1295, 2009.

[20] D. J. Langton, S. S. Jameson, T. J. Joyce, J. Webb, and A. V. F. Nargol, "The effect of component size and orientation on the concentrations of metal ions after resurfacing arthroplasty of the hip," *The Journal of Bone and Joint Surgery*, vol. 90, no. 9, pp. 1143–1151, 2008.

[21] H. Pandit, S. Glyn-Jones, P. McLardy-Smith et al., "Pseudotumours associated with metal-on-metal hip resurfacings," *Journal of Bone and Joint Surgery B*, vol. 90, no. 7, pp. 847–851, 2008.

[22] P. J. Duggan, C. J. Burke, S. Saha et al., "Current literature and imaging techniques of aseptic lymphocyte-dominated vasculitis-associated lesions (ALVAL)," *Clinical Radiology*, vol. 68, no. 11, pp. 1089–1096, 2013.

[23] B. Ollivere, C. Darrah, T. Barker, J. Nolan, and M. J. Porteous, "Early clinical failure of the Birmingham metal-on-metal hip resurfacing is associated with metallosis and soft-tissue necrosis," *Journal of Bone and Joint Surgery B*, vol. 91, no. 8, pp. 1025–1030, 2009.

[24] E. Ebramzadeh, P. Campbell, T. L. Tan, S. D. Nelson, and S. N. Sangiorgio, "Can wear explain the histological variation around metal-on-metal total hips?" *Clinical Orthopaedics and Related Research*, 2014.

# Permissions

# List of Contributors

Rachel M. Frank, Shane J. Nho, Robert C. Grumet, Brian J. Cole, Nikhil N. Verma and Anthony A. Romeo
Division of Sports Medicine, Department of Orthopaedic Surgery, Rush University Medical Center, 1611West Harrison Street, Suite 300, Chicago, IL 60612, USA

Kevin C. McGill
Department of Diagnostic Radiology, Henry Ford Hospital, Detroit, MI, USA

Melinda K. Harman
Department of Bioengineering, 301 Rhodes Engineering Research Center, Clemson University, Clemson, SC 29634-0905, USA

Stephanie J. Bonin
MEA Forensic Engineers & Scientists, 23281 Vista Grande Drive, Laguna Hills, CA 92653, USA

Chris J. Leslie
Leslie Orthopaedics & Sports Medicine, 226 East U.S. Highway 54, Camdenton, MO 65020, USA

Scott A. Banks
Department Mechanical & Aerospace Engineering, MAEA 318, University of Florida, P.O. Box 116250, Gainesville, FL 32611, USA

W. Andrew Hodge
Department of Orthopaedics, Eastern Maine Medical Center, 489 State Street, Bangor, ME 04401, USA

Burak Akan
Department of Orthopedics and Traumatology, Ufuk University Faculty of Medicine, Ankara, Turkey
Dikmen C Parkpinar Evleri, 9/B No 28 Keklikpinari Cankaya, 06420 Ankara, Turkey

Dogac Karaguven, Berk Guclu, Tugrul Yildirim, Alper Kaya and Ilker Cetin
Department of Orthopedics and Traumatology, Ufuk University Faculty of Medicine, Ankara, Turkey

Mehmet Armangil
Department of Orthopedics and Traumatology, Ankara University Faculty of Medicine, Ankara, Turkey

Michael Woods
Missoula Bone and Joint, 2360 Mullan Road, Suite C, Missoula, MT 59808, USA

Denise Birkholz and Adam Woods
Pronerve, 7600 East Orchard Road, Suite 200, Greenwood Village, CO 80111, USA

Regina MacBarb and Robyn Capobianco
SI-BONE, Inc., 3055 Olin Avenue, Suite 2200, San Jose, CA 95128, USA

Jordan H. Trafimow and Alexander S. Aruin
Department of Physical Therapy (MC 898), University of Illinois at Chicago, 1919W. Taylor Street, Chicago, IL 60612, USA

Mitsuyoshi Yamamura and Nobuo Nakamura
Center of Arthroplasty, Kyowakai Hospital, 1-24-1 Kishibekita, Suita, Osaka 564-0001, Japan

Hidenobu Miki and Takashi Nishii
Department of Orthopaedic Surgery, Osaka University Graduate School of Medicine, 2-2 Yamadaoka, Suita, Osaka 565-0871, Japan

Nobuhiko Sugano
Department of Orthopaedic Surgery, Osaka University Graduate School of Medicine, 2-2 Yamadaoka, Suita, Osaka 565-0871, Japan
Department of Orthopaedic Medical Engineering, Osaka University Graduate School of Medicine, 2-2 Yamadaoka, Suita, Osaka 565-0871, Japan

A. F. Ozer
Neurosurgery Department, Koc̦ University School of Medicine, Rumelifeneri Yolu Sarıyer, 34450 Istanbul, Turkey

F. Keskin
Neurosurgery Department, Necmettin Erbakan University Meram Medical Faculty Hospital, 42080 Konya, Turkey

T. Oktenoglu, T. Suzer and M. Sasani
Neurosurgery Department, American Hospital, 34365 Istanbul, Turkey

Y. Ataker
Physical Therapy and Rehabilitation Department, American Hospital, 34365 Istanbul, Turkey

C. Gomleksiz
Neurosurgery Department, Mengücek Gazi Training and Research Hospital, School of Medicine, Erzincan University, 24100 Erzincan, Turkey

Kushagra Sinha, Rajesh Maheshwari and Atul Agrawal
Department of Orthopaedics, Himalayan Institute of Medical Sciences, Dehradun, Uttarakhand 248140, India

Vijendra D. Chauhan
Himalayan Institute of Medical Sciences, Dehradun, Uttarakhand 248140, India

Neena Chauhan
Department of Pathology, Himalayan Institute of Medical Sciences, Dehradun, Uttarakhand 248140, India

**Manu Rajan**
Department of Plastic Surgery, Himalayan Institute of Medical Sciences, Dehradun, Uttarakhand 248140, India

**Bryan S.Moon, Patrick P. Lin and Valerae O. Lewis**
MD Anderson Cancer Center, Department of Orthopaedic Oncology, P.O. Box 301402, Houston, TX 77230-1402, USA

**Nathan F. Gilbert**
Greater Dallas Orthopaedics, 12230 Coit Road, Suite 100, Dallas, TX 75251, USA

**Christopher P. Cannon**
Polyclinic Department of Orthopaedic Surgery, 1001 Broadway, Suite 109, Seattle, WA 98122, USA

**Mario Di Silvestre, Francesco Lolli, Tiziana Greggi, Francesco Vommaro and Andrea Baioni**
Spine Surgery Department, Istituti Ortopedici Rizzoli, Via Pupilli 1, 40136 Bologna, Italy

**Milad Masjedi, Zahra Jaffry, Simon Harris and Justin Cobb**
MSk Lab, Charing Cross Hospital, Imperial College London, LondonW6 8RF, UK

**Serhat Mutlu**
Kanuni Sultan Suleyman Education and Research Hospital, Department of Orthopaedic Surgery, Istanbul, Turkey

**Mahir MahJroğullari**
Istanbul Medipol University, Istanbul, Turkey

**Olcay Güler**
Nisa Hospital, Istanbul, Turkey

**Bekir Yavuz Uçar**
Dicle University, Diyarbakır, Turkey

**HarunMutlu**
Taksim Education and Research Hospital, Istanbul, Turkey

**Güner Sönmez and Hakan Mutlu**
Gülhane Military Medical Academy Education Hospital, Istanbul, Turkey

**Li-Yu Fay, Jau-ChingWu and Henrich Cheng**
Department of Neurosurgery, Neurological Institute, Taipei Veterans General Hospital,Taipei 11217, Taiwan School of Medicine, National Yang-Ming University, Taipei 11221, Taiwan Institute of Pharmacology, National Yang-Ming University, Taipei 11221, Taiwan

**Tzu-Yun Tsai**
Department of Ophthalmology, National Taiwan University Hospital, College of Medicine, National Taiwan University, Taipei 10002, Taiwan

Department of Ophthalmology, New Taipei City Hospital, New Taipei City 241, Taiwan

**Ching-Lan Wu**
Department of Radiology, Taipei Veterans General Hospital, Taipei 11217, Taiwan

**Tsung-Hsi Tu and Wen-Cheng Huang**
Department of Neurosurgery, Neurological Institute, Taipei Veterans General Hospital,Taipei 11217, Taiwan School of Medicine, National Yang-Ming University, Taipei 11221, Taiwan

**A. Panagopoulos, P. Tsoumpos, K. Evangelou and Christos Georgiou**
Department of Shoulder & Elbow Surgery, Orthopaedic Clinic, University Hospital of Patras, Papanikolaou 1, 26504 Patras, Greece

**I. Triantafillopoulos**
Department of Shoulder & Elbow Surgery, Metropolitan Hospital Athens, Medical School, University of Athens, Ethnarxou Makariou & El. Benizelou 1, N. Faliro, 18547 Piraeus, Greece

**M. Bueschges, K. L. Mauss and C. Ottomann**
Sektion für Plastische Chirurgie und Handchirurgie, Intensiveinheit für Schwerbrandverletzte, Universitätsklinikum Schleswig Holstein Campus Lübeck, Ratzeburger Allee 160, 23560 Lübeck, Germany

**T. Muehlberger**
Abteilung für Plastische Chirurgie, DRK Kliniken Berlin, Berlin, Germany

**J. C. Bruck**
Abteilung für Plastische Chirurgie, Martin Luther Krankenhaus, Caspar-Theyß-Straße 27-31, Grunewald, 14193 Berlin, Germany

**Amir Matityahu, Meir Marmor and R. Trigg McClellan**
Department of Orthopaedic Surgery, UCSF/SFGH Orthopaedic Trauma Institute, 2550 23rd Street, 2nd Floor, San Francisco, CA 94110, USA

**Andrew H. Schmidt**
Department of Orthopaedic Surgery, University of Minnesota, Hennapin County Medical Center, Minneapolis, MN 55454, USA

**Alan Grantz and Ben Clawson**
Anthem Orthopaedics VAN, LLC, Santa Cruz, CA 95060, USA

**Monil Karia, Milad Masjedi, Barry Andrews, Zahra Jaffry and Justin Cobb**
MSK Lab, Department of Orthopaedics, Charing Cross Hospital, Imperial College London, Fulham Place Road, LondonW6 8RF, UK

**Antoine Nachanakian, Antonios El Helou and Moussa Alaywan**
Department of Neurosurgery, Saint George Hospital University Medical Center and Balamand University, Youssef Sursock Street, Rmeil, Beirut 11 00 2807, P.O. Box 166378, Lebanon

**Frank R. Avilucea, Sarah E. Greenberg,W. Jeffrey Grantham, Vasanth Sathiyakumar, Rachel V. Thakore, Samuel K. Nwosu, Kristin R. Archer, William T. Obremskey, Hassan R. Mir and Manish K. Sethi**
The Vanderbilt Orthopaedic Institute Center for Health Policy, 1215 21st Avenue S., MCE, South Tower,Suite 4200, Vanderbilt University, Nashville, TN 37232, USA

**Donald Sachs**
Center for Spinal Stenosis and Neurologic Care, P.O. Box 8815, Lakeland, FL 33806, USA

**Robyn Capobianco**
SI-BONE Inc., 3055 Olin Ave. Suite 2200, San Jose, CA 95128, USA

**N. D. Clement, A. D. Duckworth, C. M. Court-Brown and M. M. McQueen**
Department of Orthopaedics and Trauma, The Royal Infirmary of Edinburgh, Little France, Edinburgh EH16 4SA, UK

**D. K. Sengupta**
Dartmouth-Hitchcock Medical Center, One Medical Center Drive, Lebanon, NH 03756, USA

**Brandon Bucklen, Jeff Nichols, Raghavendra Angara and Saif Khalil**
Globus Medical, Inc., Valley Forge Business Center, 2560 General Armistead Avenue, Audubon, PA 19403, USA

**Paul C. McAfee**
Towson Orthopaedic Associates, P.A.—Scoliosis and Spine Center, O'DeaMedical Arts Building, Suite 104, 7505 Osler Drive, Towson, MD 21204, USA

**Dilip Sengupta**
Dartmouth-Hitchcock Medical Center, Orthopedics, One Medical Center Drive, Lebanon, NH 03756-0001, USA

**Aditya Ingalhalikar and Aditya Muzumdar**
Globus Medical Inc., Valley Forge Business Center, 2560 General Armistead Avenue, Audubon, PA 19403, USA

**Thomas B. Pace**
Department of Orthopaedics, Greenville Health System, Greenville, SC 29605, USA
University of South Carolina SOM, Greenville Health System, P.O. Box 27114, Greenville, SC 29616, USA

**Kevin C. Keith, Estefania Alvarez and John D. DesJardins**
Department of Bioengineering, Clemson University, Clemson, SC 29634, USA

**Rebecca G. Snider and Stephanie L. Tanner**
Department of Orthopaedics, Greenville Health System, Greenville, SC 29605, USA

**Arata Nakajima**
Department of Orthopaedic Surgery, Toho University Sakura Medical Center, 564-1 Shimoshizu, Sakura, Chiba 285-8741, Japan

**Masazumi Murakami**
Department of Orthopaedic Surgery, Chiba Aoba Municipal Hospital, 1273-2 Aoba-cho, Chuo-ku, Chiba 260-0852, Japan

**Yasuchika Aoki and Koichi Nakagawa**
Department of Orthopaedic Surgery, Toho University Sakura Medical Center, 564-1 Shimoshizu, Sakura, Chiba 285-8741, Japan

**Koopong Siribumrungwong, Theerasan Kiriratnikom, and Boonsin Tangtrakulwanich**
Department of Orthopedic Surgery and Physical Medicine, Faculty of Medicine, Prince of Songkla University, Hat Yai, Songkla 90110, Thailand

**Rahul Vaidya, Ndidi Onwudiwe,Matthew Roth and Anil Sethi**
Detroit Medical Center, Orthopedics Department, Wayne State School of Medicine, 4D UHC, St. Antoine Street, 540 E Canfield Street, Detroit, MI 48201, USA

**Johannes F. Plate, Sandeep Mannava, Beth P. Smith, Jason E. Lang, Gary G. Poehling and Riyaz H. Jinnah**
Department of Orthopaedic Surgery,Wake Forest School of Medicine, Medical Center Boulevard, Winston-Salem, NC 27157-1070, USA

**Ali Mofidi**
Morriston Hospital, Swansea SA6-6NL, UK

**Michael A. Conditt**
MAKO Surgical Corp., 2555 Davie Road, Fort Lauderdale, FL 33317, USA

**Olcay Eser**
Department of Neurosurgery, School of Medicine, Afyon Kocatepe University, Afyonkarahisar, Turkey

**Cengiz Gomleksiz**
Department of Neurosurgery, Ordu Medical Park Hospital, Ordu, Turkey

**Mehdi Sasani, Tunc Oktenoglu and Tuncer Suzer**
Department of Neurosurgery, American Hospital, Istanbul, Turkey

**Ahmet Levent Aydin**
Neurosurgery Department, Istanbul Physical Therapy and Rehabilitation Hospital, Istanbul, Turkey

**Yaprak Ataker**
Physical Therapy and Rehabilitation Department, American Hospital, Istanbul, Turkey

**Ali Fahir Ozer**
Department of Neurosurgery, School of Medicine, Koc University, Rumelifeneri Yolu Sarıyer, Istanbul 34450, Turkey

**Lu-Zhao Di, Vanessa Couture and Yasaman Alinejad**
Research Center of CHUS (CRCHUS), 3001, 12th Avenue North, Sherbrooke, QC, Canada J1H 5N4

**François Berthod**
Laboratoire d'Organogénèse Expérimentale (LOEX), Research Center of CHUQ, Enfant-Jésus Hospital, 1401, 18th Street, Quebec City, QC, Canada G1J 1Z4
Department of Surgery, Faculty of Medicine, Laval University, 2325 Universit´e Street, Quebec City, QC, Canada G1V 0A6

**Nathalie Faucheux,**
Research Center of CHUS (CRCHUS), 3001, 12th Avenue North, Sherbrooke, QC, Canada J1H 5N4
Department of Chemical and Biotechnological Engineering, Faculty of Engineering, University of Sherbrooke, 2500 Université Boulevard, Sherbrooke, QC, Canada J1K 2R1

**Élisabeth Leblanc, Frédéric Balg and Guillaume Grenier**
Research Center of CHUS (CRCHUS), 3001, 12th Avenue North, Sherbrooke, QC, Canada J1H 5N4
Department of Orthopedic Surgery, Faculty of Medicine and Health Sciences, University of Sherbrooke, 3001, 12th Avenue North, Sherbrooke, QC, Canada J1H 5N4

**Jean-François Beaudoin**
Research Center of CHUS (CRCHUS), 3001, 12th Avenue North, Sherbrooke, QC, Canada J1H 5N4
Sherbrooke Molecular Imaging Centre (CIMS), CRCHUS, 3001, 12th Avenue North, Sherbrooke, QC, Canada J1H5N4

**Roger Lecomte**
Research Center of CHUS (CRCHUS), 3001, 12th Avenue North, Sherbrooke, QC, Canada J1H 5N4
Sherbrooke Molecular Imaging Centre (CIMS), CRCHUS, 3001, 12th Avenue North, Sherbrooke, QC, Canada J1H5N4
Department of Nuclear Medicine and Radiobiology, Faculty of Medicine and Health Sciences, University of Sherbrooke, 3001, 12th Avenue North, Sherbrooke, QC, Canada J1H 5N4

**Metin Uzun**
Orthopaedic Department, Acıbadem Maslak Hospital, Darüşşafaka Street, Büyükdere Street No. 40,Maslak, Sarıyer, Istanbul, Turkey

**Adnan Kara**
Orthopaedic Department, Şişli Etfal Training and Education Hospital, Şişli, Istanbul, Turkey

**Müjdat Adaş**
Okmeydani Education and Training Hospital, Okmeydani, Istanbul, Turkey

**Bülent Karslioğlu**
Orthopaedic Department, Kasımpaşa Military Hospital, Istanbul, Turkey

**Murat Bülbül**
Orthopaedic Department, Medipol University, Istanbul, Turkey

**Burak Beksaç**
Orthopaedic Department, Acıbadem University, Darüşşafaka Street, Büyükdere Street No. 40, Maslak, Sarıyer, Istanbul, Turkey

**Ahmed Mabrouk**
ST2 Plastic Surgery, St. Andrews Centre for Plastic Surgery and Burns, Broomfield Hospital, Chelmsford, Essex CM1 7ET, UK

**Mysore Madhusudan, MohammedWaseem, Steven Kershaw and Jochen Fischer**
Macclesfield Hospital, Victoria Road, Macclesfield, Cheshire SK10 3BL, UK

**Tunc Oktenoglu and Mehdi Sasani**
Neurosurgery Department, American Hospital, 34365 Istanbul, Turkey

**Ali Fahir Ozer**
Neurosurgery Department, Koc University School of Medicine, 34450 Istanbul, Turkey

**Yaprak Ataker**
Physical Therapy and Rehabilitation Department, American Hospital, 34365 Istanbul, Turkey

**Cengiz Gomleksiz**
Neurosurgery Department, Mengücek Gazi Training and Research Hospital, School of Medicine, Erzincan University, 2400 Erzincan, Turkey

**Irfan Celebi**
Radiology Department, Sisli Etfal Hospital, 34360 Istanbul, Turkey

**Ignacio Carbonel, Angel A. Martínez and Jorge Ripalda**
Shoulder and Elbow Unit, Department of Orthopaedic and Trauma Surgery, Miguel Servet University Hospital, Zaragoza, Spain

**Elisa Aldea**
Emergency Department, Royo Villanova Hospital, Zaragoza, Spain

**Antonio Herrera**
Department of Orthopaedic and Trauma Surgery, Miguel Servet University Hospital and Department of Orthopaedic Surgery, School of Medicine, University of Zaragoza, Zaragoza, Spain

**Tamara Alexandrov**
Department of Orthopaedics, Los Angeles County-University of Southern California Medical Center,1200 N. State Street, GNH 3900, Los Angeles, CA 90033, USA

**Elke R. Ahlmann**
University of Southern California, Keck School of Medicine, Los Angeles County-University of Southern California Medical Center, 1200 N. State Street, GNH 3900, Los Angeles, CA 90033, USA

**Lawrence R.Menendez**
University of Southern California, Keck School of Medicine, USC University Hospital, 1510 San Pablo Street, Suite 634, Los Angeles, CA 90033-4608, USA

**William D. Bugbee**
Division of Orthopaedic Surgery, Scripps Clinic, 10666North Torrey Pines Road, MS116, La Jolla, CA 92037, USA

**Hideki Mizu-uchi, Shantanu Patil and Darryl D'Lima**
Shiley Center for Orthopaedic Research & Education at Scripps Clinic, 11025 North Torrey Pines Road, Suite 200, La Jolla, CA 92037, USA

**Breda H. F. Lau and Mark R. Lafave**
Department of Physical Education and Recreational Studies, Mount Royal University, 4825 Mount Royal Gate SW, Calgary, AB, Canada T3E 6K6

**Dale J. Butterwick**
Faculty of Kinesiology, University of Calgary, 2500 University Dr NW, Calgary, AB, Canada T2N1N4

**Nicholas G.Mohtadi**
Faculty of Medicine, Health Sciences Centre, Foothills Campus, University of Calgary, 3330 Hospital Drive NW, Calgary, AB, Canada T2N 4N1

**Michael J. Carroll and Paul Sciore**
Section of Orthopedic Surgery, Department of Surgery, University of Calgary, 3280 Hospital Drive, Calgary, AB, Canada T2N 4Z6

**Kristie D.More**
Sport Medicine Centre, University of Calgary, 2500 University Drive NW, Calgary, AB, Canada T2N 1N4

**Stephen Sohmer**
University of British Columbia, 301-909 Island Highway, Campbell River, BC, Canada V9W 2C2

**Richard Boorman, Robert Hollinshead and Ian K. Y. Lo**
Section of Orthopedic Surgery, Department of Surgery, University of Calgary, 3280 Hospital Drive, Calgary, AB, Canada T2N 4Z6
Sport Medicine Centre, University of Calgary, 2500 University Drive NW, Calgary, AB, Canada T2N 1N4

**Jenaro Fernández-Valencia, Xavier Gallart, Guillem Bori, Sebastián Garcia Ramiro, Andrés Combalía and Josep Riba**
Hip Unit, Department of Orthopaedic Surgery and Traumatology, Hospital Clínic, Universitat de Barcelona, C/Villarroel 170, 08036 Barcelona, Spain